Manual Therapy and Rehabilitation: Diagnosis and Treatment

Manual Therapy and Rehabilitation: Diagnosis and Treatment

Edited by **Esther Henson**

SYRAWOOD
PUBLISHING HOUSE
New York

Published by Syrawood Publishing House,
750 Third Avenue, 9th Floor,
New York, NY 10017, USA
www.syrawoodpublishinghouse.com

Manual Therapy and Rehabilitation: Diagnosis and Treatment
Edited by Esther Henson

International Standard Book Number: 978-1-68286-284-1 (Hardback)

Printed in China.

Contents

Preface

Every book is a source of knowledge and this one is no exception. The idea that led to the conceptualization of this book was the fact that the world is advancing rapidly; which makes it crucial to document the progress in every field. I am aware that a lot of data is already available, yet, there is a lot more to learn. Hence, I accepted the responsibility of editing this book and contributing my knowledge to the community.

Manual therapy is an essential technique of chiropractic. This book explores all the important aspects of manual therapy in the present day scenario and its success as a treatment method. Various types of manual therapy, scope of treatment, musculoskeletal framework, etc. have been explored, in an extensive manner, in this book. Coherent flow of topics and extensive use of examples make this book an invaluable source of knowledge, especially for those pursuing chiropractic and allied disciplines.

While editing this book, I had multiple visions for it. Then I finally narrowed down to make every chapter a sole standing text explaining a particular topic, so that they can be used independently. However, the umbrella subject sinews them into a common theme. This makes the book a unique platform of knowledge.

I would like to give the major credit of this book to the experts from every corner of the world, who took the time to share their expertise with us. Also, I owe the completion of this book to the never-ending support of my family, who supported me throughout the project.

Editor

1

SPECT/CT imaging of the lumbar spine in chronic low back pain: a case report

Michael H Carstensen*, Mashael Al-Harbi, Jean-Luc Urbain, Tarik-Zine Belhocine

Abstract

Mechanical low back pain is a common indication for Nuclear Medicine imaging. Whole-body bone scan is a very sensitive but poorly specific study for the detection of metabolic bone abnormalities. The accurate localisation of metabolically active bone disease is often difficult in 2D imaging but single photon emission computed tomography/computed tomography (SPECT/CT) allows accurate diagnosis and anatomic localisation of osteoblastic and osteolytic lesions in 3D imaging. We present a clinical case of a patient referred for evaluation of chronic lower back pain with no history of trauma, spinal surgery, or cancer. Planar whole-body scan showed heterogeneous tracer uptake in the lumbar spine with intense localisation to the right lateral aspect of L3. Integrated SPECT/CT of the lumbar spine detected active bone metabolism in the right L3/L4 facet joint in the presence of minimal signs of degenerative osteoarthrosis on CT images, while a segment demonstrating more gross degenerative changes was more quiescent with only mild tracer uptake. The usefulness of integrated SPECT/CT for anatomical and functional assessment of back pain opens promising opportunities both for multi-disciplinary clinical assessment and treatment for manual therapists and for research into the effectiveness of manual therapies.

Background

The concept of lumbar facet joints causing or contributing to mechanical low back pain syndromes has been debated in the health care literature for decades [1]. Practitioners of the various manual therapies commonly treat patients presenting with low back pain but are faced with the diagnostic challenge of trying to identify a tissue source of low back pain. While this complaint may be the result of any of a number of pathologies, the vast majority of low back pain falls under the diagnostic umbrella of " mechanical low back pain " [2]. We present here the case of a patient with radiological signs of marked lumbosacral junction facet joint osteoarthrosis and clinical symptoms supportive of pathology in this region but with SPECT/CT findings suggestive of an active bony lesion at a more remote spinal segment.

Case Presentation

History

The patient in question was a 45-year-old Hispanic female who had lived in Canada for the previous 11 years. She reported a long history of manual labour and subsisted on similar occupations since arriving in Canada. At the time of her presentation, her occupation required prolonged periods of standing. The patient's chief complaint was chronic low back pain. There was no antecedent trauma, bone surgery, or history of cancer. The onset of low back pain was described as insidious, with constant achy pain of at least two years duration which was progressively worsening. The pain remained localised to the central lower back in the area of the lumbosacral junction. The pain was rated at 3/10 (verbal scoring) at its best and 8/10 (verbal scoring) at its worst. An increase in pain was associated with an increased level of physical activity during the day, with the pain typically worse in the evening. During periods of increased pain, there were intermittent incidences of pain radiating to the right-sided posterior thigh and leg with "pins and needles" in the lateral toes of the right foot. Treatment to date had consisted of non-steroidal anti-inflammatory medication, which she felt had been of limited benefit. There had been no use of acupuncture, massage therapy, therapeutic exercise, or any manual therapies for this condition. The patient was referred to the department of Medical Imaging for evaluation of chronic lower back pain.

* Correspondence: docmike@nl.rogers.com
Department of Medical Imaging, St Joseph's Hospital London, Ontario, Canada

The patient reported that no spinal imaging had been performed in investigation of these complaints. This was confirmed by a review of the patient's records.

Physical Examination

Imaging specialists typically do not examine patients who are referred into an imaging department for investigation. As such, no physical examination was performed in this case. Permission was granted after the images were interpreted only to interview the patient for this case report.

Imaging Protocol

A three-phase bone scan was performed with $^{99\ m}Tc$ (Technetium)-MDP (methylene diphosphonate) including blood flow and blood pool imaging followed by a delayed whole-body scan. SPECT/CT imaging centered over the lumbar spine was subsequently performed on a Symbia T6 (Siemens), a dual-head gamma-camera incorporating a low-dose 6-slice non-contrast enhanced CT (12 mAs, 130 kVp, Effective Dose < 4 mSv). The CT scan duration was less than 1 min. Overall, the SPECT/CT scan duration was about 20 min. The SPECT/CT fused images were displayed on the e-soft 2007 workstation (Siemens) in axial, sagittal, and coronal slices.

Imaging Findings

The blood flow and pool images were unremarkable, suggesting no active inflammatory process. The delayed whole-body images showed degenerative changes in multiple sites in the axial and appendicular skeleton. Heterogeneous tracer uptake was noted at multiple spinal levels with marked increased focal tracer uptake in the right lateral aspect of L3 (Figure 1).

SPECT/CT images confirmed intense tracer uptake in the right L3/L4 facet joint (Figure 2). In the absence of other osteoblastic or osteolytic pathology, this is most consistent with active degenerative osteoarthrosis. Mild tracer uptake is also noted in the right facet joint of L5/S1 in the presence of marked degenerative arthrosis, which is consistent with limited active bony pathology. The low-dose CT images from the SPECT/CT are not of diagnostic quality but they are adequate for anatomical localisation and gross tissue evaluation. In reviewing the axial CT images, there are many abnormalities to note. At the level of the L3/L4 right facet joint, there are only mild indicators of degenerative joint disease: focal joint space narrowing and early sclerosis (Figure 3). In addition to marked degeneration of the right L5/S1 facet (Figure 4), there is a left-sided discontinuity of the pars interarticularis and an incidental spina bifida occulta at L5 (Figure 5).

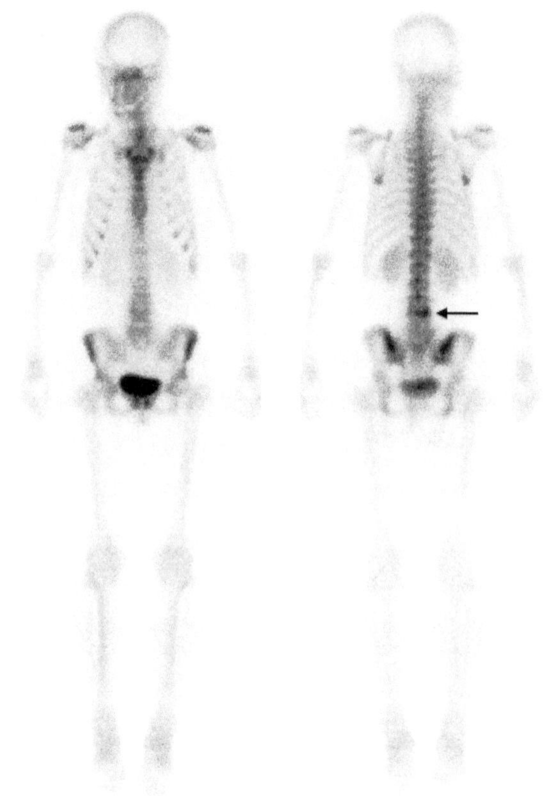

Figure 1 Delayed Whole Body images, anterior (L) and posterior showing focal tracer uptake in right L3/L4 facet joint region (continuous black arrow).

Discussion

As a category, mechanical low back pain accounts for up to 97% of low back pain diagnoses [1,2]. A diagnosis of mechanical low back pain implies that there are no vascular, infectious, inflammatory or neoplastic etiologies underlying the patient's complaints but does little to clinically isolate a specific source of pain or identify a definitive avenue of treatment. This diagnosis encompasses a broad subset of possible tissue pathologies, many of which cannot be accurately diagnosed by physical examination. This may limit a manual therapist's ability to specifically prescribe a treatment regimen or accurately predict a response to treatment.

Lumbar facet joint capsules are richly innervated with nociceptive and autonomic nerve fibers and, as such, are a potential source of low back pain [3]. Despite a broad range of reported prevalence, this position is generally accepted and is supported by investigations that have injected facet joints with corticosteroids and anesthetic agents and demonstrated success in relieving some low back pain [4].

Undifferentiated lower back pain is a well established clinical indication for planar/SPECT bone scintigraphy [5,6]. Integrated SPECT/CT imaging is useful for anatomic and functional evaluation of benign and malignant

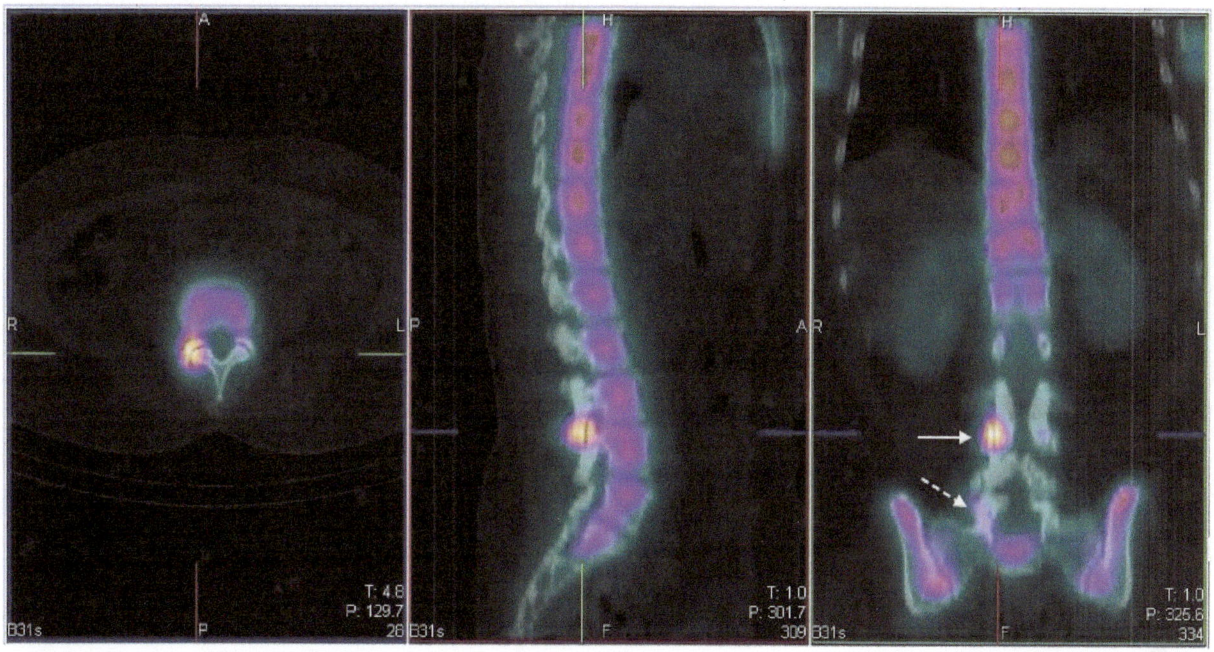

Figure 2 SPECT/CT images (axial, sagittal, coronal) localizing intense, focal tracer uptake to the right L3/L4 facet joint (continuous arrow). Note is made of mild tracer uptake in the right L5/S1 facet joint (dashed arrow).

spine bone diseases, particularly for evaluation of chronic low back pain [7-13]. The use of a low radiation dose multislice CT for 3D anatomic localisation of disk and facet degenerative disease improves the diagnostic accuracy and the specificity of planar/SPECT bone scintigraphy [11-13]. The CT images will also provide additional 3D detail about anatomic structures included in the region of interest that do not actively uptake radiotracer. The CT component of SPECT/CT provides a lower radiation dose than diagnostic multi-detector CT imaging, with an effective radiation dose of less than 4 mSv generating a radiation burden in the order of the yearly natural background exposure (approximately 3 mSv). The fast CT scanner (less than 1 min) may be used routinely for anatomic mapping in bone scintigraphy procedures [10].

This case highlights several interesting findings for the clinical setting and raises a number of potential research opportunities. Perhaps the most impressive finding is the demonstration of metabolically active bone in a facet joint with minimal overt degenerative changes that likely would not have been identified as pathological on plain radiographs. While it is well documented that clinical symptoms do not correlate well with radiographic and multidetector CT findings [2,14,15], the increased radiotracer uptake found on the SPECT part from

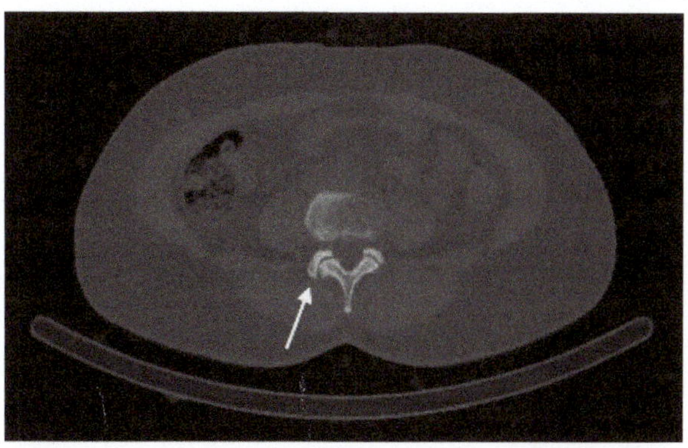

Figure 3 CT image from SPECT/CT demonstrating mild degenerative changes at right L3/L4 facet joint (white arrow).

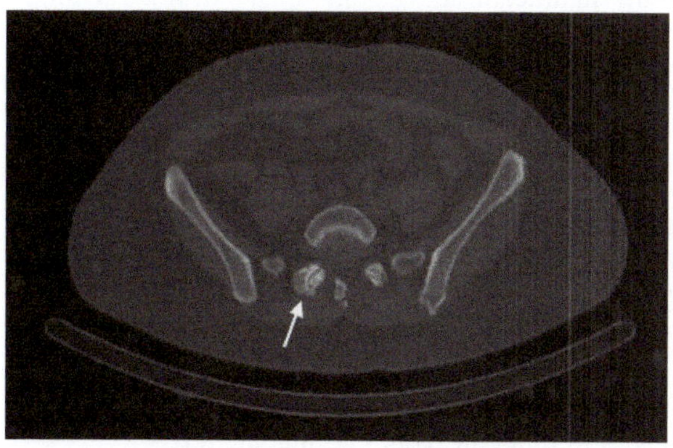

Figure 4 CT image from SPECT/CT demonstrating marked degenerative arthrosis at right L5/S1 facet (white arrow).

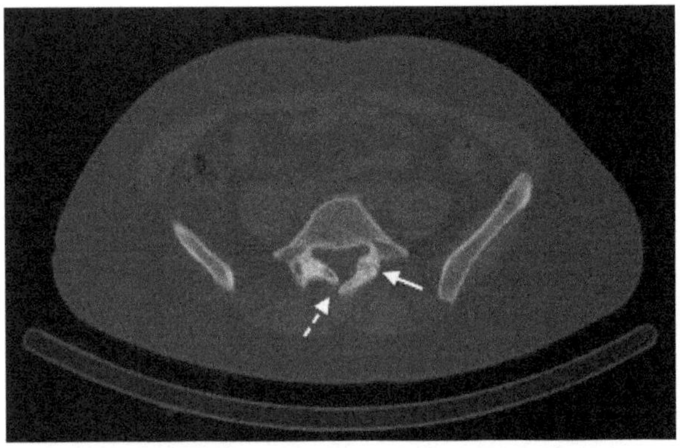

Figure 5 CT image from SPECT/CT demonstrating discontinuity of the left pars interarticularis (continuous arrow) and an incidental spina bifida occulta (dashed arrow).

SPECT/CT may be due to painful facet arthropathy, ongoing degenerative changes or the chronic sequelae of adverse mechanical loading. This case has also demonstrated that facet hypertrophy found on CT does not correlate with SPECT positivity, suggesting that facet hypertrophy has either a latent period or represents an end-point as part of the degenerative process. It is possible that by the time facet hypertrophy is notable on anatomic imaging, the metabolic activity of the bone is normalising, as demonstrated by the limited tracer uptake at the right L5/S1 facet joint. Rehabilitative treatment directed at SPECT positivity may also allow potentially corrective conservative intervention before advanced degenerative changes occur, theoretically reducing the likelihood of disability due to profound alteration of joint mechanics.

In this particular patient's clinical presentation, the CT findings of L5/S1 facet joint hypertrophy coupled with paresthesias to the right posterior thigh and leg and the lateral toes of the right foot is suggestive of a localised lesion to the L5/S1 segment, possibly affecting the right S1 nerve root. Because the SPECT findings do not reveal any significant active bony uptake in this region, any pain arising from this level may be due to non-osseous tissues being irritated, such as pain sensitive soft tissues (disc, ligament, muscle) or the exiting nerve root being affected by discal pathology and the hypertrophied facet demonstrated at this level. CT provides limited resolution of soft tissues in spine imaging and a more thorough evaluation of soft tissues would require the superior tissue resolution of MRI. However, given the findings of intense tracer uptake at the L3/L4 facet, the clinical presentation of low back pain may be due to local facet joint pathology at L3/L4 or a combination of pathologies in different tissues at multiple levels.

For manual therapists, one possible algorithm of investigation and treatment in such cases is to coordinate physical assessment with diagnostic or therapeutic facet joint injections for metabolically active facet joints found by SPECT/CT [15]. This approach can be beneficial by localizing the source of low back pain if the injection relieves the chief complaint. This approach may also be used in conjunction with manual therapies and targeted rehabilitation to improve the biomechanical function of the spine through muscle strengthening and muscle recruitment, and to improve joint mobility via mobilization and/or manipulation while the patient is experiencing pain relief from a therapeutic injection [2].

With the ability of SPECT/CT to identify sites of active bony metabolism, a role in manual therapy research becomes evident. The ability to objectively document sites of active biomechanical stress or degeneration opens up the possibility of using SPECT/CT to assess the effectiveness of manipulative and stabilization therapies. If such therapies are able to affect the biomechanics and stability of the spine, then SPECT/CT offers an avenue for objective assessment of their effectiveness. While such research may be technically and ethically difficult, SPECT/CT documentation of facet arthropathy has the potential to support the hypothesis that improving biomechanical function may both relieve pain and affect the degenerative process.

Conclusions

Facet arthropathy is a commonly accepted causative or contributing agent to low back pain syndromes. The ability of integrated SPECT/CT to precisely localise metabolically active facet joints may provide direction of treatment to manual therapies focused on improving spinal function. It is postulated here that improvements in biomechanical function, accompanied by patient subjective improvement, may demonstrate improvement or resolution of SPECT/CT findings of facet arthropathy. Research would have to be carefully designed to test this hypothesis.

Consent

Written informed consent was obtained from the patient for publication of this case report and any accompanying images. A copy of the written consent has been provided to the Editor-in-Chief of this journal.

Acknowledgements

The authors would like to thank Drs. I. Gulka, A. Leung, G. Garvin, and J. Rogers from the department of Diagnostic Radiology (St Joseph's Hospital Health Care and London Health Sciences Centre, London, Ontario) for their assistance in reviewing the CT imaging.

Authors' contributions

MC performed the literature review, interviewed the patient and prepared the manuscript. JLU, MA and TB contributed to the drafting of the manuscript as well as critical review and image interpretation. All authors approved of the final manuscript

Competing interests
The authors declare that they have no competing interests.

References

1. Kalichman L, Hunter DJ: **Lumbar Facet Joint Osteoarthritis: A Review.** *Semin Arthritis Rheum* 2007, **37(2)**:69-80.
2. Deyo RA, Weinstein JN: **Primary Care: Low back pain.** *N Engl J Med* 2001, **344(5)**:363-70.
3. Willard FH: **The lumbosacral connection: The ligamentous structure of the low back and its relationship to back pain.** In *The Integrated Function of the Lumbar Spine and Sacroiliac Joint, Proceedings of the Second International Congress on Low Back Pain* Edited by: Vleeming A, Mooney V, Dorman T, Snijders C 1995.
4. Haldeman S: **Low back pain: current physiologic concepts.** *Neurologic Clinics* 1999, **17(1)**:1-15.
5. Bombardieri E, Aktolun C, Baum RF, Bishof-Delaloye A, Buscombe J, Chatal JF, Maffioli L, Moncayo R, Mortelmans L, Reske SN: **Bone Scintigraphy Procedures guidelines for Tumour imaging.**[https://www.eanm.org/scientific_info/guidelines/gl_onco_bone.pdf].
6. Kanmaz B, Collier BD, Liu Y, Uzum F, Uygur G, Akansel G, Gunes I, Krasnow AZ, Hellman RS, Isitman AT, Carrera G: **SPET and three-phase bone scintigraphy in adult patients with chronic low back pain.** *Nucl Med Commun* 1998, **19**:13-21.
7. Schillaci O: **Hybrid SPECT/CT: a new era for SPECT imaging?** *Eur J Nucl Med Mol Imaging* 2005, **32(5)**:521-4.
8. Even-Sapir E, Flusser G, Lerman H, Lievshitz G, Metser U: **SPECT/multislice low-dose CT: a clinically relevant constituent in the imaging algorithm of nononcologic patients referred for bone scintigraphy.** *J Nucl Med* 2007, **48(2)**:319-24.
9. Belhocine T, Rachinsky I, Akincioglu C, Gambhir S, Wilcox B, Vezina W, Stitt L, Driedger A, Urbain JL: **How Useful is an Integrated SPECT/CT in Clinical Setting and Research?: Evaluation of a Low Radiation Dose 4 Slice System.** *The Open Medical Imaging Journal* 2008, **2**:80-109.
10. Buck AK, Nekolla S, Ziegler S, Beer A, Krause BJ, Herrmann K, Scheidhauer K, Wester HJ, rummeny EJ, Schwaiger M, Drzezga A: **SPECT/CT.** *J Nucl Med* 2008, **49(8)**:1305-19.
11. Gnanasegaran G, Barwick T, Adamson K, Mohan H, Sharp D, Fogelman I: **Multislice SPECT/CT in Benign and Malignant Bone Disease: When the Ordinary Turns Into the Extraordinary.** *Semin Nucl Med* 2009, **39(6)**:431-42.
12. Papathanassiou D, Bruna-Muraille C, Jouannaud C, Gagneux-Lemoussu L, Eschard JP, Leihn JC: **Single-photon emission computed tomography combined with computed tomography (SPECT/CT) in bone diseases.** *Joint Bone Spine* 2009, **76**:474-80.
13. McDonald M, Cooper R, Wang MY: **Use of computed tomography-single-photon emission computed tomography fusion for diagnosing painful facet arthropathy. Technical note.** *Neurosurg Focus* 2007, **22(1)**:E2.
14. Ryan PJ, Evans PA, Gibson T, Fogelman I: **Chronic lower back pain: Comparison of bone SPECT with Radiography and CT.** *Radiography* 1992, **182**:849-54.
15. Kalichman L, Li L, Kim DH, Guermazi A, Berkin V, O; Donnell CJ, Hoffman U, Cole R, Hunter DJ: **Facet Joint Osteoarthritis and Low Back Pain in the Community-Based Population.** *Spine* 2010, **33(23)**:2560-565.

Inexperienced clinicians can extract pathoanatomic information from MRI narrative reports with high reproducibility for use in research/quality assurance

Peter Kent[1*], Andrew M Briggs[2], Hanne B Albert[1], Andreas Byrhagen[3], Christian Hansen[4], Karina Kjaergaard[5] and Tue S Jensen[1]

Abstract

Background: Although reproducibility in reading MRI images amongst radiologists and clinicians has been studied previously, no studies have examined the reproducibility of inexperienced clinicians in extracting pathoanatomic information from magnetic resonance imaging (MRI) narrative reports and transforming that information into quantitative data. However, this process is frequently required in research and quality assurance contexts. The purpose of this study was to examine inter-rater reproducibility (agreement and reliability) among an inexperienced group of clinicians in extracting spinal pathoanatomic information from radiologist-generated MRI narrative reports.

Methods: Twenty MRI narrative reports were randomly extracted from an institutional database. A group of three physiotherapy students independently reviewed the reports and coded the presence of 14 common pathoanatomic findings using a categorical electronic coding matrix. Decision rules were developed after initial coding in an effort to resolve ambiguities in narrative reports. This process was repeated a further three times using separate samples of 20 MRI reports until no further ambiguities were identified (total n = 80). Reproducibility between trainee clinicians and two highly trained raters was examined in an arbitrary coding round, with agreement measured using percentage agreement and reliability measured using unweighted Kappa (*k*). Reproducibility was then examined in another group of three trainee clinicians who had not participated in the production of the decision rules, using another sample of 20 MRI reports.

Results: The mean percentage agreement for paired comparisons between the initial trainee clinicians improved over the four coding rounds (97.9-99.4%), although the greatest improvement was observed after the first introduction of coding rules. High inter-rater reproducibility was observed between trainee clinicians across 14 pathoanatomic categories over the four coding rounds (agreement range: 80.8-100%; reliability range *k* = 0.63-1.00). Concurrent validity was high in paired comparisons between trainee clinicians and highly trained raters (agreement 97.8-98.1%, reliability *k* = 0.83-0.91). Reproducibility was also high in the second sample of trainee clinicians (inter-rater agreement 96.7-100.0% and reliability *k* = 0.76-1.00; intra-rater agreement 94.3-100.0% and reliability *k* = 0.61-1.00).

Conclusions: A high level of radiological training is not required in order to transform MRI-derived pathoanatomic information from a narrative format to a quantitative format with high reproducibility for research or quality assurance purposes.

Keywords: MRI, narrative report, coding, spine, pathoanatomy

* Correspondence: peter.kent@slb.regionsyddanmark.dk
[1]Research Department, Spine Centre of Southern Denmark, Lillebaelt Hospital, Institute of Regional Health Services Research, University of Southern Denmark, Middelfart, Denmark
Full list of author information is available at the end of the article

Background

Magnetic resonance imaging (MRI) is considered the gold standard modality for imaging spinal structures *in vivo* [1]. Spinal pathoanatomy may be readily visualised using MRI and some pathoanatomic features, such as tumours, fractures, infections and nerve root compression, are usually clinically important. On the other hand, the clinical relevance of some other spinal pathoanatomic features, particularly their association with spinal pain and other symptoms, remains uncertain and is an ongoing topic of debate [2-4]. Although further exploration of this issue may be warranted, particularly in the context of vertebral endplate signal changes, which have shown an association with pain [5], a prerequisite for such investigations is the reliable extraction of information from MRI images.

Quantitative coding of MRI findings is important where such data are used for research and quality assurance purposes. For example, narrative MRI reports need to be routinely transformed into quantitative data within the context of clinical trials, cohort studies and health registries. Although such quantification can be performed directly by experienced radiologists who have been trained in the relevant research protocols, this is often not practical because there is a widespread shortage of experienced radiologists, especially research radiologists, and their participation is usually expensive. Therefore, an alternative pathway is for MRI findings to be quantified from narrative reports dictated by radiologists.

There are two important interpretative steps in the pathway from acquiring spinal MR images to a quantification of any identified pathoanatomic findings. Reproducibility (agreement and reliability) in each step is important for best practice research. First, radiologists need to interpret the scan images and dictate a narrative report that adequately describes the relevant normal and abnormal pathoanatomic findings. Several studies have described the inter-radiologist reliability of this process as typically being fair to substantial (Kappa's ranging from 0.21 to 0.80) [1,6-8]. Second, researchers who review narrative reports need to extract important pathoanatomic findings in a consistent manner. Although earlier research has identified comparable reproducibility between radiologists and spinal surgeons, neurosurgeons and conservative-care clinicians in reading spinal MR images [1], the reproducibility of researchers in extracting information from MRI narrative reports and transforming this information into a quantitative format has not been evaluated previously.

It remains uncertain as to what level of clinical training is required to extract pertinent pathoanatomic information from narrative reports with adequate reproducibility for research/quality assurance purposes. Therefore, the aim of this study was to quantify the reproducibility of an inexperienced group of trainee clinicians in extracting pathoanatomic information from MRI narrative reports.

Methods

Design

A repeated measures study was performed to investigate inter-rater reproducibility in transforming pathoanatomic information from narrative MRI reports into quantitative data. Two groups of three final year (third year) physiotherapy students who had received minimal training in interpreting MRI narrative reports were engaged as independent raters. They had only received two lectures introducing them to the broad array of imaging techniques. The study was covered by a quality assurance approval by the Scientific Ethics Committee of Southern Denmark and complied with the Declaration of Helsinki (2008).

Conceptually, reproducibility contains two components - agreement and reliability [9]. Agreement is about measurement error and quantifies the similarity of scores obtained by repeated measurement. This is a useful measure when the measurement tool and measurement process being examined are to be used for *monitoring change over time*. Reliability is about how well the measurement tool and measurement process are able to *distinguish between subjects or objects* (for example people or pathologies), despite the measurement error. Reliability is influenced by the variability in the scores. Therefore, reliability may vary within a study population (for example from one body region to another) or between study populations, even though the measurement error remains the same [9].

Imaging

In the MRI unit of the Spine Centre of Southern Denmark, there were narrative reports of lumbar MRIs available for a total of 4,233 community-dwelling individuals who had attended the Centre over the previous 8 years. MRIs of other body regions or repeat lumbar MRIs for individuals were not included in that sample. This spine centre is a publicly-funded secondary care outpatient facility specialising in the diagnosis and management of spinal pain, and is located on the island of Funen, Denmark. Patients were referred to the Centre by primary care chiropractors and general practitioners between the years 2000 and 2008.

A standard lumbar MRI protocol utilising a 0.2 T MRI system (Magnetom Open Viva, Siemens AG, Erlangen, Germany) was used. All patients were placed in the supine position with straightened legs. The imaging protocol consisted of one localiser and four imaging sequences - T1 and T2 sagittal and axial images (more detail is available on request from the authors).

Axial images were performed on the three lower lumbar levels. If serious pathology were present or herniations were located at higher lumbar levels, relevant supplementary sequences were performed. All images over this eight-year period were read by either one of two experienced musculoskeletal radiologists.

Coding of MRI narrative reports

An electronic coding matrix was developed for this study using FileMaker Pro 9 (FileMaker Inc, CA, USA). The coding matrix was designed to facilitate data capture for subsequent research projects. This coding matrix was used by the three raters to transform findings from narrative reports into a quantitative measure (yes/no score) of the presence of 14 possible pathologies including: intervertebral disc degeneration, disc bulge, disc herniation, nerve root compromise, Modic change type 1, Modic change type 2, spondylolisthesis (anterior or retro) with or without spondylolysis, stenosis, scoliosis, osteophytes, facet joint arthrosis, other endplate irregularities (including Scheuermann defects, irregularities), red flags (tumour, fracture, infection), and high intensity zones (Figure 1). These pathologies were chosen as they were pertinent to research undertaken in the study context. Other pathologies may have been reported in the narrative reports, but as they were not relevant to our research, they were not coded by the raters. The raters used the matrix to indicate whether pathoanatomic features were reported as present between vertebral levels T12-L5, including an option to nominate compromise of the S1 nerve root. For the purpose of coding, a vertebral segment was defined as extending from the superior vertebral endplate to the caudal aspect of the intervertebral space below, for example the T12 vertebra and T12/L1 inter-vertebral space.

An initial sample of 20 reports (0.47%) was randomly selected from all the people in the database who shared the same weekday of their date of birth. All coding was performed independently by the first group of three raters who remained blinded to each other's scores throughout the study. As each rater coded each MRI, whenever a narrative report finding was considered

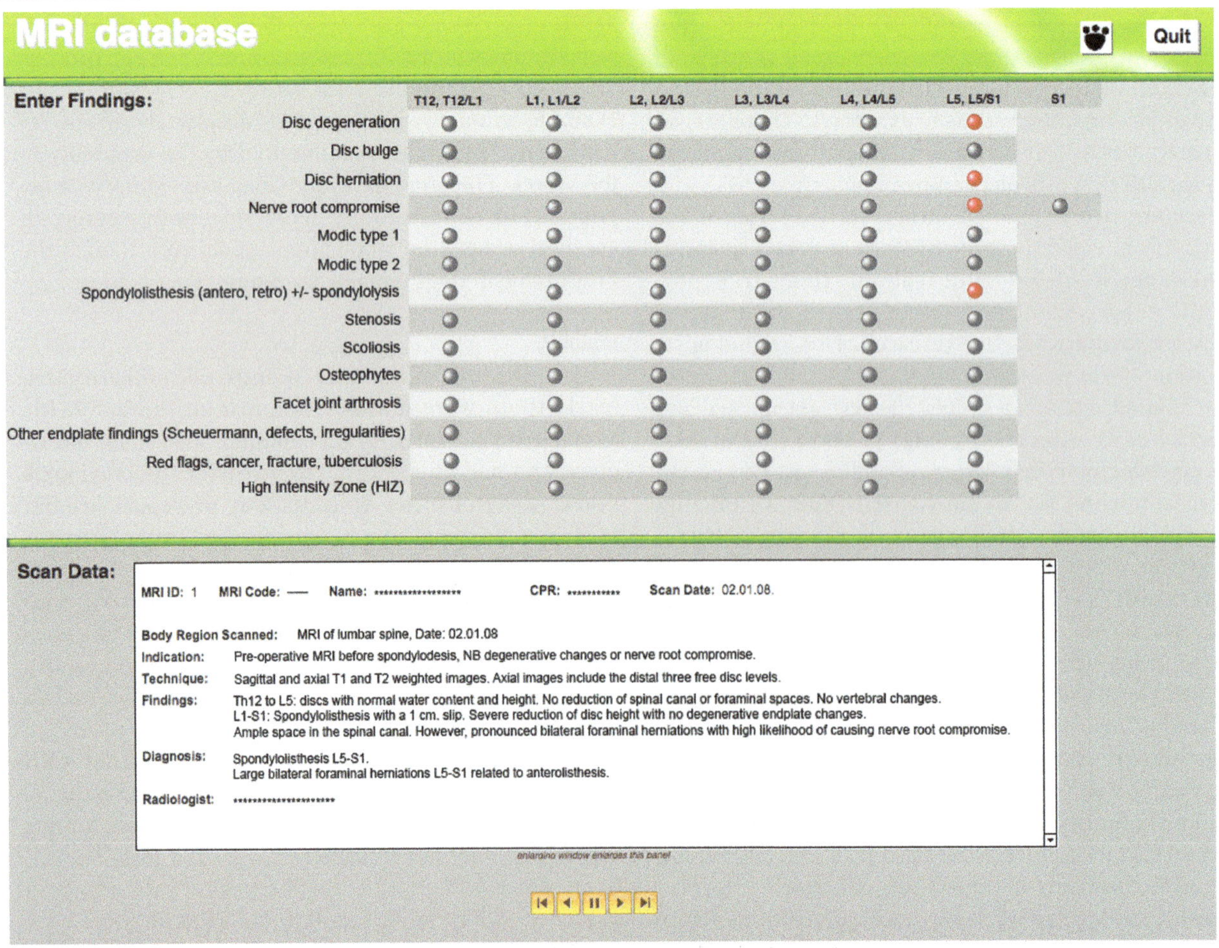

Figure 1 Screen shot of electronic coding matrix, consisting of 14 pathoanatomic categories for coding a narrative MRI report.

ambiguous, the rater(s) noted that ambiguity on a log sheet and selected the pathoanatomic feature in the coding matrix that they believed to be the most appropriate. At the completion of this initial cycle of coding 20 reports (a coding round), ambiguous report findings were collated and decision rules developed by senior researchers to provide a consistent decision-making process between raters. This group of inexperienced raters was able to contribute to the formation of the coding rules and provide feedback on their utility.

The initial coding round was undertaken without any decision rules. Another separate sample of 20 MRI reports of people who shared a different birth day was then selected and this process was repeated until no further ambiguities in reporting were identified by the raters. Three iterations of the coding rules were developed, therefore the total number of MRIs used was 80 (1.9% of the total available sample). The final set of decision rules is included as Additional file 1. In the first round of coding, three categories were not included in the matrix ('other endplate irregularities', 'red flags', and 'high intensity zones') but were added in the second round to refine the specificity of findings.

The choice of 20 MRI reports per round was arbitrary as we had no data *a priori* on which to estimate the likely reliability between raters and its variance, nor the likely proportions of positive diagnoses. Therefore, we performed a *post hoc* power calculation to determine the reliability that was statistically detectable, given the sample size, Kappa values, and observed proportion of positive diagnoses, using the method described by Sim and Wright [10].

Inter-rater reproducibility

Inter-rater reproducibility was calculated separately for coding rounds 1 to 4. Given the uncertainty as to what level of clinical training was required to achieve adequate reproducibility in extracting pathoanatomic information from the narrative reports, we compared the reproducibility of the three trainee clinicians to that of two highly trained raters during an arbitrary coding round (round two). The two highly trained raters were experienced researchers in the field of spinal MRI, including designing and conducting reproducibility studies of lumbar MRI findings [11,12]. One was a chiropractor and the other a physiotherapist, both of whose PhDs and post-doctoral experience focused on the investigation of MRI findings.

Inter-rater reproducibility was also calculated for the coding round that involved the second group of three trainee clinicians. These raters were exposed to the coding rules but did not participate in rule formation. Their training consisted solely of receiving feedback on their reproducibility when coding five randomly selected MRI reports *not used* in the coding rounds in this study. Therefore, their performance was more representative of the reproducibility that might be achievable if these coding rules were used in other clinical or research settings.

Intra-rater reproducibility (test-retest)

The second group of trainee clinicians also recoded the same 20 MRI reports one week after their initial coding round. They were blinded to their initial coding scores. These two sets of coding results were used to calculate intra-rater reproducibility.

Data Analysis

The raw coding data were exported from the Filemaker Pro 9 database into Microsoft Excel 2008 (Microsoft Corp, Redmond, WA, USA). This allowed the coding matrices for each MRI report to be aligned according to rater.

Inter-rater and intra-rater agreement were quantified using percentage agreement. Percentage agreement expresses the proportion of cases where there was agreement between the two raters' responses, that is, where both raters nominated the presence of a particular condition or concurred on the absence of a that condition. It was calculated with a method reported in other reliability studies of MRI findings [12-14] using Microsoft Excel 2008. This method involved: (a) summing the number of agreements in each paired comparison, (b) expressing that sum as a proportion (percentage) of the number of ratings, (c) repeating this for all possible pairs of raters in that coding round, and (d) calculating the mean and 95% confidence interval of those proportions to provide a single estimate of the percentage agreement for that coding round.

Inter-rater and intra-rater reliability was quantified using the unweighted Kappa statistic. The Kappa coefficient expresses reliability for nominal or ordinal ratings while accounting for chance agreement [15]. The magnitude of Kappa can be influenced by prevalence of the condition, bias and non-independence of ratings [10] Kappa coefficients were calculated using the 'kap' and 'kapci' procedures in STATA 10.1 (Stata Corp, College Station, Texas, USA). We used a STATA program (do-file) that automated the process of: (i) calculating Kappa for all the possible paired comparisons, (ii) averaging Kappa values by first transforming them into Z-scores (Fisher's transformation), (iii) finding the arithmetic mean and calculating the 95% confidence interval, and then (iv) transforming the results back into Kappa values. Consistent with recommendations in the literature [6,16,17], the program did not calculate Kappa when the prevalence of a pathoanatomic finding was less than 10% or greater than 90%, as in situations of very high or very low prevalence, the chance agreement increases and biases the value of Kappa [18]. In the current study, this restriction applied to the prevalence of the pathology at each and every vertebral level being compared, and for findings of all raters being compared.

Agreement (percentage agreement) and reliability (Kappa) were also calculated between the highly trained raters and between the highly trained raters and trainee clinicians. Comparisons between highly trained raters and trainee clinicians represent a measure of concurrent validity.

Percentage agreement and Kappa were calculated in two ways: (1) using only the ratings for each separate pathology to allow comparisons of reproducibility between pathologies, and (2) using all the ratings across all pathologies to give a global summary statistic. For the calculation of percentage agreement and Kappa for each pathology, there were between 120 (one pathology × 6 vertebral levels × 20 MRI reports) and 140 ratings (only for nerve root irritation, one pathology × 7 vertebral levels × 20 MRI reports) in each pair-wise comparison between inexperienced raters in each coding round. This method was used when determining the inter-rater or intra-rater reproducibility of either group of trainee clinicians.

To calculate a global summary statistic for either percentage agreement or Kappa, all the ratings for a coding round were used in a single comparison. This was a total of 1700 potential ratings in each pair-wise cross-pathology comparison between raters for each round ((12 pathologies × 6 vertebral levels + nerve root irritation × 7 vertebral levels) × 20 MRI reports = 1700). This method was used when determining the reproducibility between the highly trained raters and also between the highly trained raters and trainee clinicians, as although this summary statistic provides less detail, it is easier to interpret.

The prevalence for each pathology was calculated for each coding round. This was performed on a 'whole person' level, that is, where the presence of a particular pathology in a person at one or more vertebral levels was counted as a single instance.

Results

The average age of the people whose MRIs were included was 51.4 years (SD 13.1; full range 27 to 88), and 55.0% were female. The prevalence of the 14 pathoanatomic categories within each sample of 20 MRI scans ranged from 0.0% to 100.0% (Tables 1 and 2). All pathologies were present in at least one of the five coding rounds.

Reproducibility during the formation of the coding rules

Overall, the mean paired-comparison percentage agreement between the initial three trainee clinicians across the 14 pathoanatomic categories increased with each subsequent round of coding from 97.9% to 99.4%. Overall, across the 14 categories and four rounds of coding, their inter-rater agreement (percentage agreement) ranged from 80.8%-100%, and reliability (Kappa) ranged from 0.63-1.00 (Table 1). The inter-rater reproducibility between highly trained raters determined in a single coding round, expressed as percentage agreement (95% CI) was 97.3% (96.6-98.1%) and Kappa (95% CI) was 0.82 (0.77-0.86). Kappa coefficients greater than 0.80 are generally considered to represent excellent reliability [19].

For the round in which the initial trainee clinicians were compared with highly trained raters, the mean percentage agreement between the trainee clinicians and highly trained rater 1 was 97.8% (97.0%-98.7%) and with highly trained rater 2 was 98.1% (96.7%-99.5%), suggesting excellent agreement. The Kappa coefficients ranged from 0.83-0.87 for comparisons between these trainee clinicians and highly trained rater 1, and 0.83-0.91 when compared with highly trained rater 2, (Table 2).

Reproducibility in inexperienced clinicians trained with the final set of coding rules

Overall, across the 14 categories and single round of coding, the second group of inexperienced clinicians displayed an *inter-rater* agreement (percentage agreement) ranging from 96.7-100.0% and their reliability (Kappa) ranged from 0.76-1.00 (Table 3). Their test-retest reproducibility was also high, with *intra-rater* agreement ranging from 94.3-100.0% and reliability ranging from k = 0.61-1.00.

Sample size

Post-hoc observations showed that across all patient MRI reports, all pathologies and all vertebral levels, the rater endorsement of the presence of a pathology was approximately 8%. A post-hoc power calculation showed that on the basis of an observed proportion of positive diagnoses (rater endorsement) of 10%, and an assumed null hypothesis value of Kappa to be 0.40, then a sample size of 102 ratings would detect with 80% power, a statistically significant Kappa of 0.90. As the sample sizes used in this study for the calculation of Kappa usually ranged between 120 and 140 observations (within pathology comparisons), and for some calculations was as large as 1700 observations (across all pathology comparisons), there was adequate power in the sample.

Discussion

This study is the first to establish that inter-rater and intra-rater reproducibility in extracting pathoanatomic information from MRI narrative reports is excellent. Moreover, we have demonstrated that a high level of radiological experience is not required to perform this task well, even in the absence of coding rules. These

Table 1 Inter-rater reproducability results for the initial group of three trainee clinicians for 14 pathoanatomic categories across the four coding rounds, expressed as a Kappa co-efficient and percentage agreement with 95% confidence intervals (95% CI)

Pathoanatomic category	Reliability index (95%CI)	Coding round 1	Coding round 2	Coding round 3	Coding round 4
Intervertebral disc degeneration	Prevalence*	71.7% (50.2-93.1)	94.0 (92.0-96.0)	80.0 (80.0-80.0)	83.3 (80.1-86.6)
	Kappa	*0.66 (0.54-0.77)*	*0.94 (0.84-1.00)*	*n/a*	*0.91 (0.80-1.00)*
	Percentage agreement	80.8% (73.8-87.9)	95.8 (92.3-99.4)	98.2 (95.8-100.0)	97.5 (94.7-100.0)
Intervertebral disc bulge	Prevalence	73.3% (70.1-76.6)	87.0 (83.1-90.9)	70.0 (70.0-70.0)	48.3 (45.1-51.6)
	Kappa	*0.91 (0.78-1.00)*	*0.86 (0.76-0.90)*	*1.00 (0.87-1.00)*	*0.89 (0.76-1.00)*
	Percentage agreement	95.0% (94.7-100.0)	92.5 (87.7-97.2)	100.0	99.2 (97.5-100.0)
Intervertebral disc herniation	Prevalence	40.0% (34.3-45.7)	61.0 (59.0-63.0)	40.0 (40.0-40.0)	45.0 (45.0-45.0)
	Kappa	*0.91 (0.73-1.00)*	*1.00 (0.85-1.00)*	*0.98 (0.87-1.00)*	*1.00 (0.82-1.00)*
	Percentage agreement	97.5% (94.7-100.0)	100.0	96.5 (93.1-99.9)	100.0
Nerve root compromise	Prevalence	13.3% (4.7-22.0)	42.0 (31.9-52.1)	31.7 (23.0-40.3)	18.3 (15.1-21.6)
	Kappa	*n/a*	*0.74 (0.49-1.00)*	*0.63 (0.45-0.81)*	*1.00 (0.75-1.00)*
	Percentage agreement	97.5% (94.7-100.0)	94.2 (90.0-98.4)	93.0 (88.3-97.7)	99.2 (97.5-100.0)
Modic change type 1	Prevalence	26.7% (23.4-29.9)	18.0 (15.6-20.4)	20.0 (20.0-20.0)	18.3 (15.1-21.6)
	Kappa	*0.86 (0.68-1.00)*	*0.86 (0.60-1.00)*	*1.00 (0.82-1.00)*	*0.86 (0.60-1.00)*
	Percentage agreement	95.0% (91.1-98.1)	98.3 (96.0-100.0)	100.0	100.0
Modic change type 2	Prevalence	25.0% (19.3-30.7)	10.0 (5.6-14.4)	20.0 (20.0-20.0)	5.0 (5.0-5.0)
	Kappa	*0.76 (0.51-1.00)*	*n/a*	*1.00 (0.82-1.00)*	*n/a*
	Percentage agreement	97.5% (94.7-100.0)	98.3 (96.0-100.0)	100.0	100.0
Spondylolisthesis	Prevalence	20.0% (20.0-20.0)	19.0 (17.0-21.0)	10.0 (10.0-10.0)	0.0 (0.0-0.0)
	Kappa	*n/a*	*1.00 (0.75-1.00)*	*1.00 (0.82-1.00)*	*n/a*
	Percentage agreement	97.5% (94.7-100.0)	100.0	100.0	100.0
Stenosis	Prevalence	6.7% (3.4-9.9)	23.0 (20.6-25.4)	25.0 (25.0-25.0)	0.0 (0.0-0.0)
	Kappa	*n/a*	*0.84 (0.59-1.00)*	*0.95 (0.74-1.00)*	*n/a*
	Percentage agreement	97.5% (94.7-100.0)	99.2 (97.5-100.0)	99.1 (97.4-100.0)	100.0
Scoliosis	Prevalence	25.0% (25.0-25.0)	6.0 (4.0-8.0)	5.0 (5.0-5.0)	5.0 (5.0-5.0)
	Kappa	*1.00 (0.82-1.00)*	*n/a*	*n/a*	*n/a*
	Percentage agreement	100.0%	95.0 (91.1-98.9)	99.1(97.4-100.0)	100.0
Osteophytes	Prevalence	5.0% (5.0-5.0)	1.0 (0.0-3.0)	10.0 (10.0-10.0)	10.0 (10.0-10.0)
	Kappa	*n/a*	*n/a*	*n/a*	*1.00 (0.75-1.00)*
	Percentage agreement	100.0%	100.0	99.1 (97.4-100.0)	99.2 (97.5-100.0)
Facet joint arthrosis	Prevalence	0.0% (0.0)	14.0 (12.0-16.0)	20.0 (20.0-20.0)	5.0 (5.0-5.0)
	Kappa	*n/a*	*0.68 (0.42-0.93)*	*1.00 (0.82-1.00)*	*n/a*
	Percentage agreement	100.0%	95.0 (91.1-98.9)	100.0	100.0
Endplate irregularities	Prevalence	#	1.0 (0.0-3.0)	25.0 (19.3-30.7)	18.3 (11.8-24.9)
	Kappa		*n/a*	*1.00 (0.82-1.00)*	*0.74 (0.56-0.92)*
	Percentage agreement		99.2 (97.5-100.0)	98.2 (95.8-100.0)	97.5 (94.7-100.0)
Red flags	Prevalence (%)	#	0.0 (0.0-0.0)	8.3 (1.8-14.9)	0.0 (0.0-0.0)
	Kappa		n/a	*n/a*	*n/a*
	Percentage agreement		100.0	98.2 (95.8-100.0)	100.0
High intensity zone	Prevalence (%)	#	15.0 (11.9-18.1)	26.7 (20.1-33.2)	25.0 (25.0-25.0)
	Kappa		*0.84 (0.59-1.00)*	*0.85 (0.67-1.00)*	*1.00 (0.82-1.00)*
	Percentage agreement		99.2 (97.5-100.0)	98.2 (95.8-100.0)	100.0

* The prevalence estimates are calculated on a 'whole person' level. That is, the presence of a particular pathology in a person at one or more vertebral levels was counted as a single instance.

95%CI = 95% confidence interval in brackets.

not included in coding round 1.

n/a = kappa co-efficient not calculated. Calculation of kappa in STATA requires the prevalence of the pathology to be 10% to 90% at each and every vertebral level being compared. This restriction applies to the findings of all raters being compared.

findings have useful implications for conducting large-scale research and quality assurance projects that include MRI data.

Agreement between the initial group of trainee clinicians exceeded a percentage agreement of 90%, except for intervertebral disc degeneration in coding round 1 (80.8%). The greater discordance between raters for intervertebral disc degeneration may be explained by the larger number of terms used by radiologists to characterise degeneration, relative to other pathoanatomic findings. Nonetheless, with the introduction of coding rules, the percentage agreement for this category increased to a maximum of 98.2% and was comparable to that of highly trained raters (97.3%). The greatest

Table 2 Inter-rater reproducability between trainee clinicians and highly trained raters within a single coding round, expressed as a paired-comparison percentage agreement and Kappa co-efficient with 95% confidence intervals (95% CI)

Paired comparison	Percentage agreement (95% CI)	Kappa (95% CI, p value)
Highly trained rater 1 × Trainee clinician 1	98.2% (97.5%-98.8%)	0.87 (0.82-0.91)
Highly trained rater 1 × Trainee clinician 2	97.8% (97.2%-98.5%)	0.85 (0.79-0.89)
Highly trained rater 1 × Trainee clinician 3	97.5% (96.8%-98.2%)	0.83 (0.77-0.87)
Mean	*97.8% (97.0%-98.7%)*	
Highly trained rater 2 × Trainee clinician 1	98.1% (97.4%-98.7%)	0.87 (0.82-0.90)
Highly trained rater 2 × Trainee clinician 2	97.5% (96.8%-98.2%)	0.83 (0.77-0.87)
Highly trained rater 2 × Trainee clinician 3	98.6% (98.1%-99.2%)	0.91 (0.86-0.94)
Mean	*98.1% (96.7%-99.5%)*	

improvement in inter-rater agreement for intervertebral disc degeneration was observed after the first introduction of coding rules (round 2). This observation is consistent with the improvement in the mean percentage agreement across the 14 pathoanatomic categories also being largest between coding rounds 1 and 2 (0.8%). Although the mean percentage agreement continued to improve with the two subsequent iterations of the coding rules, the improvements were relatively minor (0.3-0.4%), indicating only a small additional training effect. This suggests that the initial version of coding rules was sufficient to improve reliability by the greatest extent. By the fourth coding round, the percentage agreement exceeded 99.0% in all categories except for 'intervertebral disc degeneration' and 'other endplate irregularities'. These results were reinforced by those of the second group of inexperienced clinicians who displayed a mean *inter-rater* percentage agreement of 99.0% and mean *intra-rater* percentage agreement of 98.7%.

Similarly, the levels of reliability (Kappa coefficients) achieved by the fourth coding round for the first group of inexperienced clinicians exceeded 0.85 in all categories other than for 'endplate irregularities', which would all be classified by the Landis criteria as showing excellent reliability [19]. In addition to the lower Kappa value observed for intervertebral disc degeneration in coding round 1, a lower value was also observed for nerve root compromise in coding round 3. Similar to disc degeneration, greater discordance for nerve root compromise and also for endplate irregularities might be explained by a relatively larger number of terms used to describe these findings. These results were also reinforced by those obtained by the second group of inexperienced clinicians. Their *inter-rater* Kappa coefficients all exceeded 0.92, except for 'nerve root compromise' and their *intra-rater* Kappa coefficients all exceeded 0.88, except for 'nerve root compromise' and 'disc bulge'. To our knowledge, no other studies have explored the reproducibility of this task and therefore it is not possible to compare our results with those reported in other literature.

As the level of training required to transform narrative MRI reports to quantitative data was uncertain, this study compared inter-rater reproducibility between a group of trainee clinicians and highly trained MRI coders. The results suggest that trainee clinicians displayed equal reproducibility as experienced researchers in performing this task, when trained with simple coding rules. Collectively, these data suggest that with minimal training and the introduction of basic coding rules, trainee clinicians can accurately and reliably extract pathoanatomic information from MRI narrative reports.

In the absence of radiologists being available to quantify pathoanatomic findings directly from an MRI console, having other personnel quantify these findings from narrative reports is the next best alternative, particularly in the context of workforce limitations and limited budgets for research projects. Our evidence that inexperienced clinicians can perform this task with high reproducibility has implications for the planning, feasibility and cost of research and quality assurance activities. However, these findings are derived within a research/quality assurance context and should not be inferred to have implications for clinical practice. Examination of the reliability of inexperienced clinicians at extracting *clinically relevant* information from MRI reports was not part of the current study.

Another potential alternative is to create software that could screen narrative reports for key phrases, and thereby, automate the process of coding pathoanatomic findings. However, this would need to overcome the challenge of the disparate and inconsistent ways in which radiologists report the same findings and ideally would need to be shown to have at least comparable reproducibility as human raters.

The design of this study has three strengths. First, the electronic coding matrix contained an extensive list of common pathoanatomic observations reported in MRI narrative reports. The matrix also provided an efficient and dependable mechanism to enter and store data. Second, we established reproducibility using a group of

Table 3 Inter-rater reproducability reliability results for the second group of three trainee clinicians for 14 pathoanatomic categories across a single coding round, expressed as a Kappa co-efficient and percentage agreement with 95% confidence intervals (95% CI)

Pathoanatomic category	Reliability index (95%CI)	Inter-rater Coding round 1	Inter-rater Coding round 2	Test-retest (intra-rater)
Intervertebral disc degeneration	Prevalence*	90.0% (90.0-90.0)	90.0% (90.0-90.0)	-
	Kappa	*0.99 (0.87-1.00)*	*0.93 (0.82-1.00)*	*0.88 to 1.00*
	Percentage agreement	99.3% (99.0-100.0)	96.7% (95.0-99.0)	97.3% (94.0-100.0)
Intervertebral disc bulge	Prevalence	90.0% (90.0-90.0)	85.0% (79.3-90.7)	-
	Kappa	*0.96 (0.84-1.00)*	*0.93 (0.80-1.00)*	*0.79 to 0.96*
	Percentage agreement	98.0% (97.0-99.0)	96.7% (95.0-99.0)	94.3% (91.0-97.0)
Intervertebral disc herniation	Prevalence	58.3% (55.1-61.6)	58.3% (55.1-61.6)	-
	Kappa	*0.94 (0.80-1.00)*	*0.94 (0.80-1.00)*	*0.86 to 0.91*
	Percentage agreement	98.7% (98.0-99.0)	98.7% (98.0-100.0)	97.3% (97.0-98.0)
Nerve root compromise	Prevalence	53.3% (50.1-56.6)	55.0% (49.3-60.7)	-
	Kappa	*0.76 (0.58-0.94)*	*0.81 (0.63-0.99)*	*0.61 to 0.86*
	Percentage agreement	96.0% (94.0-98.0)	97.3% (96.0-98.0)	95.3% (94.0-98.0)
Modic change type 1	Prevalence	20.0% (20.0-20.0)	21.7% (18.4-24.9)	-
	Kappa	*1.00 (0.82-1.00)*	*0.93 (0.75-1.00)*	*0.89 to 1.00*
	Percentage agreement	100.0% (100.0-100.0)	99.3% (99.0-100.0)	99.7% (99.0-100.0)
Modic change type 2	Prevalence	10.0% (10.0-10.0)	8.3% (5.1-11.6)	-
	Kappa	*1.00 (0.75-1.00)*	*n/a*	*1.00 to 1.00*
	Percentage agreement	100.0% (100.0-100.0)	99.3% (99.0-100.0)	99.7% (99.0-100.0)
Spondylolisthesis	Prevalence	20.0% (20.0-20.0)	20.0% (20.0-20.0)	-
	Kappa	*1.00 (0.75-1.00)*	*1.00 (0.75-1.00)*	*1.00 to 1.00*
	Percentage agreement	100.0% (100.0-100.0)	100.0% (100.0-100.0)	100.0% (100.0-100.0)
Stenosis	Prevalence	16.7% (13.2-19.9)	15.0% (15.0-15.0)	-
	Kappa	*n/a*	*n/a*	*n/a*
	Percentage agreement	99.3% (99.0-100.0)	100.0% (100.0-100.0)	99.7% (99.0-100.0)
Scoliosis	Prevalence	5.0% (5.0-5.0)	5.0% (5.0-5.0)	-
	Kappa	*n/a*	*n/a*	*n/a*
	Percentage agreement	100.0% (100.0-100.0)	100.0% (100.0-100.0)	100.0% (100.0-100.0)
Osteophytes	Prevalence	0.0% (0.0-0.0)	0.0% (0.0-0.0)	-
	Kappa	*n/a*	*n/a*	*n/a*
	Percentage agreement	100.0% (100.0-100.0)	100.0% (100.0-100.0)	100.0% (100.0-100.0)
Facet joint arthrosis	Prevalence	15.0% (15.0-15.0)	15.0% (15.0-15.0)	-
	Kappa	*1.00 (0.82-1.00)*	*0.92 (0.74-1.00)*	*0.88 to 1.00*
	Percentage agreement	100.0% (100.0-100.0)	98.7% (98.0-100.0)	99.3% (98.0-100.0)
Endplate irregularities	Prevalence	5.0% (5.0-5.0)	1.7% (0.0-4.9)	-
	Kappa	*n/a*	*n/a*	*n/a*
	Percentage agreement	100.0% (100.0-100.0)	99.3% (99.0-100.0)	99.3% (99.0-100.0)
Red flags	Prevalence	0.0% (0.0-0.0)	0.0% (0.0-0.0)	-
	Kappa	*n/a*	*n/a*	*n/a*
	Percentage agreement	100.0% (100.0-100.0)	100.0% (100.0-100.0)	100.0% (100.0-100.0)
High intensity zone	Prevalence	15.0% (15.0-15.0)	15.0% (15.0-15.0)	-
	Kappa	*1.00 (0.75-1.00)*	*1.00 (0.75-1.00)*	*n/a*
	Percentage agreement (%)	100.0% (100.0-100.0)	100.0% (100.0-100.0)	100.0% (100.0-100.0)

* The prevalence estimates are calculated on a 'whole person' level. That is, the presence of a particular pathology in a person at one or more vertebral levels was counted as a single instance.

95%CI = 95% confidence interval in brackets.

n/a = kappa co-efficient not calculated. Calculation of kappa in STATA requires the prevalence of the pathology to be 10% to 90% at each and every vertebral level being compared. This restriction applies to the findings of all raters being compared.

trainee clinicians in order to determine whether this task could be performed well by a relatively inexperienced group of people, as this reflects common workforce characteristics in large research projects. We then compared their level of reproducibility to that of highly trained researchers. Thirdly, we replicated the findings in a new group of trainee clinicians that did not participate in establishing the coding rules, thereby extending the generalisability of the results.

These results should, however, be considered in the context of some limitations. The number of MRI reports used in each coding round (n = 20) was chosen arbitrarily and might be considered small. However, depending on the pathologies and vertebral levels involved in each comparison between raters, this resulted in between 120 and 140 observations per rater per round for each pathology, and a total of 1700 observations per rater per round across all the pathologies combined. A post hoc power calculation showed adequate power to detect the Kappa values typically observed. Our decision to compare three trainee clinicians in each group was also arbitrary and based on these people also being part of a larger research programme. Furthermore, the trainees consisted of physiotherapy students only. It is possible that these estimates of reproducibility may vary, depending on the number of raters and their professional discipline. In this study, percentage agreement was calculated based on raters' nominating the presence of a condition by selecting a pathoanatomic category and nominating absence of a condition by not selecting a pathoanatomic category. Given there were 85 potential selections per patient, the low prevalence of some pathoanatomic findings resulted in a large proportion of 'absent findings', which may have inflated inter-rater agreement. However, this approach for calculating percentage agreement is widely reported in the literature [12-14]. Another potential limitation is that the experienced clinicians used for comparison were not radiologists. This was a pragmatic comparison, as it is not common that research radiologists are available for coding tasks in large-scale research projects. Therefore the comparison clinicians were chosen as representative of research personnel more commonly available for this task.

Conclusions

Results from this study provide evidence of very high inter-rater and intra-rater reproducibility for inexperienced clinicians in extracting pathoanatomic information from MRI narrative reports. These inexperienced clinicians also showed high reproducibility compared with researchers highly trained in this task. Small improvements in reproducibility can be achieved with the introduction of coding rules when transforming narrative information to quantitative data. These findings suggest that for research and quality assurance purposes, the quantification of pathoanatomic findings contained in narrative MRI reports can be performed by inexperienced clinicians.

Additional material

Additional file 1: The final set of decision rules used to extract pathoanatomic findings from MRI narrative reports.

Acknowledgements

We are grateful to Prof Claus Manniche for institutional support. AMB is supported by a fellowship awarded by the Australian National Health and Medical Research Council. TSJ is supported by grants from the Danish Foundation of Chiropractic Research and Postgraduate Education.

Author details

[1]Research Department, Spine Centre of Southern Denmark, Lillebaelt Hospital, Institute of Regional Health Services Research, University of Southern Denmark, Middelfart, Denmark. [2]School of Physiotherapy and Curtin Health Innovation Research Institute, Curtin University, Perth, Australia. [3]Odense Physiotherapy Sports and Fitness, Odense, Denmark. [4]Quick Care, Odense, Denmark. [5]Southwest Jutland Hospital, Esbjerg, Denmark.

Authors' contributions

All authors participated in the design of the study, its coordination, its statistical analysis, and read and approved the final manuscript. PK conceived of the study and designed the database. AMB and PK drafted the manuscript.

Competing interests

The authors declare that they have no competing interests.

References

1. Lurie JD, Doman DM, Spratt KF, Tosteson ANA, Weinstein JN: **Magnetic resonance imaging interpretation in patients with symptomatic lumbar spine disc herniations. Comparison of clinician and radiologist readings.** *Spine* 2009, **34**:701-705.
2. Dora C, Walchli B, Elfering A, Gal I, Weishaupt D, Boos N: **The significance of spinal canal dimensions in discriminating symptomatic from asymptomatic disc herniations.** *Eur Spine J* 2002, **11**:575-581.
3. Jarvik JJ, Hollingworth W, Heagerty P, Haynor DR, Deyo RA: **The longitudinal assessment of aging and disability of the back (LAIDBack) study: Baseline data.** *Spine* 2001, **26**:1158-1166.
4. Jensen MC, Brant-Zawadzki MN, Obuchowski N, Modic MT, Malkasian D, Ross JS: **Magnetic resonance imaging of the lumbar spine in people without back pain.** *N Engl J Med* 1994, **331**:69-73.
5. Jensen TS, Karppinen J, Sorensen JS, Niinimaki J, Leboeuf-Yde C: **Vertebral endplate signal changes (Modic change): a systematic literature review of prevalence and association with non-specific low back pain.** *Eur Spine J* 2008, **17**:1407-1422.
6. Arana E, Royuela A, Kovacs FM, Estremera A, Sarasibar H, Amengual G, Galarraga I, Martinez C, Muriel A, Abraira V, *et al*: **Lumbar Spine: Agreement in the Interpretation of 1.5-T MR Images by Using the Nordic Modic Consensus Group Classification Form.** *Radiology* 2010, **254**:809-817.
7. Lurie JD, Tosteson AN, Tosteson TD, Carragee E, Carrino JA, Kaiser J, Sequeiros RT, Lecomte AR, Grove MR, Blood EA, *et al*: **Reliability of readings of magnetic resonance imaging features of lumbar spinal stenosis.** *Spine* 2008, **33**:1605-1610.
8. Lurie JD, Tosteson AN, Tosteson TD, Carragee E, Carrino JA, Kaiser J, Sequeiros RT, Lecomte AR, Grove MR, Blood EA, *et al*: **Reliability of magnetic resonance imaging readings for lumbar disc herniation in the Spine Patient Outcomes Research Trial (SPORT).** *Spine* 2008, **33**:991-998.
9. de Vet HC, Terwee CB, Knol DL, Bouter LM: **When to use agreement versus reliability measures.** *J Clin Epidemiol* 2006, **59**:1033-1039.
10. Sim J, Wright CC: **The kappa statistic in reliability studies: use, interpretation, and sample size requirements.** *Phys Ther* 2005, **85**:257-268.
11. Jensen TS, Sorensen JS, Kjaer P: **Intra- and interobserver reproducibility of vertebral endplate signal (Modic) changes in the lumbar spine: the Nordic Modic Consensus Group classification.** *Acta Radiol* 2007, **48**:748-754.
12. Sorensen SJ, Kjaer P, Jensen TS, Andersen P: **Low field magnetic resonance imaging of the lumbar spine: Reliability of qualitative evaluation of disc and muscle parameters.** *Acta Radiologica* 2006, **47**:947-953.
13. Carrino JA, Lurie JD, Tosteson AN, Tosteson TD, Carragee EJ, Kaiser J, Grove MR, Blood E, Pearson LH, Weinstein JN, Herzog R: **Lumbar spine: reliability of MR imaging findings.** *Radiology* 2009, **250**:161-170.
14. Mulconrey DS, Knight RQ, Bramble JD, Paknikar S, Harty PA: **Interobserver reliability in the interpretation of diagnostic lumbar MRI and nuclear imaging.** *Spine J* 2006, **6**:177-184.

15. Altman DG: **Some common problems in medical research. Practical statistics for medical research.** London: Chapman & Hall/CRC; 1999.
16. Feinstein AR, Cicchetti DV: **High agreement but low kappa: I. The problems of two paradoxes.** *J Clin Epidemiol* 1990, **43**:543-549.
17. Kovacs FM, Royuela A, Jensen TS, Estremera A, Amengual G, Muriel A, Galarraga I, Martinez C, Arana E, Sarasibar H, *et al*: **Agreement in the Interpretation of Magnetic Resonance Images of the Lumbar Spine.** *Acta Radiologica* 2009, **50**:497-506.
18. Brennan P, Silman A: **Statistical methods for assessing observer variability in clinical measures.** *BMJ* 1992, **304**:1491-1494.
19. Landis JR, Koch GG: **The measurement of observer agreement for categorical data.** *Biometrics* 1977, **33**:159-174.

Trunk muscle fatigue during a lateral isometric hold test: what are we evaluating?

Isabelle Pagé[1] and Martin Descarreaux[2*]

Abstract

Background: Side bridge endurance protocols have been suggested to evaluate lateral trunk flexor and/or spine stabilizer muscles. To date, no study has investigated muscle recruitment and fatigability during these protocols. Therefore the purpose of our study was to quantify fatigue parameters in various trunk muscles during a modified side bridge endurance task (i.e. a lateral isometric hold test on a 45° roman chair apparatus) and determine which primary trunk muscles get fatigued during this task. It was hypothesized that the ipsilateral external oblique and lumbar erector spinae muscles will exhibit the highest fatigue indices.

Methods: Twenty-two healthy subjects participated in this study. The experimental session included left and right lateral isometric hold tasks preceded and followed by 3 maximal voluntary contractions in the same position. Surface electromyography (EMG) recordings were obtained bilaterally from the external oblique, rectus abdominis, and L2 and L5 erector spinae. Statistical analysis were conducted to compare the right and left maximal voluntary contractions (MVC), surface EMG activities, right vs. left holding times and decay rate of the median frequency as the percent change from the initial value (NMF_{slope}).

Results: No significant left and right lateral isometric hold tests differences were observed neither for holding times (97.2 ± 21.5 sec and 96.7 ± 24.9 sec respectively) nor for pre and post fatigue root mean square during MVCs. However, participants showed significant decreases of MVCs between pre and post fatigue measurements for both the left and right lateral isometric hold tests. Statistical analysis showed that a significantly NMF_{slope} of the ipsilateral external oblique during both conditions, and a NMF_{slope} of the contralateral L5 erector spinae during the left lateral isometric hold test were steeper than those of the other side's respective muscles. Although some participants presented positive NMF_{slope} for some muscles, each muscle presented a mean negative NMF_{slope} significantly different from 0.

Conclusions: Although the fatigue indices suggest that the ipsilateral external oblique and contralateral L5 erector spinae show signs of muscle fatigue, this task seems to recruit a large group of trunk muscles. Clinicians should not view this task as evaluating specifically lateral trunk flexors, but rather as providing an indication of the general endurance and stabilisation capacity of the trunk.

Keywords: Side bridge test, Muscle fatigue, Trunk muscle, Functional testing

Background

Over the past two decades, lumbar spine stability has become an integral part of the low back pain assessment and treatment strategies, especially given its potential link to injury mechanisms and the ongoing clinical efforts directed toward enhancing stability in patients [1]. Furthermore, an increasing number of researchers and clinicians consider the strategy used by patients to activate their abdominal muscles to be central to the stability theme. It has been demonstrated that bracing, defined as the increase of torso stiffness by the activation of all abdominal muscles and back extensors muscles, produces greater stability than hollowing, which consist of the activation of the transversus abdominis and internal oblique muscles in healthy subjects [1,2]. As a corollary, a variety of trunk coactivation exercise protocols are frequently used in daily clinical practice for low back pain prevention in healthy patients, rehabilitation in low back pain patients, or in order to evaluate trunk muscle function. The quadratus lumborum, external

* Correspondence: martin.descarreaux@uqtr.ca
[2]Département de chiropratique, Université du Québec à Trois-Rivières, Trois-Rivières, G9A 5H7, Canada
Full list of author information is available at the end of the article

oblique, internal oblique, iliocostalis, longissimus and intertransversalis are believed to act as spine stabilizers when contracting bilaterally and as lateral trunk flexors by pulling the rib cage toward the hip when contracting unilaterally [3].

McGill et al. [4] suggested that a difference between left and right endurance time of the trunk flexors, extensors and lateral flexors muscles would predict who is at greater risk of back problem. As no exercise can evaluate all muscles involved in lumbar spine stability, evaluation in the 3 planes has to be done separately. Side bridge exercise protocols have been suggested to evaluate torso muscles in frontal plane. Such exercises are usually executed in a position where the participant lies down sideways with support of one arm and are named after the side of the arm support (e.g. left side bridge = left arm support) [5] Variants to the protocol initially described by McGill have also been described [5-7].

A wide range of use of these exercises has been presented in the literature. Some authors proposed comparing muscle balance by evaluating holding times, whereas others assessed the use of maximal voluntary contraction or isometric contraction of short duration to evaluate muscle recruitment.

McGill et al. [8] evaluated the holding times of 75 healthy subjects (mean age of 23 years) during side bridge protocols and obtained mean times of 81 ± 34 sec and 85 ± 36 sec for right and left side bridge respectively. Other authors [9] reported similar mean times, i.e. 87.5 ± 36.4 sec and 92.0 ± 45.8 sec for right and left side bridges respectively, in a group of 24 healthy subjects (mean age of 35.3 years). McGill [10] has proposed that endurance scores during side bridges could be interpreted by using a right side to left side holding time ratio. A discrepancy of over 0.05 in the ratio would suggest unbalanced endurance. McGill et al. [8] also examined the intra-rater reliability of this test in 5 subjects on 5 consecutive days and at 8 weeks (follow-up) and got an excellent reliability coefficient of over .96. Evans et al. [9] reported high intra-rater and inter-rater reliability with the lowest coefficient being .81 and .82 respectively.A number of studies have also provided information about muscle recruitment during side bridge tests. McGill et al. [11] reported ipsilateral (left side during side bridges with left supporting arm) trunk muscle activation of the quadratus lumborum, external oblique, rectus abdominis and lumbar erector spinae during isometric side bridges. These muscles presented 54%, 40%, 22% and 24% of their maximal voluntary contraction activity (MVCA) respectively. However, the small sample (4 participants) does not allow for much generalization. Ekstrom et al. [12] evaluated muscle activation during 5-second hold side bridges and reported an activation of up to 72% of MVCA of the gluteus medius, 69% of the external oblique, between 34% and 42% of the longissimus thoracis, lumbar multifidus and rectus abdominis and less of 21% of the gluteus maximus and harmstring muscles. In 2008, Ekstrom et al. [13] used the same protocol to evaluate the longissimus thoracis and lumbar multifidus activation on both sides during side bridges. The authors reported greater activation of the ipsilateral longissimus thoracis than of the lumbar multifidus (48-49% vs. 32-33% of MVCA respectively) and greater activation on the ipsilateral side than on the contralateral side (48-49% vs 7-8% of MVCA for the longissimus thoracis and 32-33% vs 14% of MVCA for the lumbar multifidus). They also evaluated muscle activation during maximal resistance in side bridge without trunk support (legs fixed and trunk unsupported) and reported greater activation of the ipsilateral (left muscle when left side up) longissimus thoracis at L1 than of the lumbar multifidus (54-58% and 38-39% of MVCA respectively). They demonstrated a greater activation on the ipsilateral side than on the contralateral one (54-58% vs. 7-9% of MVCA for longissimus thoracis and 38-39% vs. 12-13% of MVCA for lumbar multifidus). In light of these studies, the external oblique, gluteus medius and back extensor muscles on the ipsilateral side of the side bridge seem to be the muscles with the greatest levels of activation during this exercise.

Although muscle activation during side bridge endurance and trunk lateral flexion has been described in a few studies, muscle recruitment and fatigability protocols have not been extensively studied. Therefore the purpose of our study was to quantify fatigue parameters in various trunk muscles during a modified side bridge endurance test (i.e. a lateral isometric hold test on a 45° roman chair apparatus). A second objective was to determine which primary trunk muscles are fatigued during this functional task. We hypothesized that the ipsilateral external oblique and erector spinae muscles would exhibit the highest fatigue indices during the modified side bridge protocol.

Methods

Participants

Twenty-two healthy subjects (11 men, 11 women; mean age ± SD: 24.55 ± 5.00) participated in this study. All participants were volunteers and gave their informed, written consent according to the protocol approved by the Université du Québec à Trois-Rivières (Canada) Ethics Committee.

Experimental protocol

The one hour experimental session included maximal voluntary contractions and a trunk muscle endurance task in a lateral isometric hold position. Participants' height and weight were measured prior to the experimental task.

The *Baecke-f* questionnaire was also completed by all participants in order to assess their physical activity levels (daily participation in sports and leisure activity) [14]. The experimental task was thoroughly explained and demonstrated by the experimenter before any data were recorded.

Maximal voluntary contraction

The endurance task was preceded and followed by three maximal voluntary contractions (MVC) in the same position, and participants were allowed a 2-minute rest period between the MVC pre-endurance and endurance task, and 15 minutes between post-endurance MVC and the other side pre-endurance MVC. MVC assessments, conducted 2 minutes prior to, and immediately after each endurance protocol, were performed against a force transducer that measured trunk muscle strength in the lateral position in accordance with the procedure presented by Ledoux et al. [7]. Participants were tested in the same position they held in the endurance tasks. Verbal encouragements were provided to maximize voluntary contraction. MVCs were performed against a fixed harness around the shoulders connected inline to a uni-axial force transducer on the floor (NTEP-87-057A3 class III, Artech, Riverside, CA, USA). For each MVC trial, force data were recorded at a sampling rate of 1,000 Hz and filtered digitally with a fifth-order Butterworth filter (10-Hz low-pass cutoff frequency). The higher force value obtained in 3 consecutive 10-s trials was used as the reference for MVC.

Trunk muscle endurance task

Participants were asked to perform sustained isometric contractions of the trunk muscles in a lateral position for both left and right sides named according to the side up (Figure 1). The endurance tasks (left and right) were counterbalanced across participants to control for sequence order effects. The protocol was explained and demonstrated before any experimental task was undertaken. During the left lateral isometric hold test, participants were positioned on the right side on a 45 degrees Roman chair. Ledoux et al. [7] suggested that this protocol could be used as an alternative to the side bridge test. When used to assess muscle fatigability, it yielded endurance time slightly longer than to those reported by McGill[10]. The test was developed as an alternative to the side bridge test to evaluate endurance time in older adults and adults with upper limb injuries (who could not attain support off the floor). This test also creates the possibility to assess maximal voluntary contraction in the same position. The trunk, from the anterior superior iliac spine and up, was unsupported. Arm support was allowed prior to the endurance task. On the researcher's cue, the participants removed their arms from the support and folded them across the chest with hands placed on the opposite shoulder. During the endurance task, participants were asked to keep their trunk and head in line with their lower limbs which were one above the other. The goal for all participants was to hold this position as long as they could. In order to ensure that participants abide by instructions, the same assistant observed the entire task for every participant and gave them verbal feedback to ensure proper position based on thorough observation. Failure to comply with instructions resulted in a warning by the assistant and the task was ended if the participant failed to follow instructions three times. Verbalized encouragement was provided throughout the test.

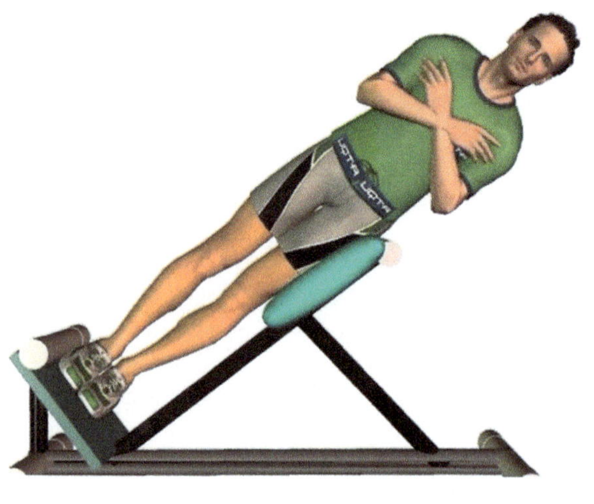

Figure 1 Apparatus and participants' positioning for right lateral isometric hold test.

Electromyography (EMG)

Surface EMG data were collected with *BiPole* disposable surface Ag-AgCl electrodes (Bortec biomedical, Calgary, Alberta, Canada) applied bilaterally on specific muscles in line with fiber direction. Inter-electrode distance was fixed at 2 cm and electrode diameter was 1 cm. Muscle activity of the external oblique, rectus abdominis, lumbar erector spinae (L2 and L5 level) was recorded according to McGill et al. [15]. A ground electrode was placed on the left olecranon of each participant. Skin impedance was reduced by (1) shaving body hair, (2) gently abrading the skin with fine-grade sandpaper (Red Dot Trace Prep, 3 M, St. Paul, MN, USA), and (3) wiping the skin with alcohol swabs. EMG activity was recorded using a single differential Delsys Surface EMG sensor with a common mode rejection ratio of 92 dB at 60 Hz, a noise level of 1.2 μV, a gain of 10 v/v ± 1%, an input impedance of $10^{15}\,\Omega$ (Model DE2.1, Delsys Inc., Boston, MA, USA) and sampled at 1,000 Hz with a 12-bit A/D converter (PCI 6024E, National Instruments, Austin, TX, USA).

The EMG data were filtered digitally by a 10- to 450-Hz band-pass, zero-lag, fifth-order Butterworth filter. They were collected by LabView (National Instruments) and processed by Matlab (MathWorks, Natick, MA, USA).

Data analysis

Maximal voluntary contraction (Newton) and maximal EMG root mean square values (RMS) (for each muscle) were obtained for every MVC trial to assess muscle fatigue. Muscular fatigue was assessed during the fatigue protocol through power spectral analysis. Median power frequency (MedF) was calculated from successive non-overlapping windows of 250 ms by Fast-Fourier transformation. Least square linear regression analysis was applied to MedF time series (MedF as a function of time) to estimate the rate of decline ($MedF_{slope}$). In order to express the decay rate of MedF as the percent change from the initial value (NMF_{slope} in%s^{-1}), $MedF_{slope}$ were divided by the initial MedF [16,17] . The equation below was used to obtained individual holding time ratios:

$$|1 - (\text{rightholdingtime}/\text{leftholdingtime})|$$

Statistical analysis

Right and left maximal voluntary contractions (Newtons) and RMS were compared between pre and post endurance tasks with 2-tailed *t*-tests for dependent samples. 2-tailed *t*-tests for dependant samples were also used to compare holding times between left and right lateral isometric hold tests. In order to test for our main hypothesis, the NMF_{slope} of antagonist muscles in both conditions (e.g. left external oblique vs. right external oblique during left lateral isometric hold test) were compared using 2-tailed *t*-tests for independent samples. *T*-tests for independent samples (1-tailed) comparing NMF_{slope} to 0 were conducted for every muscle in both conditions to determine if statistically significant decay of NMF were induced by the fatigue protocols. Simple correlation tests were performed separately for each baseline characteristic and holding times in order to evaluated the possible correlations. Statistical significance was set at $p < 0.05$ for all analyses.

Results

Participants' characteristics

Table 1 reports the mean (SD) baseline characteristics of participants (means age, weight, height, body mass index, Baecke-f questionnaire score).

Holding times and maximal voluntary contractions

T-tests for dependant samples revealed no significant difference between sides for holding times ($p > 0.88$) but showed significant decreases of MVCs between pre and post endurance task measurements for both the left and right lateral isometric hold tests ($p < 0.01$ and $p = 0.02$ respectively). No significant differences were observed between RMS pre and post endurance task values ($p > 0.05$). The calculated mean individual holding time ratio showed a 0.119 ± 0.118 discrepancy between the right and left sides. Simple correlation tests revealed no significant correlation between holding times and each baseline characteristic ($p > 0.05$). Figure 2 and Table 2 present the mean ± standard deviation for holding times and MVC statistical analysis.

Muscles recruitment during endurance task and muscle fatigue indices

Figure 3 presents the NMF_{slope} of external oblique and L5 erector spinae muscles for both sides during left and right lateral isometric hold tests. *T*-tests for independent samples comparing NMF_{slope} of antagonist muscles in both conditions (e.g. left external oblique vs. right external oblique during left lateral isometric hold test) showed a significantly greater decay rate of the NMF_{slope} of ipsilateral external oblique (i.e. left external oblique while left lateral isometric hold test comparing to right external oblique) during both conditions and of right L5 erector spinae during left lateral isometric hold test comparing to the left muscle. During right lateral isometric hold test, the left L5 erector spinae presented a trend toward a greater decay rate of the NMF_{slope} than the right one, but these differences were not significant ($p = 0.08$). No difference was observed in the other left versus right muscle comparisons (L2 erector spinae and rectus abdominis) in any of the conditions ($p > 0.05$). Table 3 presents results of *t*-tests for independent samples for NMF_{slope} of each muscle recorded during both conditions. Although some participants presented positive NMF_{slope} for some muscles, each muscle presented a mean negative NMF_{slope} significantly different from 0 at $p < 0.05$.

Discussion

This study's main objectives were to quantify fatigue parameters in various trunk muscles during a lateral isometric hold test in healthy participants and to determine which primary trunk muscles are fatigued during this functional task. The ipsilateral external oblique, during

Table 1 Participants' characteristics (mean ± SD)

	Mean ± SD
Age (years)	24.55 ± 5.00
Weight (kg)	70.62 ± 8.86
Height (m)	1.72 ± 0.09
Body mass index (kg/m^2)	23.94 ± 2.78
Sport activity indices in Baecke-f questionnaire	5.40 ± 1.51
Free-time activity indices in Baecke-f questionnaire	3.06 ± 0.79

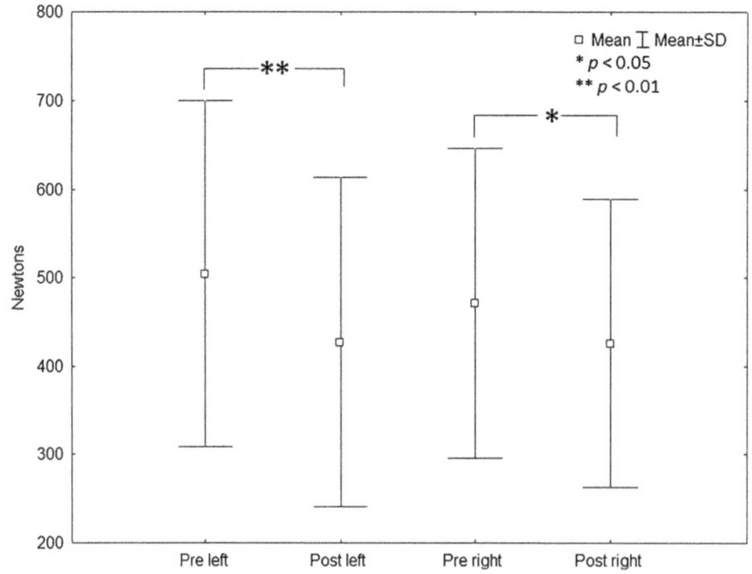

Figure 2 Left and right lateral isometric hold test MVCs before and after the endurance task.

Table 2 Left and right lateral isometric hold tests holding times and ratios (mean ± SD)

	Mean ± SD
Left lateral isometric hold test holding times (sec)	96.7 ± 24.9
Right lateral isometric hold test holding times (sec)	97.2 ± 21.5
Holding time ratio	0.119 ± 0.118
P value (between left and right lateral isometric hold tests)	0.88

both lateral isometric hold tests, and the contralateral L5 erector spinae, during the left lateral isometric hold test, showed significantly steeper negative NMF_{slope} than the other side's respective muscles. The results also showed that all recorded trunk muscles presented fatigue parameters during lateral isometric hold tests on both sides. Thereby, these results provide a preliminary understanding of the trunk muscles tested during a lateral isometric hold task.

Even if the results showed a NMF_{slope} significantly different from 0 for the 8 muscles recorded, the percentage of decay did not exceed $0.07\%s^{-1}$ which may raise questions with regard to the level of fatigue generated in individual muscles during the lateral hold. Despite the lack of normative data for fatigue parameters, other studies have reported steeper negative NMF_{slope} during trunk endurance protocols. Plamondon et al. [18] reported L3 erector spinae NMF_{slope} ($\%s^{-1} \pm SD$) of 0.10 ± 0.07 and 0.13 ± 0.05 for women and men respectively during modified Sorenson intermittent contraction tasks. Mannion et al. [16,17] reported NMF_{slope} values up to 0.46 ± 0.19 during modified Biering-Sorenson test. The results of the present study could suggest that muscles not recorded in our experiment could act as primary contributors during the lateral isometric hold task. In fact, the quadratus lumborum, which activity can be predicted with surface EMG placed on L3 erector spinae [15], has been reported to act as a trunk lateral flexor when contracted unilaterally [3,19], and some studies reported high levels of activity in this muscle during side bridges [11,20]. Lower limb muscle activity was not recorded in the present study, but gluteus medius, gluteus maximus and hamstring activation during different side bridges exercises has also been reported [6,12,13].

As often seen in motor tasks, there are certainly multiple muscle recruitment strategies (redundancy) that can be selected by the central nervous system to optimize task performance during a lateral isometric hold test [21]. During this task, more than one muscle contribute to the torque generated, and a changing combination of muscle forces to maintain the isometric contraction may be an efficient strategy to improve performance. Motor variability has been shown to be an efficient strategy to reduce the development of muscle fatigue [22]. Our results suggest that a variable trunk co-contraction strategy where numerous muscles contribute to the generation of isometric force is selected during a lateral isometric hold test. A few authors also reported global activation of trunk muscles instead of specific muscle recruitment during trunk endurance task. Page et al. [23] reported fatigue of various trunk muscles (i.e. abdominal muscles, lumbar erector spinae, biceps femoris) during sustained isometric contractions of abdominal muscles whereas Plamondon et al. [18] reported

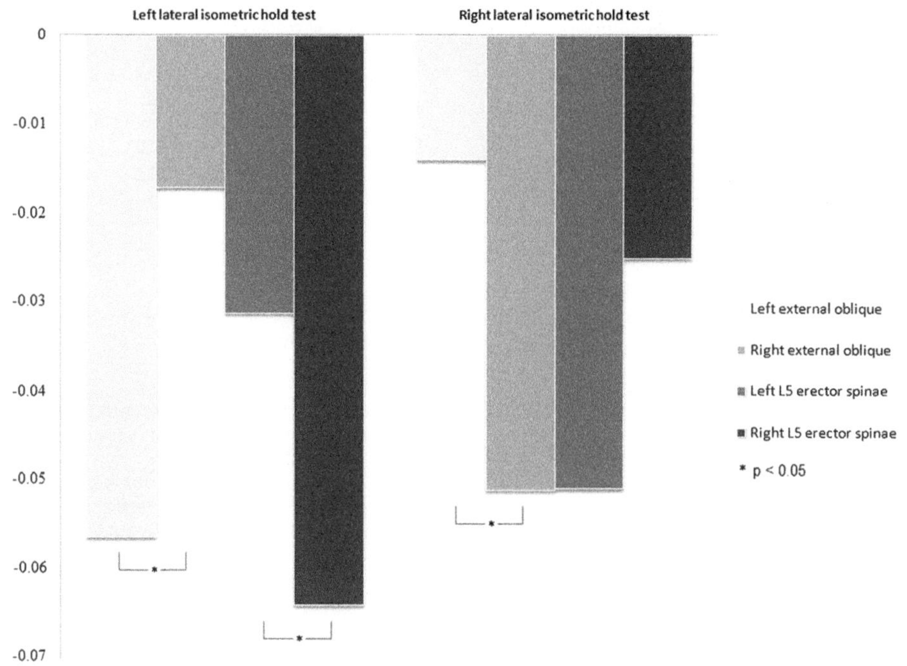

Figure 3 NMF_{slope} ($\%s^{-1}$) of external oblique and L5 erector spinae muscles during left and right lateral isometric hold tests.

Table 3 NMF_{slope} *t*-tests for left and right lateral isometric hold tests (mean ± SD)

Muscles	Left lateral isometric hold test			Right lateral isometric hold test		
	df	NMF_{slope} ($\% s^{-1}$)	*P* values	df	NMF_{slope} ($\% s^{-1}$)	*P* values
Left rectus abdominis	19	−0.025 ± 0.054	0.018	20	−0.037 ± 0.043	< 0.001
Right rectus abdominis	18	−0.032 ± 0.038	< 0.001	20	−0.026 ± 0.023	< 0.001
Left external oblique	18	−0.056 ± 0.037	< 0.001	20	−0.014 ± 0.026	0.0106
Right external oblique	19	−0.017 ± 0.030	0.009	20	−0.051 ± 0.039	< 0.001
Left L2 erector spinae	20	−0.023 ± 0.031	< 0.001	20	−0.034 ± 0.054	0.0041
Right L2 erector spinae	20	−0.043 ± 0.051	< 0.001	20	−0.025 ± 0.029	< 0.001
Left L5 erector spinae	20	−0.031 ± 0.053	0.0011	17	−0.051 ± 0.031	< 0.001
Right L5 erector spinae	18	−0.064 ± 0.048	< 0.001	20	−0.025 ± 0. 055	0.022

fatigue of lumbar erector spinae and hip extensor muscles (hamstring and gluteus maximus) during an intermittent modified Sorenson contraction task. Furthermore, other studies have reported the recruitment of several trunk muscles (e.g. quadratus lumborum, external oblique, rectus abdominis, lumbar and thoracis erector spinae, gluteus medius, lumbar multifidus, gluteus maximus and hamstrings) during side bridge tasks [11-13].

Our participants showed mean holding times similar to the ones reported in previous studies where lateral flexors endurance was evaluated using the side bridge position [8,9]. However, although only healthy participants were included in the study, a mean difference of more than 5% between both side holding times was observed. According to McGill, such differences in holding times during the side bridge position would suggest trunk muscle imbalance [10]. The relatively high variability of the right on left holding time ratio (i.e. a standard deviation of 11.8%) suggests a wide variation of this ratio in healthy populations. Differences in testing protocols (isometric lateral hold versus side bridge) may explain these differences. However, one might question the clinical value of the proposed criteria suggesting that differences of more than 5% between right and left holding times characterize individuals with a history of disabling back troubles or an increased risk of back trouble [10]. Others studies are necessary to validate the use of a holding time ratio derived from the lateral isometric hold test as a normative data to evaluate muscle balance and function.

A few limitations need to be considered when interpreting the present results. For this study, only healthy young adults were recruited, and consequently generalization to other healthy or clinical populations may be limited. Only eight trunk muscles (surface EMG) were recorded, and other studies are necessary to evaluate the possible contribution and fatigue of several other trunk or lower limb muscles that could be recruited during lateral isometric hold task.

Conclusions

This study was conducted in order to identify muscles evaluated during a lateral isometric hold task. Although the fatigue indices suggest that ipsilateral external oblique and contralateral L5 erector spinae are significant contributors, all recorded muscles were active during the lateral isometric hold task. The lateral isometric hold, while different from the side bridge assessment for endurance because it does not involve support of the floor, seems to be adequate for the evaluation of lateral trunk flexors. Studies involving individuals with low back pain are needed to evaluate the clinical relevance of this procedure.

Competing interests

The author(s) declare that they have no competing interests.

Acknowledgements

The study was funded by the Chaire de Recherche en Chiropratique FRCQ, the Fonds de Recherche en Santé du Québec (FRSQ), the Institut de Recherche Robert-Sauvé en Santé et en Sécurité du Travail (IRSST) and the Canadian Chiropractic Association. Other contributors: Marie-Pierre Harvey and Maude Carroll who contributed to the experimentation.

Author details

[1]Département des sciences de l'activité physique, Université du Québec à Trois-Rivières, Trois-Rivières, G9A 5H7, Canada. [2]Département de chiropratique, Université du Québec à Trois-Rivières, Trois-Rivières, G9A 5H7, Canada.

Authors' contributions

IP participated in the study design, experimentation and manuscript writing. MD participated in study design, data analysis, manuscript writing and revision. All authors read and approved the final manuscript.

References

1. Grenier SG, McGill SM: **Quantification of lumbar stability by using 2 different abdominal activation strategies.** *Arch Phys Med Rehabil* 2007, **88** (1):54–62.
2. Richardson CA, Snijders CJ, Hides JA, Damen L, Pas MS, Storm J: **The relation between the transversus abdominis muscles, sacroiliac joint mechanics, and low back pain.** *Spine (Phila Pa 1976)* 2002, **27**(4):399–405.
3. Wiatt E, Flanagan SP: **Lateral trunk flexors and low back pain: endurance and bilateral asymmetry.** *Athl10etic Therapy Today* 2009, **14**(3):10–12.
4. McGill SM, Grenier S, Kavcic N, Cholewicki J: **Coordination of muscle activity to assure stability of the lumbar spine.** *J Electromyogr Kinesiol* 2003, **13**(4):353–359.
5. McGill SM: **Low back exercises: evidence for improving exercise regimens.** *Phys Ther* 1998, **78**(7):754–765.
6. Konrad P, Schmitz K, Denner A: **Neuromuscular evaluation of trunk-training exercises.** *J Athl Train* 2001, **36**(2):109–118.
7. Ledoux E, Dubois JD, Descarreaux M: **Physical and psychosocial predictors of functional trunk capacity in older adults with and without low back pain.** *JMPT* 2012 (In press).
8. McGill SM, Childs A, Liebenson C: **Endurance times for low back stabilization exercises: clinical targets for testing and training from a normal database.** *Arch Phys Med Rehabil* 1999, **80**(8):941–944.
9. Evans K, Refshauge KM, Adams R: **Trunk muscle endurance tests: reliability, and gender differences in athletes.** *J Sci Med Sport* 2007, **10**(6):447–455.
10. McGill S: *Low back disorders: evidence-based prevention and rehabilitation.* Champaign, IL: Human Kinetics; 2002.
11. McGill S, Juker D, Kropf P: **Quantitative intramuscular myoelectric activity of quadratus lumborum during a wide variety of tasks.** *Clin Biomech (Bristol, Avon)* 1996, **11**(3):170–172.
12. Ekstrom RA, Donatelli RA, Carp KC: **Electromyographic analysis of core trunk, hip, and thigh muscles during 9 rehabilitation exercises.** *J Orthop Sports Phys Ther* 2007, **37**(12):754–762.
13. Ekstrom RA, Osborn RW, Hauer PL: **Surface electromyographic analysis of the low back muscles during rehabilitation exercises.** *J Orthop Sports Phys Ther* 2008, **38**(12):736–745.
14. Bigard AX, Duforez F, Portero P, Guezennec CY: **Détermination de l'activité physique par questionnaire: validation du questionnaire autoadministrable de Baecke.** *Sciences and Sports* 1992, **7**:215–221.
15. McGill S, Juker D, Kropf P: **Appropriately placed surface EMG electrodes reflect deep muscle activity (psoas, quadratus lumborum, abdominal wall) in the lumbar spine.** *J Biomech* 1996, **29**(11):1503–1507.
16. Mannion AF, Connolly B, Wood K, Dolan P: **The use of surface EMG power spectral analysis in the evaluation of back muscle function.** *J Rehabil Res Dev* 1997, **34**(4):427–439.
17. Mannion AF, Dolan P: **Electromyographic median frequency changes during isometric contraction of the back extensors to fatigue.** *Spine (Phila Pa 1976)* 1994, **19**(11):1223–1229.
18. Plamondon A, Trimble K, Lariviere C, Desjardins P: **Back muscle fatigue during intermittent prone back extension exercise.** *Scand J Med Sci Sports* 2004, **14**(4):221–230.
19. Huang QM, Andersson E, Thorstensson A: **Intramuscular myoelectric activity and selective coactivation of trunk muscles during lateral flexion with and without load.** *Spine (Phila Pa 1976)* 2001, **26**(13):1465–1472.
20. Kavcic N, Grenier S, McGill SM: **Determining the stabilizing role of individual torso muscles during rehabilitation exercises.** *Spine (Phila Pa 1976)* 2004, **29**(11):1254–1265.
21. Latash ML, Scholz JP, Schoner G: **Toward a new theory of motor synergies.** *Mot Control* 2007, **11**(3):276–308.
22. Madeleine P: **On functional motor adaptations: from the quantification of motor strategies to the prevention of musculoskeletal disorders in the neck-shoulder region.** *Acta Physiol (Oxf)* 2010, **199**(Suppl 679):1–46.
23. Page I, Dubois JD, Descarreaux M: **A comparison of 2 assessment protocols to specifically target abdominal muscle endurance.** *J Manipulative Physiol Ther* 2011, **34**(3):188–194.

4

Feasibility of the STarT back screening tool in chiropractic clinics: a cross-sectional study of patients with low back pain

Alice Kongsted[1,2*], Else Johannesen[3] and Charlotte Leboeuf-Yde[2]

Abstract

The STarT back screening tool (SBT) allocates low back pain (LBP) patients into three risk groups and is intended to assist clinicians in their decisions about choice of treatment. The tool consists of domains from larger questionnaires that previously have been shown to be predictive of non-recovery from LBP. This study was performed to describe the distribution of depression, fear avoidance and catastrophising in relation to the SBT risk groups. A total of 475 primary care patients were included from 19 chiropractic clinics. They completed the SBT, the Major Depression Inventory (MDI), the Fear Avoidance Beliefs Questionnaire (FABQ), and the Coping Strategies Questionnaire. Associations between the continuous scores of the psychological questionnaires and the SBT were tested by means of linear regression, and the diagnostic performance of the SBT in relation to the other questionnaires was described in terms of sensitivity, specificity and likelihood ratios.

In this cohort 59% were in the SBT low risk, 29% in the medium risk and 11% in high risk group. The SBT risk groups were positively associated with all of the psychological questionnaires. The SBT high risk group had positive likelihood ratios for having a risk profile on the psychological scales ranging from 3.8 (95% CI 2.3 - 6.3) for the MDI to 7.6 (95% CI 4.9 - 11.7) for the FABQ. The SBT questionnaire was feasible to use in chiropractic practice and risk groups were related to the presence of well-established psychological prognostic factors. If the tool proves to predict prognosis in future studies, it would be a relevant alternative in clinical practice to other more comprehensive questionnaires.

Background

Low back pain (LBP) is common and most cases of LBP are handled either without any contact to the health care system or in primary care [1,2]. However, some LBP patients develop severe or long-lasting pain with far-reaching consequences both personally and socioeconomically [3]. It is widely accepted that patients at risk of lasting back disability should be identified early in their course of LBP in order to prevent chronicity, and much effort has been put into investigating factors that predict non-recovery in LBP [4,5]. Although variability in research methods and quality limits what can be concluded about useful predictors in LBP, it seems that self-reported information on symptoms and beliefs about LBP is as valuable from a prognostic angle as data from the clinical examination [4,5]. It is therefore worthwhile to construct questionnaires focusing on such established prognostic indicators that can easily be filled in directly by patients.

The STarT back screening tool (SBT) was introduced as a tool that can assist general practitioners' decision-making concerning initial treatment options in primary care [6]. It consists of nine questions covering aspects of fear avoidance beliefs, depression, disability and presence of leg pain and neck/shoulder pain. Patients are allocated into one of three subgroups (low, medium or high risk of chronicity) based on the obtained score. The authors suggest that the low risk group only needs a 'light' intervention with e.g. analgesics and advice, the medium group requires treatments involving elements such as exercises or manual therapy, and that a combination of physical and cognitive-behavioral approaches should be considered for the high risk group [6].

* Correspondence: a.kongsted@nikkb.dk
[1]Nordic Institute of Chiropractic and Clinical Biomechanics, University of Southern Denmark, Odense. Part of Clinical Locomotion Network, Denmark
Full list of author information is available at the end of the article

The SBT has been validated against well-established questionnaires regarding disability and psychological parameters and its psychometric performance was shown to be similar to that of the longer Orebro Musculoskeletal Pain Screening Questionnaire [7]. So far, the tool has not been tested outside the United Kingdom and it has not been validated in relation to identifying patients with different treatment needs.

The aims of this study were 1) to test whether chiropractic patients in Denmark were able and willing to fill in a Danish version of the SBT, 2) to find out whether this tool is able to identify the three subgroups also in this cohort, and 3) to examine whether patients in the three expected subgroups differ regarding gender, age, symptoms, depression, fear avoidance beliefs, and catastrophising coping strategies.

Methods

A cross-sectional study was conducted with data collection in 19 chiropractic clinics that constitute the practice-research unit organized under the Nordic Institute of Chiropractic and Clinical Biomechanics. These clinics are geographically scattered throughout Denmark and have volunteered to participate in data collection upon invitation. In Denmark there is no requirement of a referral for chiropractic care and most patients see a chiropractor on their own initiative. The state pays some of the fee through a collective agreement with the chiropractic profession, but most (approximately 80%) is paid by the patient. The project was presented for the local ethical committee who stated that it did not need approval.

Procedures

The objectives of the project as well as practical procedures were described to the participating chiropractors at a meeting. Questionnaires and project procedures in writing were handed over at the meeting. On the first day of the data-collection the clinicians or their secretaries were contacted by phone to clarify any questions about the procedures. Another call was made at the end of the first week of data-collection to make sure they were all well underway, and this was repeated in weeks two and three, if considered necessary.

Patients with LBP were invited to participate when presenting to the clinics, and those who agreed to fill in a questionnaire were asked to do so in the waiting room. Afterwards, the completed questionnaire was put into a sealed envelope and returned to the chiropractor or secretary. Once a week the questionnaires were sent to the research unit. In a few cases the questionnaires were filled in by patients at home and afterwards returned to the clinic.

Patients

All patients between 18 and 67 years of age, who were consulting the chiropractor because of a LBP problem and were able to read and speak Danish, were qualified for participation.

Questionnaires

The questionnaire package consisted of the STarT back screening tool (SBT)[6], the Major Depression Inventory (MDI) [8], the Fear Avoidance Beliefs Questionnaire (FABQ) [9], and the Coping Strategies Questionnaire (CSQ) [10]. The allocation of patients into the three SBT risk groups is described in Figure 1. The purpose and scoring of the questionnaires are summarized in Table 1. The dichotomizing of the MDI and the FABQ were based on previous recommendations [8,9]. The CSQ consists of six subscales, each identifying the use of one coping strategy. For the present study we used only the subscale related to catastrophising. There is no consensus about a cut-point on the catastrophising subscale of the CSQ, therefore, based on the distribution in our study, we decided to consider scores of 16 or more to indicate a high use of catastrophising strategies, as this was considered the point for the split between the majority of observations and the right hand tail of the estimates.

In addition to the above described questionnaires, patients were asked about demographic factors, pain duration of the present episode (0 - 2 weeks, 2 weeks - 3 months, > 3 months), total number of pain days the preceding 12 months (< 30 days, ≥ 30 days), and number of days with LBP during the previous two weeks (0 - 14).

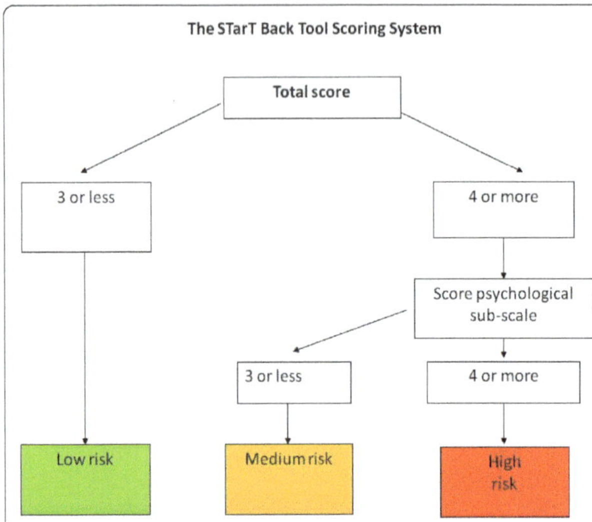

Figure 1 Allocation of patients into risk groups according to their SBT-scores. The illustrating was adapted from http://www.keele.ac.uk/research/pchs/pcmrc/dissemination/tools/startback/.

Table 1 Overview of the questionnaires used in the study

Questionnaire	Intended to evaluate	Possible range of scores	Sub-divisions used
SBT	Risk of chronicity	0 - 9 (overall)	Low risk: Overall < 4
		0 - 5 (psychological sub score)	Medium risk: Overall ≥ 4 and psych. sub scale < 4
			High Risk: Psych. sub scale ≥ 4
MDI	Depression	0 - 50	> 24: depressed
FABQ	Fear Avoidance Beliefs	0 - 66	> 48: high fear avoidance
CSQ	Use of six coping strategies. Catastrophising was the only domain used for the present study	Catastrophising: 0 - 36	≥ 16: high use of catastrophising

SBT: STarT back screening tool. MDI: Major depression inventory.
FABQ: Fear avoidance beliefs questionnaire. CSQ: Coping strategies questionnaire.

Data Analysis

The SBT questionnaire

Since the SBT holds only nine items that represent different domains, strict criteria for completion were defined. If an item was missing from the SBT, the missing value was replaced with the most frequent answer (0 or 1) to the remaining questions. If more than one item were missing, the entire scale was excluded.

User friendliness was established by noting the number and nature of unanswered questions. Whether the three SBT subgroups existed in the cohort was examined by noting the proportions of patients allocated into these groups.

The other questionnaires

Missing scores on the MDI and the FABQ scales were replaced by the average of the completed ones, if no more than two items were missing. Since the catastrophising domain of the CSQ only consisted of 6 questions, we used the average value on that scale to impute the missing value, if only one item was missing. In case of more missing values the scales were excluded. Imputation was performed in four, twenty-five and four scales of the MDI, FABQ, and CSQ respectively.

Associations between the SBT and the other questionnaires

Associations between the SBT risk groups and the MDI, FABQ, and CSQ were tested by means of linear regression with robust variance estimation using the SBT risk groups as a categorical variable. Prior to the regression analyses it was tested whether age and gender were equally distributed in the SBT groups. Since this was the case, the analyses were conducted without any adjusting. The dichotomised MDI, FABQ, and CSQ scores were used to calculate the sensitivity, specificity and likelihood ratios in relation to the SBT's diagnostic performance. Furthermore, prior and posterior probabilities of high scores on these scales were calculated to evaluate how knowledge of the SBT categories would alter a patient's "risk profile".

Data were double entered into Epidata (The EpiData Association, Odense, Denmark), corrected when necessary and transmitted to STATA 10.1 (StataCorp, Texas, USA) for the analyses.

Results

Study Population

A total of 607 questionnaires were distributed to the chiropractic clinics, and 543 questionnaires were completed between the 23rd of November and the 15th of December 2009. Twenty-four of these questionnaires were discarded because the respondents were not within the age-limits defined in the inclusion criteria, and the participants hence consisted of 519 subjects (255 females, 207 males, 57 did not report gender). The involved clinics recruited from seven to forty patients each (median = 31, IQR 29 - 35). The mean age was 43 years (67 subjects did not report age).

The participating patients were almost equally distributed among acute (30%), sub acute (36%), and chronic LBP (34%). Fifty-seven percent reported to have had pain for more than 30 days during the preceding year, and during the past two weeks a median of 8 days with LBP was reported (Interquartile range 4 - 14). Daily pain during the last two weeks was reported by 31% of the participants, and 43% reported that pain has spread to the leg(s) within the preceding two weeks.

Completion of the SBT

A total of 451/519 (87%) of the SBT questionnaires were complete. One item was missing in 24 questionnaires, and another 44 patients, who were hence excluded, had missed more than one item. Hence, the SBT was adequately completed by 475/519 (92%) of the patients; 244 females, 194 males, 37 sex not reported. The mean age in this final study sample was 43 (range 18 - 67).

When only one item was missing, it was most frequently the answer to 'Worrying thoughts have been going through my mind a lot of the time in the last 2 weeks' (5 cases) or to 'In general in the last 2 weeks, I have not enjoyed all the things I used to enjoy' (5 cases).

Distribution of patients on the SBT groups

The overall SBT scores ranged from 0 to 9 (median 3, IQR 1 - 5). The proportions of patients in the three risk groups were 59% (95% CI 55 - 64%) in low risk, 29% (95% CI 25 - 33%) in medium risk, and 11% (95% CI 8 - 14%) in high risk. The proportion of low risk patients varied between the data collecting clinics from 52% to 73%, and the proportion of high risk patients from 4% to 33%.

Patient characteristics in the SBT groups

Gender, age and symptom characteristics

Associations between the risk groups and the baseline characteristics appear from Table 2. The high risk patients had more days with LBP both the preceding year and the preceding two weeks, and tended to have had a longer duration of the present episode. Regarding duration the low and medium risk groups were very similar, whereas number of LBP days during the past two weeks increased for each SBT risk level. Fewer patients in the low risk group reported leg pain as compared to the other groups, which is partly explained by leg pain being one of the SBT items. Gender and age were equally distributed over the risk groups.

Associations between the STarT Back Screening Tool and the Major Depression Inventory

The MDI was adequately completed by 471 patients. The scores ranged from 0 to 42 (median 9), and 10% had a score of > 24 indicating the possibility of at least a moderate depression. The continuous MDI scores were positively associated with the SBT risk groups showing a dose-response relation (Table 3). The proportions of patients with signs of depression increased from 5% in the low risk group to 31% in the high risk SBT group (Figure 2). The low risk group had a lower post-test risk of being depressed than the prior probability, whereas the posterior risk of the medium risk group did not differ from the risk of the entire population (Table 4). The high risk group had a high specificity for depression and an almost four times increased likelihood of depression, but the sensitivity was only 33% (Table 4).

Table 3 Associations between continuous scores on psychological questionnaires and three SBT risk groups

	Regression coefficients (95% CI)	
MDI		p < 0.001
Low risk*	0	
Medium Risk	6.6 (5.1 - 8.2)	
High Risk	12.2 (9.5 - 15.0)	
FABQ		p < 0.001
Low risk*	0	
Medium Risk	5.7 (3.1 - 8.3)	
High Risk	17.7 (13.0 - 22.3)	
Catastrophising		p < 0.001
Low risk*	0	
Medium Risk	3.8 (2.5 - 5.1)	
High Risk	9.8 (8.0 - 11.6)	

* Reference category. CI: Confidence interval. MDI: Major depression inventory. FABQ: Fear avoidance beliefs questionnaire.

Associations between the STarT Back Screening Tool and the Fear Avoidance Beliefs Questionnaire

The FABQ scores, from 465 patients who completed the scale, ranged from 0 to 66 (median 22) and 6% had high fear avoidance beliefs. This proportion ranged from 1% - 31% in the SBT risk groups (Figure 2), and fear avoidance scores were positively associated with risk group (Table 3). As for depression, the high risk group had a high diagnostic performance, the low risk group increased the likelihood of non-fear avoidance, and the medium group had a profile similar to that of the total population (Table 4).

Associations between the STarT Screening Back Tool and catastrophising

The catastrophising sub-scale of the CSQ was available from 463 of the patients. Scores were 0 - 36 (median 8), with 15% categorized as high on catastrophising. Catastrophising was positively associated with risk group (Table 3), and the proportions with high scores ranged from 7% in the low risk group to 55% in the high risk SBT group (Figure 2). The diagnostic properties of the SBT groups in relation to catastrophising resembled what was seen for fear-avoidance (Table 4).

Table 2 Distribution of findings in 475 chiropractic patients in relation to the three STarT back screening tool risk groups.

	Low Risk n = 282	Medium Risk n = 139	High Risk n = 54	p-value
Duration, %				0.2
< 2 weeks	32	34	17	
- 3 months	34	36	44	
> 3 months	34	30	39	
> 30 days LBP preceding year, %	51	59	76	< .01
Leg pain, %	26	64	69	< .01
Number of LBP days during the last 2 weeks, median (IQR)	7 (3 - 12)	10 (6 - 14)	14 (10 - 14)	< .001

IQR = Interquartile range.

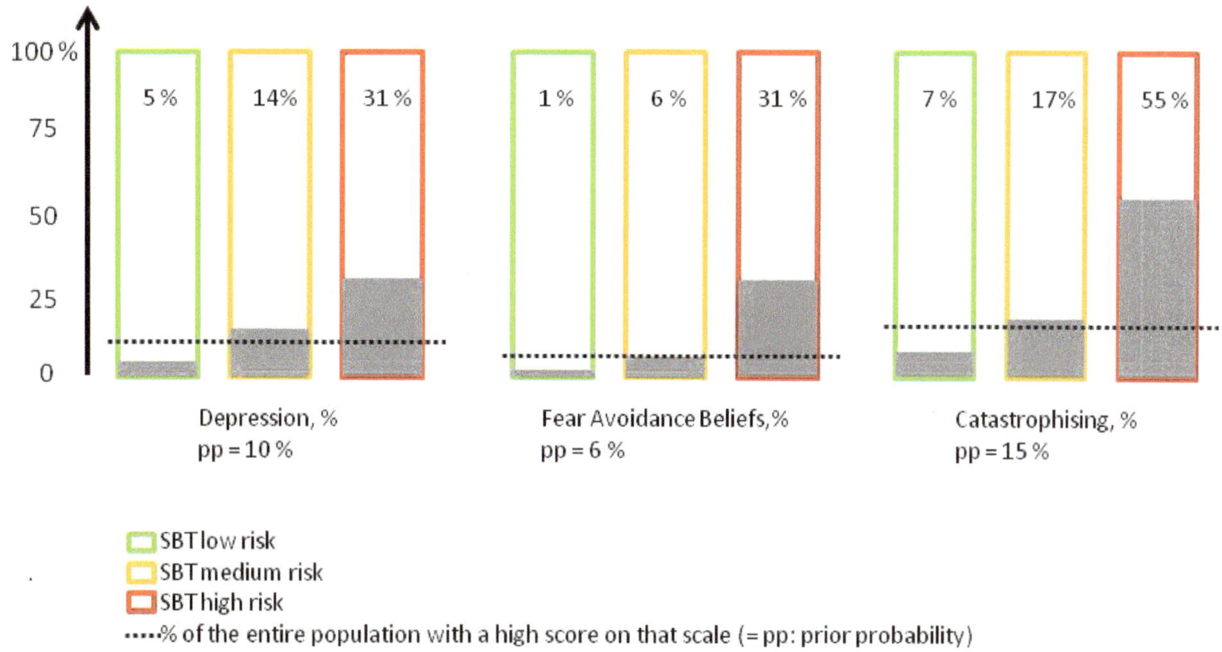

Figure 2 The proportion of patients with high scores on depression, fear-avoidance or catastrophising within the three SBT risk groups in 475 chiropractic patients.

Co-existing psychological factors

Data were available from all questionnaires in 453 patients. Among these, 76% had none of the three measured psychological factors, 17% had one, 5% two and 2% (7 patients) had high scores on all three scales. In the low, medium and high risk SBT groups 12%, 28%, and 76%, respectively, had high scores on at least one of the other scales. The number of positive scores on psychological factors increased from the low risk to the medium and high risk groups (Figure 3).

Discussion

This study tested the 9-item SBT and compared it to three large and well-known psychological questionnaires in a cohort of Danish primary care patients. The SBT is appealing to primary care clinicians since most patients would be able to complete it in short time and it can be scored easily on the spot by the clinician. The studied cohort was able to complete the SBT with very few missing values, and patients were distributed on the three predefined risk groups. The proportion of patients with a

Table 4 Llikelihood ratios, sensitivities, and specificities for the three SBT groups' diagnostic performance in relation to identifying patients with high scores on three more comprehensive questionnaires

	Pretest risk of high scores, % (95% CI)	Neg. LHR (95% CI)	Pos. LHR (95% CI)	Sensitivity % (95% CI)	Specificity % (95% CI)
MDI	10 (8 - 14)				
Low risk		2.01 (1.63 - 2.48)	.42 (.26 - .67)	27 (15 - 41)	37 (32 - 41)
Medium Risk		.82 (.65 - 1.04)	1.46 (1.01 - 2.11)	41 (27 - 56)	72 (68 - 76)
High Risk		.74 (.61 - .90)	3.83 (2.30 - 6.37)	33 (20 - 48)	92 (88 - 94)
FABQ	6 (4 - 8)				
Low risk		2.35 (1.96 - 2.81)	.18 (.06 - .52)	11 (2 - 29)	38 (33 - 43)
Medium Risk		1.00 (.78 -	1.00 (.55 - 1.82)	30 (14 - 52)	70 (66 - 75)
High Risk		1.29) .44 (.28 - .70)	7.21 (4.63 - 11.2)	59 (39 - 78)	92 (89 - 94)
Catastrophising	15 (12 - 19)				
Low risk		2.10 (1.72 - 2.55)	.41 (.28 - .61)	27 (17 - 39)	35 (30 - 40)
Medium Risk		.95 (.80 - 1.13)	1.12 (.78 - 1.63)	32 (22 - 45)	71 (66 - 76)
High Risk		.63 (.52 - .77)	6.67 (4.14 - 10.8)	41 (29 - 53)	94 (91 - 96)

LHR: Likelihood ratio

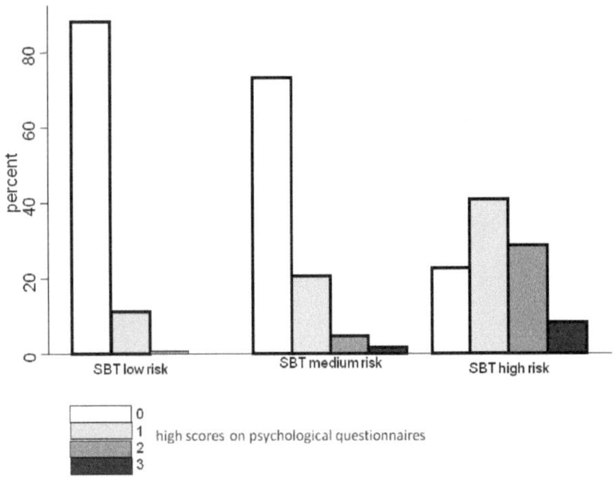

Figure 3 Proportions of patients within the three SBT risk groups with high scores on 0, 1, 2, and 3 psychological questionnaires.

"risk profile" was rather low both on the SBT and regarding depression, fear- avoidance beliefs, and catastrophising from 6% with high scores on fear avoidance beliefs to 15% expressing a catastrophising coping strategy. Still, close to 25% of the study population had high scores on at least one of the psychological questionnaires. If the investigated factors are important prognostic factors in this population, it would be highly relevant to identify such patients. This remains to be clarified.

Distribution of patients on SBT subgroups

Compared to the population used for the initial validation of the SBT [6], a larger proportion of our population was in the low risk group (59% versus 47%). This difference may be a result of the two populations being recruited from different settings, general vs. chiropractic practice, or of one being from the UK and the other from Denmark. There is presently an ongoing validation of the SBT-cut points in Danish primary care that will reveal whether the scale should be interpret differently in these patients (Morsø, L. Personal communication).

Since almost 60% of the present population was in the low risk group, there is potentially a high number of patients seeking chiropractic care, who need only advice and "minimal care". If validation studies support the use of the established cut-points in Danish patients, and if randomised trials confirm the hypothesis that the low risk group only needs minimal care, this could be important for allocation of resources within back care.

Does the SBT identify patients with a psychological risk profile?

We tested the SBT against three comprehensive questionnaires regarding psychological prognostic factors and found significant associations between the SBT risk groups and scores on the other scales. The presence of high scores on depression, fear avoidance beliefs, or catastrophising increased significantly from the SBT low risk group, over the medium group to the high risk group. A patient in the SBT high risk group had a 10-fold increased likelihood of having a high score on at least one of the three psychological questionnaires as compared to the probability prior to knowing the SBT risk group. Both the low and the high risk group had useful diagnostic properties as compared to the chosen questionnaires. *Not* being in the low risk group increased the likelihood of psychological risk factors to some extent and *being* in the high risk group was related to a marked increased likelihood of a risk profile.

These results support the assumption that the SBT can assist clinicians' detection of patients for whom a psychological assessment is likely to be relevant. The questionnaires that we used to measure depression, fear avoidance beliefs and catastrophising differed from those used in the original validation of the SBT, and the present results adds to the impression that the SBT actually distinguishes between patients with truly different profiles.

Do the SBT groups differ in relation to symptom characteristics?

The intention of the SBT is not to detect those patients who have a certain psychological profile, but rather to identify the patients, who have the most severe back pain complaints, and who, therefore, possibly have a special need for care. The present study did not compare SBT groups to pain severity or disability scores, but we found that patients in the high risk group more often reported a high number of LBP days the preceding year, that the present episode had more often lasted for more than two weeks, and that they were more likely to have had daily pain during the preceding two weeks as compared to patients in the low and medium risk groups. A higher number of LBP days during the previous year was earlier shown to be a negative prognostic factor in primary care LBP patients [11], and the larger proportion of patients with > 30 LBP days the preceding year in the high risk group as compared to the other groups supports the notion that the predictive value of the risk groups is worth investigating.

Strengths and limitations of the study

The study was carried out in a large population recruited from nineteen clinics and we believe that this cohort represents Danish chiropractic patients well. The questionnaires were well completed and only a very small number was not included in the analyses due to missing values. We only tested the SBT in relation to the psychological domains and did not include pain intensity or disability scales. Therefore our study is limited to describe the distribution of a few known risk factors, which are not very prevalent in the present study population. Ongoing work will describe the relationship between other health domains and the SBT risk groups in Danish chiropractic patients.

It should be noted that there is no documentation for the chosen catastrophising cut-point, and the proportion found to be catastrophisers should be interpret with caution. If we had instead considered patients with an above-median score to be catastrophisers this definition would obviously include a much higher number of patients.

Clinical relevance

Results on the predictive value of the SBT have to our knowledge only been published from one study so far [6]. In UK general practitioner patients, the SBT risk groups did relate to risk of non-recovery after 6 months. If the domains included in the SBT are modifiable, as they instinctively would be, this is a promising tool to guide the intervention offered to patients. The potential gain from offering targeted treatment as guided by the SBT is presently studied by Foster et al. [12]

It is still to be tested whether the SBT is useful as a predictor of prognosis in other populations and on the mere basis of cross-sectional studies such as this one it is not possible to recommend whether clinicians should use the SBT. What we can conclude based on the present study is that the SBT is feasible to use in chiropractic clinics, and with the low prevalence of psychological risk factors in this population, it is most relevant to screen for these risk factors with a short and general tool instead of having to use three large questionnaires that would be irrelevant to most patients.

Future research needs

There is a need for testing the prognostic value of the SBT in different patient populations. Thereafter RCTs, specifically designed for testing if treatment effects differ in the SBT subgroups, should be conducted to evaluate if interventions can be delivered more efficiently when clinical decisions are guided by the SBT risk groups. This study was a small step towards testing a tool that may in coming studies show helpful when deciding which patients we should spend the most resources on.

Acknowledgements

The authors want to thank the participating chiropractic clinics (appears from http://www.nikkb.dk/enheden-for-kiropraktisk-praksisforskning-kip) for a fast and well-conducted data collection. No external funding was provided.

Author details

[1]Nordic Institute of Chiropractic and Clinical Biomechanics, University of Southern Denmark, Odense. Part of Clinical Locomotion Network, Denmark. [2]Research Department, Spine Centre of Southern Denmark, Hospital Lillebaelt Middelfart, Institute of Regional Health Research, University of Southern Denmark. Part of Clinical Locomotion Network, Denmark. [3]Master of Science in Public Health, Institute of Public Health, University of Southern Denmark, Esbjerg, Denmark.

Authors' contributions

All the authors participated in planning of the study. EJ coordinated the data collection. AK was responsible for the design, did the data analyses, and drafted the manuscript. EJ and CLY have critically revised the manuscript and all authors have read and approved the final manuscript.

Competing interests

The authors declare that they have no competing interests.

References

1. Kjaer P, Leboeuf-Yde C, Korsholm L, Sorensen JS, Bendix T: **Magnetic resonance imaging and low back pain in adults: a diagnostic imaging study of 40-year-old men and women.** *Spine* 2005, **30**:1173-1180.
2. Molano SM, Burdorf A, Elders LA: **Factors associated with medical care-seeking due to low-back pain in scaffolders.** *Am J Ind Med* 2001, **40**:275-281.
3. Maniadakis N, Gray A: **The economic burden of back pain in the UK.** *Pain* 2000, **84**:95-103.
4. Kent PM, Keating JL: **Can we predict poor recovery from recent-onset nonspecific low back pain? A systematic review.** *Man Ther* 2008, **13**:12-28.
5. Chou R, Shekelle P: **Will this patient develop persistent disabling low back pain?** *JAMA* 2010, **303**:1295-1302.
6. Hill JC, Dunn KM, Lewis M, Mullis R, Main CJ, Foster NE, Hay EM: **A primary care back pain screening tool: identifying patient subgroups for initial treatment.** *Arthritis Rheum* 2008, **59**:632-641.
7. Hill JC, Dunn KM, Main CJ, Hay EM: **Subgrouping low back pain: a comparison of the STarT Back Tool with the Orebro Musculoskeletal Pain Screening Questionnaire.** *Eur J Pain* 2010, **14**:83-89.
8. Bech P, Rasmussen NA, Olsen LR, Noerholm V, Abildgaard W: **The sensitivity and specificity of the Major Depression Inventory, using the Present State Examination as the index of diagnostic validity.** *J Affect Disord* 2001, **66**:159-164.
9. Waddell G, Newton M, Henderson I, Somerville D, Main CJ: **A Fear-Avoidance Beliefs Questionnaire (FABQ) and the role of fear- avoidance beliefs in chronic low back pain and disability.** *Pain* 1993, **52**:157-168.
10. Swartzman LC, Gwadry FG, Shapiro AP, Teasell RW: **The factor structure of the Coping Strategies Questionnaire.** *Pain* 1994, **57**:311-316.
11. Axen I, Jones JJ, Rosenbaum A, Lovgren PW, Halasz L, Larsen K, Leboeuf-Yde C: **The Nordic Back Pain Subpopulation Program: validation and improvement of a predictive model for treatment outcome in patients with low back pain receiving chiropractic treatment.** *J Manipulative Physiol Ther* 2005, **28**:381-385.
12. Foster NE, Mullis R, Young J, Doyle C, Lewis M, Whitehurst D, Hay EM: **IMPaCT Back study protocol. Implementation of subgrouping for targeted treatment systems for low back pain patients in primary care: a prospective population-based sequential comparison.** *BMC Musculoskelet Disord* 2010, **11**:186.

5

The use of diagnostic coding in chiropractic practice

Cecilie D Testern[1], Lise Hestbæk[1] and Simon D French[2,3*]

Abstract

Background: Diagnostic coding has several potential benefits, including improving the feasibility of data collection for research and clinical audits and providing a common language to improve interdisciplinary collaboration. The primary aim of this study was to determine the views and perspectives of chiropractors about diagnostic coding and explore the use of it in a chiropractic setting. A secondary aim was to compare the diagnostic coding undertaken by chiropractors and an independent coder.

Method: A codin exercise based on the International Classification of Primary Care version 2, PLUS extension (ICPC-2 PLUS) provided the 14 chiropractors with some experience in diagnostic coding, followed by an interview on the topic. The interviews were analysed thematically. The participating chiropractors and an independent coder applied ICPC-2 PLUS terms to the diagnoses of 10 patients. Then the level of agreement between the chiropractors and the coder was determined and Cohen's Kappa was used to determine the agreement beyond that expected by chance.

Results: From the interviews the three emerging themes were: *1) Advantages and disadvantages of using a clinical coding system in chiropractic practice, 2) ICPC-2 PLUS terminology issues for chiropractic practice* and *3) Implementation of a coding system into chiropractic practice.* The participating chiropractors did not uniformly support or condemn the idea of using diagnostic coding. However there was a strong agreement that the terminology in ICPC-2 PLUS would not be applicable or desirable for all practice types. In the coding exercise the chiropractors in total coded 202 diagnoses for 135 patients. The overall percentage agreement between the chiropractors and the coder was 52% (17% expected by chance) with a Kappa score of 0.4 (95% CI 0.3-0.7). Agreement was lower for more detailed coding (percentage agreement 35%; Kappa score of 0.3 (95% CI 0.2-0.5)).

Conclusion: It appears that implementation of diagnostic coding would be possible in the majority of the chiropractic practices that participated in this study. However for those chiropractors who do not focus on symptoms in their approach to clinical care, it could be challenging to use the ICPC-2 PLUS coding system, since ICPC-2 PLUS is a symptom-based classification.

Keywords: Diagnostic coding, Chiropractors

Background

Diagnostic coding in chiropractic practice has several potential benefits. These benefits include improving the feasibility of data collection for research and clinical audits, improving the clinical applicability of research, and providing a common clinical language to help improve interdisciplinary collaboration. Diagnostic coding allows for systematic classification of clinical information in clinical practice and assists with the conduct of clinical audits and data collection for research purposes. Use of the same classification system by different clinical groups creates a common language between different healthcare professions and sectors and could enhance interdisciplinary collaboration. This could lead to better communication, improved continuity of care as well as simplifying the process of referring patients [1].

* Correspondence: Simon.french@queensu.ca
[2]General Practice and Primary Health Care Academic Centre, University of Melbourne, Melbourne, VIC, Australia
[3]School of Rehabilitation Therapy, Faculty of Health Sciences, Queen's University, Kingston, Ontario, Canada
Full list of author information is available at the end of the article

The International Classification of Primary Care (ICPC) is an example of a diagnostic coding system that could be relevant for chiropractic practice [2]. The ICPC consists of 17 chapters based on body systems following the principle that localisation has precedence over aetiology. A second version of the diagnostic code system, International Classification of Primary Care, Version 2 (ICPC-2), was published in 1998. Originally ICPC was designed for paper based data collection and analysis, but it has spread to electronic clinical and research systems. ICPC has gradually received increasing recognition and use, especially in Europe and Australia [2].

Diagnostic coding is not commonly undertaken in chiropractic practice, and the choice of an appropriate coding system is important as the profession moves towards this. A study in Danish general medical practice showed that the ICPC has a good reliability and validity at the chapter level for musculoskeletal conditions [3]. Thus, it would appear that ICPC is a good choice for diagnostic coding in chiropractic practice since most conditions treated are musculoskeletal [4]. Additionally, the ICPC-2 is already integrated in several healthcare systems [3], as well as into the International Classification of Disease (ICD-10), a coding system used in hospital settings [2].

ICPC-2 classifies clinical information using three character codes called a *rubric* [5]. The first character, a letter, represents a chapter or a body system (such as Musculoskeletal, Cardiovascular or Neurological), and the two additional characters, a number, represent a concept within this body system (a symptom/complaint, problem/diagnosis or process of care). To allow for greater detail and specificity, the ICPC-2 PLUS terminology was developed. ICPC-2 PLUS is a clinical terminology (*terms*) classified to the ICPC-2. ICPC-2 PLUS has been developed for the Bettering the Evaluation And Care of Health (BEACH) research project, which is an ongoing Australian national study of general medical practice activity [6]. ICPC-2 PLUS is also used in Australia in age-sex disease registers, morbidity registers and electronic health records in primary care.

New ICPC-2 PLUS codes are created by aligning a *term* with the description of the specific problem/diagnosis, or type of care, with the most appropriate ICPC-2 *rubric*. For each of the ICPC-2 PLUS *terms* a three digit code is assigned. This provides ICPC-2 PLUS with a six-character identifier as oppose to the three digits identifier for ICPC-2. As such, the final three digits of the six character ICPC-2 PLUS code identify the specific *term* within the *rubric*. For example, the three character ICPC-2 code L01 represents 'Neck Symptom or Complaint'. In ICPC-2 PLUS there are 11 neck-related *terms* in the L01 rubric to describe patient problems. For example 'Pain;neck' is represented in ICPC-2 PLUS as L01 004 and the 'Cervicalgia' as L01 006 [2].

Knowledge of who receives chiropractic care and what care they receive is important to understand contemporary chiropractic practice [3]. The Chiropractic Observation and Analysis STudy (COAST) [4] was a cross sectional observational study that described the clinical practice of chiropractors in Victoria, Australia. COAST explored why people seek chiropractic care, what diagnoses chiropractors make and what treatment chiropractors provide. The research method used in COAST was based on the BEACH study methods [6]. In coding the chiropractic clinical information, some new *terms* were required to describe chiropractic clinical practice. In developing the chiropractic specific ICPC-2 PLUS (Chiro), researchers followed the BEACH coding rules [7].

The long-term aim of this area of work is to implement diagnostic coding into chiropractic clinical practice. We are not aware of any previous research exploring the use of diagnostic coding in the chiropractic profession. This project explored chiropractors' attitudes towards diagnostic coding to provide important information about how coding will be received in this setting. Specifically, the primary purpose was to investigate the views among practising chiropractors in relation to feasibility, applicability and future perspectives of diagnostic coding in chiropractic clinical practice. A secondary aim was to compare the diagnostic coding undertaken by chiropractors to that undertaken by an independent coder.

Method

Summary

This study consisted of quantitative and qualitative components. Each of the chiropractors took part in a coding exercise and this exercise then formed the basis for the subsequent interview. The coding exercise primarily provided the chiropractors with some experience in diagnostic coding for them to describe in the interview. The coding exercise also provided the opportunity to compare the diagnostic coding undertaken by chiropractors to diagnostic coding undertaken by an independent coder. We aimed to determine how accurate the coding process was by determining if an independent coder used the same codes, (in this case *terms*) that chiropractors used, considering the chiropractors had more information available to them. The interviews were analysed qualitatively and the coding exercise was analysed quantitatively.

Participants and recruitment

Chiropractors approached for this study had all participated in the COAST project in 2011 [4] and were currently in clinical practice in Victoria. Chiropractors had already received training in completing the COAST encounter forms and they were familiar with the background for the study. Fifty-two chiropractors participated in COAST and they were all approached for this study. The chiropractors received an invitation pack in the post, including an invitation letter for the study, a Plain Language Statement describing what participation in the study consisted of, and a consent form. Chiropractors opted into the study by returning a signed consent form via post or fax/email.

After two weeks the chiropractors who had not responded to the invitation letter were sent a follow up letter. After two additional weeks, non-responders were contacted by telephone until 15 chiropractors agreed to participate.

Patients were invited to participate in the study when they attended the practices of participating chiropractors during the recording period. Patients were approached if they were 18 years or older and had spinal pain (neck or back pain). Patients received a Plain Language Statement with information about the study and the chiropractors were trained to obtain verbal consent from patients wishing to participate.

Sample size

The number of chiropractors chosen (15) was by convenience. This number of interviews was feasible to complete considering resources and time available. Further, we are not aware of any similar studies conducted in this setting so this preliminary data would provide important information that can be used for future, larger studies.

For the quantitative analysis, we assumed the agreement on the choice of codes between the coder and the chiropractors would be around 50% with an intra-cluster correlation of 0.1. Therefore a sufficient sample size to provide a 95% confidence interval with a margin of error of 11% was 150 encounters or 10 patients per chiropractor.

Data collection and analysis

First, the 15 chiropractor participants were asked to complete encounter forms for 10 consecutive patients with neck or back pain. The encounter form used for the data collection was a slightly modified version of the encounter form used in COAST and included patient demographics, up to three reasons for encounter, relevant health information, presenting pain, diagnosis and care given (see Additional file 1 for a copy of the form).

After the chiropractor had completed their patient data collection, face-to-face semi-structured interviews were conducted between the chiropractor and the first author (CT). During the interviews the first author presented the chiropractors with a short introduction to ICPC-2 PLUS. Chiropractors were then asked to choose the ICPC-2 PLUS *terms* most relevant for the diagnoses of the patients. In order to make the coding decision, the chiropractors were asked to use their memory of the patient encounter, the patient's clinical file and the encounter recording form they had completed at the time of the consultation. The chiropractor could document up to three diagnoses for each patient encounter and therefore also choose up to three ICPC-2 PLUS *terms* per patient encounter.

To make the coding exercise feasible and relevant to back and neck pain problems/diagnoses, the chiropractor was provided with a shortened list of ICPC-2 PLUS *terms* to choose from. The list only included *terms* relevant to neck and back pain from the ICPC-2 PLUS musculoskeletal chapter (254 *terms*).

The face-to-face interview consisted of open-ended questions about the chiropractors' perspective and views on the use of diagnostic coding in chiropractic practice. The questions enquired about the chiropractors' views on diagnostic coding, the potential role of a diagnostic coding system in chiropractic practice, the chiropractors' views on using the ICPC-2 PLUS *terms* in chiropractic practice, and finally the facilitators and barriers the chiropractors faced when trying to use ICPC-2 PLUS. All interviews were audio recorded and transcribed verbatim.

The patient encounter forms completed by the chiropractors, together with the chiropractors' choice of ICPC-2-PLUS *terms*, were collected at the end of the interviews. An independent hospital trained coder examined the encounter forms and assigned relevant ICPC-2 PLUS *terms* to the diagnosis recorded by the chiropractor on the forms. The coder used the "Demonstrator" function on the ICPC-2 PLUS website to select the appropriate *terms* for the diagnosis provided by the chiropractors [8]. The Demonstrator is an online search tool that allows access to all of the ICPC-2 PLUS *terms*. This coder searched an extensive keyword list with keywords linking the ICPC-2 PLUS six-character codes. When selecting a keyword, the coder was presented with all the available associated *terms*. The coder then selected the *term* that most closely reflected the chiropractors' exact wording of the diagnosis written on the encounter forms. The only information available about the patient for the coder was the information on the encounter forms, as is the case for the BEACH and COAST studies. Encounters were excluded from agreement analysis where the ICPC-2 PLUS *term* chosen by the coder was not included on the list provided to the chiropractors.

For the qualitative analysis, all interviews were examined by the first author (CT) by reading through and listening to each of the transcripts/audio files and labeling paragraphs with descriptive and interpretive codes as suggested by King [9]. After the first read through commonly repeating patterns were identified for each transcript. The same process was performed by the third author (SF) for the interview transcripts of three chiropractors, each with a different type of clinical practice. Descriptive and interpretive codes were then compared between the first and third author for the three interview transcripts, and divergent views between the two authors were resolved through discussion. The first author then re-examined the remaining 11 transcripts in light of this discussion.

For each of the interviews the repeating patterns were merged to define broader themes [10]. The interview were then finally analysed by looking for common themes across all of the 14 interviews, as well as areas of differences in the views and perspectives of the participants [11].

For the quantitative analysis of the coding exercise, the agreement between the independent coder and the chiropractors for their choices of ICPC-2 PLUS *terms* was determined at two levels: ICPC-2 *Rubric level*, three-character code; and also ICPC-2 PLUS *term level*, six-character code. The analysis was undertaken at two levels to determine whether more specific coding at the *term level* resulted in lower agreement. The overall percentage agreement was calculated, as well as the percentage agreement for each practitioner. Cohen's Kappa was used to determine the agreement beyond that expected by chance, using the statistical software Stata. Kappa was derived by comparing whether each chiropractor and the coder agreed (or not) on the choice of codes, and a mean Kappa value with 95% confidence intervals was determined. The guidelines of Landis and Koch [12] were used for interpreting the Kappa values. Finally, the time taken for the chiropractors to make a choice about a diagnostic code was determined from the audio recordings.

Ethics approval

The project received full approval from the Human Ethics Subcommittee at the University of Melbourne on 20th of June 2012 (ID1237727) as a Minimal Risk Project following the ethical guidelines described by the Australian National Health and Medical Research Council, NHMRC [13]. All participants (chiropractors and patients) gave informed consent to participate.

Results

Fourteen chiropractors completed the study and their demographic characteristics are described in Table 1. One chiropractor did not have the encounter forms available at the time of the coding exercise and was therefore not included in the study. Most of the chiropractors were males practising in metropolitan Melbourne. All participated in the COAST project, but typically did not have any other experience participating in research.

Table 1 Characteristics of participating chiropractors

Chiropractor characteristics (N = 14)		
Chiropractor characteristics	**Average**	***Range***
Age in years	46	30-57
Years in practice	19	5-32
	No.	**%**
Gender		
Female	1	7
Male	13	93
Location		
Metropolitan*	10	72
Rural	4	28
Graduated in Australia	13	92
Holds Postgraduate qualification	5	35
Involved in Teaching	3	20
Membership:		
CAA	6	42
COCA	5	35
Other **	6	42
Computer use in clinic:		
Do not have computer in practice	2	14
Clinical records paperless	1	7
Clinical records partially paperless	5	35
Clinical records paper only	7	50

*Determined from Australian Standard Geographical Classification - Remoteness Area (ASGC-RA).
**Other includes: The Australasian College of Chiropractors, Gonstead Chiropractic group, Australian Spinal Research Foundation, CAA sports.
CAA = Chiropractors' Association of Australia; COCA = Chiropractic and Osteopathic College of Australasia.

The characteristics of the 135 participating patients are described in Table 2. The majority of the patients were between 46 and 70 years of age. There were more female than male patients but the difference in the distribution was only 10% (4 missing). Most patients (58%) presented with one reason for encounter and the most common reason was back pain.

The interview themes

Three overall themes emerged from the interview data: *1) Advantages and disadvantages of using a clinical coding system in chiropractic practice, 2) ICPC-2 PLUS terminology issues for chiropractic practice, and 3) Implementation of a coding system into chiropractic practice.* The themes are described in the following section along with illustrative quotes from the participating chiropractors. For additional quotes see Additional file 2.

Table 2 Patient demographics and encounter reasons

Patient characteristics (N = 135)	No.	%
Age [missing]	[7]	5
18-30	24	18
31-45	38	28
46-70	61	45
70+	5	4
Gender [missing]	[5]	4
Male	58	43
Female	72	53
Number of reasons for encounter per patient: [missing]	[3]	2
1	77	57
2	40	30
3	15	11
Reasons for encounter: [missing]	[7]	5
Neck pain	46	22
Back pain	76	38
Check up/maintenance	27	13
Other*	53	26
Total number of reasons for encounter	202	
Total number of diagnoses provided by the chiropractors	167	

*Examples of other: Headache, shoulder pain, arm pain, leg pain.
Note: The number of patients, the number of reasons for encounter and the number of diagnoses varied. Patients could report up to three reasons for encounter, which meant that some patients could have multiple diagnoses. In other cases the chiropractor combined some of a patient's reasons for encounter into one diagnosis thus for these patients there could be more reasons for encounter than diagnoses.

Theme 1) Advantages and disadvantages of using a clinical coding system in chiropractic practice

Most of the chiropractors were positive towards to the idea of using diagnostic coding in chiropractic practice and they suggested many possible advantages. Some talked about how this could streamline their own clinical practice. Many suggested the possibility of creating a database of coded clinical practice information. They suggested that this database could be used to produce research more efficiently and to ensure the clinical relevance of the research produced.

However, some of the chiropractors did not see the relevance or purpose of ICPC-2 PLUS in chiropractic practice. An issue mentioned by many was that the terminology would not fit into what they called the "wellness-based approach" of some chiropractors. Some chiropractors suggested that the use of ICPC-2 PLUS in chiropractic practice could "medicalise" the profession. On the other hand many chiropractors discussed how diagnostic coding could create a common language that could facilitate better communication between the different musculoskeletal health professions. Some chiropractors also mentioned how this could lead to integration into the mainstream healthcare system. Some illustrative quotes demonstrating these issues follows:

> *"The advantages are quite evident, what it can create is a very good database for epidemiological studies and for further research and getting a better appreciation of the type of presentations and you got a lot of data that then could be stored, collected and accessed and drawn upon for future research"* [ID1, 48 years old, 16 years in practice, Metro].

> *"The minute I start doing this* [coding exercise] *with trying to match their reported reason for encounter that then assumes that what you are doing on that day is a treatment for that reason for encounter right? And I can understand why you would have this if you are in medicine because that is what they do right? But that's not what we do. So someone might have a presenting complaint: "okay let's check you, let's see if you are subluxated, if you are then I'll adjust you, whether or not you've got that presenting complaint, it's irrelevant okay.. So I don't know how you could fit this* [ICPC-2 PLUS] *into the way I have just explained it, if there was a way that would be great."*[ID8, 43 years old, 19 years in practice, Metro].

> *"If it's going to create a language that helps through - not just the chiropractic profession communicating well with each other, but chiropractic profession communicating with the rest of the medical industry - medical - well, rather, the health world. Then that's good for everybody. So, that's a great role and if we're talking about chiropractic - getting a larger level of research towards it and integrating itself into a mainstream system more. I think that would be actually essential. So, yeah there's certainly a role for it."*[ID13, 30 years old, 5 years in practice, Metro].

Theme 2) ICPC-2 PLUS terminology issues for chiropractic practice

The terminology in ICPC-2 PLUS was a topic mentioned frequently by the chiropractors. Many of the chiropractors mentioned that there were too many *terms* to choose from, but also that the *terms* were not specific enough to reflect chiropractic clinical practice. They believed that there were not enough relevant *terms* for the stage of the problem/diagnosis, for example the limited possibilities to describe if a problem/diagnoses was acute or chronic or somewhere between the two. Some illustrative quotes demonstrating these issues follows:

> *"Obviously they are not specific enough, it doesn't tell you the state of whether it's acute, chronic or what have you. Again it might tell you the region you are*

looking at but not the anything specific of what you are looking at" [ID2, 50 years old, 28 years in practice, Metro]

"It wasn't easy cause 27000 things for the same thing (laughs) almost, yes too many choices and not specific enough or they are trying to be too specific which then makes it a bit harder to find exactly what is going on." [ID6, 46 years old, 11 years in practice, Rural]

Theme 3) Implementation of a coding system into chiropractic practice

Many chiropractors thought that implementation of ICPC-2 PLUS into chiropractic clinical practice would be feasible after some practice. Some of the issues mentioned were getting ICPC-2 PLUS into the existing electronic clinical record systems and that not all chiropractors use electronic clinical practice records. Some chiropractors mentioned that implementing a system like ICPC-2 PLUS would have to start at the undergraduate level. One chiropractor stated that the idea was good but the motivation for clinicians was not great enough to make implementation of ICPC-2 PLUS possible. Some illustrative quotes demonstrating these issues follows:

It got easier. I guess part of it is just being familiar with what your options are. " [ID12, 38 years old, 16 years in practice, Rural]

"When you familiarize yourself with it, it would be great."[ID1, 48 years old, 16 years in practice, Metro] *"I really think it's gotta start at the undergraduate level. To start teaching people this is the way of the future. And through training sessions and seminars disseminating it to the field practitioners."*[ID7, 49 years old, 25 years in practice, Metro]

Coding exercise and agreement analysis

The 135 included patients provided 202 reasons for encounter. The chiropractors spent between 30 seconds to 20 minutes choosing a code for a particular diagnosis/problem.

Each of the 14 participating chiropractors recorded 10 patient encounters. For each of these patient encounters, the chiropractor could list up to 3 diagnoses. The total number of diagnostic codes provided by the chiropractors, and used in the agreement analysis, was 167 (Table 3). See Figure 1 for flow of participant and data in the study.

As presented in Table 3 the overall percentage agreement between the coder and the chiropractors on the ICPC-2 *Rubric level* (three-character code) was just over 50% agreement. On ICPC-2 PLUS *term level* (six-character code) the agreement was just over 30%. The level of agreement beyond chance was moderate with a Kappa score 0.4 (95% CI 0.3-0.7) on the ICPC-2 *Rubric level*, and fair with a Kappa score 0.3 (95% CI 0.2-0.5) on the ICPC-2 PLUS *term level.*

Table 3 Level of agreement

Chiropractor ID	Number of diagnoses coded	Agreement on *rubric level* (%)	Agreement on **term level* (%)
1	9	89	67
2	20	15	10
3	12	92	50
4	15	60	0
5	14	29	29
6	9	67	56
7	14	29	7
8	10	100	100
9	16	44	31
10	11	82	73
11	10	100	10
12	11	27	18
13	12	0	0
14	4	75	0
Overall agreement %		52	35
Agreement expected by chance		17	6
Overall agreement (Cohen's Kappa)	**Total number of codes:** 167	0.4 (95% CI 0.3-0.7)***	0.3 (95% CI 0.2-0.5)***

**Rubric level*: ICPC-2 classifies symptoms/complaints, problems/diagnoses and process of care using three character codes called a rubric. The first character, a letter, represents a chapter or a body system and the two additional characters, a number, represent a concept within this body system.

***Term level*: To allow for greater specificity, the ICPC-2 PLUS terminology was developed. Each PLUS *term* is classified to ICPC-2. ICPC-2 PLUS uses a six-character identifier by adding another three digits (a code) to the ICPC-2 rubric, to which the *term* has been classified.

***CI = 95% confidence interval.

Discussion

This paper provides a first insight into views and perspectives of chiropractors about diagnostic coding in chiropractic practice. ICPC-2 PLUS was chosen as the example of a diagnostic coding system in this study because it has been proven to have a good reliability and validity for musculoskeletal diagnosis, which is the most common conditions treated in chiropractic practice. Also, it is already used in hospital settings/ secondary sector, the COAST data was coded with this particular classification and alongside the process a set of *terms* for chiropractic practice is under development ICPC-2 PLUS (Chiro) [7].

Most chiropractors were positive toward using a diagnostic coding system in their daily practice but some of

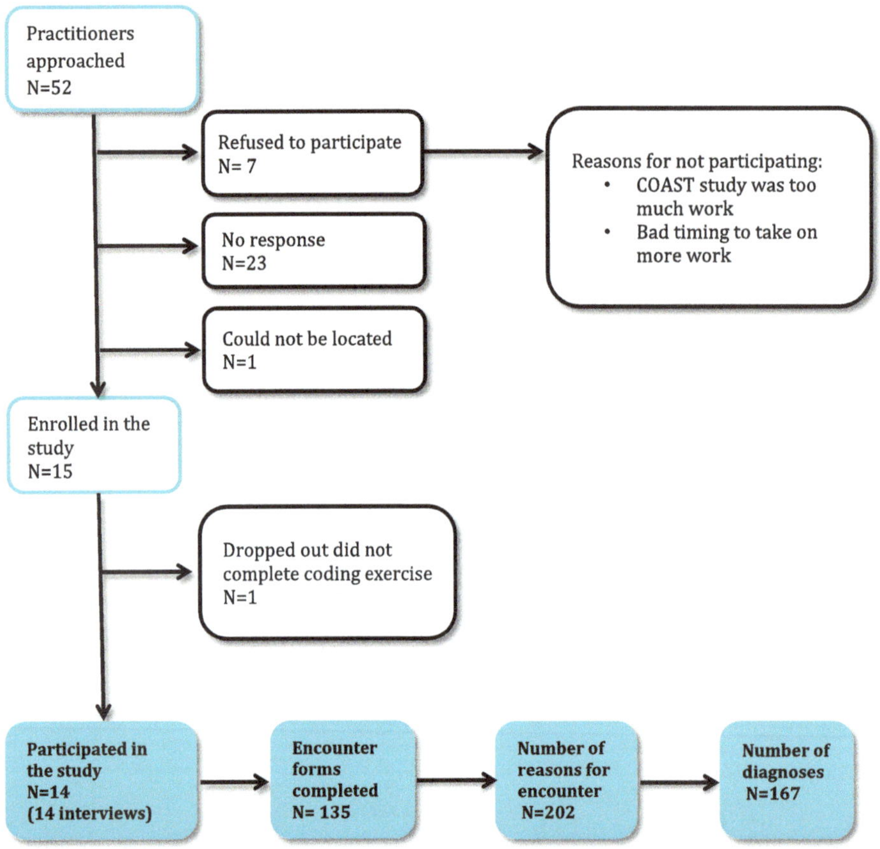

Figure 1 Flow of participants and data in the study.

those chiropractors did not see the relevance of the ICPC-2 PLUS for their practice. The chiropractors who described themselves as *wellness chiropractors* typically expressed the view that the terms available were not adequate to describe their clinical practice. The main issue here was the fact that they did not have a particular focus on specific symptoms. They said that it was obvious that ICPC-2 PLUS terms were made for medical practice, and that it would be better to make a new system for chiropractic practice with more relevant terms. Coding with the current terms in ICPC-2 PLUS may therefore not be relevant for all practice types. The terminology issue was also addressed alongside the conduct of COAST and resulted in a chiropractic-specific coding system being developed, ICPC-2 PLUS (Chiro) [7]. Many however agreed that with some training, ICPC-2 PLUS might be a useful system to have in chiropractic practice, especially to facilitate producing more clinically relevant research.

For the coding exercise if agreement between the chiropractor and coder was high, this would provide some support that ICPC-2 PLUS was potentially a good choice for diagnostic coding in chiropractic practice. If the agreement was low it would tell us that something needed improvement. Either ICPC-2 PLUS was not a good fit for chiropractic practice, or the encounter forms the chiropractors completed did not provide enough information for the coder to agree with the chiropractors' choice of code.

The agreement between the coder and the chiropractors was higher than agreement expected by chance at both the ICPC-2 *Rubric level* and the ICPC-2 PLUS *term level*. However, the agreement was only fair to moderate and this could be due to a number of reasons. First, none of the chiropractors were familiar with the *terms* available for coding when they completed the encounter forms. The amount of time spent to get familiar with the *terms* available before the coding exercise differed considerably. The practitioners spent between 30 seconds to 20 minutes choosing a *term* for a particular diagnosis/problem. Some of the participating chiropractors mentioned that they would have preferred some prior knowledge about the available *terms* before filling out the encounter forms. To avoid adding to the burden for the participating chiropractors, we decided not to include the list of *terms* in the study materials they received prior to the interviews. We do not know whether this would have improved the level of agreement or had an influence on their overall view on the idea of diagnostic coding in chiropractic practice.

For the agreement on ICPC-2 *rubric* level two chiropractors had 100% agreement with the coder, eight chiropractors had over 50% agreement with the coder. But the two chiropractors who achieved 100% agreement with the coder had only chosen one *term* for all the diagnoses. Despite a variation in their patients' reasons for encounter, the diagnoses, written by the chiropractor on the encounter form, were all the same. All other chiropractors had used at least three different *terms* when coding. In order to conduct the agreement analysis the participating chiropractors had to choose a *term* for every one of their diagnoses. They were asked to choose the *term* that came closest to describing the diagnosis, rather than being given an option of not choosing a *term*. This might have resulted in these two chiropractors choosing the same *term* for all the diagnoses.

Even the chiropractor who did not agree with the coder on any of the *terms* chosen was positive to using ICPC-2 PLUS in practice. Another chiropractor had an 82% agreement rate with the coder but was negative to the idea of using ICPC-2 PLUS in practice and emphasized a lack of relevance of the coding system to their clinical work and therefore lacked of motivation to implement the system. This chiropractor did not have a wellness practice.

Limitations and strengths

The sample size for both chiropractors and patient participants were smaller than planned. We did not reach our intended number of practitioners (14 instead of 15) and therefore also less patient participants. This meant one interview less than expected and less data for the agreement analysis. However, this study being the first of its kind and therefore exploratory we do not know what effects this would have had on the results. Qualitative research is not meant to be representative, it is meant to provide in-depth information and this study offers some insight to what possibilities and challenges diagnostic coding could bring to chiropractic practice.

The qualitative interviews, as well as the analysis, were completed with an awareness of the first author's (CT) personal background as a chiropractic student with minimal clinical experience, and a preconception that diagnostic coding could potentially improve patient care. Being aware of this a neutral approach was emphasized when interviewing and when conducting the analysis.

Suggestions for further studies

This study was the first to examine the role of diagnostic coding using an established primary care coding system in chiropractic practice. To determine the applicability of ICPC-2 PLUS or another diagnostic coding system in chiropractic practice, more research is needed. A study with a bigger sample would provide further information on this topic.

In Denmark an introduction of the Danish version of ICPC-2, ICPC-2-DK to chiropractic practice is currently underway. ICPC-2-DK has been part of the electronic medical records in Danish general medical practice since 2009 [1]. A similar study to this with a sample of Danish chiropractors to evaluate the use of ICPC-2-DK in chiropractic practice would provide valuable information and potentially ease the implementation process.

Conclusion

Most of the chiropractors in this study found the use of diagnostic coding both feasible and applicable in their practices but recommended specific training for chiropractors in the use of the coding system. However, there was a strong agreement that the terminology in ICPC-2 PLUS would not be applicable or desirable for those members of the chiropractic profession who do not focus on symptoms in their approach to clinical care. Clinically relevant research opportunities and further integration in the mainstream health care system were mentioned as some of the future perspectives of diagnostic coding.

Thus, this first insight into the use of diagnostic coding in chiropractic practice is encouraging, but more research is needed to determine if these results are applicable to chiropractic practice in other countries and to investigate possibilities for improving the chiropractic relevance of the terminology.

Additional files

Additional file 1: The encounter form.

Additional file 2: Additional quotes.

Competing interests

LH is a member Editorial Board of Chiropractic & Manual Therapies, and SF is an Associate Editor, however neither had any involvement in the editorial process of this manuscript. Otherwise the authors declare no competing interests.

Authors' contributions

The study was conducted as part of a one-year pre-graduate research project undertaken by CT. SF was the main supervisor on location and overlooked every step of the process. SF and LH conceived the study. All authors were responsible for the study design. CT performed the data collection. CT and SF undertook the analyses. CT was responsible for drafting the manuscript. All authors read and approved the final manuscript.

Acknowledgements

We thank the participating chiropractors and patients, including Peter Werth and Tini Pham who participated in a pilot of the study. We would also like to thank the team in the Department of General Practice, at the University of Melbourne for their invaluable support, especially Melanie Charity and Patty Chondros for their help with the quantitative component as well as Victoria Palmer for her help with the qualitative component. Funding support for the first author (CT) to travel to Melbourne and conduct this study came from the Nordic Institute for Chiropractic and Clinical Biomechanics (NIKKB). The University of Southern Denmark funded the vast majority of interview transcription and the Department of General Practice, the University of Melbourne, funded the transport to and from the clinics.

Author details

[1]Nordic Institute of Chiropractic and Clinical Biomechanics and Institute of Sports Science and Biomechanics, University of Southern Denmark, Odense, Denmark. [2]General Practice and Primary Health Care Academic Centre, University of Melbourne, Melbourne, VIC, Australia. [3]School of Rehabilitation Therapy, Faculty of Health Sciences, Queen's University, Kingston, Ontario, Canada.

References

1. Rosendal M, Falkoe E. Diagnostic classification in Denmark with emphasis on general practice. Ugeskr Laeger. 2009;171(12):997–1000. Danish.
2. ICPC-2 PLUS: The BEACH coding system Sydney, University of Sydney [updated 5 September 2012]. Available from: http://sydney.edu.au/medicine/fmrc/classifications/index.php.
3. Nielsen MN, Aaen-Larsen B, Vedsted P, Nielsen CV, Hjollund NH. Diagnosis coding of the musculoskeletal system in general practice. Ugeskr Laeger. 2008;170(37):2881–4.
4. French SD, Charity MJ, Forsdike K, Gunn JM, Polus BI, Walker BF, et al. Chiropractic Observation and Analysis Study (COAST): providing an understanding of current chiropractic practice. Med J Aust. 2013;199 (10):687–91.
5. Classification Committee of the World Organization of Family Doctors (WONCA) ICPC-2. International classification of primary care. Oxford: Oxford University Press; 1998.
6. Britt H, Miller GC, Henderson J, Charles J, Valenti L, Harrison C et al. General practice activity in Australia 2011–12. 2012;General practice series no. 31.
7. Charity MJ, French SD, Forsdike K, Britt H, Polus B, Gunn J. Extending ICPC-2 PLUS terminology to develop a classification system specific for the study of chiropractic encounters. Chiropr Man Therap. 2013;21(1):4.
8. ICPC-2 PLUS - Demonstrator Sydney, Australia: University of Sydney; 2002–2013 [updated 20 January 2013]. Available from: http://sydney.edu.au/medicine/fmrc/icpc-2-plus/demonstrator/index.php.
9. Kings N, Horrocks C. Interviews in Qualitative Research: SAGE Publications. 2010.
10. Patton M. Qualitative research and evaluation methods. 3rd ed. California, USA: Sage Publications, Inc.; 2002.
11. Hansen E. Successful qualitative health research. NSW, Australia: Allen and Unwin; 2006.
12. Landis JR, Koch GG. The measurement of observer agreement for categorical data. Biometrics. 1977;33(1):159–74.
13. National Statement on Ethical Conduct in Human Research Australia: National Health and Medical Research Council, NHMRC; 2013 [cited 2013 20 December 2013]. Available from: http://www.nhmrc.gov.au/guidelines/publications/e72.

6

Effects of massage therapy and occlusal splint therapy on electromyographic activity and the intensity of signs and symptoms in individuals with temporomandibular disorder and sleep bruxism: a randomized clinical trial

Cid André Fidelis de Paula Gomes[1,3*], Yasmin El Hage[2,3], Ana Paula Amaral[2], Fabiano Politti[2,3] and Daniela Aparecida Biasotto-Gonzalez[2,3]

Abstract

Introduction: Temporomandibular disorder (TDM) is the most common source of orofacial pain of a non-dental origin. Sleep bruxism is characterized by clenching and/or grinding the teeth during sleep and is involved in the perpetuation of TMD. The aim of the present study was to investigate the effects of massage therapy, conventional occlusal splint therapy and silicone occlusal splint therapy on electromyographic activity in the masseter and anterior temporal muscles and the intensity of signs and symptoms in individuals with severe TMD and sleep bruxism.

Methods: Sixty individuals with severe TMD and sleep bruxism were randomly distributed into four treatment groups: 1) massage group, 2) conventional occlusal splint group, 3) massage + conventional occlusal splint group and 4) silicone occlusal splint group. Block randomization was employed and sealed opaque envelopes were used to conceal the allocation. Groups 2, 3 and 4 wore an occlusal splint for four weeks. Groups 1 and 3 received three weekly massage sessions for four weeks. All groups were evaluated before and after treatment through electromyographic analysis of the masseter and anterior temporal muscles and the Fonseca Patient History Index. The Wilcoxon test was used to compare the effects of the different treatments and repeated-measures ANOVA was used to determine the intensity of TMD.

Results: The inter-group analysis of variance revealed no statistically significant differences in median frequency among the groups prior to treatment. In the intra-group analysis, no statistically significant differences were found between pre-treatment and post-treatment evaluations in any of the groups. Group 3 demonstrated a greater improvement in the intensity of TMD in comparison to the other groups.

Conclusion: Massage therapy and the use of an occlusal splint had no significant influence on electromyographic activity of the masseter or anterior temporal muscles. However, the combination of therapies led to a reduction in the intensity of signs and symptoms among individuals with severe TMD and sleep bruxism.

Trial registration: This study is registered in August, 2014 in the ClinicalTrials.gov (NCT01874041).

Keywords: Physical therapy modalities, Temporomandibular joint disorders, Massage therapy, Occlusal splint

* Correspondence: cid.andre@gmail.com
[1]Postgraduate Program in Biophotonics Applied to Health Sciences, Universidade Nove de Julho (UNINOVE), Av. Dr. Adolfo Pinto,109, Água Branca, 05001-100 São Paulo, SP, Brazil
[3]Department of Physical Therapy, Universidade Nove de Julho (UNINOVE), Av. Dr. Adolfo Pinto,109, Água Branca, 05001-100 São Paulo, SP, Brazil
Full list of author information is available at the end of the article

Background

Temporomandibular disorder (TMD) is considered the most common source of orofacial pain of a non-dental origin and constitutes a heterogeneous group of conditions that affect the temporomandibular joint and/or masticatory muscles [1]. Sleep bruxism is characterized by clenching and/or grinding one's teeth during sleep and may be involved in triggering and/or perpetuating TMD [2]. Treatment strategies for both conditions are founded on minimally invasive, reversible interventions involving a multidisciplinary team [3].

In recent years, physiotherapists have employed different resources, such as electrotherapy [4], phototherapy [5], mobilization [6] and massage therapy [7,8,3], with the aim of improving symptoms related to TMD and sleep bruxism through the reestablishment of local blood flow and consequent improvement in muscle function and local analgesia [9]. In dentistry, occlusal splint therapy has been used for this purpose and is founded on the notion that a bite plate promotes relaxation of the masticatory muscles, protects the teeth and jaws from the adverse effects of bruxism, normalizes proprioception of the periodontal ligament and repositions the condyles and jaws into their correct alignment (centric relation) [10].

Despite the large number of randomized clinical trials addressing TMD and sleep bruxism, systematic reviews of the literature [7,11] point out the need for further investigations due to the low degree of methodological quality in previously published papers, such as failures regarding blinding and the use of reliable measures. Moreover, the multifactor etiology of both TMD and sleep bruxism suggests that it may be advantageous to investigate the effects of different resources used either alone or in combination.

The aim of the present study was to investigate the effects of massage therapy, traditional occlusal splint therapy and silicone occlusal splint therapy on electromyographic activity in the masseter and anterior temporal muscles and the intensity of signs of symptoms in individuals with severe TMD and sleep bruxism. The hypothesis tested was that the combination of massage therapy and a muscle-relaxing oral appliance would lead to a decrease electromyographic activity in the masticatory muscles as well as a reduction in the intensity of signs and symptoms of TMD.

Methods

Subjects

A blinded, randomized, clinical trial was conducted. The procedures of the present study received approval from the Human Research Ethics Committee of Nove de Julho University, Sao Paulo, Brazil (protocol number 133012). This study is registered in August, 2014 in the ClinicalTrials.gov (NCT01874041). Prior to participation, all volunteers signed a statement of informed consent.

Individuals diagnosed with TMD and sleep bruxism aged 18 to 40 years were recruited from the university community of the city of Sao Paulo, Brazil, through notices placed on information boards located in general areas of the university and the Internet between June 2011 and December 2012. Neither the examiner in charge of the surface electromyography (EMG) nor the researcher in charge of the data analysis was aware of the allocation of the volunteers to the different groups.

The volunteers received an intra-oral examination by an experienced dentist for signs of sleep bruxism. Those with incisal and/or occlusal tooth wear and clinical signs in the buccal mucosa and tongue of clenching or grinding were diagnosed with bruxism based on the criteria of the American Academy of Sleep Medicine [12] and a positive self-report of awake bruxism [13].

The Fonseca Patient History Index was used to diagnose the presence and intensity of TMD, which is an adequately valid, reliable measure for identifying individuals with TMD that has been widely used in recent studies [14-18]. This Portuguese-language measure for the assessment of TMD severity has 10 items, each with three response options: "yes" (scored as 10 points), "sometimes" (5 points) and "no" (0 points). The sum of the points for all items gives the overall score and allows the following classification: absence of TMD (0 to 15 points), mild TMD (20 to 45 points), moderate TMD (50 to 65 points), and severe TMD (70 to 100 points) [18]. Only individuals with severe TMD and bruxism for at least one year were included in the present study.

The following were the exclusion criteria: occurrence of missing teeth (except third molars); current use of an orthodontic appliance; history of neuromuscular disease; current use of analgesic, anti-inflammatory agent or muscle relaxant; and currently undergoing physical therapy for TMD.

One hundred nine male and female individuals were consecutively recruited and screened based on the eligibility criteria. During this process, 49 volunteers were excluded. Thus, the final sample was made up of 60 volunteers with severe TMD and sleep bruxism. Block randomization was employed and opaque envelopes were used to conceal the allocation of the volunteers to the four treatment groups described below (Additional file 1: Figure S1).

The massage group (MG) (n =15; 13 women and 2 men; mean age: 29.32 ± 4.31 years) was submitted to three weekly 30-minute sessions of massage therapy performed by a physiotherapist who had undergone a training exercise for the administration of sliding and kneading maneuvers of the masseter and anterior temporal muscles, bilaterally, over four consecutive weeks (total: 12 sessions) [19]. Sliding consisted of a unidirectional movement in which part of the therapist's hand (mainly the fingertips) was used, moving from the proximal to the distal portion of the face with constant, progressive pressure compatible with the status of each tissue. The degree of pressure varied depending on the level of pain, sensitivity and tension in each individual. Kneading consisted of a gripping maneuver of a muscle group or portion of a muscle, with intermittent movements of compression and decompression. The therapist performed circular movements with the fingertips such that the skin and subcutaneous tissues were moved over the subjacent structures. A facial massage cream was used to facilitate the manual procedures [15].

The conventional occlusal splint group (COSG) (n =15; 12 women and 3 men; mean age: 27.89 ± 5.82 years) was submitted to treatment with an occlusal splint for four weeks. The aim of this form of treatment was to promote greater stability of the joint components, establish a more favorable occlusal relationship, promote the reorganization of neuromuscular activity, reduce hyperactivity of the masticatory muscles and reestablish balanced muscle function. After a clinical examination by a dentist, the upper arch of each volunteer was molded with irreversible hydrocolloid for the fabrication of a Michigan-type occlusal splint with canine and protrusive guides as well as a flat occlusal surface for contact with the antagonist teeth. The volunteers were instructed to wear the splint while sleeping. Adjustments were made after two weeks by the same dentist in charge of the evaluation and splint fabrication [20,21,15].

The massage + conventional occlusal splint group (MCOSG) (n = 15; 14 women and 1 man; mean age: 26.05 ± 3.32 years) was submitted to combined treatment with massage and occlusal splint as described in the previous two paragraphs.

The silicone occlusal splint group (SOSG) (n = 15; 10 women and 4 men; mean age: 28.92 ± 6.78 years) was submitted to treatment with a silicone splint for four weeks fabricated from a 3-mm soft polyvinyl sheet in a vacuum pressure molding device with a thermally controlled infrared heater. This machine performed vacuum suctioning of the warmed sheet of thick, resilient mouth-guard material over the maxillary cast. When the sheet had properly adapted to the cast in the vacuum former, the splint was separated from the cast with a laboratory knife/scissors, the edges were smoothed and the palatal area was removed. Chair-side occlusal fitting was made by evenly warming the occlusal surface of the splint with an alcohol torch before placement in the patient's mouth. The soft splint was then polished with pumice, disinfected and placed in the oral cavity. The soft, resilient material is believed to help distribute the load during parafunctional activity (bruxism) [22]. The volunteers were instructed to wear the splint while sleeping.

Electromyographic analysis

The right and left masseter and anterior temporal muscles were analyzed using surface EMG. EMG signals were obtained using an eight-channel module (EMG System do Brasil Ltda®) consisting of conditioner with a band pass filter with cut-off frequencies at 20–1000 Hz, an amplifier gain of 1000 and a common mode rejection ratio >120 dB. All data were acquired and processed using a 16-bit analog to digital converter (EMG System do Brasil Ltda®) with a sampling frequency 2 kHz. The system was composed of active bipolar electrodes with a pre-amplification gain of 20 x.

The volunteer was instructed to remain seated in a chair, feet apart, shoulders relaxed and hands resting on thighs, with the head on the Frankfurt parallel to the ground and no visual feedback of the signals registered on the computer. The sites for the electrodes were cleaned with a cotton ball soaked in alcohol to diminish impedance between the skin and electrodes. Disposable circular electrodes (Ag/AgCl – Medical Trace©) measuring 10 mm in diameter were attached to the belly of the muscle in the region with the greatest tonus after the volunteer performed moderate clenching. Bandage tape was used to secure the electrodes further, with care taken to avoid micro-movements. The inter-electrode distance was 20 mm from center to center, as suggested by the European Recommendations for Surface Electromyography [23]. A rectangular metallic electrode measuring 3 x 2 cm coated with Lectron II conductive gel (Pharmaceutical Innovations®) to increase the conduction capacity and impede interference from external noise was attached to the left wrist of the volunteers for reference [23].

Three EMG readings were taken before and after treatment in all groups during maximum voluntary clenching for 10 seconds, with a five-minute rest period between readings. To avoid direct occlusal contact between the dental cusps, a strip of Parafilm M® (American National Can TM, Chicago, USA) with texture and dimensions similar to commercial chewing gum was folded into five parts and positioned in the molar region bilaterally.

The initial two seconds and final three seconds of the EMG signal were discarded. Thus, a five-second reading was considered for each test. The signal was analyzed using Fast Fourier Transform computed with a 2048-point hamming window processing (50% overlap). The median frequency (MDF) of the power spectrum was calculated for each five-second period analyzed. All EMG signal processing was performed using specific routines carried out in the Matlab program, version 7.1 (The MathWorks Inc., Natick, Massachusetts, USA).

Data analysis

The sample size was calculated with the aid of the Ene software, version 3.0 (Barcelona, Spain) and based on the findings of a pilot study. The data were collected during maximum voluntary clenching for eight seconds before (T0) and after five sessions of massage therapy (T1). Considering an 80% test power and α of 0.05, the suggested sample size was 13 individuals (T0 = 1.19; T1 = 1.08; SD =0.14) per group.

As the Shapiro-Wilk test revealed that the MDF was not normally distributed ($p < 0.05$), the data were analyzed using nonparametric tests and expressed as median and interquartile range (25% and 75%). The Kruskal-Wallis test used to determine the similarity in the MDF among the groups (MG, COSG, MCOSG, SOSG) before treatment (baseline). The Wilcoxon test was used to evaluate the effects of the treatments. TMD intensity before and after treatment was determined using the Fonseca Patient History Index and verified through repeated-measures analysis of variance (ANOVA) considering two factors: group (MG vs. COSG vs. MCOSG vs. SOSG) and treatment (pre-treatment vs. post-treatment). Specific differences were analyzed using Tukey's post hoc test. The significance level was set to 5% ($p < 0.05$). All data were analyzed using the Statistical Package for the Social Sciences, version 17.

Results

Inter-group analysis of variance revealed no statistically significant differences in the MDF among the MG, COSG, MCOSG and SOSG prior to treatment, thereby excluding the possibility that any group was more or less susceptible to the influence of the treatment employed (Figure 1).

In the intra-group analysis, no statistically significant differences were found between the pre-treatment and post-treatment evaluations of the left and right masseter and anterior temporal muscles in any group (Table 1).

Table 2 displays the results of the group-treatment interactions regarding TMD intensity based on the Fonseca Patient History Index. Significant differences were found between the pre-treatment and post-treatment evaluations in the MG, COSG and MCOSG, the latter of which exhibited greater improvement in comparison to the other groups.

Discussion

The lack of significant differences in the MDF during the pre-treatment evaluation demonstrated the similarity among the groups at baseline. Moreover, no statistically significant reductions in EMG activity were found in any of the groups after treatment, even when treatment involved the combination of massage and occlusal splint therapy. These findings are in agreement with data reported in previous studies on massage therapy [24-26] and occlusal splint therapy [27,28], which also found no reduction in EMG activity among individuals with TMD.

Hyperactivity of the masseter muscles and constant activity of the anterior temporal muscles even when the mandible is in the resting position is a common characteristic among individuals with sleep bruxism and TMD [29]. Such individuals exhibit reduced blood flow to the masticatory muscles due to vasoconstriction stemming from muscle hyperactivity, which impedes the transport of nutrients and metabolites and can cause the buildup of by-products, thereby triggering pain [30].

Massage therapy has been shown to stimulate parasympathetic activity by engaging the relaxation response,

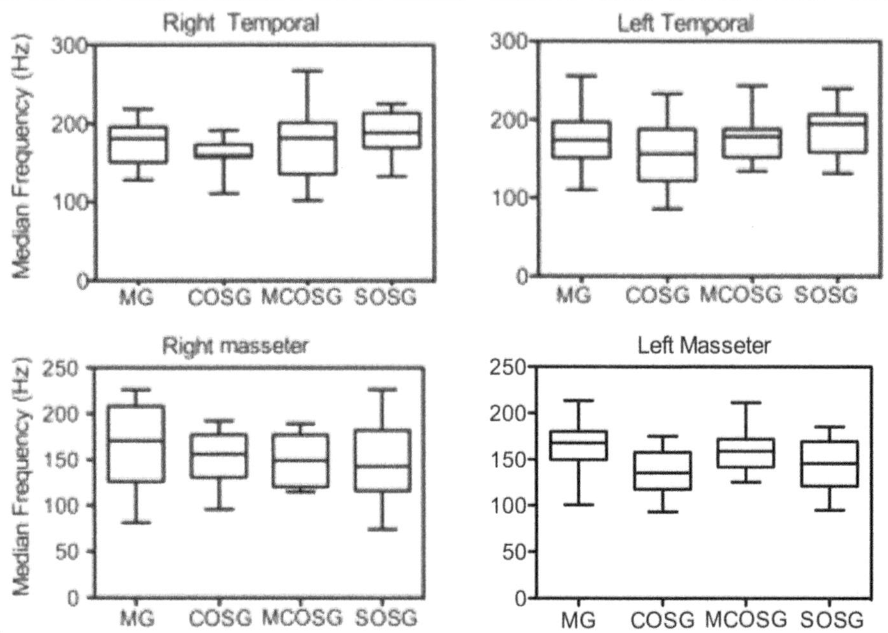

Figure 1 Median (25% and 75% quartile) of median frequency (Hz) in right and left anterior temporal and masseter muscles during maximum voluntary clenching in each group (non-significant differences, *p* > 0.05; Kruskal-Wallis test).

Table 1 Pre-treatment and post-treatment MDF in right temporal (RT), right masseter (RM), left temporal (LT) and left masseter (LM) during maximum voluntary clenching in different groups (Wilcoxon signed rank test)

		MG	COSG	MCOSG	SOSG
RT	**Pre**	181.9 [136.2-201.4]	188.7 [169.9-213.6]	189,5 [140.9-203.1]	159.7 [157.7-173.6]
	Post	173.1 [133.3-189.5]	195.8 [182.9-210.1]	198.0 [138.4-206.1]	168.7 [156.5-180.2]
	p	0.65	0.69	0.73	0.44
RM	**Pre**	170.9 [150.9-185.5]	151.6 [116.9-168,9]	142.8 [116.8-182.1]	156.5 [130.6-177.5]
	Post	155.3 [113.3-187.3]	160.4 [135.7-183,8]	149.2 [120.4-177.2]	148.7 [121.3-167.5]
	p	0.22	1.00	0.86	0.91
LT	**Pre**	178.7 [152.3-188.2]	194.8 [158.9-206.8]	176.1 [143.6-193.8]	156.7 [122.1-188.2]
	Post	168.7 [147.2-199.7]	193.4 [158.4-206.3]	183.4 [136.4-196.9]	170.4 [145.5-208.7]
	p	0.82	0.91	0.36	0.60
LM	**Pre**	157.5 [140,6-169.4]	145.8 [120.8-169.4]	142.1 [118.2-171.6]	135.0 [117.4-158.0]
	Post	142.3 [123.5-170.4]	154.3 [122.3-179.7]	152.6 [124.3-157.5]	143.8 [90.09-155.8]
	p	0.60	0.67	0.82	0.15

MG: massage therapy group; COSG: conventional occlusal splint group; MCOSG: massage therapy + conventional occlusal splint group; SOSG: silicone occlusal splint group.

which, in turn, reduces hormonal and autonomic indicators and has an analgesic effect caused by the activation of a pain-gate mechanism, which disables pain signals travelling to central nervous system through larger, faster conductive nerve fibers [9,29,31,32]. Thus, massage can lead to an increase in mandibular function [15] as well as a reduction in the frequency and intensity of bruxism and symptoms of TMD [33]. However, contrary to expectations, massage therapy, occlusal splint therapy or a combination of the two was insufficient to reduce muscle activity in the present study, as demonstrated by the analysis of the masseter and anterior temporal muscles. This may have been related to the severe, chronic characteristics of the participants in the present study, who had sleep bruxism and TMD for at least five years.

The use of occlusal splints for individuals with bruxism and TMD is a common practice in dentistry. However, the mechanism of action has not yet been fully clarified. Indeed, an occlusal splint does not cure TMD or sleep bruxism, but can contribute to improving quality of life [34], increasing maximum mouth opening [22] and reducing myofascial pain [28]. A number of hypotheses may explain the mechanism of action of this type of treatment: 1) a reduction in EMG activity of the masticatory muscles (which did not occur in the present study); 2) the repositioning of the condyle and/or joint disc; 3) a change in the occlusion; and 4) a change in oral habits [35].

Despite being one of the hypotheses for the function of occlusal splint therapy, considerable variation is found in the literature regarding the reduction in EMG activity of the masticatory muscles. Some studies indicate only immediate reductions in EMG activity after the use of an occlusal splint, whereas no reductions occur after long-term use of an occlusal splint [25,26]. These findings suggest the effect of occlusal splints, including silicone splints indicated to control parafunctional activity, is not maintained for a long time due to the adaptive mechanisms of the muscles. Thus, the benefits seem to be temporary and non-cumulative and continual daily use seems to be required to maintain the effect, which may explain the present results, as evaluations were only performed before and after four weeks of occlusal splint use.

Table 2 Mean e standard deviation and the results of interactions between groups (ANOVA) pre e post treatment relative intensity according to Fonseca Patient History Index

	Treatment (Mean ± SD)		ANOVA		
Groups	**Pre**	**Post**	**Interactions**	**F**	**P**
MG	67±12,5	50,33 ±10,76[a]	Treatment (Pré x Post)	32,41	<0,0001
COSG	52 ±15,44	44 ±13,78[a]	Groups (MG x COSG x MCOSG x SOSG)	8,88	<0,0001
MCOSG	54,33±21,03	29,33±10,83[a,b]			
SOSG	56±16,16	59,33±13,21			

[a]Significant difference between pre e post treatment (ANOVA, Bonferroni corrections).
[b]Significant difference between groups MCOSG > MG, COSG, SOSG (Test post hoc de Tukey).

TMD and sleep bruxism treatment should be performed by a multidisciplinary team [36] involving a combination of therapeutic resources. The present study involved both massage therapy and occlusal therapy. However, the findings demonstrated no changes in EMG activity among individuals with a diagnosis of chronic, severe TMD and sleep bruxism. Thus, EMG activity is not the best variable for the evaluation of improvements in such individuals and preference should be given to clinical characteristics, such as pain and vertical mandibular movement. Indeed, massage therapy is reported to achieve positive results regarding a reduction in pain and an increase in mandibular function.

Occlusal splint therapy can lead to a reduction in fatigue of the masticatory muscles, as demonstrated in a study by Zhang et al. [37], who found EMG changes in the masticatory muscles following occlusal splint therapy employed for the same period of time as that used in the present study. However, the individuals in the present investigation had a greater intensity and longer duration of signs and symptoms of TMD, which may explain the lack of EMG changes in the sample.

Among individuals with TMD and bruxism, surface EMG is fundamentally employed to demonstrate dysfunction in the masticatory muscles. However, divergent opinions are found regarding its use as a diagnostic tool and parameter of clinical improvement [38]. Moreover, a weak correlation is reported between symptoms of TMD, such as pain, and electrical activity in the masticatory muscles [39], which makes EMG questionable when used as the main reference for the determination of clinical improvement, especially in individuals with signs and symptoms of severe TMD.

The present results regarding the intensity of TMD following the different forms of therapy are in agreement with data reported in a previous study [37] and underscore the importance of the clinical history and physical exam based on signs and symptoms. The improvement found when massage therapy and occusal splint therapy were combined indicates that this combination of treatment modalities is highly desirable when there is a need to diminish clinical signs and symptoms, such as pain in the masticatory muscles, when treating individuals with chronic characteristics associated with sleep bruxism and severe mandibular limitations, as found in the present sample.

There are a number of limitations in the present study that should be recognized. A convenience sample was used and was limited to the university community, which may not be representative of the entire population of individuals with bruxism and TMD. Due to the demand and need for urgent care for the individuals who seek our laboratory, which is a reference service for the treatment of TMD and sleep bruxism, it was not possible to form a control group in an attempt to structure this group with the formation of a silicone occlusal splint, which is a procedure used only for emergencies or as a temporary measure until a conventional occlusal splint can be fabricated. Moreover, only the long-term results of massage therapy and occlusal therapy were investigated. The massage therapy protocol did not involve intraoral (pterygoid) massage, which may have exerted a direct influence on the findings. Considering the improvement in signs and symptoms of TMD reported in a recent study [3], further studies involving the release of intraoral structures are suggested. Moreover, due to the variations in the effects of different therapies on EMG activity, future studies should be carried out to compare immediate and long-term effects.

Conclusion

In summary, massage therapy and the use of an occlusal splint did not lead to statistically significant changes in electromyographic activity in the masseter and anterior temporal muscles. However, the combination of therapies led to a reduction in the intensity of signs and symptoms among individuals with severe TMD and sleep bruxism.

Additional file

Additional file 1: Figure S1. Flowchart of the study.

Abbreviations

TMD: Temporomandibular disorder; EMG: Electromyography; MG: Massage group; COSG: Conventional occlusal splint group; MCOSG: Massage + conventional occlusal splint group; SOSG: Silicone occlusal splint group; MDF: Median frequency.

Competing interests

The authors declare that they have no competing interests.

Authors' contributions

CAFPG: conception and design, data collection and analysis, manuscript writing and final approval of the manuscript. YEH: data collection and analysis, critical revision and final approval of the manuscript. APA: data collection and analysis, critical revision and final approval of the manuscript. FP: data collection and analysis, critical revision and final approval of the manuscript. DABG: conception and design, financial support, manuscript writing, final approval of manuscript. All authors read and approved the final manuscript.

Acknowledgments

The authors are grateful to all involved in the study, the team and participants. This study had no financial support. However, we appreciate Nove de Julho University for infrastructure and equipment available for this study.

Author details

[1]Postgraduate Program in Biophotonics Applied to Health Sciences, Universidade Nove de Julho (UNINOVE), Av. Dr. Adolfo Pinto,109, Água Branca, 05001-100 São Paulo, SP, Brazil. [2]Postgraduate Program in Rehabilitation Sciences, Universidade Nove de Julho (UNINOVE), Av. Dr. Adolfo Pinto,109, Água Branca, 05001-100 São Paulo, SP, Brazil. [3]Department of Physical Therapy, Universidade Nove de Julho (UNINOVE), Av. Dr. Adolfo Pinto,109, Água Branca, 05001-100 São Paulo, SP, Brazil.

References

1. Manfredini D1, Piccotti F, Ferronato G, Guarda-Nardini L: **Age peaks of different RDC/TMD diagnoses in a patient population.** *J Dent* 2010, **38**(5):392–399. doi:10.1016/j.jdent.2010.01.006.
2. McNeill C: **Management of temporomandibular disorders: concepts and controversies.** *J Prosthet Dent* 1997, **77**(5):510–522.
3. Kalamir A, Graham PL, Vitiello AL, Bonello R, Pollard H: **Intra-oral myofascial therapy versus education and self-care in the treatment of chronic, myogenous temporomandibular disorder: a randomised, clinical trial.** *Chiropr Man Therap* 2013, **5**:21. 17. doi:10.1186/2045-709X-21-17.
4. Monaco A, Sgolastra F, Ciarrocchi I, Cattaneo R: **Effects of transcutaneous electrical nervous stimulation on electromyographic and kinesiographic activity of patients with temporomandibular disorders: a placebo-controlled study.** *J Electromyogr Kinesiol* 2012, **22**(3):463–468. doi:10.1016/j.jelekin.2011.12.008.
5. Pereira TS, Flecha OD, Guimarães RC, de Oliveira D, Botelho AM, Ramos Glória JC, Aguiar Tavano KT: **Efficacy of red and infrared lasers in treatment of temporomandibular disorders–a double-blind, randomized, parallel clinical trial.** *Cranio* 2014, **32**(1):51–56.
6. De Vocht JW, Long CR, Zeitler DL, Schaeffer W: **Chiropractic treatment of temporomandibular disorders using the activator adjusting instrument: a prospective case series.** *J Manipulative Physiol Ther* 2003, **26**(7):421–425.
7. Medlicott MS, Harris SR: **A systematic review of the effectiveness of exercise, manual therapy, electrotherapy, relaxation training, and biofeedback in the management of temporomandibular disorder.** *Phys Ther* 2006, **86**:955–973.
8. Pierson MJ: **Changes in temporomandibular joint dysfunction symptoms following massage therapy: a case report.** *Int J Ther Massage Bodywork* 2011, **4**:37–47.
9. Holey LA, Dixon J, Selfe J: **An exploratory thermographic investigation of the effects of connective tissue massage on autonomic function.** *J Manipulative Physiol Ther* 2011, **34**(7):457–462.
10. Dylina TJ: **A common-sense approach to splint therapy.** *J Prosthet Dent* 2001, **86**(5):539–545.
11. McNeely ML, Armijo Olivo S, Magee DJ: **A systematic review of the effectiveness of physical therapy interventions for temporomandibular disorders.** *Phys Ther* 2006, **86**:710–725.
12. Buysse DJ, Young T, Edinger JD, Carrol J, Kotagal S: **Clinicians use of the international classification of sleep disorders: results of a national survey.** *Sleep* 2003, **26**:48–51.
13. Pintado MR, Anderson GC, DeLong R, Douglas WH: **Variation in tooth wear in young adults over a two-year period.** *J Prosthet Dent* 1997, **77**:313–320.
14. Gomes CAFPG, Dibai-Filho AV, da Silva JR, Oliveira PM: **Correlation between severity of temporomandibular disorder and mandibular range of motion.** *J Bodyw Mov Ther* 2014, **18**(2):306–310.
15. Gomes CA, Politti F, Andrade DV, de Sousa DF, Herpich CM, Dibai-Filho AV, Gonzalez T d O, Biasotto-Gonzalez DA: **Effects of massage therapy and occlusal splint therapy on mandibular range of motion in individuals with temporomandibular disorder: a randomized clinical trial.** *J Manipulative Physiol Ther* 2014, **37**(3):164–169. doi:10.1016/j.jmpt.2013.12.007.
16. Campos JADB, Gonçalves DAG, Camparis CM, Speciali JG: **Reliability of a questionnaire for diagnosing the severity of temporomandibular disorder.** *Rev Bras Fisioter* 2009, **13**:38–43.
17. Nomura K, Vitti M, Oliveira AS, Chaves TC, Semprini M, Siéssere S, Hallak JE, Regalo SC: **Use of the Fonseca's questionnaire to assess the prevalence and severity of temporomandibular disorders in Brazilian dental undergraduates.** *Braz Dent J* 2007, **18**(2):163–167.
18. Bevilaqua-Grossi D, Chaves TC, de Oliveira AS, Monteiro-Pedro V: **Anamnestic index severity and signs and symptoms of TMD.** *Cranio* 2006, **24**(2):112–118.
19. El Hage Y, Politti F, de Sousa DF, Herpich CM, Gloria IP, Gomes CA, Amaral AP, de Melo NC, da Silva TC, Arruda EE, Amorim CF, Gadotti IC, Gonzalez TO, Berzin F, Bussadori SK, Garcia MB, Barbosa BR, Biasotto-Gonzalez DA: **Effect of mandibular mobilization on electromyographic signals in muscles of mastication and static balance in individuals with temporomandibular disorder: study protocol for a randomized controlled trial.** *Trials* 2013, **1**:14. 316. doi:10.1186/1745-6215-14-316.
20. Ash MM Jr, Ramfjord SP: **Reflections on the Michigan splint and other intraocclusal devices.** *J Mich Dent Assoc* 1998, **80**(8):32–35. 41-6.
21. Dao TT, Lavigne GJ: **Oral splints: the crutches for temporomandibular disorders and bruxism?** *Crit Rev Oral Biol Med* 1998, **9**:345–361.
22. Naikmasur V, Bhargava P, Guttal K, Burde K: **Soft occlusal splint therapy in the management of myofascial pain dysfunction syndrome: a follow-up study.** *Indian J Dent Res* 2008, **19**:196–203.
23. Ferrario VF, Sforza C, Tartaglia GM, Dellavia C: **Immediate effect of a stabilization splint on masticatory muscle activity in temporomandibular disorder patients.** *J Oral Rehabil* 2002, **29**(9):810–815.
24. Albertin A, Kerppers II, Amorim CF, Costa RV, Ferrari Corrêa JC, Oliveira CS: **The effect of manual therapy on masseter muscle pain and spasm.** *Electromyogr Clin Neurophysiol* 2010, **50**(2):107–112.
25. Harada T, Ichiki R, Tsukiyama Y, Koyano K: **The effect of oral splint devices on sleep bruxism: a 6-week observation with an ambulatory electromyographic recording device.** *J Oral Rehabil* 2006, **33**(7):482–488.
26. Nascimento LL, Amorim CF, Giannasi LC, Oliveira CS, Nacif SR, Silva Ade M, Nascimento DF, Marchini L, de Oliveira LV: **Occlusal splint for sleep bruxism: an electromyographic asso- ciated to Helkimo Index evaluation.** *Sleep Breath* 2008, **12**(3):275–280.
27. Weggen T, Schindler HJ, Kordass B, Hugger A: **Clinical and electromyographic follow-up of myofascial pain patients treated with two types of oral splint: a randomized controlled pilot study.** *Int J Comput Dent* 2013, **16**(3):209–224.
28. Villalón P1, Arzola JF, Valdivia J, Fresno MJ, Santander H, Gutiérrez MF, Miralles R: **The occlusal appliance effect on myofascial pain.** *Cranio* 2013, **31**(2):84–91.
29. Piquero K, Sakurai K: **A clinical diagnosis of diurnal (non- sleep) bruxism in denture wearers.** *J Oral Rehabil* 2000, **27**(6):473–482.
30. Barão VA, Gallo AK, Zuim PR, Garcia AR, Assunção WG: **Effect of occlusal splint treatment on the temperature of different muscles in patients with TMD.** *J Prosthodont Res* 2011, **55**(1):19–23.
31. Delaney JP, Leong KS, Watkins A, Brodie D: **The short-term effects of myofascial TrPTs massage therapy on cardiac autonomic tone in healthy subjects.** *J Adv Nurs* 2002, **37**(4):364–371.
32. Field T, Hernandez-Reif M, Diego M, Schanberg S, Kuhn C: **Cortisol decreases and serotonin and dopamine increase following massage therapy.** *Int Jl Neurosci* 2005, **115**(10):1397–1413.
33. Eisensmith LP: **Massage therapy decreases frequency and intensity of symptoms related to temporomandibular joint syndrome in one case study.** *J Bodyw Mov Ther* 2007, **11**(3):223–230.
34. Magdaleno F, Ginestal E: **Side effects of stabilization oeclusal splints: a report of three ca.ses and literature review.** *J Craniomandih Pract* 2010, **28**(2):128–135.
35. Botelho AL, Silva BC, Gentil FH, Sforza C, da Silva MA: **Immediate effect of the resilient splint evaluated using surface electromyography in patients with TMD.** *Cranio* 2010, **28**(4):266–273.
36. Felicio CM, Mazzetto MO, da Silva MA R, Bataglion C, Hotia TH: **A preliminary protocol for multi-professional centers for the determination of signs and symptoms of temporomandibular disorders.** *J Craniomandih Pract* 2006, **24**:258–264.
37. Zhang F-y, Wang X-g, Dong J, Zhang J-f, Lu Y-l: **Effect of occlusal splints for the management of patients with myofascial pain: a randomized, controlled, double-blind study.** *Chin Med J* 2013, **126**:2270–2275.
38. Machado MB, Nitsch GS, Pitta NC, Oliveira AS: **Muscle activation time during chewing in temporomandibular disorder patients.** *Audiol Commun Res* 2014, **19**:202–207.
39. Almeida FL, Silva AMT, Correa ECR, Busanello AR: **Relation between pain and electric activity in the presence of bruxism.** *Rev CEFAC* 2011, **13**:399–406.

7

Diagnostic challenges in the older patient

Lisa Zaynab Killinger

Abstract

Older patients often present with a long, complex history and a clinical picture that frequently includes co-morbidities. It is essential that health professionals caring for older patients become familiar with common age-related changes, and the specific clinical factors that complicate the diagnostic process. A case-based approach is taken in this article to explore the diagnostic challenges in caring for older patients. Three areas of focus are used: a) polypharmacy, b) cognitive issues such as delirium, dementia and depression, and c) increased odds of pathologies and chronic illnesses.

Keywords: Diagnosis, Geriatrics, Polypharmacy, Cognitive health, Delirium, Dementia, Depression, Pathologies, Chiropractic

Background

One of the greatest challenges in caring for older adult patients is formulating an accurate and appropriate diagnosis [1,2]. Older adult patients bring complex health histories and clinical scenarios into our practices, and it takes a skilled practitioner to overcome the related diagnostic challenges. These challenges have been discussed in the chiropractic and other health literature, often with an emphasis on improving patient care outcomes [2-5].

The fastest growing subset of the US population is the 75+ age category [6] and currently, about 15% of chiropractic patients are over 65. Most industrialized nations are seeing similar trends of rapid growth in the aging population. Many patients [in the US] seek chiropractic care for a chief complaint of musculoskeletal pain [7]. This is not surprising, considering that recent research shows that nearly one quarter of patients over the age of 75 experience non-disabling back pain, and another 6% report disabling back pain [8-11]. Chiropractors are well-suited to manage many patients with spinal complaints since chiropractic or spinal manipulative therapy is one of several efficacious evidence-based interventions for patients with back pain [12-19]. However, further research needs to be done to assess the efficacy and safety of chiropractic in the management of older back pain patients.

Correspondence: lisa.killinger@palmer.edu
Director of Diagnosis and Radiology, Palmer College of Chiropractic, 1000 Brady Street, 52803, Davenport, IA, USA

Due to this confluence of an aging world and the complex nature of geriatric health, it is essential that chiropractors thoroughly assess their older patients for concomitant health issues that may impact clinical decision making and patient prognosis. In this article a case-based approach will be taken to explore several important clinical problem solving examples. These cases are fictitious, based on an amalgam of previous clinical experiences, therefore no IRB or ethics approvals were required. The focus will be on three major confounding areas that create diagnostic challenges in managing older adult patients: Polypharmacy, cognitive issues, and increased risk of a co-morbid pathology or chronic illness.

Main text

Common age-related changes in older patients

In spite of the frequency in which chiropractic patients present with a musculoskeletal pain complaint, there is no doubt that common age related changes impact older patients profoundly. Such changes include [20]:

- A decline in all five senses [vision, hearing, touch, taste and smell]
- Lower muscle mass, bone density, and ligament elasticity
- Some amount of atherosclerosis
- Increased risk of co-morbid conditions [higher incidences of cancers, etc.]

- ➢Greater likelihood of chronic disease, like heart disease and arthritis,
- ➢Potential cognitive changes

It is with these changes in mind that examination of older patients should occur with a heightened vigilance for co-morbid conditions that may require medical care or concomitant care. One goal of a health professional in geriatric care should be to identify the diagnosis or to have a high index of suspicion of an important health concern.

Case: Sophie's sniffle and slip

Sophie, age 80, has a little cold. She takes an over the counter fizzy tablet [as she describes it] She reports that it helps with her cold symptoms. Unfortunately, last night Sophie got up to go to the bathroom and she got dizzy and fell. She comes to see you because she twisted her back and hurt her wrist in the fall. A careful examination strongly suggests that Sophie did not break any bones, and her aching back and wrist appear to be simple strains. The dizziness concerns you, so, you ask a local pharmacist if the cold medication she took the night before may have dizziness as a side effect. The pharmacist cautions that this particular medication can increase the risks of falls in older patients. She suggests several alternate over the counter medications that would be safer for Sophie. Subsequently, you may manage this patient with gentle chiropractic care, if indicated.

Medication issues

According to Healthy People 2020, polypharmacy is the principle drug safety issue in the US, particularly in older patients [21]. Polypharmacy is defined in a number of ways including: too many medications, inappropriate medications, bad combinations of medications, or medications being used to treat the side effects of other medications [21,22]. While prescription medication falls outside the scope of chiropractic practice, we do see patients who are taking many different medications. In fact, the average person over the age of 65 in America is taking 6–8 medications, often including several over the counter forms [23].

In the USA adverse drug events cause over 700,000 emergency department visits each year. Nearly 120,000 patients [all ages] each year need to be hospitalized for further treatment after emergency visits for adverse drug events. As more and more people take more medicines, the frequency of adverse events may increase. Older adults [65 years or older] are twice as likely as others to come to emergency departments for adverse drug events [over 177,000 emergency visits each year] and nearly seven times more likely to be hospitalized after an emergency visit [22,24,25]. Chiropractors must carefully note patient's medications, and be vigilant for adverse events, which may even present simply as muscle or joint pain.

Several resources are available related to medication information [22,24-26]. Chiropractors may also want to consider teaming up with a local pharmacy to sponsor "Brown Bag Events"; when patients bring in all their medications in a brown bag, and take a list of medications to the local pharmacist to identify problems or concerns with their medications. If issues are detected, the patient [or pharmacist, or chiropractor] can request that their prescribing doctor conduct a medication review which may result in potential changes to the medication regimen.

The 3 D'S: cognitive issues in the aging patient

Delirium: the first of the 3Ds

Delirium or *acute* confusion is fairly common in older adult patients and may be frightening for both chiropractor and patient. Delirium is common and is a transient state, and nearly always resolves once the cause is determined and underlying issue is addressed [27]. Acute confusion may make it difficult to diagnose and care for the delirious chiropractic patient. Three major contributing factors in delirium stand out and each will be illustrated by a case below [27,28]:

Case: George's bad day

George, age 73, has been your patient for years, but today, he says it was the craziest thing. He got lost coming to your office, something he has done a hundred times. His brother, Bill, who is visiting, comes to George's appointment with him, and is worried. He tells you in private that George has been acting strangely since he arrived, although he had been fine over the phone just a few days ago. George had a recent medical appointment, but now he seems "off". He forgot to pick Bill up at the airport, seemed confused when Bill showed up at the house, seems to not know that his sister recently passed away, and has been "in a daze." This sort of thing has never occurred before. George is usually as sharp as a tack.

Discussion

this change in cognitive status prompts a focused examination and renewed history. George's vital signs are all normal and he has not suffered any recent injury or emotional trauma. He does not drink alcohol and his diet has not changed. In further discussion with George, he reports that one of his anti-anxiety medications was changed a few days ago. With a quick call to the pharmacist about the new medication, the concern is raised that the new medication may be causing acute confusion [confusion is a common side effect of several common medications taken by older adults.]. A call is made to the prescribing doctor, and George is given the first available appointment. After a medical review and a change in the medications, George is back to his old self again in a few days and Bill is glad to have his brother back.

Medications

One of the most common causes of delirium is medications. Both over the counter medications and medications taken as prescribed may become toxic in older patients, resulting in confusion [27,28]. The only way to eliminate the delirium is to have the prescribing doctor or pharmacist identify and eliminate the medication or combination of medications which caused the confusion. Since many commonly used medications in older adults are taken for life-threatening diseases, medication evaluation should be overseen by a family medical doctor or a medical geriatrician/gerontologist and in consultation with a pharmacist where necessary.

Case: Hugh's bump in the road

You witness a minor car accident up ahead, so you stop to see if anyone was hurt. An older gentleman rear ended a man in his 30's who appears to be very upset about the damage to his newer car. He approaches the older driver angrily as you peek into the driver's window. Hugh, who looks to be in his 80's is looking around nervously in the car and fumbling with the door. You help him to open the door and you see that he has a bad cut on his forehead. He's bleeding and when you ask him if he is okay, he speaks unintelligibly, something about a horse and then says he has to get some milk. He gets out of the car with some unsteadiness then starts to walk out into the street, despite oncoming cars. When you try to stop him, he curses and takes a swing at you.

Trauma

Acute injury may result in acute confusion. For example, a minor bump on the head may result in delirium, and create a confused and maybe even violent and unpredictable patient. It is essential to get immediate emergency treatment for an injured older adult, and to be aware that acute confusion will regress once the injury is resolved. Patients who present for chiropractic care due to a musculoskeletal injury may be difficult to properly assess due to delirium.

Case: Bill's pain in the back

Bill's family is concerned. Bill, at age 75, is normally a mentally sharp man. Lately, however, Bill seems confused and has also been complaining of a "back ache" for 2 weeks. During your history and exam, you determine that he has had no change in medications, and no recent injury, however Bill's back pain seems to be more than just musculoskeletal pain. He has an achy vague pain in his back, pelvic area and lower abdomen. Since he is over 50, with a high fat diet, and has a family history of prostate cancer, you know he is also at increased risk for prostate cancer. Even though you had encouraged him to have a baseline Prostate Specific Antigen [PSA] blood test and prostate exam several years ago, he has not had one for years. You ask the related history questions: "Do you have any changes in urination, defecation or sexual function?" His wife, who is in the room with Bill, chimes in, reporting that Bill has been getting up to urinate several times a night, which wakes her up. Bill confesses to having some burning and frequency of urination. Urinalysis reveals a bladder infection, so you inform Bill and his wife and send a copy of Bill's urinalysis results to his doctor. The doctor requests to see Bill that day, and Bill's wife takes him in. One day after Bill starts taking his antibiotics, his urinary frequency and pain is resolved, along with the suprapubic pain. His wife calls to tell you his confusion has completely gone away.

Infection

A simple bladder infection or respiratory infection may have a unique presentation in elderly patients. In fact, all other symptoms may be eclipsed by the erratic, confused behavior. In the case above Bill had a simple bladder infection, secondary to benign prostatic hypertrophy [BPH]. It is important to note that an estimated 50% of men demonstrate histopathologic BPH by age 60 years. This number increases to 90% by age 85 years [29]. Missing this diagnosis may result in delirium that may not resolve until the infection has been resolved. Long term confusion may be mistaken for dementia, one example of a very serious misdiagnosis.

Dementia: the 2nd of the 3Ds

Dementia is a collection of symptoms including slow, gradual onset memory loss, intellectual impairment, loss of emotional control and problem solving ability. One type, Alzheimer's Dementia [AD] leads to a progressive loss of mental functions, and often includes disruption of speech or difficulty finding words [30-32]. It is estimated that 5 million people are currently living in the

US with AD, and about 360,000 people are diagnosed each year with over 50,000 death attributed to AD annually [32]. The case below may present to chiropractors showing a gradual onset of several of the main symptoms of AD. In recent years, research has shown that heart health and brain health are related, and patients may slow the progression of AD by making heart healthy lifestyle choices [31,32]. Chiropractors should consider assessing confused patients with the Mini-Mental Status Exam [MMSE] and discussing the patient's score with his or her medical provider [33].

Case: Henry is lost

Henry, age78, has been your patient for a decade, but you have noticed his mental sharpness has been in decline over the past few years. He remarks that he got lost coming to your office today, and he confesses that he got lost going to the grocery store twice in the past 2 months. As he speaks, he verbally wanders and seems to have difficulty finding the words to complete his sentences. He says he has good and bad days, but lately there have been more and more bad days. Henry becomes emotional as he tells you for the second time about getting lost today. He is noticeably shaken up. Henry has a history of cardiovascular health issues and does little, if any, physical activity.

Discussion

While a chiropractor can potentially treat Henry for his musculo-skeletal problems, medical oversight is required to further assess his dementia. It is essential that his cardiac health be monitored, so it is important for the chiropractor to regularly take blood pressure and to make certain that Henry is regularly consulting his medical physician. Dementia can be devastating for both patient and family, so it is important that the family identify resources related to dementia such as the Alzheimer's Association (USA) [34].

Depression: the 3rd of the 3Ds

Depression is a common mental health concern in older adults. One in 5–10 elderly adults suffer from depression and 80% of all depression is completely treatable, once detected. Detection is of utmost importance since suicide is one of the top 10 causes of death in older patients [35]. Suicide among white males aged 85 and older was nearly six times the national U.S. rate, making this a serious concern for all health professionals. Older adults often have significant risk factors for depression such as chronic illness and/or chronic pain. Poor diet and poor absorption of B vitamins in the aging body, may also contribute to depression [28,35]. Older adults are often faced with the death of a spouse, friends or peers. Significant life events such as these, combined with all the factors above, create fertile ground for depression to take hold in the elderly patient. Chiropractors may see depressed older patients since depression often magnifies symptoms of musculoskeletal pain [28,35].

It is important that all health professionals caring for the older adults be aware of the diagnostic criteria for depression [36]. Further, if a patient reports being sad or depressed it is important to assess the patient more thoroughly using a Geriatric Depression Scale [37] or similar assessment tool, which takes only a minute or two for patients to complete. Online versions can readily be downloaded. Scores on such forms should be discussed with their treating medical doctor, a psychologist or psychiatrist to determine an appropriate and safe course of care, and improve patient outcomes.

Common co-morbidities and pathologies

The heart of the matter

According to World Health Organization statistics, heart disease is the number one cause of death worldwide, accounting for 7.2 million deaths annually [38]. Cerebrovascular disease [a related disorder] is the second leading cause of death with another 3 million deaths annually. In Australia, heart disease is also the leading cause of death with nearly 50,000 deaths annually [39]. Using America as another example, heart disease is the top killer of both men and women, with most deaths in patients over age 60 [40]. About 18 million Americans currently have heart disease, and about half of those are over age 60 [41]. The 2011 published statistics from the American Heart Association, state that from 1997 to 2007, the total number of inpatient cardiovascular operations and procedures increased by 27 percent. The estimated total cost from heart disease and stroke in the United States for 2007 [including health expenditures and lost productivity] was $286 billion, which is higher than for any other diagnosis [40].

The case below will illustrate why heart disease should be on the mind of chiropractors every day in practice. Nearly all chiropractors, if they are in practice long enough will have a patient present for chiropractic care while they are having a heart attack. It is essential that chiropractors be good diagnosticians, so as to avoid a delay in emergency care for patients experiencing a cardiac event.

Inez's bad day

Inez is 65 years old. She cares for 3 of her grandchildren at home on a regular basis, getting two of them ready for school, and one to day care each morning. One morning, in the midst of her busy routine, Inez started feeling queasy and uncomfortable. By the time she dropped the 3rd child off at daycare, Inez also started having neck and jaw pain. She headed straight to your chiropractic clinic, as she has been a patient there before for her occasional neck pain. Today, you examine her and decide to take her blood pressure and pulse since her blood pressure has increased over the past few years and she reported last year that her doctor had mentioned that she may need to go on medication. She is not currently taking any anti-hypertensives, but is taking oral medications for type 2 diabetes. Her blood pressure was high [150/100] and her pulse was fast. In evaluating her neck and jaw, movement did not make it worse. You ask her to march in place with high steps for 1 minute to see if exertion makes it worse, and sure enough, she has to stop due to "feeling sick". You call for emergency services and arrange an ambulance. Inez was having a heart attack, and she calls you once she is out of the hospital to thank you for "saving her life."

Discussion

Heart attacks in women don't always follow the rules. Heart attacks, after all, are supposed to present as crushing chest pain, and left arm pain. But, female heart attacks often result in vague pain, no pain, discomfort or just an uneasy feeling [39]. While awareness among doctors is improving, women used to have twice the chance of dying from a heart attack than a man, in part due to missed diagnoses in the emergency room [27,39]. However, since the symptoms are so subtle and unpredictable, many women fail to go to the hospital during a heart attack, making treatment impossible. It is important that chiropractors be aware of the way cardiac events mimic musculoskeletal pain in many cases.

Notes on care of the older patient with back pain

Among older adults, back pain is one of the leading causes of a trip to the doctor [8-10]. It is essential that a chiropractor know some of the factors that make back pain more challenging in older adults. Older adults often have stiffness as a chief complaint, along with limits in their range of motion and functional ability. For many older patients, the most worrying factor about musculoskeletal pain is that it might rob them of their independence. Not being able to turn one's neck may translate into "having to give up driving." Not being able to bend, may translate into, "not being able to pick up the grandkids." Not being able to stand up from a seated position comfortably, may translate to "needing help in the bathroom." As you can see, functional outcomes may be more important to the older adult than any other patient age group.

It is beyond the scope of this article to point out the specifics of care and assessment of patients with back pain, but excellent literature has been presented elsewhere including in this journal's series on the elderly.

Increased risk of pathology

For many younger patients, musculoskeletal pain may be a simple as a sprain or strain, including the common presentation of uncomplicated back pain [7,13-15]. In fact, a high percentage of the cases chiropractors see [in all ages of patients], it is likely that a simple course of chiropractic care may address the problem and the patient's functional status and pain will improve [11,13,14]. While older patients also may enjoy good results with chiropractic care, the odds of complicating factors and comorbidities are much higher. Some examples of co-morbidities that complicate the care of older adults are [38-44]:

1. Arthritic changes
2. Spinal stenosis [narrowing of the vertebral canal]
3. Osteoporosis with possible compression fractures
4. Pathologies [metastasis of cancer from other sites, other bone tumors]
5. Organ dysfunction causing back pain symptoms [prostate, heart, lung]

The table below indicates some of the incidences of common health concerns in older adults using the United States as an example [40-43]:

All of these disease processes are more likely in the older adult [38-45]. These statistics help emphasize the need for diagnostic imaging of the older patient when the history, examination, and symptoms indicate something beyond uncomplicated back pain.

The odds of pathology are higher in the older patient than in any other age group. Sixty per cent of the metastases to the spine are from the prostate [almost exclusively

Health concern	# of American older adults affected	Annual cost
Osteoarthritis	27 million people total	$185 billion
Osteoporosis	10 million plus 50 million with osteopenia [low bone mass]	$17-20 billion
Back Pain	60 million people total	$50 billion
Ischemic Heart Disease	9 million people over age 60 [18 million total]	$286 billion
Cancers	7 million people over age 60 [11 million total]	$260 billion

in patients over 50] and another 25% of metastases are from the lung [also more common in older patients with a history of smoking.] Breast cancer metastases to the spine are also predominantly seen in older patients [43,45].

Recent imaging prior to initiating manual therapy for older patients may be useful to avoid damaging anatomical structures that contain underlying pathology. Although the definition of "older" in the case of routine imaging is controversial, with some now recommending 65 and older as the age of concern for low back pain [46]. Incidental findings, such as osteoporosis, degenerative joint disease, hiatal hernias, abdominal aortic aneurisms, stenosis, and so on, are all more likely in the older patient. Some of these findings may indicate the need for medical co-management, while others may influence the chiropractor's choice of management strategies.

Discussion and conclusion

In this article we have explored just a few cases that highlight the diagnostic challenges in the older adult patient. As the baby boomers reach their golden years, it is essential that all health professionals learn more about normal aging, and common health related concerns in older patients. Excellent resources for providers are available at the National Institute on Aging at www.nia.nih.gov [47] and the American Geriatric Society http://www.healthinaging.org/agingintheknow/ [48] These and other resources can be utilized to stay abreast of the latest health information related to caring for the older adult patient.

Competing interest

The author declares no competing interests or financial interests.

Author details

Director of Diagnosis and Radiology, Palmer College of Chiropractic, 1000 Brady Street, 52803, Davenport, IA, USA.

References

1. Gleberzon BJ: **Chiropractic geriatrics: the challenges of assessing the older patient.** *J Am Chiropractic Assoc* 2000, **43**:6–37.
2. Bowers L: **Clinical assessment of geriatric patients: unique challenges.** *Top Clin Chiropr* 1996, **3**(2):10–21.
3. Killinger LZ, Morley J, Kettner N, Kauric E: **Integrated care of the older patient.** *Top Clin Chiropr* 2001, **8**(2):46–54.
4. Hawk CK, Schneider M, Dougherty P, Gleberzon BJ, Killinger LZ: **Best practices recommendations for chiropractic care for older adults: results of a consensus process.** *J Manipulative Physio Ther* 2010, **33**:464–473.
5. Coulter ID, Hurwitz EL, Aronow HU, Cassata DM, Beck JC: **Chiropractic patients in a comprehensive home-based geriatric assessment, follow-up and health promotion program.** *Topics in Clin Chiropr* 1996, **3**(2):46–55.
6. Day JC: ***National population projections. U.S. Census Bureau***: www.census.gov/population/www/pop-profile/natproj.html.
7. Christiansen MG, Kollasch MW, Hyland JK: *Practice Analysis of Chiropractic, 2010: A project report, survey analysis and summary of chiropractic practice within the United States.* Greeley, CO: National Board of Chiropractic Examiners; 2010.
8. Docking RE, Fleming J, Brayne C, Zhao J, Macfarlane GJ, Jones GT: **Epidemiology of back pain in older adults: prevalence and risk factors for back pain onset.** *Rheumatology (Oxford)* 2011, **50**:1645–1653.
9. Bressler H, Keyes W, Wochon P, Bradley E: **The prevalence of low back pain in the elderly: a systematic review of the literature.** *Spine* 1999, **24**(17):1813–1819.
10. Evans MW: **Use of chiropractic or osteopathic manipulation by adults aged 50 and older: an análisis of data from the 2007 National Health Interview Survey.** *Topics in Integrative Health Care* 2010, **1**(2):1–16.
11. Beyerman KL, Palermion MB, Zohn Le, *et al*: **Efficacy of treating low back pain and dysfuntion secondary to osteoarthritis: chiropractic care compared with moist heat alone.** *J Manipulative Physiol Ther* 2006, **29**(2):107–114.
12. Hondras MA, Long CR, Cao Y, Rowell RM, Meeker WC: **A randomized controlled trial comparing 2 types of spinal manipulative therapy and minimal conservative medical care for adults 55 years and older with subacute or chronic low back pain.** *J Manipulative Physiol Ther* 2009, **32**:330–343.
13. Giles LGF, Muller R: **Chronic spinal pain: A randomized controlled trial comparing medication, acupuncture and spinal manipulation.** *Spine* 2003, **28**(14):1490–1503.
14. Shekelle PG, Adams AH, Chassin MR: **Spinal manipulation for low back pain.** *Annals Intern Med* 1992, **117**:590–598.
15. Descareaux M, Blouin JS, Drolet M, Papaditriou S, Teasdale N: **Efficacy of preventive spinal manipulation for chronic low back pain and related disabilities: a preliminary study.** *J Manipulative Physiol Ther* 2004, **27**(8):509–517.
16. Murphy DR, Hurwitz EL, Gregory AA, Clary R: **A non-surgical approach to the management of lumbar spinal stenosis: a prospective observational cohort study.** *BMC Musculoskelet Disord* 2006, **7**:16.
17. Bigos S, Bowyer O, Braen G, Brown K, Deyo R, Haldeman S: *Acute low back pain problems in adults. Clinical Practice Guideline No. 14.* Rockville MD: AHCPR publication no. 95–00642; 1994.
18. Koes BW, Assendelft WJ, van der Heijden GJ, Bouter LM, Knipschild PG: **Spinal manipulation and mobilization for back and neck pain: a blinded review.** *British Med J* 1991, **363**:1298–1303.
19. Van Tulder MW, Koes BW, Bouter LM: **Conservative treatment of acute and chronic nonspecific low back pain.** *Spine* 1997, **22**:2128–2156.
20. Kane R, Ouslander J, Abrass I, Resenter B: *Essentials of clinical geriatrics: 6th Edition.* New York, NY: McGraw Hill Publishers; 2008.
21. *Healthy People*; 2020. http://www.cdc.gov/nchs/healthy_people/hp2020.htm.
22. The Center for Disease Control and Prevention: *Medication Safety*; http://www.cdc.gov/medicationsafety/.
23. Gurwitz JH, Field TS, Harrold LR, Harrold LR, Rothschild J, Debellis K, Seger AC, Cadoret C, Fish LS, Garber L, Kelleher M, Bates DW: **Incidence and preventability of adverse drug events among older persons in the ambulatory setting.** *JAMA* 2003, **289**:1107–1116.
24. Hamilton H, Gallagher P, Ryan C, Byrne S, O'Mahony D: **Potentially inappropriate medications defined by STOPP Criteria and the risk of adverse drug events in older hospitalized patients.** *Arch Intern Med* 2011, **171**:1013–1019.
25. Avorn J: **Medication use in older patients: better policy could encourage better practice.** *JAMA* 2010, **304**(14):1606–1607.
26. Budnitz DS, Shehab N, Kegler SR, Richards CL: **Medication use leading to emergency department visits for adverse drug events in older adults.** *Annals Int Med* 2007, **147**(11):755–765.
27. Robnett RH, Chop WC: ***Medications***. *In Gerontology for the Health Care Professional.* 2nd edition. Boston: Jones and Bartlett publishers; 2010:119.
28. Dillon P: *In Nursing Health Assessment: A Critical Thinking Case Studies Approach.* 2nd edition. Philadelphia: F.A. Davis Publishers; 2007:117–118.
29. Fick DM, Cooper JW, Wade WE, Waller JL, Maclean JR, Beers MH: **Updating the beers criteria for potentially inappropriate medication use in older adults: results of a US consensus panel of experts.** *Arch Intern Med* 2003, **163**:2716–2724.
30. Dieters LV, Kim D: *Benign Prostatic Hypertrophy*; http://emedicine.medscape.com/article/437359-overview.
31. Hybels CF, Blazer DG: **Epidemiology of late-life mental disorders.** *Clin Geriatr Med* 2003, **19**:663–696.
32. National Institute of Health's National Institute of Neurological Disorders and Stroke: *The Dementias. Publication No. 04–2252.* Bethesda, MD:; 2004.
33. Flostein MF: **The Mini Mental Status Exam [MMSE].** In *Assessment in geriatric psychopharmacology.* Edited by Powley M, Crook T, Ferris R, Bartus R, New Canan CT.; 1983:50–51.

34. The Alzheimer's Association: 2012, www.alz.org.
35. The National Institute of Health: **Older Adults Depression and Suicide Facts Sheet.**, [http://www.nimh.nih.gov/health/publications/older-adults-depression-and-suicide-facts-fact-sheet/index.shtml]
36. U.S. Surgeon General:, http://www.surgeongeneral.gov/library/mentalhealth/chapter4/sec3.html.
37. **Geriatric Depression Scale.**, http://www.chcr.brown.edu/GDS_SHORT_FORM.PDF.
38. **World Health Organization Statistics Mortality.**, http://apps.who.int/whosis/database/mort/table1_process.cfm.
39. World Health Organization: *Global Burden of Disease.[2004 cohort; publ.2008;* http://www.who.int/healthinfo/global_burden_disease/GBD_report_2004update.
40. American Heart Association: **Statistical Update Heart Disease and Stroke Statistics—2011 Update: A Report from the American Heart Association.** *Circulation* 2011, http://circ.ahajournals.org/content/123/4/e18.
41. American Society on Aging: *Heart Health*; http://www.agingsociety.org/agingsociety/pdf/heart.pdf.
42. Docking R, Fleming J, Brayne C, Zhao J, Macfarlane GJ, Jones GT: **Epidemiology of back pain in older adults: prevalence and risk factors for back pain onset.** *Rheumatology* 2011, **50**(9):1645–1653.
43. Becker DJ, Kilgore ML, Morrisey MA: **The societal burden of osteoporosis.** *Curr Rheumatol Rep* 2010, **12**(3):186–91.
44. Simmons ED, Guyer RD, Graham-Smith A, Herzog R: **Radiograph assessment for patients with low back pain.** *Spine J* 2003, **3**:3–5.
45. Centers for Disease Control and Prevention: *U.S. Cancer Statistics Working Group*. Atlanta, GA: United States Cancer Statistics: 1999–2007 Incidence and Mortality; 2010. http://www.cdc.gov/uscs.
46. Kotlarz H, Gunnarsson CL, Fang H, Rizzo JA: **Insurer and out-of-pocket costs of osteoarthritis in the US: evidence from national survey data.** *Arthritis Rheum* 2009, **60**(12):3546–53.
47. **The National Institute on Aging; National Institute of Health.**, www.nia.nih.gov.
48. The American Geriatric Society; [http://www.healthinaging.org/agingintheknow/]

Relationship between STarT Back Screening Tool and prognosis for low back pain patients receiving spinal manipulative therapy

Jonathan Field[1*] and Dave Newell[2]

Abstract

Background: Low back pain (LBP) is common and costly and few treatments have been shown to be markedly superior to any other. Effort has been focused on stratifying patients to better target treatment. Recently the STarT Back Screening Tool (SBT) has been developed for use in primary care to enable sub grouping of patients based on modifiable baseline characteristics and has been shown to be associated with differential outcomes. In the UK the SBT is being recommended to assist in care decisions for those presenting to general practitioners with LBP. In the light of growing recommendation for widespread use of this tool, generalisability to other LBP populations is important. However, studies to date have focused only on patients attending physiotherapy whereas LBP patients seeking other treatment have not been investigated.

Aims: This study aims to investigate the utility of the SBT to predict outcomes in LBP patients presenting for chiropractic management.

Methods: A total of 404 patients undergoing chiropractic care were asked to complete the SBT before initial treatment. Clinical outcomes were collected at 14, 30 and 90 days following this initial consultation. The clinical course was described comparing SBT categories and logistic regression analysis performed to examine the tool's prognostic utility.

Results: Although the high-risk categories had greater pain at baseline this difference rapidly faded, with both change in composite outcome scores and pain scores being statistically insignificant between the risk groups at 30 and 90 days follow up. In addition, both univariate and adjusted analysis showed no prognostic utility of the SBT categorisations to differentiate clinical outcomes between risk groups.

Conclusion: Whilst the SBT appears useful in some back pain populations it does not appear to differentiate outcomes in LBP patients seeking chiropractic care.

Keywords: Start back tool, Low back pain, Prognosis, Spinal manipulative therapy

Introduction

Low back pain (LBP) is a common symptom causing health-seeking behavior in up to half of those who experience it [1,2]. Between six and nine percent of the UK population consult their general practitioner (GP) for LBP each year, accounting for 5 million GP consultations annually [3,4]. For most of these patients a low back pain episode will most likely be a temporary inconvenience, yet for a minority who have sought care (approximately 28%) it becomes an enduring and disabling problem [5,6].

The extent of the costs to society of this syndrome have led to the call for identification of potential subgroups of non specific low back pain (nsLBP) in the belief that this group consists of a heterogeneous mix of presentations and etiologies. Identification of groups of back pain that respond better with specific interventions would facilitate targeted treatment [7]. In addition, evidence-based guidelines highlight the need to consider prognostic factors when deciding the management of nsLBP [8-10], where early identification of potential

* Correspondence: jonathanfield@me.com
[1]Private practice Back2Health, 2 Charles Street, Petersfield, Hants, UK
Full list of author information is available at the end of the article

barriers to recovery may help guide treatment aimed at secondary prevention of persistent back pain [11,12].

In the absence of serious pathology, recovery from back pain in individuals from the general back pain population as well as those seeking help from chiropractors is only weakly related to physical findings [13-17], with only a small number of condition specific factors associated with poor prognosis [13,18,19]. However, psychological factors are found to influence future disability, pain and self reported improvement in LBP patients presenting to GPs, secondary care services and surgery [20-23]. This has led to guidelines recommending that non-physical factors be considered when setting the treatment for LBP patients [8-10]. In chiropractic LBP populations the significance of psychological factors is less certain as exploratory studies have found little or no correlation with outcomes [14,24-26].

The STarT Back Tool (SBT) has recently been developed to help primary care practitioners make care decisions about the likely need LBP patients have for secondary prevention based on modifiable risk factors for poor outcome [20]. The SBT places patients into one of three categories (Low, Medium and High) of risk for having persisting LBP with disability. In a recent trial, patients whose care had been stratified using the SBT to receive either advice alone, 'standardised' physiotherapy or psychologically based care with physiotherapy had lower disability at 4 and 12 months than those patients undergoing usual care as directed by the clinical judgment of a physiotherapist [27]. As a consequence of those studies the SBT is being recommended by commissioning services in the UK NHS to guide care pathways for those presenting to GP with LBP. Whilst the feasibility of using the SBT in a chiropractic patient population has been demonstrated [28], as yet, no appraisal of the prognostic utility of grouping individuals seeking chiropractic care has been published.

This paper investigated whether nsLBP patients classified in the high-risk (complex psychosocial) group by the SBT do less well with chiropractic care than those either at low risk or medium risk groups.

Methods

Subjects and procedure

Consecutive patients aged over 16 presenting with nsLBP to one of six chiropractic clinics in the south of England were asked, as part of normal practice to complete the Bournemouth Questionnaire (BQ) [29] either at the clinic or on-line before their first visit. Those doing so on line were additionally asked to complete the SBT. Patients were presented with a consent form when they completed pre-examination forms online, via a web page. In these practices patients who start treatment are emailed outcome assessment questionnaires consisting of the BQ and a Patients Global Impression of Change (PGIC), at 14, 30 and 90 days following their initial visit.

Outcomes

For this study, the primary outcome was the PGIC. In addition we also measured pain as derived from the pain sub-scale of the BQ and total BQ scores. Patients were categorised into the three SBT risk groups using the method as described by Hill et al. [20,30]. For each of the follow up points, all outcomes were dichotomized. Thus poor outcome was defined by a PGIC response of better or much better (score of <6) [31], a change in pain of less than or equal to ($\leq$)2 points [32] and a change in total BQ of $\leq 46\%$ [33]. Recently, both the PGIC and BQ have been recommended as preferred measurements by the 'Any Qualified Provider Resource Centre' (UK, NHS) for monitoring outcomes in low back pain patients [34].

Analysis

General characteristics of the patient sample were calculated as means and proportions with appropriate measures of variance. Differences between categorical baseline characteristics were determined using χ^2, or Pearson χ^2 test for trend. Further, a Kolmogorov-Smirnov test revealed significant deviation from Gaussian distributions for pain and total BQ data, despite using logarithmic transformation. Consequently differences within these variables across SBT categories were analysed using Kruskal Wallis tests, whereas change scores revealed a Gaussian distribution and were analysed using a one-way ANCOVA adjusted for baseline scores.

To determine any associations between baseline SBT categorisation and the outcomes univariate logistic regression analysis was carried out using the SBT categorisation as the independent variable and the dichotomised outcomes (PGIC, change in pain and change in total BQ) as dependent variables at each of the follow up time points. This analysis was repeated after sub grouping by gender, but only for the PGIC as a dependent variable. Finally, adjusted models for predicting poor outcome as defined by the PGIC were constructed with an entry criterion for significant variables of $p < 0.15$ and retention at $p < 0.05$ using a binary logistic analysis forward LR procedure. All statistical analyses were performed using statistical software SPSS (v17.0, SPSS Inc., Chicago IL).

Ethics

Ethics for this study were sought and approved by the Research and Ethics subcommittee of the Anglo-European College of Chiropractic Research Committee.

Results

A total of 819 patients presented with nsLBP between March and November 2011. Four hundred and five were ineligible to participate in the study, as they did not complete the initial forms online. There was no difference ($p > 0.05$) in gender, duration, or BQ scores at presentation or in pain and BQ scores at 90 days follow up between those submitting the forms online and those doing so at the clinic. However at presentation those completing the forms online and so being included in this study had slightly less pain (mean (SD) 6.2(2.0) versus 6.6(2.2), p0.04) and were younger (44.7 (15) versus 48.9(15.4) years, $p < 0.01$). Four hundred and four individuals completing the forms online were categorized by the SBT at the study inception. Of these 168 (41.6%), 129 (31.9%) and 107 (26.5%) were at low, medium or high risk of poor outcome at baseline respectively. Numbers of participants at follow up within each SBT group and percentage response rates are shown in Figure 1. The number of treatments received across the three SBT categories were; low (4.1(2.4)); medium (4.3 (2.4)) and high (4.4 (2.6)). There were no significant differences in treatment visits between SBT categories ($p = 0.54$).

Table 1 shows the demographic and condition specific characteristics within each SBT risk group. Only the proportions of those patients with pain above the knee, higher baseline pain and greater total BQ scores differed between the SBT categories. The distribution of duration of back pain in the complete sample was 56.2%, 12.4% and 31.4% for less than 1 month, 1–3 months and greater than 3 months respectively. These proportions were similar across the SBT risk groups.

Table 1 Descriptive analysis of baseline variables across Start Back Tool (SBT) categories

Variables	SBT Category		
	Low (n = 168)	Medium (n = 129)	High (n = 107)
Mean age (SD)	45.4 (15.1)	45.9 (15.0)	45.8 (14.1)
Female	54.8%	52.7%	50.5%
Seen practitioner before	47.0%	59.7%	33.6%
Leg Pain			
Above the knee *	25.5%	23.3%	35.5%
Below the knee	6.0%	10.9%	12.1%
>30 days pain in year	41.1%	41.1%	38.3%
Recurring	69.6%	65.9%	59.8%
Duration			
< 1 month	54.8%	53.5%	61.7%
1–3 months	14.3%	14.0%	7.5%
>3 months	31.0%	32.6%	30.8%
Median Pain (25, 75) **	5 (4–7)	7 (6–8)	7 (6–9)
Median BQ (25, 75) **	24 (14–33)	36 (30–44)	45 (34–54)

*$P < 0.05$ (Chi^2 test for trend). **$p < 0.001$, (Kruskal-Wallis).

Table 2 shows the total BQ and pain scores over time for each of the SBT categories. Pain and total BQ scores differed significantly between the SBT risks groups at

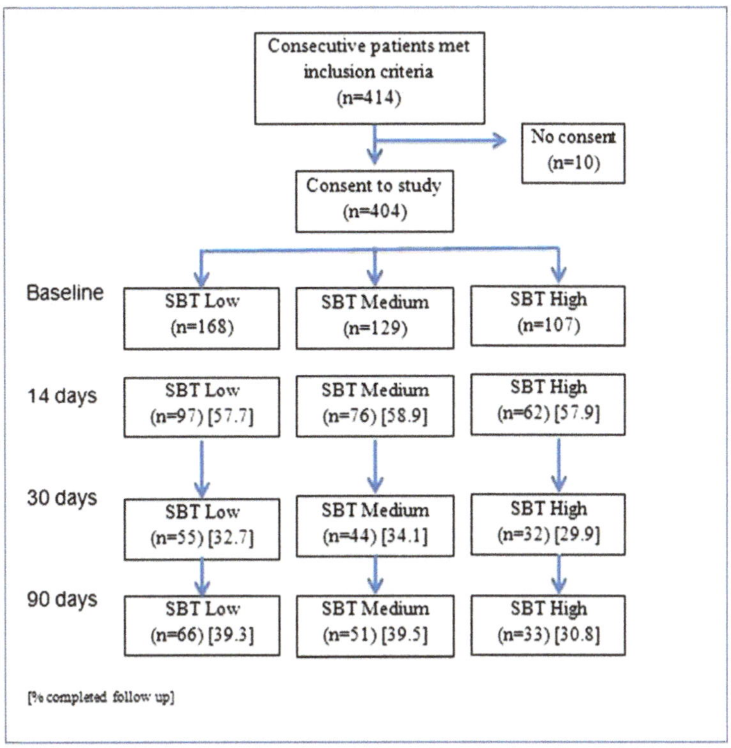

Figure 1 Numbers in study at each follow up point in each Start Back Tool category.

Table 2 Pain, total BQ scores and proportion of subjects with a poor outcome across Start Back Tool (SBT) categories at 14, 30 and 90 days follow up

SBT Category	14 days (n = 235)		30 days (n = 131)		90 days (n = 150)	
	Median Pain (25, 75)	Median BQ (25, 75) **	Median Pain (25, 75)	Median BQ (25, 75)	Median Pain (25, 75)	Median BQ (25, 75)
Low	2 (1–3)	10 (3–18)	1 (1–3)	6 (2–14)	1 (1–2)	5 (0–15)
Medium	2 (1–5)	12 (3–26)	2 (1–4)	10 (5–21)	1 (1–4)	8 (0–18)
High	3 (1–5)	20 (8–33)	2 (0–3)	6 (2–20)	2 (0–3)	10 (3–22)

**p < 0.001, (Kruskal-Wallis), ¥Patients Global Impression of Change < 6.

baseline, where high-risk groups started with higher scores ($p < 0.001$). The total BQ scores also differed at 14 days follow up ($p < 0.001$). However, any differences between the risk groups were absent by 30 days with all groups achieving very similar scores by 90 days. Mean residual change scores for total BQ and pain are illustrated in Figure 2. These changes are not significantly different between risk categories at any of the follow up time points (Change in Pain: 14 days (ANCOVA. $F = 1.1$, $p = 0.32$); 30 days (ANCOVA. $F = 1.4$, $p = 0.25$); 90 days (One way ANCOVA. $F = 0.5$, $p = 0.62$) Change in total BQ: 14 days (ANCOVA. $F = 0.8$, $p = 0.46$); 30 days (ANCOVA. $F = 0.2$, $p = 0.83$); 90 days (ANCOVA. $F = 0.2$, $p = 0.83$)).

Table 3 shows the proportion of patients with poor outcome in each SBT group at each follow up point as defined by three dichotomized outcomes. A univariate logistic regression analysis revealed that SBT categorisations were not statistically associated with the primary outcome (PGIC) at any of the follow up points (Table 4) However, the utility of the SBT to discriminate poor outcome using the PGIC did increase over time, with both medium and high risk groups being around 1.7 times the odds of poor outcome by 90 days compared to low risk groups, albeit not statistically significant. A further analysis using this outcome but sub grouping by gender revealed a similar, but again statistically insignificant association. In this analysis only male patients showed any marked association between baseline categorisation by SBT and poor outcome, where those in the medium and high risk groups had 3 times the odds of experiencing poor outcome compared to low risk groups at 90 days. In females however, the SBT had little predictive utility at any follow up point. (Table 5).

Categorising poor outcome as ≤2 points drop in pain, a further analysis revealed no significant association between the SBT and an absence of meaningful change in pain at any follow up point (Table 6). This result was also apparent when using dichotomized total BQ change scores as the dependent variable (Table 7).

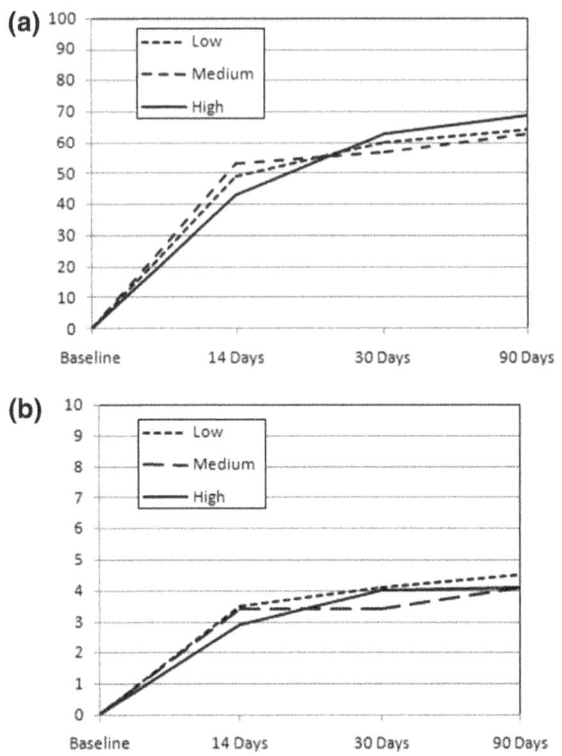

Figure 2 Resdualised* change scores compared between SBT risk groups for Total BQ (a) and Pain (b).

Table 3 Proportions (%) of patients with a poor outcome across Start Back Tool categories defined by cut-off points for each outcome

Outcomes	14 days (n)	30 days (n)	90 days (n)
PGIC			
Low	36.1 (35)	29.1 (16)	18.2 (12)
Medium	30.3 (23)	29.5 (13)	27.5 (14)
High	33.9 (21)	28.1 (9)	27.3 (9)
≤2 on NRS			
Low	37.9 (33)	24.0 (12)	23.0 (14)
Medium	24.7 (18)	26.2 (11)	24.5 (12)
High	32.8 (19)	32.3 (10)	18.8 (6)
≤47% on BQ			
Low	28.9 (24)	20.4 (10)	14.0 (8)
Medium	29.4 (20)	25.6 (10)	19.6(9)
High	41.5 (22)	29.0 (9)	18.2 (6)

PGIC = Patient Global Impression of Change; *NRS* = Numerical Rating Scale; *BQ* = Bournemouth Questionnaire.

Table 4 Predicting poor outcome (PGIC) at 14, 30 and 90 days for the whole group (n = 404)

SBT Category	14 days (n = 235)	30 days (n = 131)	90 days (n = 150)
	OR (95% CI)	OR (95% CI)	OR (95% CI)
Low	1.0	1.0	1.0
Medium	0.8 (0.4 to 1.5)	1.0 (0.4 to 2.4)	1.7 (0.7 to 4.1)
High	0.9 (0.5 to 1.8)	0.9 (0.4 to 2.5)	1.7 (0.6 to 4.5)

PGIC = Patient Global Impression of Change; *SBT* = Start Back Tool.

Table 6 Predicting poor outcome (Change in pain ≤ 2 points) at 14, 30 and 90 days

SBT Category	14 days (n = 218)	30 days (n = 123)	90 days (n = 142)
	OR (95% CI)	OR (95% CI)	OR (95% CI)
Low	1.0	1.0	1.0
Medium	0.5 (0.3 to 1.1)	1.1 (0.4 to 2.9)	1.1 (0.4 to 2.6)
High	0.8(0.4 to 1.6)	1.5 (0.5 to 4.1)	0.8 (0.3 to 2.2)

SBT = Start Back Tool.

A forward LR logistic analysis adjusting for all potential baseline predictors (Enter: $p \leq 0.15$, Retain $p \leq 0.05$) resulted in few variables remaining as independent predictors of outcome at the follow up points, with baseline SBT categorisations failing to be retained in any of the models (Table 8). Only duration, reoccurrence of the problem and pain for greater than 30 days in the last year provided any prognostic utility and even here the degree of variance explained remained relatively low as did the predictive accuracy.

Discussion

In this study those categorised by the SBT as being at low risk of having a poor prognosis were somewhat more likely to do well compared to those placed in the medium or high risk groups. However this difference was small and failed to reach any statistical significance in a univariate analysis. In addition the adjusted models at each follow up did not include the SBT tool as a significant predictor of outcome. This result suggests that, in this population at least, the proportion of high-risk patients that improve is not significantly different from those at medium or low risk.

Patients placed in the SBT high-risk group had more adverse BQ and pain scores at presentation. However, there was a greater improvement in these scores in the high-risk group with the result that by the 30-day assessment this difference was no longer evident. These results are partially corroborated by Fritz et al. [35] who showed that despite high risk patients starting with more pain and disability at baseline they experienced greater improvement over a course of care.

The SBT has been developed to better stratify LBP patients for targeted treatment. Hill et al. (2008) [20] showed the discriminative ability of this tool to differentiate those who clinically changed on the RMDQ. This was largely based on differences in barriers to recovery, with the high-risk group being defined as having psychological barriers and the medium as having physical barriers. These authors went on to show that the SBT was able to support treatment choice more efficiently than physiotherapists' clinical experience alone. Although this approach has potential to improve outcomes and cost in LBP the generalisability of their results may not be supported by this study.

There may be a number of reasons why this is so. Firstly, this LBP population differs from previous studies in that they were largely self-selecting and sought chiropractic care privately. In addition to this, around 41% of this sample had experienced chiropractic care from the same practitioner previously. This may have led to higher expectations of success which may have impacted on the psychological response of people in this sample. Another possibility is that patients in the various SBT categories within our cohort study received different types of care and that this influenced their recovery. However, communicating with the participating clinicians indicated that they had not accessed the SBT category data, and there were no differences in the number of treatments provided between SBT categories. Despite this, differences in treatment approach cannot be ruled out. It is possible that those placed in the high risk SBT category received care that was consciously or unconsciously delivered by the chiropractor in a way so as to address the patient's psychological requirements. As a development of this idea, the treatment interventions in this study may inherently be similar to the treatment intervention given in Hill et al. (20) for their SBT high-

Table 5 Predicting poor outcome (PGIC) at 14, 30 and 90 days follow up split by gender

SBT Category	14 days		30 days		90 days	
	OR (95% CI)		OR (95% CI)		OR (95% CI)	
	Male (n = 117)	Female (n = 118)	Male (n = 66)	Female (n = 65)	Male (n = 71)	Female (n = 79)
Low	1.0	1.0	1.0	1.0	1.0	1.0
Medium	1.2 (0.5 to 3.0)	0.5 (0.2 to 1.3)	0.7 (0.2 to 2.7)	1.2 (0.3 to 4.0)	3.0 (0.9 to 10.0)	0.9 (0.2 to 3.3)
High	1.8 (0.7 to 5.0)	0.5 (0.2 to 1.2)	0.7 (0.2 to 3.2)	1.0 (0.3 to 4.1)	3.0 (0.6 to 16.0)	1.1 (0.3 to 4.0)

PGIC = Patient Global Impression of Change; *SBT* = Start Back Tool.

Table 7 Predicting poor outcome (Change in total BQ ≤47%) at 14, 30 and 90

SBT Category	14 days (n = 204)	30 days (n = 119)	90 days (n = 136)
	OR (95% CI)	OR (95% CI)	OR (95% CI)
Low	1.0	1.0	1.0
Medium	1.0 (0.5 to 2.1)	1.3 (0.5 to 3.6)	1.5 (0.5 to 4.2)
High	1.7 (0.8 to 3.6)	1.6 (0.6 to 4.5)	1.4 (0.4 to 4.3)

BQ = Bournemouth Questionnaire; *SBT* = Start Back Tool.

risk group. This would mean that all groups in this study may have received the treatment reserved in the Hill et al. study (20) exclusively for the high risk group, thus masking any initial prognostic information given by the SBT at baseline. However, any treatment effects must be viewed as strongly speculative due to this study's purely observational design.

It has been suggested that patients presenting to chiropractors are a psychologically healthy subgroup with few individuals having levels of adverse psychological factors sufficient to influence their prognosis [24]. In support of this, a narrative review comparing reports of psychological questionnaires applied to chiropractic populations and non-chiropractic populations where the same test tools have been used [36], concluded that those seeing chiropractors were less likely to have adverse scores across a range of psychological domains that have previously been linked to poor prognosis in other LBP populations. In this study 26.5% of patients were categorised by the SBT as in the high-risk group. This suggests that either a significant proportion had potentially adverse psychology, or that the SBT is inappropriately categorizing some of those in this population.

The failure of SBT categorisation in this LBP population to identify those less likely to improve may be because, as a self-selecting subgroup, these individual possess features that negate the impact of otherwise adverse psychology. The possible existence of 'protective' factors in some populations is supported by the presence of higher pain related self-efficacy reducing the impact of raised fear avoidance beliefs in patients with chronic LBP [37]. Reports from one chiropractic study that has looked at this found more favorable levels of self-efficacy than other reported populations, and higher levels of self-efficacy were found to relate to a better prognosis [26,36].

Alternatively a reduction in levels of adverse psychological variables may have occurred during care, therefore reducing their effect on treatment response. In support of this, a systematic review of psychological outcomes from studies involving manipulation describes significantly greater reduction in adverse scores on psychological questionnaires in populations having manipulation when compared to groups receiving verbal interventions (advice, education or handout) or other physical treatments (exercise, electrotherapy, sham manipulation or acupuncture) [38]. In addition to this, a small study found that a statistically significant reduction in fear avoidance beliefs and catastrophisation as well as improvement in self-efficacy occurred shortly after an initial visit with a chiropractor. Despite baseline levels of these variables not relating to self-reported outcome at one month, post-visit scores did display a weak but significant relationship to outcomes, with those retaining two or more higher variables post-visit having increased odds of a poor outcome [26].

Caution however, must be used when interpreting these findings. Firstly, this was not a clinical trial investigating treatment effects and as such it is not possible to ascertain any treatment impact on changes in patients' psychology or symptoms. In addition this population of patients had been drawn from a group of six linked practices and as such may not be representative of the wider population seeking privately funded treatment for LBP.

Table 8 Adjusted models for predicting poor outcome (PGIC) at 14, 30 and 90 days follow up

Follow up point	Variables in the equation	OR (95% CI)	Nagelkerke*	sn/sp
14 days (n = 235)	Pain for >30 days in year	3.2 (1.9 to 5.6)	0.26	90/25
	Pain (for every 1 point increase)	0.8 (0.8 to 0.9)		
30 days (n = 131)	Duration		0.32	92/29
	< 1 month	1.0		
	1–3 months	5.6 (1.8 to 17.0)		
	>3 months	2.4(1.1 to 5.5)		
90 days (n = 150)			0.45	94/23
	Duration			
	< 1 month	1.0		
	1–3 months	9.3 (3.0 to 29.0)		
	>3 months	3.0(1.3 to 7.0)		

* = variance explained by model; *sn* = sensitivity; *sp* = specificity; *PGIC* = Patient Global Impression of Change.

Additionally, there are some differences in response rates between the SBT categories, particularly at 90 days and the potential remains for selection bias through differential attrition. However, comparisons of baseline demographics (age, pain, duration and BQ score) for each of the three SBT categories demonstrated no statistically significant differences between responders and non responders, as was the number of treatments received at 90 days. Although this cannot rule out the possibility that those responding experienced different outcomes to non responders it provides some support for the contention that responders were more likely to be a representative sample based upon care received and baseline factors.

Lastly, comparisons of the results here with other studies are problematic due to differences in follow up times, outcome instruments and other methodological differences.

Conclusion

This study has shown that LBP patients seeking treatment for chiropractic and categorised by SBT at baseline show no differential risk of poor outcome between categorisation groups. Although this tool does differentiate LBP patients in terms of baseline pain and baseline total BQ scores, these differences disappeared by 30 days. At the present time, it is unclear whether the SBT is transferable to LBP populations outside of those it was originally developed for.

Competing interests

The author(s) declare that they have no competing interests.

Authors' contribution

JF conceived of the study, and was involved with its design, data collection, statistical analysis, interpretation and drafting the manuscript. DN performed the statistical analysis and was involved with its interpretation and in drafting the manuscript. Both authors read and approved the final manuscript.

Author details

[1]Private practice Back2Health, 2 Charles Street, Petersfield, Hants, UK.
[2]Anglo-European College of Chiropractic, 13-15 Parkwood Rd, Bournemouth, UK.

References

1. Hillman M, Wright A, Rajaratnam G, Tennant A, Chamberlain MA: **Prevalence of low back pain in the community: implications for service provision in Bradford, UK.** *J Epidemiol Community Health* 1996, **50**(3):347–352.
2. Waxman R, Tennant A, Helliwell P: **Community survey of factors associated with consultation for low back pain.** *BMJ* 1998, **317** (7172):1564–15647.
3. Croft PR, Macfarlane GJ, Papageorgiou AC, Thomas E, Silman AJ: **Outcome of low back pain in general practice: a prospective study.** *BMJ* 1998, **316** (7141):1356–1359.
4. Dunn K: **Classification of low back pain in primary care: using "bothersomeness" to identify the most severe cases.** *Spine* 2005, **30** (16):1887–1892.
5. Hestbaek L, Leboeuf-Yde C, Manniche C: **Low back pain: what is the long-term course? A review of studies of general patient populations.** *Eur Spine J* 2003, **12**(2):149–165.
6. Henschke N, Maher CG, Refshauge KM, Herbert RD, Cumming RG, Bleasel J, *et al*: **Prognosis in patients with recent onset low back pain in Australian primary care: inception cohort study.** *BMJ* 2008, **337**:171.
7. Bouter LM, Pennick V, Bombardier C: **Cochrane back review group.** *Spine* 2003, **28**(12):1215.
8. vanTulder M, Becker A, Bekkering T, Breen A, Gil del Real M, Hutchinson A, *et al*: **European guidelines for the management of acute nonspecific low back pain in primary care.** *Eur Spine J* 2006, **15**:169–15. 16.
9. Chou R, Quseem A, Snow V, Casey D, Cross T, Shekelle P, *et al*: **Diagnosis and Treatment of Low Back Pain: A Joint Clinical Practice Guideline from the American College of Physicians and the American Pain Society.** *Ann Intern Med* 2007, **2**:147–478. 147.
10. NICE, Savigny P, Watson P, Underwood MR, Guideline Development Group: **Early management of persistent non-specific low back pain: summary of NICE guidance.** *BMJ* 2009, **338**.
11. Jellema P, Van Der Windt D: **Prediction of an unfavourable course of low back pain in general practice: comparison of four instruments.** *Br J General Practice* 2007, **57**(534):15–22.
12. Melloh M, Elfering A, EgliPresland C, Roeder C, Barz T, RolliSalathh C, *et al*: **Identification of prognostic factors for chronicity in patients with low back pain: a review of screening instruments.** *International Orthopaedics (SICOT)* 2009, **33**(2):301–301.
13. Leboeuf-Yde C, Greboeuf-Y A, Borge JA, Lothe J, Magnesen E, Nilsson Nilssoal: **The nordic back pain subpopulation program: demographic and clinical predictors for outcome in patients receiving chiropractic treatment for persistent low back pain.** *JMPT* 2004, **27**(8):493–502.
14. Newell D, Field J: **Who will get better? Predicting clinical outcomes in a chiropractic practice.** *Clin Chiropr* 2008, **13**(1):108.
15. Lakke S, Soer R, Takken T, Reneman M: **Risk and prognostic factors for non-specific musculoskeletal pain: A synthesis of evidence from systematic reviews classified into ICF dimensions.** *Pain* 2009, **147**(3):153–164.
16. Chou R, Shekelle P: **Will this patient develop persistent disabling low back pain?** *JAMA* 2010, **303**(13):1295–1302.
17. Ramond A, Bouton C, Richard I, Roquelaure Y, Baufreton C, Legrand E, *et al*: **Psychosocial risk factors for chronic low back pain in primary care--a systematic review.** *Fam Pract* 2011, **28**(1):12–21.
18. Thomas E, Silman AJ, Croft PR, Papageorgiou AC, Jayson MIV, Macfarlane GJ: **Predicting who develops chronic low back pain in primary care: a prospective study.** *BMJ* 1999, **318**:1662–1667.
19. Bolton JE, Hurst H: **Prognostic factors for short-term improvement in acute and persistent musculoskeletal pain consulters in primary care.** *Chiropr Man Therap* 2011, **19**:27.
20. Hill JC, Dunn KM, Lewis M, Mullis R, Main CJ, Foster NE, *et al*: **A primary care back pain screening tool: identifying patient subgroups for initial treatment.** *Arthritis Rheum* 2008, **59**(5):632–641.
21. Celestin J, Edwards RR, Jamison RN: **Pretreatment Psychosocial Variables as Predictors of Outcomes Following Lumbar Surgery and Spinal Cord Stimulation: A Systematic Review and Literature Synthesis.** *Pain Medicine* 2009, **10**(4):639–653.
22. Kamper SJ, Maher CG, Hancock MJ, Koes BW, Croft PR, Hay EM: **Treatment-based subgroups of low back pain: a guide to appraisal of research studies and a summary of current evidence.** *Best Practice & Research Clinical Rheumatology* 2010, **24**(2):181–191.
23. Grotle M, Foster NE, Dunn KM, Croft P: **Are prognostic indicators for poor outcome different for acute and chronic low back pain consulters in primary care?** *Pain*, 2010, **151**(3):790–797.
24. Langworthy J, Breen A: **Psychosocial factors and their predictive value in chiropractic patients with low back pain: a prospective inception cohort study.** *ChiroprOsteopat* 2007, **15**:5.
25. Leboeuf-Yde C, Rosenbaum A, Axen I, Lövgren P, Jørgensen K, Halasz L, *et al*: **The Nordic Subpopulation Research Programme: prediction of treatment outcome in patients with low back pain treated by chiropractors - does the psychological profile matter?** *ChiroprOsteopat* 2009, **17**:14.
26. Field J, Newell D, McCarthy PW: **Preliminary study into the components of the fear-avoidance model of LBP: change after an initial chiropractic visit and influence on outcome.** *ChiroprOsteopat* 2010, **18**:21.
27. Hill JC, Whitehurst DG, Lewis M, Bryan S, Dunn KM, Foster NE, *et al*: **Comparison of stratified primary care management for low back pain with current best practice (STarT Back): a randomised controlled trial.** *Lancet* 2011, **378**(9602):1560–1571.

28. Kongsted A, Johannesen E, Leboeuf-Yde C: **Feasibility of the STarT Back Screening Tool in chiropractic clinics: A cross-sectional study of patients with low back pain.** *Chiropr Man Therap* 2011, **19**:10.
29. Bolton JE, Breen A: **The Bournemouth Questionnaire: a short-form comprehensive outcome measure. I. Psychometric properties in back pain patients.** *JMPT* 1999, **22**(8):503–510.
30. Hill JC, Vohora K, Dunn KM, Main CJ, Hay EM: **Comparing the STarT back screening tool's subgroup allocation of individual patients with that of independent clinical experts.** *The Clinical journal of pain* 2010, **26**(9):783–787.
31. Newell D, Bolton JE: **Responsiveness of the Bournemouth Questionnaire in determining minimal clinically important change in subgroups of low back pain patients.** *Spine* 2010, **35**(19):1801–1806.
32. Ostelo RW, Deyo RA, Stratford P, Waddell G, Croft P, Von Korff M, Bouter LM, de Vet HC: **Interpreting change scores for pain and functional status in low back pain: towards international consensus regarding minimal important change.** *Spine* 2008, **33**(1):90–94.
33. Hurst H, Bolton J: **Assessing the clinical significance of change scores recorded on subjective outcome measures.** *J Manipulative PhysiolTher* 2004, **27**(1):26–35.
34. *Extension of Patient choice of Any Qualified Provider in MSK Services for Back and Neck Pain.* http://www.supply2health.nhs.uk.
35. Fritz JM, Beneciuk JM, George SZ: **Relationship Between Categorization With the STarT Back Screening Tool and Prognosis for People Receiving Physical Therapy for Low Back Pain.** *Phys Ther* 2011, **91**(5):722–732.
36. Field J, Newell D, McCarthy P: **Are chiropractic patients a psychologically self defining subgroup?** *Clin Chiropr* 2011, **14**(2):72–73.
37. Woby SR, Urmston M, Watson PJ: **Self-efficacy mediates the relation between pain-related fear and outcome in chronic low back pain patients.** *Eur J Pain* 2007, **11**(7):711–718.
38. Williams N, Hendry M, Lewis R, Russell I, Westmoreland A, Wilkinson C: **Psychological response in spinal manipulation (PRISM): A systematic review of psychological outcomes in randomised controlled trials.** *Complementary Therapies in Medicine* 2007, **15**(4):271–283.

9

The correlation of radiographic findings and patient symptomatology in cervical degenerative joint disease: a cross-sectional study

Iris Sun Rudy, Alexandra Poulos, Laura Owen, Ashlee Batters, Kasia Kieliszek, Jessica Willox and Hazel Jenkins*

Abstract

Background: There are few known studies investigating the correlation of symptomatology with the specific subtypes of cervical spine degenerative joint disease demonstrated on radiograph. The aim of this study was to assess the correlation and diagnostic test accuracy of specific symptoms in determining the presence, type and severity of degenerative joint disease on radiograph.

Methods: A retrospective cross-sectional design was used to correlate cervical radiographic findings with neck pain and related symptomatology. Radiographs of 322 patients from April 2010 to June 2012 were assessed and evidence of radiographic cervical degenerative joint disease was extracted. Clinical data for each patient was obtained from their patient files including: pain using a VAS, presence of neck stiffness, presence of headaches, presence of shoulder referral, presence of hand radiculopathy and presence of hand numbness. Measures of diagnostic test accuracy and regression analysis were used to assess for any correlation between symptoms and radiographic findings.

Results: Referral of pain to the shoulder and neck stiffness showed small degrees of correlation with cervical degenerative joint disease, however, these correlations were not maintained when age was accounted for. Only age showed consistent statistical significance as a predictor for degree of disc degeneration (correlation coefficient (95% confidence interval): 0.06 (0.055, 0.066)); the presence of facet hypertrophy (odds ratio (95% confidence interval): 1.12 (1.09, 1.15)); or uncinate process hypertrophy (odds ratio (95% confidence interval): 1.15 (1.12, 1.18)). Neck stiffness demonstrated a small degree of diagnostic test accuracy for the degree of cervical disc degeneration (area under the curve (95%CI): 0.62 (0.56, 0.68)) and the presence of either facet (diagnostic OR (95%CI):1.69 (1.04, 2.76)) and uncinated process hypertrophy (LR+ (95%CI): 1.17 (1.00, 1.38)).

Conclusion: The results of this study indicate that clinical symptoms such as pain level, headaches, shoulder referral and hand radiculopathy or numbness are not reliably correlated with radiographic findings of degenerative joint disease in the cervical spine. A small increase in diagnostic accuracy between the presence of neck stiffness and all forms of cervical degenerative joint disease is shown, however, this increase is not at the level expected to change clinical practice.

Keywords: Degenerative joint disease, Osteoarthritis, Cervical spine, Neck pain, Neck stiffness, Sensitivity and specificity

* Correspondence: hazel.jenkins@mq.edu.au
Macquarie University, Sydney, Australia

Background

Neck pain is a widespread entity that affects a large majority of the population. The prevalence is greatest amongst middle-aged people, with approximately 66% of individuals experiencing neck pain and related symptoms at some stage in their lives [1,2]. Neck pain is also the second most frequent musculoskeletal complaint presenting to primary healthcare practitioners [3] and most people with neck pain do not experience a complete resolution of symptoms [4]. Although there is a large prevalence of neck pain, neck pain is difficult to diagnose [4] and therefore, to treat.

Among the many causes of neck pain, degenerative joint disease of the cervical spine is a common condition affecting the synovial joints [5] with a prevalence of 3.3 cases per 1000 people [6]. It is characterised by a series of degenerative changes comprising intradiscal tears with subsequent disc space loss, osteophytic growths and spur formation, ligamentous hypertrophy and capsular thickening [7]. Cervical spine degenerative joint disease occurs mostly in 4th and 5th decades and is associated with the natural aging process [8]. It also varies in presentation, with the most common complaints consisting of neck pain, activity related neck stiffness, headaches and upper limb referral [7].

Magnetic resonance imaging (MRI) remains the most advanced assessment tool to evaluate degenerative changes, however the costs and accessibility to this type of imaging requires clinicians to differentiate those patients that require this level of investigation. Plain film radiography is the most commonly used modality to diagnose degenerative joint disease [9], however the literature indicates that radiographic findings do not correlate well with pain and symptoms [10,11]. It also has been suggested that the use of plain film radiography based solely on the suspicion of detecting degenerative changes is not clinically justified [12,11].

Marchiori and Henderson [13] compared radiographic findings of spinal degeneration with severity and chronicity of cervical pain and any resulting lifestyle changes in 700 consecutive patients referred for a cervical radiographic examination. The authors concluded that increasing levels of spinal degeneration are related to increased chronicity of patient complaints. Gore et al. [14] in 1987 completed an investigation in 205 patients previously seen for a neck complaint. A follow up radiographic examination was conducted after a minimum of ten years to assess for subsequent spinal degeneration. The results concluded no significant relationship between the degree of spinal degeneration and patient symptoms at either initial presentation or at follow up. Heller et al. [11] examined the relation between symptoms and changes seen on radiograph in a hospital setting. Using the symptoms of pain in the arm or shoulder, shoulder blade, neck, and back of the head and stiffness in the neck, they concluded that there were few and inconsistent relationships between symptoms and changes on radiograph. However, they did not examine whether hallmark symptoms could be predicting factors in diagnosing the severity or grade of cervical degenerative joint disease.

The aim of this study was to assess for correlation and the diagnostic test accuracy of hallmark symptoms in determining the presence, type and severity of cervical degenerative joint disease on radiograph.

Methods

Sample selection

The subjects included in this study were patients attending one of three Macquarie University Chiropractic Teaching Clinics who had cervical radiographs taken between April 2010 to June 2012. Of the 502 studies taken in this period, 180 were excluded, as they were: under 18 years of age, had incomplete or absent patient files or the cervical radiographic quality was too poor to interpret (non-diagnostic). This study complies with national research ethics guidelines and was approved by the Macquarie University Human Research Ethics Committee (HREC), approval number: 5201300294.

Data collection

Two members of the research team accessed the chiropractic clinic's radiographic report database to find all cervical spine radiographs taken within the selected time period. The radiographic reports were assessed and the following information was recorded: name, date of birth, gender and presence of degenerative joint disease (Yes/No) on cervical anteroposterior (AP) and lateral views. The AP and lateral radiographs reported to have signs of cervical degenerative joint disease were then accessed and graded using the Kellgren and Lawrence Osteoarthritis Severity Grading System [15-17] by the same two research members. The presence of facet hypertrophy and uncinate process hypertrophy was also recorded (Yes/No). The assessed radiographic reports were reported by chiropractic radiologists at the time of imaging. The two members of the research team assessing the radiographs for the grading of degenerative joint disease were both in their final year of chiropractic studies.

The names of the included patients were then provided to three other research team members, also in their final year of chiropractic studies, uninvolved with the radiographic data collection to preserve blinding. These researchers located the corresponding patient files in the clinics and extracted clinical data taken at the time of cervical radiographic referral, relating to the following: cervical pain levels (measured on the visual analogue scale (VAS)); the presence (Yes/No) as reported by the patient of: headaches, neck stiffness, pain referral to shoulders, radicular symptoms to the hands and numbness in the hands. Data pertaining to initial consultation, previous treatment or management plans was not recorded.

The recorded data was allocated to an independent group member, also in their final year of chiropractic studies, with no involvement in the radiographic or clinical data collection processes, to analyse and compare the results. Intra- and inter-observer reproducibility on the radiographic evaluations and extraction of clinical data was not performed, however, the radiographic evaluations were performed independently by two members of the research team. Results were compared and any discrepancies were discussed and arbitrated by the group supervisor, a chiropractic radiologist. Extraction of clinical data was from standardised files used in a chiropractic teaching institution. Files were excluded from analysis if they had incomplete or ambiguous data with respect to the symptoms being assessed.

Instruments

Kellgren and Lawrence osteoarthritis severity grade

Disc degeneration is a component of cervical degenerative joint disease. Kellgren developed certain criteria to classify and grade disc degeneration in the spine [15-17]. It uses the presence and severity of osteophytes, disc space narrowing and sclerosis to grade the level of degenerative disc disease present within a vertebral level on a grade of 1to 4 as outlined in Table 1. This assessment tool was selected based on its accuracy, reproducibility and recent validation for osteoarthritis in the cervical spine [18].

Presence of facet joint hypertrophy and uncinate process hypertrophy

These radiographic findings are also components of cervical degenerative joint disease [5]. Disc degeneration, facet joint hypertrophy and uncinate process hypertrophy may occur independently or in combination with each other. There is no known grading scale for facet joint and uncinate process hypertrophy, therefore the presence or absence of these findings was assessed (Yes/No).

Visual Analogue Scale (VAS)

The VAS is a subjective measurement of a person's pain intensity on a scale of 0 (no pain) to 10 (worst pain you have ever felt). This scale was used as it's a commonly implemented tool for patients presenting at the student clinics. The VAS is also considered valid, reliable and appropriate for clinical use [19,20].

Presence of headaches, neck stiffness, referral to shoulder, radicular symptoms in hands and numbness in hands

These symptoms are common complaints associated with cervical degenerative joint disease which are well described in the literature [5]. The presence of these symptoms was recorded (Yes/No) as reported in the clinical files at the time of radiographic referral.

Data analysis

Linear or logistic regression analysis was used to assess for correlations between radiographic findings of cervical degenerative joint disease as the dependent variable and independent predictor variables. The independent predictor variables assessed were: gender, age, VAS, presence of neck stiffness, presence of headache, presence of shoulder referral and presence of hand radiculopathy or numbness.

Diagnostic accuracy testing was used to assess dichotomous data. Dichotomous data included the presence of facet hypertrophy and uncinate hypertrophy as dependent variables. These were tested for positive and negative correlations to the presence or absence of headache, neck stiffness, shoulder referral, hand radiculopathy and hand numbness as predictor variables. Sensitivity, specificity, positive predictive value (PPV), negative predictive value (NPV), positive likelihood ratio (LR+), negative likelihood ratio (LR-) and diagnostic odds ratios (OR) were calculated with 95% confidence intervals (95%CI).

ROC curves were used to assess for the diagnostic test accuracy of continuous data compared to dichotomous data. Comparisons were made between the grade of disc degeneration as a dependent variable and the presence of headache, shoulder pain, neck stiffness, hand radiculopathy or hand numbness as independent predictor variables. The area under the ROC curve with 95%CI was calculated to assess for statistical significance of the diagnostic test accuracy.

Results

322 subjects were included in the study. Of these, 162 (50.3%) subjects were male, the mean age was 40.5 (standard deviation 17.4) and 78 (24.2%) subjects had no radiographic signs of cervical degenerative joint disease.

Table 1 Kellgren-Lawrence grading scale [15]

Grade 0	No signs of degenerative disc disease
Grade 1	Minimal anterior osteophytes
Grade 2	Definite anterior osteophytosis with possible narrowing of the disc space and some sclerosis of vertebral plates
Grade 3	Moderate narrowing of the disc space with definite sclerosis of vertebral plates and osteophytes
Grade 4	Severe narrowing of the disc space with definite sclerosis of vertebral plates and multiple large osteophytes

Table 2 outlines the distribution of radiographic findings degenerative joint disease in the cervical spine.

Kellgren Lawrence grade of cervical disc degeneration

Linear regression analysis was conducted to examine the relationship between the Kellgren Lawrence grade of disc degeneration and the independent predictor variables. A significant trend could only be extrapolated for age as an independent variable. As demonstrated in Figure 1, the correlation coefficient (95%CI) of 0.06 (0.055, 0.066) shows a positive trend and variation around the regression line is acceptable as indicated by the R^2-value of 0.61. This indicates that for every 16.7 years a person ages, their grade of cervical disc degeneration is expected to increase by 1 on the Kellgren Lawrence grading scale.

Assessment of diagnostic accuracy between the Kellgren Lawrence grade of disc degeneration and specified symptomatologies was performed using ROC curves. The presence of neck stiffness and the presence of shoulder referral did show mild evidence of diagnostic accuracy in predicting disc degeneration as depicted in Figures 2 and 3. The area under the curve (95%CI) measured 0.62 (0.56, 0.68) and 0.60 (0.54, 0.67) respectively. Although these values were statistically significant the clinical significance is uncertain as these values do not represent high levels of diagnostic accuracy. The area under the curve (Area under curve (95%CI)) for headaches (0.43 (0.36, 0.50)), hand radiculopathy (0.57 (0.47, 0.67)) and hand numbness (0.57 (0.47, 0.68)) did not exhibit statistical significance. Therefore, the presence of headaches, hand radiculopathy and hand numbness did not predict the grade of disc degeneration on cervical radiograph.

Presence of cervical facet joint hypertrophy

Logistic regression analysis was conducted to examine the relationship between presence of facet joint hypertrophy and the independent predictor variables. Only age showed a significant relationship with an odds ratio (95%CI) of 1.12 (1.09, 1.15). Therefore, for every year increase in age the odds of having facet hypertrophy increase by 1.12.

Table 3 depicts the diagnostic accuracy outcomes for the presence of facet joint hypertrophy and the presence of specified symptomatologies. The presence of neck stiffness was the only symptom to demonstrate statistically significant diagnostic accuracy with diagnostic OR (95% CI) of 1.69 (1.04, 2.76). Despite being statistically significant, however, this only represents a small increase in the odds of having facet hypertrophy on radiograph in the presence of neck stiffness. Hand radiculopathy and hand numbness both exhibited a high specificity for the presence of facet joint hypertrophy on radiograph at 0.89 (0.84, 0.93) and 0.90 (0.85, 0.94) respectively. Therefore, if there is no facet joint hypertrophy on radiograph then it is unlikely that the patient will have presented with hand radiculopathy or hand numbness.

Presence of cervical uncinate process hypertrophy

Logistic regression analysis was conducted to examine the relationship between presence of uncinate process hypertrophy and the independent predictor variables. Only age showed a significant relationship with an odds ratio (95% CI) of 1.15 (1.12, 1.18). Therefore, for every year increase in age the odds of having uncinate process hypertrophy increase by 1.15.

Table 4 depicts the diagnostic accuracy outcomes for the presence of uncinate process hypertrophy and the presence of specified symptomatologies. Neck stiffness demonstrated a small positive correlation with the presence of uncinate process hypertrophy with a sensitivity (95% CI) of 0.70 (0.61, 0.77) and LR+ (95% CI) of 1.17 (1.00, 1.38). Therefore, the presence of neck stiffness correlates with a mild increase in the odds of having uncinate process hypertrophy on radiograph. Hand radiculopathy and hand numbness both exhibited a high specificity for the presence of uncinate process hypertrophy on radiograph at 0.91 (0.85, 0.94) and 0.92 (0.87, 0.95) respectively. Therefore, if there is no uncinate process hypertrophy on radiograph then it is unlikely that the patient will have presented with hand radiculopathy or hand numbness.

Discussion

In this study, symptomatology was not correlated with the presence of cervical degenerative joint disease. The only independent predictor to show consistent significant

Table 2 Distribution of radiographic findings of cervical spine degenerative joint disease

Disc degeneration		Facet hypertrophy		Uncinate process hypertrophy	
Kellgren Lawrence grade	No. (%)	Presence (Y/N)	No. (%)	Presence (Y/N)	No. (%)
0	78 (24.2)	Y	118 (36.6)	Y	141 (43.8)
1	101 (31.4)	N	204 (63.4)	N	181 (56.2)
2	54 (16.8)				
3	45 (14)				
4	44 (13.7)				
Total	322 (100)	Total	322 (100)	Total	322 (100)

No.: Number of subjects exhibiting the finding; Y: Yes; N: No.

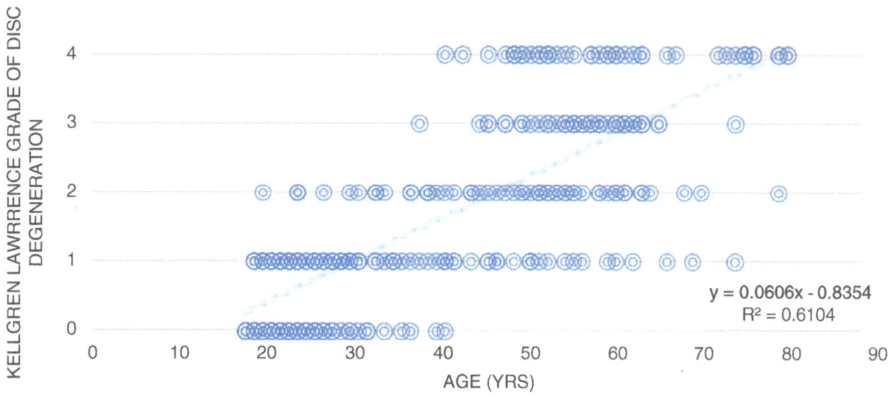

Figure 1 Correlation of disc degeneration vs age.

correlation with radiographic findings of degenerative joint disease was age. Cervical pain levels, measured by VAS, and the presence of headaches did not provide any increase in diagnostic accuracy for the presence of cervical degenerative joint disease. Hand radiculopathy and hand numbness did not show any correlations with grade of degenerative disc disease, however they did exhibit high specificity for the presence of facet joint or uncinate process hypertrophy. Although a correlation between radiographic findings and symptomatology is evident here, clinically this result does not aid the clinician in predicting the presence or absence of cervical degenerative joint disease from the presence or absence of these symptoms.

The presence of pain referring to the shoulder exhibited statistically significant but low diagnostic test accuracy with the grade of degenerative disc disease in the cervical spine. The area under the ROC curve, despite being statistically significant at 0.60 (95%CI: 0.54, 0.67), only represents a low level of accuracy in predicting radiographic findings of degenerative disc disease from the presence of shoulder referral. Similarly the accuracy of the presence of neck stiffness in predicting cervical disc degeneration also had an area under the ROC curve of 0.62 (95%CI: 0.55, 0.68), indicating a statistically significant result but of low diagnostic accuracy.

As a symptom, the presence of neck stiffness showed mild diagnostic test accuracy with all radiographic findings associated with degenerative joint disease of the cervical spine. The correlation of the presence of neck stiffness with radiographic evidence of cervical degenerative joint disease is plausible considering the combination of hypertrophic changes to the articular surfaces of

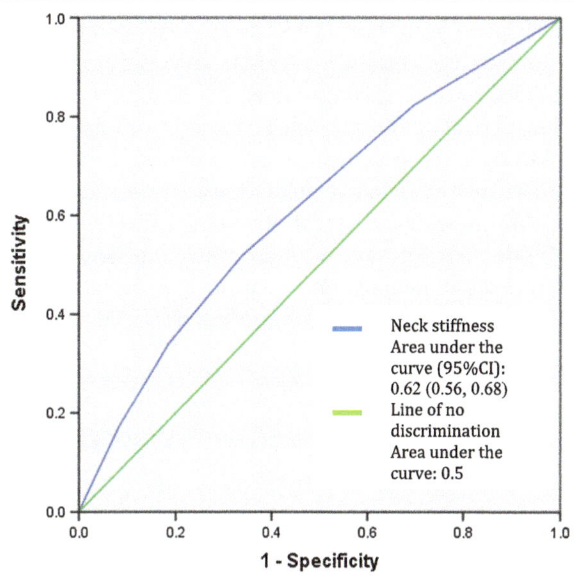

Figure 2 ROC curve for presence of neck stiffness vs grade of disc degeneration.

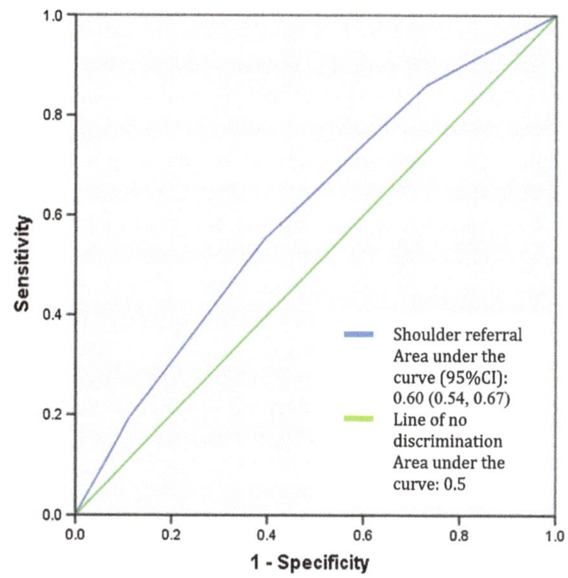

Figure 3 ROC curve for presence of shoulder referral vs grade of disc degeneration.

Table 3 Diagnostic accuracy of specified symptomatologies for facet joint hypertrophy

	Sensitivity (95%CI)	Specificity (95%CI)	PPV (95%CI)	NPV (95%CI)	LR+ (95%CI)	LR- (95%CI)
Headache	0.28 (0.21, 0.37)	0.65 (0.59, 0.71)	0.32 (0.24, 0.42)	0.61 (0.54, 0.67)	0.81 (0.57, 1.14)	1.1 (0.95, 1.28)
Neck stiffness	0.71 (0.63, 0.79)	0.4 (0.34, 0.47)	0.41 (0.34, 0.48)	0.71 (0.62, 0.78)	1.2 (1.02, 1.41)	0.71 (0.51, 0.98)
Shoulder referral	0.41 (0.32, 0.5)	0.64 (0.57, 0.7)	0.4 (0.31, 0.49)	0.64 (0.57, 0.71)	1.13 (0.85, 1.5)	0.93 (0.77, 1.11)
Hand Radiculopathy	0.14 (0.09, 0.21)	0.89 (0.84, 0.93)	0.42 (0.28, 0.58)	0.64 (0.58, 0.69)	1.26 (0.69, 2.3)	0.99 (0.89, 1.06)
Hand Numbness	0.1 (0.06, 0.17)	0.9 (0.85, 0.94)	0.36 (0.22, 0.53)	0.63 (0.58, 0.69)	0.99 (0.5, 1.94)	1.0 (0.93, 1.08)

the joints, osteophyte formation and resulting muscle tension that can cause neck stiffness [21]. However, the LR+ for both facet joint and uncinate process hypertrophy, despite exhibiting statistical significance, were at values associated with low levels of diagnostic accuracy that would not be expected to change clinical practice [22]. In addition, when regression analysis was performed, and age and gender were also accounted for, neck stiffness did not show statistically significant correlation with any form of cervical spine degenerative joint disease.

The results of this study agree with previous studies that the severity of cervical degeneration is not correlated with the degree of pain perceived [3,10,12,14]. This study adds to the body of evidence in this area by assessing the different radiographic findings associated with cervical degenerative joint disease individually and by grading the extent of degenerative disc disease using established grading criteria. Symptoms associated with cervical degenerative joint disease were also assessed individually for diagnostic accuracy. Although results were similar between disc degeneration, facet joint hypertrophy and uncinate process hypertrophy, some statistically significant differences were noted. The grade of disc degeneration correlated most significantly with the presence of neck stiffness or referral of pain to the shoulder, whereas, facet joint and uncinate process hypertrophy showed correlation with the presence of neck stiffness and high specificity with upper limb radicular symptoms.

The main limitation of this study is the retrospective study design. Only subjects who had been referred for cervical imaging were assessed and this would have skewed the sample towards subjects with symptomatology. In addition, clinical files were accessed to obtain data regarding presenting symptoms and, therefore, inter-practitioner inconsistencies when recording symptomatic data at the time of presentation could not be accounted for. Any files with missing data were excluded from the study to limit the associated bias. A prospective study would control for these limitations, however, the results of this study do not provide compelling evidence that a prospective study in this field would produce results that would lead to a change in clinical practice. Finally, this study only assessed for the presence of degeneration in any one of cervical discs, facet joints or uncovertebral joints. It did not account for presentations of multi-level or concomitant degenerative findings. These additional findings may help differentiate between levels of severity of cervical degeneration, however, a validated scale for this assessment could not be found in the current literature. Validation of a more precise scale to grade the severity of cervical degeneration may allow for further research into this area and a better understanding of any association between symptomatology and cervical degenerative joint disease.

Conclusion

In conclusion, the results of this study indicate that clinical symptoms such as pain level (VAS), headaches, shoulder referral and hand radiculopathy or numbness do not correlate with radiographic findings of degenerative joint disease in the cervical spine. A small increase in diagnostic accuracy between the presence of neck stiffness and all forms of cervical degenerative joint disease was shown. However, this increase is not at the level expected to change clinical practice. Age was the only independent predictor variable to demonstrate a statistically significant correlation with radiographic findings of cervical spine degenerative joint disease.

Table 4 Diagnostic accuracy of specified symptomatologies for uncinate process hypertrophy

	Sensitivity (95% CI)	Specificity (95% CI)	PPV (95% CI)	NPV (95% CI)	LR+ (95% CI)	LR- (95% CI)
Headache	0.3 (0.24, 0.39)	0.66 (0.59, 0.73)	0.42 (0.33, 0.51)	0.55 (0.48, 0.61)	0.91 (0.66, 1.26)	1.05 (0.9, 1.22)
Neck stiffness	0.7 (0.61, 0.77)	0.41 (0.34, 0.48)	0.48 (0.41, 0.55)	0.63 (0.54, 0.71)	1.17 (1.0, 1.38)	0.75 (0.55, 1.01)
Shoulder referral	0.44 (0.36, 0.52)	0.66 (0.59, 0.73)	0.5 (0.42, 0.59)	0.6 (0.53, 0.66)	1.23 (0.98, 1.7)	0.85 (0.71, 1.02)
Hand Radiculopathy	0.15 (0.1, 0.22)	0.91 (0.85, 0.94)	0.55 (0.4, 0.7)	0.58 (0.52, 0.63)	1.59 (0.87, 2.89)	0.94 (0.86, 1.02)
Hand Numbness	0.13 (0.08, 0.19)	0.92 (0.87, 0.95)	0.55 (0.38, 0.7)	0.57 (0.52, 0.63)	1.54 (0.81, 2.95)	0.95 (0.88, 1.03)

Consent

Written informed consent was obtained from the patient for the publication of this report and any accompanying images.

Abbreviations

AP: Anteroposterior; VAS: Visual analogue scale; PPV: Positive predictive value; NPV: Negative predictive value; LR+: Positive likelihood ratio; LR-: Negative likelihood ratio; OR: Odds ratio; 95%CI: 95% confidence intervals.

Competing interests

The authors declare that they have no competing interests.

Authors' contributions

IR was involved in the conception and design of the research, collection and interpretation of the data, and drafting and editing of the final manuscript. AP was involved in the conception and design of the research, data collection and drafting and editing of the final manuscript. LO was involved in design of the research, statistical analysis and interpretation of the data and drafting and editing of the final manuscript. AB was involved in design of the research, data collection and drafting and editing of the final manuscript. KK was involved in design of the research, data collection and editing of the final manuscript. JW was involved in design of the research, data collection and editing of the final manuscript. HJ was involved in conception, design and supervision of the research, statistical analysis and interpretation of the data and editing of the final manuscript. All authors read and approved the final manuscript.

References

1. Binder AI. Cervical spondylosis and neck pain. Br Med J. 2007;334:527–31.
2. Feder R, Hartvigsen J. Neck pain and disability due to neck pain: what is the relation? Eur Spine J. 2008;17:80–8.
3. Bovim G, Schrader H, Sand T. Neck pain in the general population. Spine (Phila Pa 1976). 1994;19(12):1307–9.
4. Abhishek A, Doherty M. Diagnosis and clinical presentation of osteoarthritis. Rheum Dis Clin North Am. 2013;39(1):45–66.
5. Haldeman S, Carroll K, Cassidy DJ, Schubert J, Nygren A. The bone and joint decade 2000–2010 task force on neck pain and its associated disorders: executive summary. Eur Spine J. 2008;17 Suppl 1:S5–7.
6. Cassidy JD, Cote P, Carrol L. The Saskatchewan health and back pain survey. The prevalence of neck pain and related disability in Saskatchewan adults. Spine (Phila Pa 1976). 1998;23(17):1860–6. discussion 1867.
7. Butler JS, Oner FC, Poynton AR, O'Byrne JM. Degenerative cervical spondylosis: a natural history, pathogenesis and current management strategies. Advances in Orthopedics. 2012;2012:916–87.
8. Lestini WF, Wiesel SW. The pathogenesis of cervical spondylosis. Clin Orthop Relat Res. 1989;239:69–93.
9. Ory PA. Radiography in the assessment of musculoskeletal conditions. Best Practice and Research Clinical Rheumatology. 2003;17(3):495–512.
10. Laplante BL, DePalma MJ. Spine osteoarthritis. Am Acad Physical Medicine and Rehabilitation. 2012;4(5 Suppl):S28–36.
11. Heller CA, Stanley P, Lewis-Jones B, Heller RF. Value of x ray examinations of the cervical spine. Br Med J (Clin Res Ed). 1983;287(6401):1276–8.
12. French SD, Walker BF, Cameron M, Pollard HP, Vitiello AL, Reggars JW, et al. Risk management for chiropractors and osteopaths: imaging guidelines for conditions commonly seen in practice. Aust Chir Osteo. 2003;11(2):41–8.
13. Marchiori DM, Henderson CNR. A cross-sectional study correlating degenerative findings to pain and disability. Spine (Phila Pa 1976). 1996;21(23):2747–51.
14. Gore DR, Sepie SB, Gardner GM, Murray PM. Neck pain: a long-term follow up of 205 patients. Spine (Phila Pa 1976). 1987;12(1):1–5.
15. Kellgren JH, Lawrence JS. Radiological assessment of osteo-arthrosis. Ann Rheum Dis. 1957;16:494–501.
16. Chapman JR, Dettori JR, Norvell DC. Spine Classifications and Severity Measures. New York: Thieme Verlag; 2009. p. 186–7.
17. Kellgren JH, Ball J. Atlas of standard radiographs: the epidemiology of chronic rheumatism, vol II. Oxford, England: Blackwell Scientific; 1963.
18. Ofiram E, Garvey TA, Schwender JD. Cervical degenerative index: a new quantitative radiographic scoring system for cervical spondylosis with interobserver and intraobserver reliability testing. J Orthop Traumatol. 2009;10(1):21–6.
19. Williamson A, Hoggart B. Pain: a review of three commonly used pain rating scales. J Clin Nurs. 2005;14:798–804.
20. Misailidou V, Paraskevi M, Beneka A, Karagiannidis A, Godolias G. Assessment of patients with neck pain: a review of definitions, selection criteria, and measurement tools. J Chiropr Med. 2010;9(2):49–59.
21. Hunter DJ. In the clinic: osteoarthritis. Ann Intern Med. 2007;147(3):ITC8-1–ITC8-16.
22. Fischer J, Bachmann L, Jaeschke R. A readers' guide to the interpretation of diagnostic test properties: clinical example of sepsis. Intensive Care Med. 2003;29:1043–51.

Public health engagement: detection of suspicious skin lesions, screening and referral behaviour of UK based chiropractors

Sara Glithro[1*], David Newell[2], Lorna Burrows[3^], Adrian Hunnisett[1] and Christina Cunliffe[1]

Abstract

Background: UK morbidity and mortality rates from skin cancer are increasing despite existing preventative strategies involving education and early detection. Manual therapists are ideally placed to support these goals as they see greater quantities of exposed patient skin more often than most other healthcare professionals. The purpose of this study therefore was to ascertain the ability of manual therapists to detect, screen and refer suspicious skin lesions.

Method: A web-based questionnaire and quiz was used in a sample of UK chiropractic student clinicians and registered chiropractors to gather data during 2011 concerning skin screening and referral behaviors for suspicious skin lesions.

Results: A total of 120 questionnaires were included. Eighty one percent of participants agreed that screening for suspicious skin lesions was part of their clinical role, with nearly all (94%) assessing their patients for lesions during examination. Over 90% of the participants reported regularly having the opportunity for skin examination; with nearly all (98%) agreeing they would refer patients with suspicious skin lesions to a medical practitioner. A third of respondents had referred a total of 80 suspicious lesions within the last 12 months with 67% warranting further investigation.

Conclusions: Nearly all respondents agreed that screening patients for suspicious skin lesions was part of their clinical role, with a significant number already referring patients with lesions.

Keywords: Skin lesion, Skin cancer, Screening, Referral behaviour, Prevention, Detection, Dermatology, Chiropractor, Manual therapist

Background

Malignant melanoma incidence rates have increased more than fivefold since the mid-1970s and continue to rise [1]. In 2002, the UK paid over £240 million in total costs associated with skin cancer; of which 42% were direct costs to the NHS [2]. Of the various forms of skin cancer, melanoma treatment was directly responsible for 63% of this total. Early detection of pre-cancerous and cancerous lesions not only improves patient mortality rates [3-5] it also substantially reduces this economic burden by enabling faster, cheaper and less-invasive interventions as out-patients in comparison to the otherwise high costs associated with in-patient care required to treat advanced lesions. Yet, in a study of US patients, 75% reported having never been advised by their medical practitioner or any other medical professional in their medical practice, to examine their skin for growths or changes in spots or moles. Furthermore, most participants (58% and 83% respectively) reported that their medical practitioner 'never' or 'rarely' looked at the skin on their back or on the backs of their legs [6].

However, in the UK, in addition to medical practitioners, a diverse group of clinical practitioners are in a position to detect, screen and refer suspicious skin lesions [6-10]. Of these, a smaller number regularly see patients unclothed and particularly see areas of the body inaccessible to visual inspection by the patient themselves. Of those that do, manual therapists such as masseurs, osteopaths and chiropractors are ideally placed to regularly screen the skin for suspicious lesions. Chiropractic practice is concerned with the diagnosis and treatment of musculoskeletal syndromes, including low back, neck pain,

* Correspondence: sglithro@bournemouth.ac.uk
^Deceased
[1]McTimoney College of Chiropractic, Abingdon, UK
Full list of author information is available at the end of the article

headaches and peripheral joint problems [11]. Despite 42% of chiropractors regularly examining patients who were in their underwear [12], little if any research exists that has attempted to determine whether chiropractors in the field take advantage of this opportunity to perform basic skin screening. Of that research already carried out, this was restricted to a student population only and recommended that further research should test the ability of chiropractors to identify pathological moles on a broader, evaluative basis [13]. In view of this we investigated the accuracy with which chiropractic student clinicians and registered chiropractors were able to recognise as suspicious or benign, a variety of common skin lesions from images chosen by a dermatologist. More generally we also examined attitudes towards skin screening and the screening and referral patterns within this sample. For the purpose of this article the term 'chiropractic student clinicians' has been adopted to describe chiropractic students or interns in their final year of clinical study.

Methods

Dissemination

A web based, self-administered questionnaire was emailed to the chiropractic student clinicians of both participating UK colleges. These participants were in their final clinical year of study when the survey was distributed in 2011 (n = 154). The questionnaire was also emailed to a sample of 250 practising UK registered chiropractors who were randomly selected by the McTimoney Chiropractic Association from their members list. Finally, a link to the questionnaire was published in the United Chiropractic Association's regular members' e-newsletter. The questionnaire contained closed questions and images designed to gather descriptive information on the participants' frequency and accuracy of detecting suspicious skin lesions.

Inclusion/exclusion criteria

Students were those in their final clinical year of chiropractic study at a UK college or university which on completion of their course, allowed registration with the General Chiropractic Council (GCC). The chiropractors were all registered with the GCC at the time the questionnaire was issued. For inclusion within the data analysis, respondents must have confirmed whether they were either a student or a registered chiropractor. In addition, they had to provide a response to the question concerning whether or not they considered screening patients for suspicious skin lesions to be part of their role as a chiropractor. Only subjects that responded either 'Yes' or 'No' were included as failure to answer this question meant the subject had exited the questionnaire without answering any further questions. Questionnaire completion was advised and taken as consent.

Questionnaire design

The questionnaire had four sections: 1) Participant demographics, 2) Willingness and attitudes towards examination of patients for skin lesions, 3) Skills associated with lesion detection and 4) Identification of training needs associated with lesion detection.

Likert scales were used to evaluate participants' knowledge of risk factors involved with and identification of, suspicious skin lesions. The second part of the questionnaire established participants' skills in identifying lesions. A dermatologist advised on and approved a set of images of commonly occurring skin lesions, including some where early detection could have substantial impact on prognosis and decrease costs to health services. In an attempt to prevent participants from searching for the images online prior to answering questions; a statement encouraging the participants to resist using any reference material was displayed at the beginning of the questionnaire; image references were only revealed to the participants on questionnaire completion and an on-demand document providing all the images, references and correct diagnoses was also provided to participants on questionnaire completion. Face validity and piloting of the questionnaire took place prior to finalising the questionnaire design. Anonymous responses were accepted for a period of four weeks, with emailed reminders sent at pre-identified points during this period.

Sampling

The aim was to capture responses from a sample group reflective of the UK chiropractic profession and a final year pre-registration student chiropractic population. Invitations to take part were made to the four UK chiropractic associations; British Chiropractic Association (BCA), McTimoney Chiropractic Association (MCA), Scottish Chiropractic Association (SCA), United Chiropractic Association (UCA) and all three UK chiropractic colleges; Anglo-European College of Chiropractic (AECC), McTimoney College of Chiropractic (MCC) and the Welsh Institute of Chiropractic (WIOC).

The final sample included 62 UK based registered chiropractors who were members of the MCA and 58 final year students from two UK teaching institutions. Of these, 34 (58%) were from AECC and 25 (42%) were from the MCC.

Analysis

Questionnaire data was analysed using a descriptive approach. Continuous variables where normally distributed were described using means and standard deviations, while non-parametric distributions were described with medians and percentiles. Categorical variables were described using proportions.

Ethics

Ethical approval was granted by the McTimoney College Research Ethics Committee on the 21st of November 2010, prior to commencement of the study.

Results

From the 404 questionnaires that were issued, a total of 139 questionnaires were returned. Nineteen failed to meet the inclusion criteria, leaving 120 included in the analysis and giving a successful response rate of 30%. Eighty (67%) participants were female and 40 (33%) were male. Sixty two (52%) were registered chiropractors and the remaining 58 (48%) were chiropractic students. In the registered chiropractor group, the mean number of years qualified was 5.8 years (SD ± 8.0) and the mean number of patients treated per month was 89 (SD ± 70.3) (Table 1).

Table 1 Demographic characteristics of sample

Variable		n	%	Mean (SD)	Range
Gender	Female	80	67		
Age (years)	21-30	36	30		
	31-40	27	23		
	41-50	31	26		
	51-60	16	13		
	>60	10	8		
Practicing category	Chiropractic student clinician	58	48		
	Registered Chiropractor	62	52		
Years qualified				5.8 (8)	0-35
	Not yet qualified	58	48		
	Less than 5 years	14	12		
	5-9 years	15	13		
	10-14 years	15	13		
	15-19 years	7	6		
	20-24 years	6	5		
	25-35 years	5	4		
New patients per month				12.8 (13)	0-108
	1-4	50	42		
	5-9	18	15		
	10-19	25	21		
	20-39	21	18		
	Over 40	5	4		
Repeat patients per month				76.1 (65)	13-347
	1-49	58	48		
	50-99	28	23		
	100-199	27	23		
	200-799	7	6		

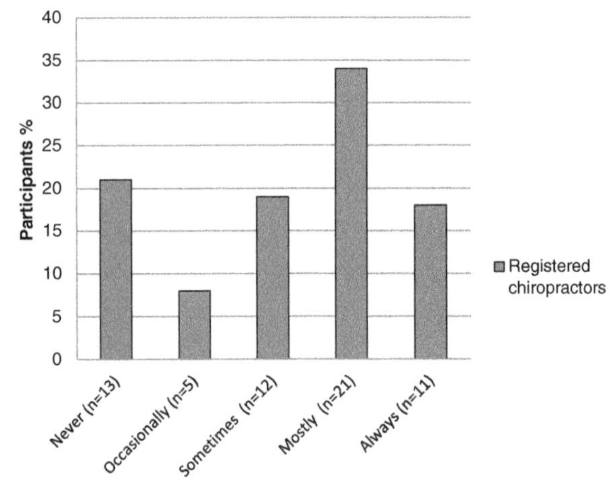

Figure 1 Percentage of registered chiropractor participants who performed chiropractic examinations with patients wearing only their underwear thus having the opportunity to examine at least some of their skin.

As the chiropractic student clinicians approach to examination of patients was likely to be dictated by their college policy on patient gowning, skin exposure analysis was evaluated from the data provided by participating registered chiropractors. Figure 1 shows the degree of patient skin exposure during the examination and treatment by the registered chiropractor. Fifty two percent (n = 32) agreed they 'always' or 'mostly' examined patients in their underwear during the examination. In another question, over half, (71%, n = 44) indicated that their patients were 'never' or 'occassionally' fully clothed during the examination, implying regular opportunities to examine at least some of their patients' skin.

Most chiropractic student clinician and registered chiropractor participants (81%, n = 97) agreed that screening patients for skin lesions was part of their clinical role (Table 2). Of these, 94% (n = 91) indicated they screened each new patient, 53% (n = 51) screened existing patients

Table 2 Screening attitude and behaviours of participants

Question posed		Answered 'Yes' %	n
Do you consider screening patients for suspicious skin lesions to be part of your role as a chiropractor?		81	97
If 'Yes', is this part of your normal patient assessment for...	New patients?	94	91
	Repeat patients at every visit?	53	51
	Repeat patients during regular assessments?	73	71

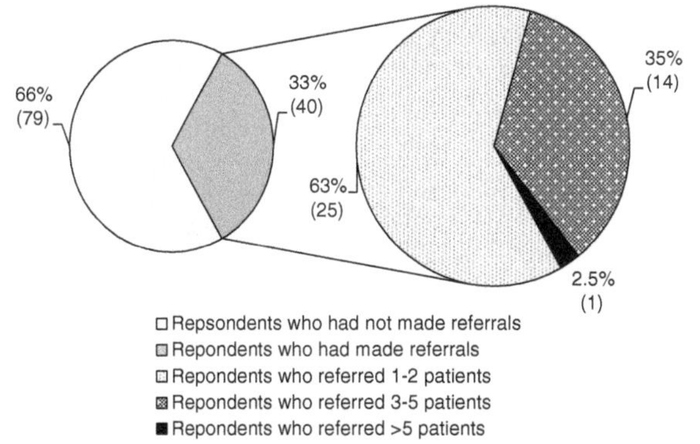

Figure 2 **Participants (all) referral rates of patients with suspicious skin lesions within the previous 12 months %(n).**

at every visit and 73% (n = 71) at visits scheduled specifically for patient re-assessments.

Registered chiropractors and final year chiropractic students already identify and refer patients with suspicious skin lesions. Within the previous 12 months, 33% (n = 40) of the participants had referred a total of 104 patients with skin lesions they felt warranted further investigation (Figure 2).

Of the 104 referrals made, referrers declared they were aware of 80 outcomes via feedback from their patients or medical practitioners. Over two-thirds of the 80 outcomes known (67%, n = 54), warranted further secondary healthcare investigation by a medical professional. Of these 80 outcomes; 29% (n = 23), were diagnosed as Basal Cell Carcinoma, Malignant Melanoma or Squamous Cell Carcinoma. A further 17% (n = 9) of patients were still awaiting the outcome and 9% (n = 5) were diagnosed with other conditions requiring medical care. Almost a third (31%, n = 17) of those referred required no further treatment following examination by their medical practitioner (Figure 3).

The participants generally demonstrated a good understanding of the risk factors associated with developing skin cancers, although some frequently occurring features were less understood (Table 3). Few respondents identified having blue/green eyes (10%, n = 12), red hair/freckles (37%, n = 36) or an unprotected balding head (45%, n = 53) as risk factors for developing skin cancer. Yet over 88% recognised an increased risk with having an outdoor occupation, repeated sunburn as a child or history of using UV tanning beds. When assessing whether a lesion should be considered suspicious, over 90% agreed or strongly agreed the importance of a change in the appearance or behavior of a lesion. Furthermore, over 70% agreed or strongly agreed that the recent appearance, an uneven colour or lesion asymmetry should also be looked out for. Additionally, 55% deemed a raised surface to be important although this is not a major feature for all suspicious lesions. The majority practiced a proactive approach in the detection and referral of lesions however, less than 40% advised their patients on preventative strategies in avoiding or reducing risk.

Figures 4a to d document the responses to questions asked about the ten images of skin lesions shown to the subjects. As is shown, with reference to identification of suspicious lesions, over 75% of participants correctly labeled examples of malignant melanoma and squamous cell carcinoma. However, less than 45% did so for superficial basal cell carcinoma and actinic keratosis. Interestingly,

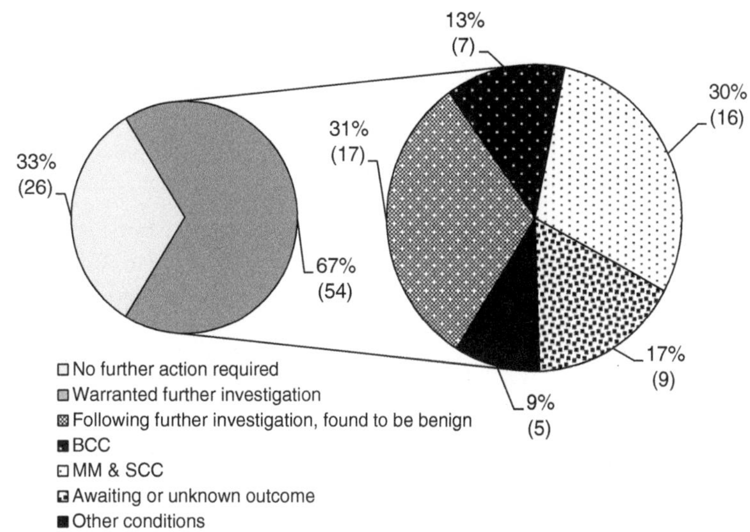

Figure 3 **Patient outcomes following referral %(n).**

Table 3 Respondents knowledge of the risk factors associated with developing skin cancer and the advice they offer patients

	%	n
The risk of developing skin cancer increases with...'		
An outdoor occupation		
Strongly agree/agree	76	89
Neutral	20	23
Disagree/strongly disagree	4	5
An indoor occupation and holidays in the sun once or twice a year (beach, skiing, outdoor etc.)		
Strongly agree/agree	71	82
Neutral	21	24
Disagree/strongly disagree	8	9
Repeated incidents of having sunburn as a child		
Strongly agree/agree	88	104
Neutral	11	13
Disagree/strongly disagree	1	1
A history of using UV tanning beds		
Strongly agree/agree	93	110
Neutral	6	7
Disagree/strongly disagree	1	1
More than 50 moles		
Strongly agree/agree	56	65
Neutral	38	45
Disagree/strongly disagree	6	7
More than 100 moles		
Strongly agree/agree	69	78
Neutral	27	31
Disagree/strongly disagree	4	4
A history of at least one pre-cancerous or cancerous skin lesion		
Strongly agree/agree	92	109
Neutral	6	7
Disagree/strongly disagree	2	2
A first degree relative with a history of at least one pre-cancerous or cancerous skin lesion		
Strongly agree/agree	69	82
Neutral	22	26
Disagree/strongly disagree	8	10
Freckles and/or red hair		
Strongly agree/agree	37	36
Neutral	51	49
Disagree/strongly disagree	12	12
Blue or green eyes		
Strongly agree/agree	10	12
Neutral	65	75
Disagree/strongly disagree	25	29
Fair skin		
Strongly agree/agree	58	69
Neutral	34	40
Disagree/strongly disagree	8	9
A history of long-term use of drugs with known side-effects of photosensitivity		
Strongly agree/agree	66	77
Neutral	32	37
Disagree/strongly disagree	3	3
Thinning or balding hair		
Strongly agree/agree	45	53
Neutral	42	50
Disagree/strongly disagree	13	15
A skin lesion should be considered 'suspicious' if...	**%**	**n**
It has uneven colour		
Strongly agree/agree	72	84
Neutral	23	27
Disagree/strongly disagree	4	5
It is asymmetrical		
Strongly agree/agree	73	85
Neutral	22	25
Disagree/strongly disagree	5	6
It has changed in size (growing)		
Strongly agree/agree	95	114
Neutral	2	2
Disagree/strongly disagree	3	4
It has changed in shape (irregular border)		
Strongly agree/agree	97	113
Neutral	2	2
Disagree/strongly disagree	1	1
It has changed in colour (including several different colours)		
Strongly agree/agree	93	112
Neutral	4	5
Disagree/strongly disagree	3	3
It has a crusty keratinised surface		
Strongly agree/agree	71	82
Neutral	22	26
Disagree/strongly disagree	7	8
It bleeds		
Strongly agree/agree	95	110
Neutral	3	3
Disagree/strongly disagree	3	3
It appeared recently		
Strongly agree/agree	71	82

Table 3 Respondents knowledge of the risk factors associated with developing skin cancer and the advice they offer patients *(Continued)*

Neutral	24	28
Disagree/strongly disagree	5	6
It has a raised surface		
Strongly agree/agree	55	66
Neutral	32	38
Disagree/strongly disagree	13	15
It itches		
Strongly agree/agree	78	91
Neutral	17	20
Disagree/strongly disagree	4	5
The patient is concerned about it		
Strongly agree/agree	73	85
Neutral	25	29
Disagree/strongly disagree	3	3
Do you advise your patients on...	**%**	**n**
The risks of sun exposure		
Yes	33	39
No	67	78
The risks of using UV sunbeds		
Yes	37	43
No	63	74
Using sunscreen with an SPF of at least 15		
Yes	32	36
No	68	78
Other factors that can increase photosensitivity (E.g. some antibiotics, anti-depressants, anti-malarial medications etc.)		
Yes	14	16
No	86	96
Have you ever been asked for advice on preventing skin cancer by your patients?		
Yes	7	8
No	93	108

whilst confident to label these lesions as suspicious, less than 10% diagnosed the lesions correctly (Figure 4d). Over 60% incorrectly labeled the benign seborrhoeic wart as suspicious, however more participants correctly labeled the haemangioma and junctional naevus as not suspicious. The majority, 75% (n = 90) correctly identified the intradermal naevus as not suspicious.

Participant's referral rates were slightly greater (<11%) than those declaring the corresponding lesion as 'suspicious' (Figure 4b). Whilst not wanting to over-refer, perhaps this degree of caution demonstrates respondents recognising when to request help beyond their own expertise. Participant's confidence in their ability to diagnose the images correctly mirrored the actual number of correct diagnoses; however both were low at less than 20%.

Participants were asked whether they had completed any skin lesion identification training as part of their undergraduate course and whether they would be interested in receiving more. The majority (68%, n = 81) had received some form of undergraduate training and 75% (n = 90) of all respondents were interested in receiving further training.

Discussion

A position paper decrying the less than main stream position of chiropractic within the wider health care system and using podiatry as a model to describe how a similar profession has navigated a course toward greater acceptance, cited podiatrists traditional dedication to public health issues as one of the major reasons why they became influential members of the healthcare community [14]. They urged the chiropractic profession to *'...openly embrace, and become actively involved in public health initiatives'.*

In the context of these discussions this study investigated the degree to which chiropractors were engaging in an important key public health issue, namely early detection of skin cancer.

As long ago as 2003, Mahon [15] concluded that given skin cancer remaining as a major public health problem, efforts following those associated with primary prevention, such as sun screen use and judicial reductions in exposure to UV, should also include secondary prevention such as professional skin examinations. This author went on to suggest that nurses have a major role to play in these secondary preventative efforts.

A recent article by Ramcharan et al. [13] using a cross sectional design, reported that over 80% of chiropractic student clinicians thought that recognising skin cancer in their patients was important or very important in their practice, concluding that chiropractic education should emphasize the opportunity to detect and assess atypical moles as a routine part of primary prevention in clinical education.

Similarly in this study, the majority of participants agreed that screening patients was part of their clinical role and felt they already had the skills to recognise suspicious lesions and refer patients for further investigation. Within this small sample (n = 120), 40 practitioners had referred 80 patients for further investigation within the previous 12 months and at least 23 were found to have skin cancer. Extrapolating to the UK registered chiropractic population of approximately 2827,

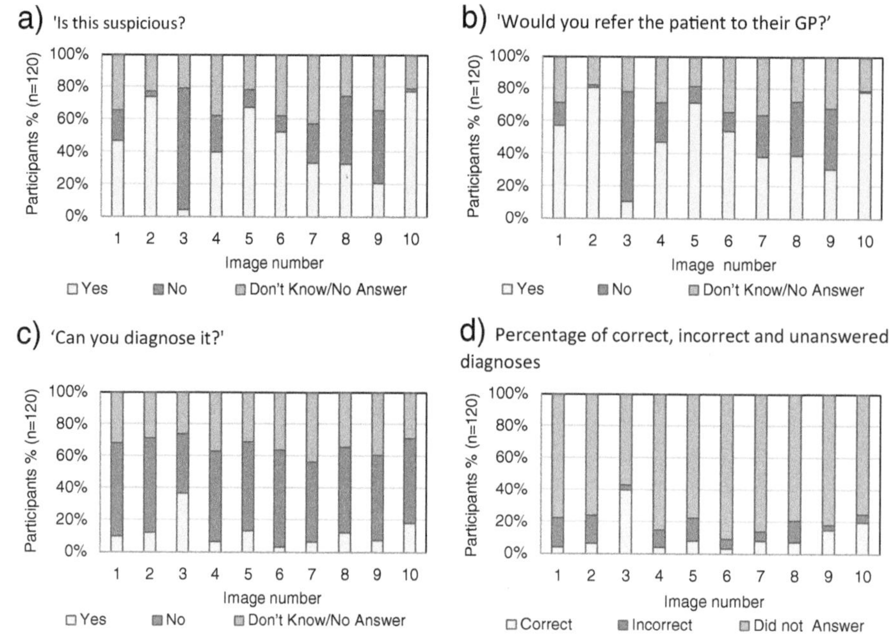

Figure 4 Participants response to questions concerning images. For **a)** to **d)**: n = 120; Images, 1: Superficial Basal Cell Carcinoma, 2: Squamous Cell Carcinoma, 3: Intradermal Naevus, 4: Actinic Keratosis, 5: Seborrhoeic Wart, 6: Bowen's Disease, 7: Nodular Basal Cell Carcinoma, 8: Haemangioma, 9: Junctional Naevus and 10: Malignant Melanoma. NB: for the purposes of this study, images 1,2,4,6,7 and 10 were considered 'suspicious' by the researchers.

one could estimate that the chiropractic profession might identify and refer 1866 patients annually for further investigation and of these 29% (541) could have skin cancer.

This research indicates that detecting and referring patients with suspicious skin lesions is already taking place, yet patient education in primary prevention by chiropractors is lacking during these consultations. A need and willingness to undertake further training was identified which, if put in place, may improve patient education and contribute to improving outcomes in skin cancer.

Clearly the study has limitations. Firstly, generalizability is limited with the inclusion of participants from only two of the three UK chiropractic educational institutions and only one chiropractic association. This means the results may not be representative of the whole UK chiropractic population, although the one association included does comprise 19% of the UK chiropractic practitioner population. Secondly, whilst every effort was made in the research design to discourage participants, the possibility that reference material was used while completing the questionnaire cannot be overlooked.

Conclusion

Visual screening is an important weapon in the arsenal against the rise of malignant skin lesions and is also highly cost effective [16]. Chiropractors serve to positively contribute to this public health problem and the role of the profession should both be articulated and improved in this respect.

This study has shown that not only do chiropractic student clinicians and registered chiropractors feel this screening to be an important part of their role but it also indicates that significant numbers of patients are referred on to specialist care with the potential to importantly reduce mortality and morbidity together with the substantial costs associated with these lesions.

With focused undergraduate training and further post graduate opportunities, chiropractors may feel more confident in detecting suspicious skin lesions and subsequently prove to be increasingly important advocates in the early detection of skin cancer.

Competing interests

The authors declare that they have no competing interests.

Authors' contributions

SG and DN conceived the study. SG collected data and produced first draft. DN provided statistical advice. LB provided advice and assistance on lesion images. AH reviewed and amended initial draft. All authors read and approved the final manuscript.

Author details

[1]McTimoney College of Chiropractic, Abingdon, UK. [2]Anglo European College of Chiropractic (AECC) and Bournemouth University, Dorset, UK. [3]Salisbury NHS Foundation Trust, Salisbury, UK.

References

1. Cancer Research. Cancer Statistics. http://info.cancerresearchuk.org/Cancerstats/Types/Skin 2011a; [Accessed 22/09/11].
2. Morris S, Cox B, Bosanquet N. Cost of skin cancer in England. Eur J Health Econ. 2009;10(3):267–73.
3. Karakousis CP, Emrich LJ, Rao U. Tumor thickness and prognosis in clinical stage I malignant melanoma. Cancer. 1989;64(7):1432–6.
4. Mackie R, Bray C, Leman J. Effect of public education aimed at early diagnosis of malignant melanoma: cohort comparison study. BMJ. 2003;326:367.
5. Rossi C, Vecchiato A, Bezze G, Mastrangelo G, Montesco M, Mocellin S, et al. Early detection of melanoma: an educational campaign in Padova, Italy. Melanoma Res. 2000;10:181–7.
6. Weinstock M, Martin R, Risica P, Berwick M, Lasater T, Rakowski W, et al. Thorough skin examination for the early detection of Melanoma. Am J Prev Med. 1999;17(Issue 3):169–75.
7. Boiko P, Colleagues in Skin Cancer Prevention. The family practitioner, pediatrician, internist, gynaecologist, physician assistant and nurse. Clin Dermatol. 1998;16:467–75. Elsevier Science Inc, New York.
8. Cummings SR, Tripp MK, Herrmann NB. Approaches to the prevention and control of skin cancer. Cancer Metastasis Rev. 1997;16(3):309–27.
9. Greenly L. Guide to detecting skin cancer – Part one. Chiropr Tech. 1997.
10. Greenly L. Guide to detecting skin cancer – Part two. Chiropr Tech. 1998.
11. General Chiropractic Council. Code of Practice and Standard of Proficiency. Gen Chiropr Council. 2005.
12. General Chiropractic Council. Consulting the profession: A survey of UK chiropractors. Gen Chiropr Council. 2004.
13. Ramcharan M, Evans MW, Ndetan H, Beddard J. Knowledge, perceptions, and practices of chiropractic interns in the early detection of atypical moles. J Chiropr Med. 2011;10:77–85.
14. Murphy D, Schneider M, Seaman D, Perle S, Nelson C. How can chiropractic become a respected mainstream profession? The example of podiatry. Chiropr Osteopat. 2008;16:10.
15. Mahon S. Skin cancer prevention: education and public health issues. Semin Oncol Nurs. 2003;19(1):52–61.
16. Losina E, Walensky RP, Geller A, Beddingfield FC, Wolf LL, Gilchrest BA, et al. Visual screening for malignant melanoma: a cost-effective analysis. Arch Dermatol. 2007;143(1):21–8.

11

Application of a diagnosis-based clinical decision guide in patients with low back pain

Donald R Murphy[1,2,3*] and Eric L Hurwitz[4]

Abstract

Background: Low back pain (LBP) is common and costly. Development of accurate and efficacious methods of diagnosis and treatment has been identified as a research priority. A diagnosis-based clinical decision guide (DBCDG; previously referred to as a diagnosis-based clinical decision rule) has been proposed which attempts to provide the clinician with a systematic, evidence-based means to apply the biopsychosocial model of care. The approach is based on three questions of diagnosis. The purpose of this study is to present the prevalence of findings using the DBCDG in consecutive patients with LBP.

Methods: Demographic, diagnostic and baseline outcome measure data were gathered on a cohort of LBP patients examined by one of three examiners trained in the application of the DBCDG.

Results: Data were gathered on 264 patients. Signs of visceral disease or potentially serious illness were found in 2.7%. Centralization signs were found in 41%, lumbar and sacroiliac segmental signs in 23% and 27%, respectively and radicular signs were found in 24%. Clinically relevant myofascial signs were diagnosed in 10%. Dynamic instability was diagnosed in 63%, fear beliefs in 40%, central pain hypersensitivity in 5%, passive coping in 3% and depression in 3%.

Conclusion: The DBCDG can be applied in a busy private practice environment. Further studies are needed to investigate clinically relevant means to identify central pain hypersensitivity, poor coping and depression, correlations and patterns among the diagnostic components of the DBCDG as well as inter-examiner reliability and efficacy of treatment based on the DBCDG.

Keywords: low back pain, diagnosis, therapeutics, practice-based research

Background

Low back pain (LBP) affects approximately 80% of adults at some time in life [1] and occurs in all ages [2,3]. Despite billions being spent on various diagnostic and treatment approaches, the prevalence and disability related to LBP has continued to increase [4]. There has been a recent movement toward comparative effectiveness research [5], i.e., research that determines which treatment approaches are most effective for a given patient population. In addition, there is increased recognition of the importance of practice-based research which generates data in a "real world" environment as a tool for conducting comparative effectiveness research [6,7]. This movement calls for greater participation of private practice environments in clinical research [7].

One of the reasons often given for the meager benefits that have been found with various LBP treatments is that these treatments are generally applied generically, without regard for specific characteristics of each patient, whereas the LBP population is a heterogeneous group, requiring individualized care [8]. Developing a strategy by which treatments can be targeted to the specific needs of patients has been identified as a research priority [9,10].

In recent years there has been a movement away from the biomedical model for understanding the LBP experience toward a biopsychosocial model [11-15]. That is, LBP has increasingly been recognized as involving somatic, neurophysiological and psychological factors

* Correspondence: rispine@aol.com
[1]Rhode Island Spine Center, 600 Pawtucket Avenue, Pawtucket, RI 02860 USA
Full list of author information is available at the end of the article

that all contribute to the clinical picture clinicians encounter. In addition, it has been recognized in recent years that, while there are several individual treatments for LBP that have evidence of effectiveness, the effects sizes of these treatments are generally small [4]. It was been argued that this is likely because patients with LBP have individual needs and taking an approach that identifies the key features in each case, so that treatment can be tailored to those key features, provides the greatest benefit to the patient [16]. However little information is available on the relative efficacy of any particular systematic approach to applying the biopsychosocial model in clinical practice.

A diagnosis-based clinical decision guide (DBCDG) has been proposed for the purpose of guiding clinicians in applying biopsychosocial concepts to the diagnosis and management of patients with LBP [16]. This has been referred to in previous publications as a diagnosis-based clinical decision rule. The approach evolved from the evidence regarding the somatic, neurophysiological and psychological factors that have been found to contribute to suffering in patients with LBP, along with those treatments that have been found to be effective in patients with LBP [17]. It attempts to respond to the challenge of applying the biopsychosocial model and providing individualized treatment programs based on the particular features of each patient.

Cohort studies documenting the outcome of treatment of subsets of LBP patients have been published and the results appear promising [18-20]. However, more research is needed to determine the generalizability of these findings as well as whether they can be replicated in controlled studies. The primary purpose of this study is to document the types of working diagnoses in patients with LBP that are formed by clinicians trained in the use of the DBCDG. This will serve as the basis for further refining the approach in an attempt to improve diagnostic accuracy.

Methods

The study protocol was approved by the Institutional Review Board of New York Chiropractic College (protocol #09-04). It was also reviewed by the Health Insurance Portability and Accountability Act (HIPAA) compliance officer of the facility at which the data were gathered and was deemed to be in compliance with HIPAA regulations. All subjects signed informed consent forms, agreeing to have their data included in the study.

Data were gathered prospectively in consecutive patients seen at the Rhode Island Spine Center between 2/7/08 and 2/26/09.

Participants

Patients were included in the study if they 1) had LBP (defined as pain between the thoracolumbar junction and the buttocks, with or without lower extremity pain; 2) were age 18 years or older; 3) provided informed consent; 4) were able to communicate well in English; 5) had a Bournemouth Disability Questionnaire (BDQ) score of 15 or higher.

Clinical Examination

All examinations were carried out by one of two chiropractic physicians, one with over 20 years experience and the other with over 9 years experience, or by a physical therapist with over 10 years experience. All had a minimum of 50 hours of postgraduate training in the McKenzie method. The physical therapist also had 80 hours of postgraduate training in manual therapy. Several discussions between the examiners took place over the course of five years prior to commencing data gathering on the application of the DBCDG. This occurred in the form of monthly clinical meetings in which the application of the DBCDG in particular patients was discussed as well as recent developments in the literature related to the evaluation and management of patients with LBP. History and examination were performed according to the usual course of patient care at the Rhode Island Spine Center.

Details of the DBCDG are published elsewhere [16,17] but the approach is based on three questions of diagnosis:

1. Are the symptoms with which the patient is presenting reflective of a visceral disorder or a serious or potentially life-threatening disease?
The purpose of this question is to identify signs and symptoms suggestive of non-musculoskeletal problems for which LBP may be among the initial symptoms. Gastrointestinal and genitourinary disorders are included in addition to such "red flag" disorders as infection and malignancy.
2. From where is the patient's pain arising?

With this question the clinician investigates distinguishable characteristics of the pain that may allow treatment decisions to be made. In most cases, the exact tissue of origin cannot be unequivocally determined, however several studies have found that patients can be distinguished based on historical and examination characteristics [21-27] and treatment decisions can be made based on these characteristics [28].

3. What has gone wrong with this person as a whole that would cause the pain experience to develop and persist?

With this question the clinician attempts to identify factors that may serve to perpetuate the ongoing pain experience. These factors may involve somatic, neurophysiologic or psychological processes [16].

Following each new patient encounter the answers to the three questions of diagnosis were documented on a standardized form (see Additional file 1). These data, along with patient demographic data and data from standardized outcome measurement instruments were then entered on a spreadsheet by a chiropractic intern.

The answers to the three questions of diagnosis allows for the development of a working diagnosis (Figure 1) upon which a trial of treatment can be based (Figure 2). The working diagnosis is often multifactorial and may include a combination of biological and psychological processes as well as the social context in which these occur.

In seeking an answer to the first question of diagnosis (rule out visceral or serious disease) standard history and examination procedures were used. In cases in which it was warranted, special tests such as radiographs, MRI or blood tests were ordered.

In seeking answers to the second question of diagnosis (source of the pain), four signs were considered [16,17]:

1. Centralization signs, detected through historical factors that are associated with disc pain [23] and by using the end-range loading examination procedure of McKenzie [29].
2. Segmental pain provocation signs, detected through historical factors that are associated with lumbar facet or sacroiliac pain [23] and through the pain provocation tests of Laslett, et al [22,23,25,30]. Evidence suggest that centralization signs must be ruled out prior to consideration of segmental pain provocation signs [22,30]. Therefore, segmental pain provocation signs were only considered relevant if centralization signs were absent.
3. Neurodynamic signs, detected through historical factors associated with radiculopathy and neurodynamic tests designed to provoke nerve root pain [31-34].
4. Myofascial signs, detected through palpation of myofascial tissues [35]. These signs were only considered relevant if the clinician felt they were separate and distinct from the other signs.

In seeking answers to the third question of diagnosis (perpetuating factors), three factors were considered [16]:

1. Dynamic instability, detected through clinical tests of motor control for the lumbopelvic spine [36-43].
2. Central pain hypersensitivity, detected through observation of pain behavior in response to stimuli as well as through Waddell's nonorganic signs [44]. A threshold of 3/5 nonorganic signs was used as this is the threshold that has been used in previous studies as being significant for the presence of nonorganic pain behavior [45].
3. Psychological factors. Fear beliefs were measured using the 11-item Tampa Scale for Kinesiophobia (TSK) [46]. A score of 27 was considered indicative of clinically meaningful fear beliefs. This number was adapted from Vlaeyen, et al [47] who used a cutoff score 40 using a previous 17-item version of the TSK and Woby (personal communication 3 August, 2009) whose unpublished data suggested a score of 26 to 27 to be associated with clinically meaningful fear beliefs. In addition, two questions from the Coping Strategies Questionnaire [48] which have previously been found to be predictive of changes in disability in LBP patients [49] were used to measure patients' perception of their control over the pain. At the time this study was conducted no data were available regarding whether a particular score with these questions constitutes a threshold for clinically meaningful difficulty with coping strategies. The depression subscale of the BDQ [50] was used to measure depression. As with the coping strategies questions, no data were available at the time of the study by which to determine a threshold for clinical significance with this question.

Each patient completed the full BDQ [50] and the total score from this questionnaire score was recorded. The initial subscale of the BDQ consists of a Numerical Rating Scale for pain intensity (NRS) [51], a scale in which the patient is asked to rate the average intensity of the pain over the past week on a 0-10 scale with "0" representing "no pain" and "10" representing "worst possible pain". This score was also recorded.

Treatments

Treatment was left to the discretion of the primary treating clinician based on the diagnosis, and in general a "team approach" was taken. In the context of the DBCDG, these are the treatments that were applied:

In response to the findings or the second question of diagnosis (source of the pain):

Centralization signs: End range loading maneuvers in the direction that produced centralization [29]. Because centralization signs are believed to reflect disc pain [21], distraction manipulation [52] was also used, as this has been found to decrease intradiscal pressure [53] and has been shown to be helpful in patients with LBP in general [54].

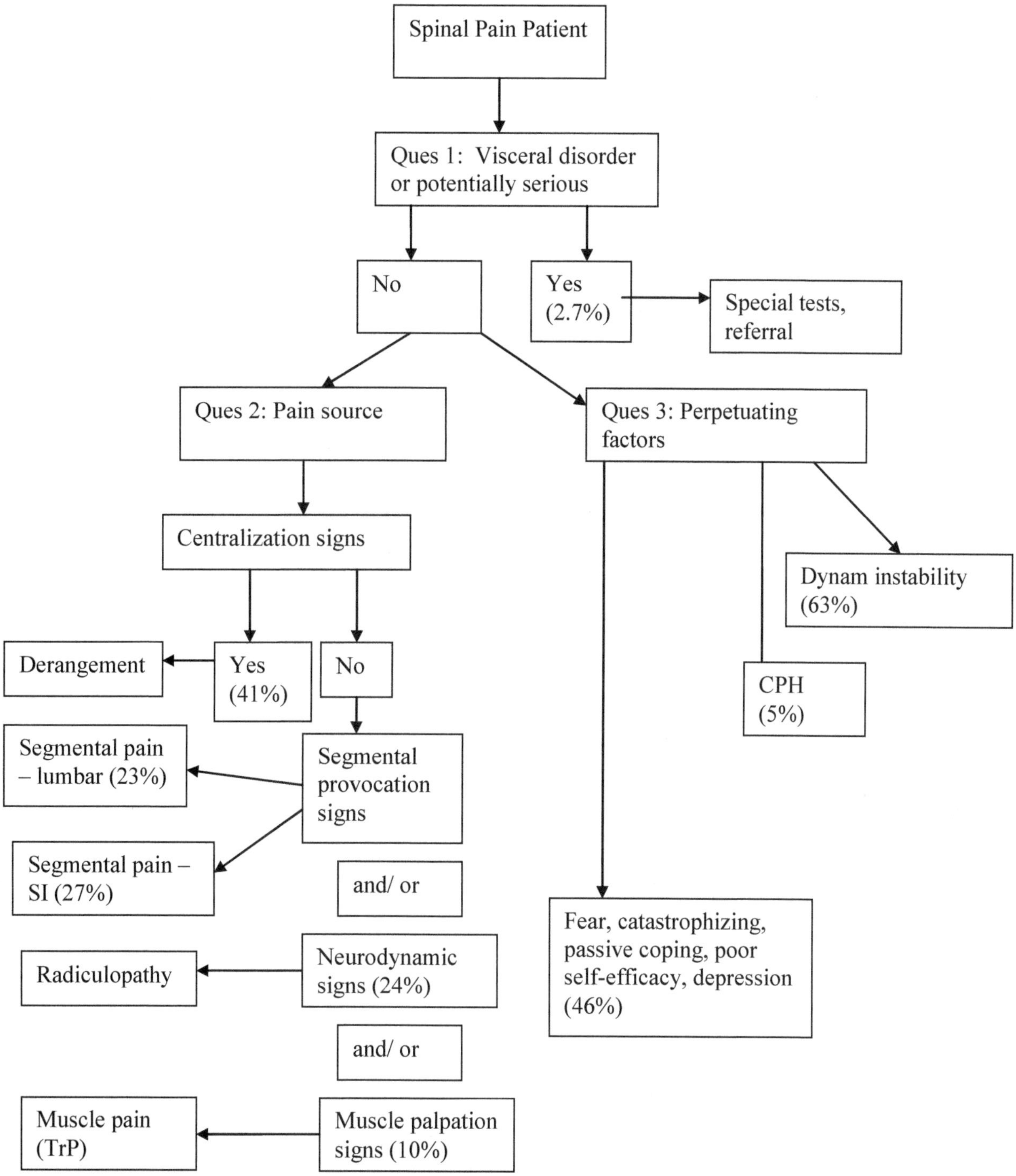

Figure 1 Diagnostic algorithm for the application of the DBCDG. Reprinted with permission from: Murphy DR, Hurwitz EL. A theoretical model for the development of a diagnosis-based clinical decision guide for the management of patients with spinal pain. BMC Musculoskelet Disord 2007;8:75. cerv = cervical; thor = thoracic; lumb = lumbar; SI = sacroiliac; TrP = trigger point; CPH = central pain hypersensitivity; dysfx = dysfunction; catastroph = catastrophizing.

Segmental pain provocation signs: As joint manipulation has been shown to have both neurological [55] and biomechanical [56] segmental effects and has been found to be beneficial in patients with LBP in general [57], this was applied as the treatment of choice in patients with segmental pain provocation signs.

Neurodynamic signs: In the acute stage, anti-inflammatory measures were pursued via referral. This was in

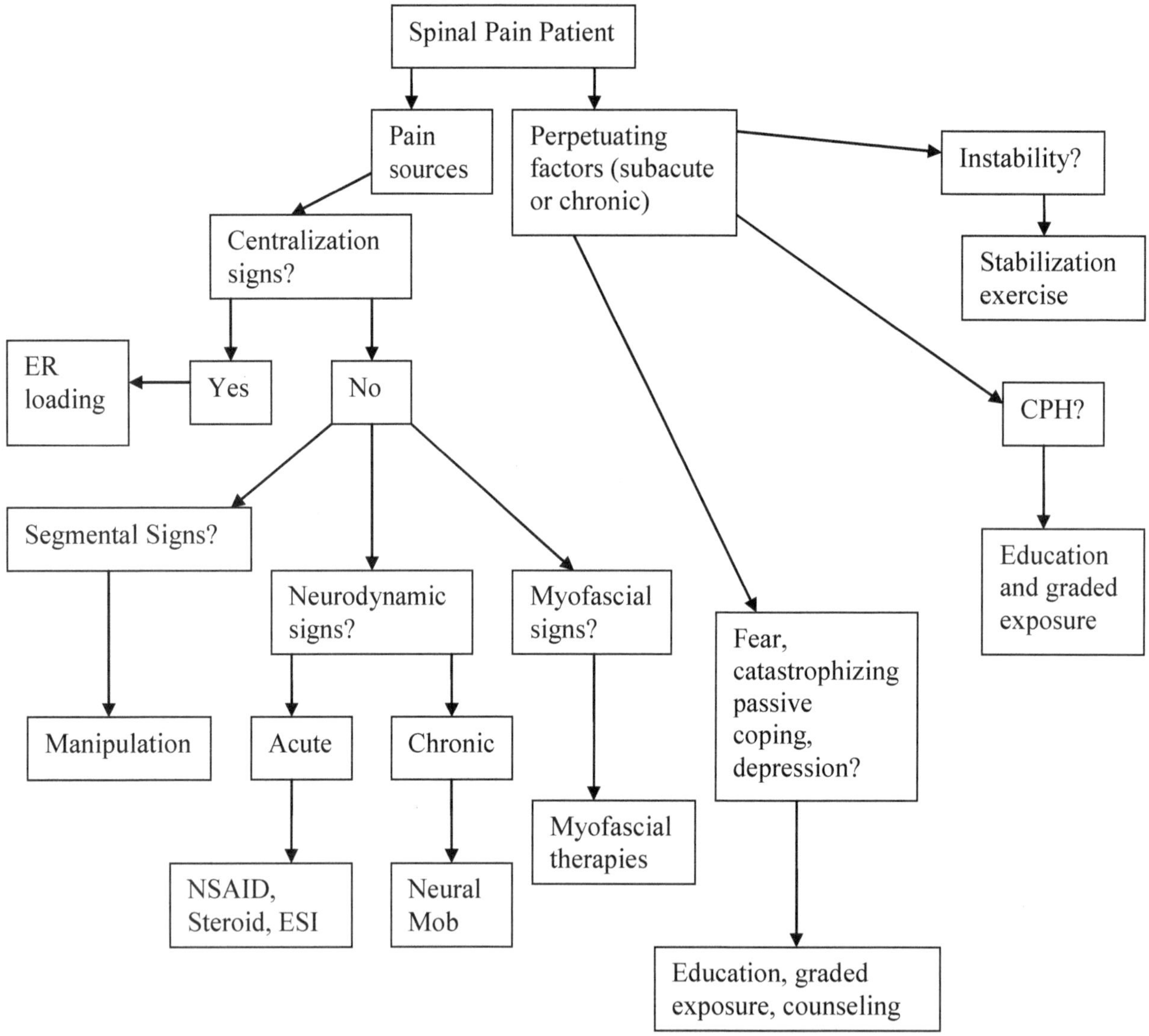

Figure 2 Management algorithm for the application of the DBCDG. Reprinted with permission from: Murphy DR, Hurwitz EL. A theoretical model for the development of a diagnosis-based clinical decision guide for the management of patients with spinal pain. BMC Musculoskelet Disord 2007;8:75. ER = end range; NSAID = non-steroidal anti-inflammatory drugs; ESI = epidural steroid injection; mob = mobilization; CPH = central pain hypersensitivity.

the form of non-steroidal anti-inflammatory medications, oral steroids or epidural steroid injections [58], depending on the diagnosis. In the subacute or chronic stage, neural mobilization was used [59].

Myofascial signs: Myofascial therapies such as ischemic compression and post-isometric relaxation [60] were used if the myofascial signs were deemed clinically relevant by the treating clinician.

In response to the third question of diagnosis (perpetuating factors):

Dynamic instability: Patients diagnosed with dynamic instability were treated with stabilization exercise [61,62].

Central pain hypersensitivity: Education was provided regarding the nature of pain for the purpose of helping the patient understand that the intensity of pain was not related to extensive "tissue damage" [63,64]. In addition, graded exposure [65] was applied in which patients were exposed to movements, positions and activities that provoked their pain to a level they could handle and the stimulus was continued until habituation occurred [66]. Graded exposure was only applied in the subacute or chronic stage, not in acute patients.

Fear, catastrophizing, passive coping, depression, poor self-efficacy: Education was provided for the purpose of correcting misperceptions regarding the nature of pain

[63]. In addition, graded exposure was applied [67]. Occasionally patients were referred for cognitive-behavioral therapy [68].

The treatment algorithm can be found in Figure 2.

Statistical analysis

Descriptive statistics were used to characterize the study population. Frequencies, percentages, and 95% confidence intervals were computed for categorical variables; means, standard deviations, medians, and ranges were computed for continuous variables. Data management and statistical analyses were conducted with Microsoft Excel and SAS (version 9.1, Cary, NC).

Results

Data were gathered on 264 patients, 63% of whom were female. The mean BDQ score was 40 and the mean pain intensity was 7/10. Baseline characteristics are presented in Table 1.

Regarding the first question of diagnosis (rule out visceral or serious disease), 2.7% of patients were positive. Data regarding the second (source of the pain) and third (perpetuating factors) questions of diagnosis are provided in tables 2 and 3, respectively. The most common sign under the second question of diagnosis was centralization (41.1%) followed by sacroiliac segmental pain provocation signs (27.0%). The most common sign under the third question of diagnosis was dynamic instability (63.3%) followed by fear (39.8%).

Discussion

In recent years, spending on the diagnosis and management of patients with LBP has dramatically increased, yet this has not resulted in improved outcomes in terms of patient suffering and disability rates [4]. As such, there is a great need for improved decision making in the care of patients with LBP. Specifically, there is a need to identify characteristics of each individual's condition that allow clinicians to make treatment decisions. In addition there is a great need for research that documents the clinical processes and outcomes that occur in the "real-world" environment of clinical practice as a contributor to comparative effectiveness research [6,7]. This study was part of a broad research strategy to respond to the need for practice-based research by investigating and refining the clinical utility of the DBCDG for patients with LBP. The purpose was to document the types of diagnostic features identified and the frequency of the clinical findings.

Centralization signs were found in 41% of patients. This is similar but slightly lower than the 45-50% prevalence of this sign found in other studies of patients with LBP [21,69,70]. It is substantially lower than the 61.5% prevalence found by Murphy, et al [20] in a population of patients with radiculopathy secondary to herniated disc. In the present study data were only gathered at the initial visit. It has been found that when the determination of the centralization response occurs over the course of several visits, the process is more accurate [71]. Thus, the percentage of patients who were centralizers may be underestimated in the present study.

The prevalence of segmental signs involving the SI joint was 27%. This is similar to the 31% reported by DePalma, et al [72] but substantially higher than the 13% reported by Maigne, et al based on diagnostic injections [73]. This is interesting in that the means of identifying these signs have been found to have high sensitivity and specificity when using injection as a Gold Standard [23,25]. However, these validity studies used single, rather than double, joint blocks. The prevalence of 23% for segmental signs related to the facet joints was within the range of 15-40% reported previously [74] and very similar to the 18% reported by DePalma, et al

Table 1 Baseline characteristics

Variable	Mean (SD)	Median (IQR)	Range
Age (years)	49.0 (16.2)	48.0 (24)	18-86
Duration (days)	912.8 (2639.4)	106.0 (337)	1 day - 54 years
BDQ	40.5 (13.4)	39.0 (20)	14-70
NRS	6.9 (1.9)	7.0 (2)	2-10
Tampa	25.1 (6.1)	25.0 (8)	11-42
Coping	5.6 (2.5)	6.0 (3)	0-12
Depression	4.3 (3.2)	5.0 (6)	0-10

SD = Standard deviation; IQR = Interquartile range; BDQ = Bournemouth Disability Questionnaire; NRS = Numerical Rating Scale (pain); Tampa = Tampa Scale for Kinesiophobia

Table 2 Responses to the second question of diagnosis

Diagnostic sign	Percent (95% CI)
Centralization sign	41.1 (35.1 - 47.0)
Segmental pain provocation sign (lumbar)	23.3 (18.2 - 28.4)
Segmental pain provocation sign (sacroiliac)	27.0 (21.6 - 32.4)
Neurodynamic sign	23.9 (18.7 - 29.0)
Myofascial sign	10.3 (6.6 - 13.9)

CI = confidence interval

Table 3 Responses to the third question of diagnosis

Diagnostic sign	Percent (95% CI)
Dynamic instability (lumbar)	46.6% (95% CI 40.6 - 52.6)
Dynamic instability (pelvic)	16.7 (12.2 - 21.2)
Central pain hypersensitivity	5.3 (2.6 - 8.0)
Fear	39.8 (33.9 - 45.7)
Passive coping	3.0 (1.0 - 5.1)
Depression	3.0 (1.0 - 5.1)

CI = confidence interval

[72]. The prevalence of the diagnosis of muscle palpation signs was low (10%). No prevalence data on myofascial pain is found in the literature, but it is the perception of the clinicians involved in this study, based on discussions over the five years prior to the gathering of these data, that muscle palpation signs are very common but often do not require specific treatment, and that applying treatment based on these signs does not positively impact outcome. This may explain why these signs were deemed clinically relevant in only a small percentage of patients. Further research is needed to investigate this perception. The relatively low prevalence of muscle palpation signs may also reflect the fact that the reliability of palpation to identify myofascial trigger points in the lumbar spine is relatively low [75-77].

There were three factors under the third question of diagnosis (perpetuating factors) for which the prevalence was quite low. Only 5% of patients were identified to have central pain hypersensitivity and only 3% were identified to have each of passive coping and depression. As these factors have been found to be significant in the development of chronic LBP [78-80], it is likely that the low prevalence of the diagnosis of these factors in this study represents under-recognition. However, as the mean duration of pain was only 109 days, it may be that the prevalence would naturally be higher in a cohort of patients with more long-standing pain. Another possibility is that this cohort did not display these features or that a sampling error led to low prevalence. It also may be that the means used in this study to identify these factors were suboptimal. In the case of central pain hypersensitivity, there is no well-established means of identification. Utilizing Waddell's non-organic signs with a threshold of a score of 3/5 may be of insufficient sensitivity to be used as a screening tool for central pain hypersensitivity. In addition, there may be other methods, such as pressure algometry [81], that may be useful in the detection of central pain hypersensitivity. Criteria have been developed by Smart, et al using a Delphi process [82], three factors of which have been found to have discriminative validity for the identification of central pain [83]. This may be a more useful approach than the one taken here and further research is required to investigate this. In the case of passive coping and depression, the scales used to identify these factors had no established threshold score that identifies the presence of clinically meaningful problematic coping strategies and depression. The mean score on the coping strategies questions was 5.6 out of a possible 12 and on the depression subscale on the BDQ was 4.3 out of a possible 10. A recent study found that a baseline coping score of less than 8 had the highest sensitivity and score of less than 4 had the greatest specificity in identifying a LBP patient who is not likely to experience clinically meaningful improvement in pain and disability [84]. These data will be used as the basis for further investigation that attempts to establish thresholds for clinical meaningful coping problems. It is expected that this knowledge will increase the validity of these questions when attempting to identify patients with problematic coping

strategies and depression. Other important psychological factors that are of importance in patients with LBP, such as catastrophizing [85], poor self-efficacy [85], hypervigilance for symptoms [86] and cognitive fusion [87] were not specifically measured. There is some evidence that the various psychological factors interact, rather than occurring in isolation [88-91] and that identification of more than one factor, but not necessarily all factors is adequate [92]. As this was a practice-based research project that is part of the investigation of identification of key elements in the perpetuation of LBP in a "real-world" environment, it was decided that fear, coping and depression would be measured rather than attempting to measure all potentially relevant factors. Further work is needed to determine whether this is a worthwhile approach for clinicians.

This study had several limitations. First, the sample size was only 264 patients. A larger sample would have increased the study's scientific rigor. In addition, all data were gathered at a single clinic and thus it is not known whether the information is generalizable. Also the design was observational and the practitioners were not blinded to the findings on each patient. Finally, because this was a pragmatic study in which data were gathered during the normal course of clinical care detailed information regarding psychological factors was not obtained as this would have required patients to fill out several questionnaires. On the other hand, the fact that this study was carried out in a real-world environment may be a strength, in that it suggests that the information applies to the environment in which patients are most commonly cared for as opposed to the controlled environment of a research center.

Future studies will seek to determine correlations and patterns among the various diagnostic factors, the utility of the coping strategies and depression questions that were used, the inter-examiner reliability of the diagnostic strategy, and ultimately efficacy of the approach. Preliminary data suggests that outcomes in select patients groups may be favorable [18-20,93], but this is based on observational studies without randomization or control.

Conclusion

The DBCDG can be applied in a private practice setting. It appears that patients with LBP can be distinguished on the basis of the findings of this approach, and treatment plans can be formulated based on the diagnosis by utilizing this strategy. Future research is needed to investigate the validity of the questions used in this study to identify problematic coping strategies and depression and to seek improved means of identifying central pain hypersensitivity. Further research is also needed to investigate correlations between the diagnostic findings, reliability of the diagnoses and efficacy of treatment based on the DBCDG.

Additional material

Additional file 1: Standardized form on which the answers to the three questions of diagnosis were documented.

Acknowledgements

This work was originally presented at the Research Agenda Conference, Las Vegas, NV 19 March 2010.

Author details

[1]Rhode Island Spine Center, 600 Pawtucket Avenue, Pawtucket, RI 02860 USA. [2]Department of Health Services, Policy and Practice, Alpert Medical School of Brown University, Providence, RI USA. [3]Department of Research, New York Chiropractic College, Seneca Falls, NY USA. [4]Department of Public Health Sciences, John A. Burns School of Medicine, University of Hawaii at Mānoa, Hawaii USA.

Authors' contributions

DRM originally conceived of the study and served as an examiner. He was also the main writer of the manuscript. ELH was responsible for statistical analysis and writing and editing the manuscript. Both authors read and approved the final manuscript.

Competing interests

The authors declare that they have no competing interests.

References

1. Deyo RA, Phillips WR: **Low back pain a primary care challenge.** *Spine* 1996, **21(24)**:760-765.
2. Hartvigsen J, Christensen K: **Pain in the back and neck are with us until the end: a nationwide interview-based survey of Danish 100-year-olds.** *Spine* 2008, **33(8)**:909-913.
3. Pellise F, Balague F, Rajmil L, Cedraschi C, Aguirre M, Fontecha CG, Pasarin M, Ferrer M: **Prevalence of low back pain and its effect on health-related quality of life in adolescents.** *Arch Pediatr Adolesc Med* 2009, **163(1)**:65-71.
4. Deyo RA, Mirza SK, Turner JA, Martin BI: **Overtreating chronic back pain: time to back off?** *J Am Board Fam Med* 2009, **22(1)**:62-68.
5. Barnett D, Chalkidou K, Rawlins M: **Comparative effectiveness research: a useful tool.** *Health Aff (Millwood)* 2009, **28(2)**:600-601, author reply 601.
6. Horn SD, Gassaway J: **Practice-based evidence study design for comparative effectiveness research.** *Med Care* 2007, **45(10 Supl 2)**:S50-57.
7. Giffin RB, Woodcock J: **Comparative effectiveness research: who will do the studies?** *Health Aff (Millwood)* 2010, **29(11)**:2075-2081.
8. Leboeuf-Yde C, Manniche C: **Low back pain: Time to get off the treadmill.** *J Manipulative Physiol Ther* 2001, **24(1)**:63-66.
9. Borkan JM, Cherkin DC: **An agenda for primary care research on low back pain.** *Spine* 1996, **21(24)**:2880-2884.
10. Bouter LM, van Tulder MW, Koes BW: **Methodologic issues in low back pain research in primary care.** *Spine (Phila Pa 1976)* 1998, **23(18)**:2014-2020.
11. Jones M, Edwards I, Gifford L: **Conceptual models for implementing biopsychosocial theory in clinical practice.** *Man Ther* 2002, **7(1)**:2-9.
12. Pollard H, Hardy K, Curtin D: **Biopsychosocial model of pain and its relevance to chiropractors.** *Chiropr J Aus* 2006, **36(3)**:92-96.
13. Burton AK: **Back injury and work loss: biomechanical and psychosocial influences.** *Spine* 1997, **22(21)**:2575-2580.
14. Peters ML, Vlaeyen JWS, Weber WEJ: **The joint contribution of physical pathology, pain-related fear and catastophizing to chronic back pain disability.** *Pain* 2005, **113(1-2)**:45-50.
15. Waddell G: **The Back Pain Revolution.** Edinburgh: Churchill Livingstone;, 2 2004.
16. Murphy DR, Hurwitz EL: **A theoretical model for the development of a diagnosis-based clinical decision rule for the management of patients with spinal pain.** *BMC Musculoskeletal Disorders* 2007, **8**:75.
17. Murphy DR, Hurwitz EL, Nelson CF: **A diagnosis-based clinical decision rule for patients with spinal pain. Part 2: Review of the literature.** *Chiropr Osteop* 2008, **16**:8.
18. Murphy DR, Hurwitz EL, Gregory AA, Clary R: **A non-surgical approach to the management of lumbar spinal stenosis: a prospective observational cohort study.** *BMC Musculoskelet Disord* 2006, **7**:16.
19. Murphy DR, Hurwitz EL, McGovern EE: **Outcome of pregnancy related lumbopelvic pain treated according to a diagnosis-based clinical decision rule: A prospective observational cohort study.** *J Manipulative Physiol Ther* 2009.
20. Murphy DR, Hurwitz EL, McGovern EE: **A non-surgical approach to the management of patients with lumbar radiculopathy secondary to herniated disc: A prospective observational cohort study with follow up.** *J Manipulative Physiol Ther* 2009, **32(9)**:723-733.
21. Donelson R, Aprill C, Medcalf R, Grant W: **A prospective study of centralization of lumbar and referred pain a predictor of symptomatic discs and anular competence.** *Spine* 1997, **22(10)**:1115-1122.
22. Laslett M, Young SB, Aprill CN, McDonald B: **Diagnosing painful sacroiliac joints: A validity study of a McKenzie evaluation and sacroiliac provocation tests.** *Aus J Physiother* 2003, **49**:89-97.
23. Young S, Aprill C, Laslett M: **Correlation of clinical examination characteristics with three sources of chronic low back pain.** *Spine J* 2003, **3(6)**:460-465.
24. Laslett M, Oberg B, April CN, McDonald B: **Zygapophysial joint blocks in chronic low back pain: a test of Revel's model as a screening test.** *BMC Musculoskel Disord* 2004, **5**:43.
25. Laslett M, Aprill CN, McDonald B, Young SB: **Diagnosis of sacroiliac joint pain: validity of individual provocation tests and composites of tests.** *Man Ther* 2005, **10**:207-218.
26. Laslett M, Birgitta O, Aprill CN, McDonald B: **Centralization as a predictor of provocation discography results in chronic low back pain, and the influence of disability and distress on diagnostic power.** *Spine J* 2005, **5(4)**:370-380.
27. Laslett M, Aprill CN, McDonald B, Oberg B: **Clinical predictors of lumbar provocation discography: a study of clinical predictors of lumbar provocation discography.** *Eur Spine J* 2006, **15(10)**:1473-1484.
28. Long A, Donelson R, Fung T: **Does it matter which exercise? A randomized control trial of exercise for low back pain.** *Spine* 2004, **29(23)**:2593-2602.
29. McKenzie RA, May S: **The Lumbar Spine: Mechanical Diagnosis and Therapy.** Waikenae, NZ: Spinal Publications;, 2 2003.
30. Laslett M, McDonald B, Aprill CN, Tropp H, Oberg B: **Clinical predictors of screening lumbar zygopophyseal joint blocks: development of clinical prediction rules.** *Spine J* 2006, **6(4)**:370-379.
31. Vroomen PCAJ, de Krom CTFM, Knottnerus JA: **Consistency of history taking and physical examination in patients with suspected lumbar nerve root involvement.** *Spine* 2000, **25(1)**:91-97.
32. Hunt DG, Zuberbier OA, Kozlowski AJ, Robinson J, Berkowitz J, Schultz IZ, Milner RA, Crook JM, Turk DC: **Reliability of the lumbar flexion, lumbar extension, and passivve straight leg raise test in normal populations embedded within a complete physical examination.** *Spine* 2001, **26(24)**:2714-2718.
33. Vroomen PCAJ, de Krom MCTFM, Kester ADM, Knottnerus JA: **Diagnostic value of history and physical examination in patients suspected of lumbosacral nerve root compression.** *J Neurol Neurosurg Psychiatry* 2002, **72**:630-633.
34. Lurie J: **What diagnostic tests are useful for low back pain?** *Best Pract Res Clin Rheumatol* 2005, **19(4)**:557-575.

35. Simons DG, Travell JG, Simons LS: **Myofascial Pain and Dysfunction: The Trigger Point Manual.** Baltimore: Williams and Wilkens; 19991.
36. Hicks GE, Fritz JM, Delitto A, Mishock J: **Interrater reliability of clinical examination measures for identification of lumbar segmental instability.** *Arch Phys Med Rehabil* 2003, **84**:1858-1864.
37. Murphy D, Byfield D, McCarthy P, Humphreys K, Gregory A, Rochon R: **Interexaminer reliability of the hip extension test for suspected impaired motor control of the lumbar spine.** *J Manipulative Physiol Ther* 2006, **29(5)**:374-377.
38. Mens JMA, Vleeming A, Snijders CJ, Stam HJ, Ginai AZ: **The active straight leg raising test and mobility of the pelvic joints.** *Eur Spine J* 1999, **8.**
39. Mens JMA, Vleeming A, Snijders CJ, Koes BJ, Stam HJ: **Reliability and validity of the active straight leg raise test in posterior pelvic pain since pregnancy.** *Spine* 2001, **26(10)**:1167-1171.
40. Mens JMA, Vleeming A, Snijders CJ, Koes BW, Stam HJ: **Validity of the active straight leg raise test for measuring disease severity in patients with posterior pelvic pain after pregnancy.** *Spine* 2002, **27(2)**:196-200.
41. Mens JMA, Vleeming A, Snijders CJ, Stam HJ: **Active straight leg raising test: a clinical approach to the load transfer function of the pelvic girdle.** In *Movement, Stability and Low Back Pain The Essential Role of the Pelvis.* Edited by: Vleeming A, Mooney V, Snijders CJ, Dorman TA, Stoeckart R. New York: Churchill Livingstone; 1997:425-431.
42. Roussel NA, Nijs J, Truijen S, Smeuninx L, Stassijns G: **Low back pain: clinimetric properties of the Trendelenburg test, active straight leg raise test, and breathing pattern during active straight leg raising.** *J Manipulative Physiol Ther* 2007, **30(4)**:270-278.
43. O'Sullivan PB, Beales DJ, Beetham JA, Cripps J, Graf F, Lin IB, Tucker B, Avery A: **Altered motor control strategies in subjects with sacroiliac joint pain during the active straight-leg-raise test.** *Spine (Phila Pa 1976)* 2002, **27(1)**:E1-8.
44. Fishbain DA, Cole B, Cutler RB, Lewis J, Rosomoff HL, Rosomoff RS: **A structured evidence-based review on the meaning of nonorganic physical signs (Waddell Signs).** *Pain Med* 2003, **4(2)**:141-181.
45. Kummell BM: **Nonorganic signs of significance in low back pain.** *Spine* 1996, **21(9)**:1077-1081.
46. Woby SR, Roach NK, Urmston M, Watson PJ: **Psychometric properties of the TSK-11: a shortened version of the Tampa Scale for Kinesiophobia.** *Pain* 2005, **117(1-2)**:137-144.
47. Vlaeyen JW, de Jong J, Geilen M, Heuts PH, van Breukelen G: **Graded exposure in vivo in the treatment of pain-related fear: a replicated single-case experimental design in four patients with chronic low back pain.** *Behav Res Ther* 2001, **39(2)**:151-166.
48. Koleck M, Mazaux JM, Rascle N, Brichon-Schweitzer M: **Psycho-social factors and coping strategies as predictors of chronic evolution and quality of life in patients with low back pain: A prospective study.** *Eur J Pain* 2006, **10**:1-11.
49. Woby SR, Watson PJ, Roach NK, Urmston M: **Are changes in fear-avoidance beliefs, catastrophizing, and appraisals of control, predictive of changes in chronic low back pain and disability?** *Eur J Pain* 2004, **8(3)**:201-210.
50. Bolton JE, Breen AC: **The Bournemouth Questionnaire. A short-form comprehensive outcome measure I: Psychometric properties in back pain patients.** *J Manipulative Physiol Ther* 1999, **22(8)**:503-510.
51. Farrar JT, Young JP, LaMoreaux L, Werth JL, Poole RM: **Clinical importance of changes in chronic pain intensity measured on an 11-point numerical pain rating scale.** *Pain* 2001, **94(2)**:149-158.
52. Cox JM: **Low back pain: mechanisms, diagnosis and treatment.** Baltimore: Williams and Wilkens;, 6 1999.
53. Gudavalli MR, Cox JM, Cramer GD, Baker JA, Patwardhan AG: **Intervertebral disc pressure changes during low back treatment procedures.** *BED-Advances in Bioengineering* 1998, **39.**
54. Gudavalli MR, Cambron JA, McGregor M, Jedlicka J, Keenum M, Ghanayem AJ, Patwardhan AG: **A randomized clinical trial and subgroup analysis to compare flexion-distraction with active exercise for chronic low back pain.** *Eur Spine J* 2006, **15(7)**:1070-1082.
55. Pickar JG: **Neurophysiological effects of spinal manipulation.** *Spine J* 2002, **2(5)**:357-371.
56. Cramer GD, Gregerson DM, Knudsen JT, Hubbard BB, Ustas LM, Cantu JA: **The effects of side posture positioning and spinal adjusting on the lumbar Z joints a randomized controlled trial with sixty-four subjects.** *Spine* 2002, **27(22)**:2459-2466.
57. Bronfort G, Haas M, Evans R, Kawchuk G, Dagenais S: **Evidence-informed management of chronic low back pain with spinal manipulation and mobilization.** *Spine J* 2008, **8(1)**:213-225.
58. Abdi S, Datta S, Trescot AM, Schultz DM, Adlaka R, Atluri SL, Smith HS, Manchikanti L: **Epidural steroids in the management of chronic spinal pain: A systematic review.** *Pain Physician* 2007, **10(1)**:185-212.
59. Shacklock M: **Clinical Neurodynamics. A New System of Musculoskeletal Treatment.** Edinburgh: Elsevier; 2005.
60. Vernon H, Schneider M: **Chiropractic management of myofascial trigger points and myofascial pain syndrome: a systematic review of the literature.** *J Manipulative Physiol Ther* 2009, **32(1)**:14-24.
61. Richardson C, Jull G, Hodges P, Hides J: **Therapeutic Exercise For Spinal Segmental Stabilization In Low Back Pain. Scientific Basis and Clinical Approach.** Edinburgh: Churchill Livingstone; 1999.
62. McGill S: **Low Back Disorders. Evidence-Based Prevention and Rehabilitation.** Champaign, IL: Human Kinetics; 2002.
63. Moseley L: **Unraveling the barriers to reconceptualization of the problem in chronic pain: the actual and perceived ability of patients and health professionals to understand the neurophysiology.** *J Pain* 2003, **4(4)**:184-189.
64. Henrotin Y, Cedraschi C, Duplan B, Bazin T, Duquesnoy B: **Information and low back pain management: a systematic review.** *Spine* 2006, **31(11)**: E326-E334.
65. George SZ, Zeppieri G: **Physical therapy utilization of graded exposure for patients with low back pain.** *The Journal of orthopaedic and sports physical therapy* 2009, **39(7)**:496-505.
66. Bingel U, Schoell E, Herken W, Buchel C, May A: **Habituation to painful stimulation involves the antinociceptive system.** *Pain* 2007, **131(1-2)**:21-30.
67. Vlaeyen JW, de Jong J, Geilen M, Heuts PH, van Breukelen G: **The treatment of fear of movement/(re)injury in chronic low back pain: further evidence on the effectiveness of exposure in vivo.** *Clin J Pain* 2002, **18(4)**:251-261.
68. Hoffman BM, Papas RK, Chatkoff DK, Kerns RD: **Meta-analysis of psychological interventions for chronic low back pain.** *Health Psychol* 2007, **26(1)**:1-9.
69. Werneke MW, Hart DL: **Centralization: association between repeated end-range pain responses and behavioral signs in patients with acute non-specific low back pain.** *J Rehabil Med* 2005, **37**:286-290.
70. Long AL: **The centralization phenomenon. Its usefulness as a predictor or outcome in conservative treatment of chronic law back pain (a pilot study).** *Spine (Phila Pa 1976)* 1995, **20(23)**:2513-2520, discussion 2521.
71. Werneke M, Hart DL: **Discriminant validity and relative precision for classifying patients with nonspecific neck and back pain by anatomic pain patterns.** *Spine* 2003, **28(2)**:161-166.
72. Depalma MJ, Ketchum JM, Saullo T: **What is the source of chronic low back pain and does age play a role?** *Pain Med* 2011, **12(2)**:224-233.
73. Maigne JY, Aivaliklis A, Pfefer F: **Results of sacroiliac joint double block and value of sacroiliac pain provocation tests in 54 patients with low back pain.** *Spine (Phila Pa 1976)* 1996, **21(16)**:1889-1892.
74. Bogduk N: **The anatomical basis for spinal pain syndromes.** *J Manipulative Physiol Ther* 1995, **18(9)**:603-605.
75. Njoo KH, Van der Does E: **The occurrence and inter-rater reliability of myofascial trigger points in the quadratus lumborum and gluteus medius: a prospective study in non-specific low back pain patients and controls in general practice.** *Pain* 1994, **58(3)**:317-323.
76. Nice DA, Riddle DL, Lamb RL, Mayhew TP, Rucker K: **Intertester reliability of judgements of the presence of trigger points in patients with low back pain.** *Arch Phys Med Rehabil* 1992, **73**:893-898.
77. Hsieh CY, Hong CZ, Adams AH, Platt KJ, Danielson CD, Hoehler FK, Tobis JS: **Interexaminer reliability of the palpation of trigger points in the trunk and lower limb muscles.** *Arch Phys Med Rehabil* 2000, **81(3)**:258-264.
78. Mercado AC, Carroll LJ, Cassidy D, Cote P: **Passive coping is a risk factor for disabling neck or low back pain.** *Pain* 2005, **117(1-2)**:51-57.
79. DeLeo JA: **Basic science of pain.** *J Bone Joint Surg* 2006, **88-A(Suppl 2)**:58-62.
80. Carroll LJ, Cassidy JD, Cote P: **Depression as a risk factor for onset of an episode of troublesome neck and low back pain.** *Pain* 2004, **107(1-2)**:134-139.
81. Wolfe F, Smythe HA, Yunus MB, Bennett RM, Bombardier C, Goldenberg DL, Tugwell P, Campbell SM, Abeles M, Clark P, *et al*: **The American College of**

Rheumatology 1990 Criteria for the Classification of Fibromyalgia. Report of the Multicenter Criteria Committee. *Arthritis Rheum* 1990, **33(2)**:160-172.
82. Smart KM, Blake C, Staines A, Doody C: **Clinical indicators of 'nociceptive', 'peripheral neuropathic' and 'central' mechanisms of musculoskeletal pain. A Delphi survey of expert clinicians.** *Man Ther* 2010, **15(1)**:80-87.
83. Smart KM, Blake C, Staines A, Doody C: **The Discriminative Validity of "Nociceptive," "Peripheral Neuropathic," and "Central Sensitization" as Mechanisms-based Classifications of Musculoskeletal Pain.** *Clin J Pain* 2011, **27(8)**:655-663.
84. Murphy DR, Hurwitz EL: **Usefulness of a 2-question coping screening tool in patients with low back pain.** *American Academy of Pain Management 21st Annual Clinical Meeting, Exploring the Science Practicing The Art* Las Vegas, NV; 2010.
85. Woby SR, Roach NK, Urmston M, Watson PJ: **The relation between cognitive factors and levels of pain and disability in chronic low back pain patients presenting for physiotherapy.** *Eur J Pain* 2007, **11(8)**:869-877.
86. Leeuw M, Goossens ME, Linton SJ, Crombez G, Boersma K, Vlaeyen JW: **The fear-avoidance model of musculoskeletal pain: current state of scientific evidence.** *J Behav Med* 2007, **30(1)**:77-94.
87. Wicksell RK, Lekander M, Sorjonen K, Olsson GL: **The Psychological Inflexibility in Pain Scale (PIPS)–statistical properties and model fit of an instrument to assess change processes in pain related disability.** *Eur J Pain* 2010, **14(7)**:771, e771-714.
88. Vlaeyen JWS, Kole-Snijders AMJ, Boeren RGB, van Eek H: **Fear of movement/reinjury in chronic low back pain and its relation to behavioral performance.** *Pain* 1995, **62**:363-372.
89. Boersma K, Linton S: **Psychological processes underlying the development of a chronic pain problem. A prospective study of the relationship between profiles of psychological variables in the fear-avoidance model and disability.** *Clin J Pain* 2006, **22**:160-166.
90. Woby SR, Urmston M, Watson PJ: **Self-efficacy mediates the relation between pain-related fear and outcome in chronic low back pain patients.** *Eur J Pain* 2007, **11(7)**:711-718.
91. Turk DC: **Understanding pain sufferers: the role of cognitive processes.** *Spine J* 2004, **4(1)**:1-7.
92. Murphy DR, Hurwitz EL: **The usefulness of clinical measures of psychological factors in patients with spinal pain.** *J Manipulative Physiol Ther* 2011.
93. Murphy DR, Hurwitz EL, Gregory AA, Clary R: **A nonsurgical approach to the management of patients with cervical radiculopathy: A prospective observational cohort study.** *J Manipulative Physiol Ther* 2006, **29(4)**:279-287.

12

Brief screening questions for depression in chiropractic patients with low back pain: identification of potentially useful questions and test of their predictive capacity

Alice Kongsted[1,2*], Benedicte Aambakk[2], Sanne Bossen[2] and Lise Hestbaek[1,2]

Abstract

Background: Depression is an important prognostic factor in low back pain (LBP) that appears to be infrequent in chiropractic populations. Identification of depression in few patients would consequently implicate screening of many. It is therefore desirable to have brief screening tools for depression. The objective of this study was to investigate if one or two items from the Major Depression Inventory (MDI) could be a reasonable substitute for the complete scale.

Methods: The MDI was completed by 925 patients consulting a chiropractor due to a new episode of LBP. Outcome measures were LBP intensity and activity limitation at 3-months and 12-months follow-up. Single items on the MDI that correlated strongest and explained most variance in the total score were tested for associations with outcome. Finally, the predictive capacity was compared between the total scale and the items that showed the strongest associations with outcome measures.

Results: In this cohort 9% had signs of depression. The total MDI was significantly associated with outcome but explained very little of the variance in outcome. Four single items performed comparable to the total scale as prognostic factors. Items 1 and 3 explained the most variance in all outcome measures, and their predictive accuracies in terms of area under the curve were at least as high as for the categorised complete scale.

Conclusions: Baseline depression measured by the MDI was associated with a worse outcome in chiropractic patients with LBP. A single item (no. 1 or 3) was a reasonable substitute for the entire scale when screening for depression as a prognostic factor.

Keywords: Chiropractic, Depression, Questionnaires, Low back pain, Primary health care

Introduction

Pain and depression often co-exist [1-3], and although the causal relation between the two is not clear [4,5], evidence suggests that pain negatively affects outcome in depression as well as vice versa [6].

Low back pain (LBP) is a highly frequent pain condition with a substantial impact on global health [7] for which the risk of a poor prognosis is increased in the presence of depression [8,9]. It is a condition for which there is no generally effective treatment, but non-pharmacological treatment addressing psychological symptoms in addition to the physical symptoms has been demonstrated to improve outcome in LBP patients with high scores on psychological questions [10].

Chiropractors see a large number of LBP patients who appear to be a population with relatively low frequency of severe psychological distress [11-13]. Nevertheless, a substantial proportion with borderline depressive scores has been observed [12]. Therefore, to improve care and to predict prognosis, it may be important to identify psychological factors, including depression, among those

* Correspondence: a.kongsted@nikkb.dk
[1]The Nordic Institute of Chiropractic and Clinical Biomechanics, Campusvej 55, 5230 Odense, M, Denmark
[2]Department of Sports Science and Clinical Biomechanics, University of Southern Denmark, Odense, Denmark

seeking care for LBP, also in chiropractic practice. For that purpose screening instruments generally perform better than clinical impressions [14,15], and a number of questionnaires screening for depression exist [16]. The Major Depression Inventory is thoroughly validated as a diagnostic screening instrument [17,18] and has been shown to be feasible in chiropractic care [13]. However, it is unknown if the MDI predicts outcome in chiropractic patients.

Despite the potential implications for management and prognosis, routine screening for psychological factors is not widely implemented [19] and has met some resistance from clinicians [20]. One reason might be that the questionnaires are too extensive for routine clinical use where information on a variety of other prognostic factors is also relevant to collect. This is especially true in chiropractic practice where the subpopulation with depressive symptoms is small [11-13], and therefore the identification of these relatively rare cases involves screening of many for whom it has no relevance.

If systematic screening for depression is to be implemented, there is a need for a very short and easily completed tool. Fair to good diagnostic accuracies of one- and two-item screening tools with full questionnaires for depression as reference standards have been demonstrated [21-23]. It is unknown whether observed variations are due to differences between screening questions or between screened populations, and it is possible that suitable screening questions differ between populations. Furthermore, the usefulness of brief screening questions for prediction of prognosis is unrevealed.

The aim of this study was to investigate whether the MDI is predictive of outcome in chiropractic practice and if so, whether one or two items from the MDI could potentially be used as an ultra-short tool for capturing depressive symptoms in LBP patients seeking chiropractic care. To obtain that we tested whether the total MDI was associated with 3- and 12-months outcomes, explored which single items of the MDI correlated best with the total score, and compared the predictive capacity of these items to that of the total MDI.

Method

The study was incorporated in a previously described cohort study with data collection occurring at seventeen chiropractic clinics in the research network of the Nordic Institute for Chiropractic and Clinical Biomechanics in Denmark [24]. Patients completed questionnaires in the reception area prior to the first consultation due to a new episode of LBP. Follow-up questionnaires were mailed after 3 and 12 months. Treatment was unaffected by study participation and the chiropractors were free to choose the treatment they found appropriate. It was confirmed by The Regional Scientific Ethical Committees for Southern Denmark that the study did not need ethics approval according to Danish rules [25].

Participants

Consecutive patients aged 18–65 years attending chiropractic practice for the first time due to their current episode of LBP, and who could read Danish were potential participants. Patients were not included if inflammatory or pathological pain were suspected, in case of nerve root involvement requiring acute referral to surgery, if pregnant, or if having had more than one health care consultation due to LBP within the previous 3 months. Patients were excluded if pathology was diagnosed as the reason for LBP during the course of the study.

Measurements

Depression was measured by the MDI consisting of twelve items answered by choosing one of 6 response options from 'At no time' (= 0) to 'All the time' (= 5) [17] (Additional file 1). When using the MDI as a depression rating scale ten of the twelve items are used for the total score. Only the highest score on the items 8a and 8b is included since these are considered opposites (feeling restless and feeling slowed down) and similarly only the highest score on items 10a and 10b (reduced appetite and increased appetite) is included. This results in a sum score ranging from 0 to 50 that are categorised into 'no depression' (score of 0 – 19), 'mild depression' (score of 20 – 24), 'moderate depression' (score of 25 – 29), and 'severe depression' (score of 30 – 50) [18].

At baseline, patients also responded to questions regarding LBP duration (0–2 weeks, 2–4 weeks, 1–3 months, >3 months), number of previous episodes (0, 1–3, >3), LBP intensity (Numeric rating scale (NRS) 0–10 [26]), leg pain intensity (NRS 0–10), and activity limitation (Roland Morris Disability Questionnaire (RMDQ) proportional score 0–100 [27,28]).

Outcome measures were LBP intensity (NRS 0–10) and the RMDQ proportional score (0–100) after 3 and 12 months.

Data analysis

Data were entered twice in EpiData [29]. Analyses were performed in STATA/SE 12.1 (STATA Corp, College Station, Texas, USA). No imputations were made, and sixteen subjects (1.7%) were excluded from the analyses due to missing values on one or more MDI items.

Associations between the MDI and outcome were investigated in linear regression models after categorisation of MDI since the sum score had a non-linear relation with outcome measures.

The identification of potential prognostic screening items was performed in two steps: (1) We identified the single items that best reflected the sum score of the scale by calculating the Spearman correlation between each item and the total score and the variance explained (R-squared) in a linear regression model with the MDI sum score as dependent variable and the single item as the independent variable. These were considered 'candidate items'. (2) The associations between the candidate items and outcomes at 3-months and 12-months follow-up were then tested by means of linear regression, and the prognostic capacity was compared in terms of effect sizes (β-coefficients) and amount of variance in the outcome explained by the item (R-squared). Responses "Most of the time" and "All the time" were collapsed for this purpose due to few observations in these categories.

To report more clinically interpretable results the predictive abilities of the two preferred candidates, quantified as area under the ROC curve (AUC) and likelihood ratios (LH+/LH-), were compared to that of the total MDI when predicting 'persistent pain' (LBP intensity > 0) and 'persistent activity limitation' (RMDQ >8% corresponding to >2 points on the 24-item RMDQ [30]. For the total MDI, we considered all of mild, moderate, and severe depression as a positive test, since these categories were quite small. On the single items scores 2–5 were considered signs of depression based on ROC-curves and favouring a high sensitivity. Each single item was tested by itself, and the two best screening questions were combined defining a patient as depressed if scoring 2–5 on any of the two questions.

Results

Participants

The study cohort consisted of 925 patients (45% females, mean age 43 years) who had completed the MDI. Those excluded because of missing MDI items were 3.6 years older than participants, more often females, and their LBP had less frequently lasted for more than 4 weeks. No differences were observed on LBP severity or on the completed MDI items. Follow-up was completed by 731 (79%) and 684 (74%) after 3 and 12 months, respectively. Non-responders were more often males, were on average 5 years younger, and had slightly higher MDI scores (1.5 points) than those participating in follow-up. Patient characteristics are summarised in Table 1.

MDI scores

Scores on the MDI were generally low (median 6, IQR 3–11) and 91% were categorised as non-depressed. The mild, moderate, and severe depression categories included respectively 4%, 3%, and 2% of participants. Single items were answered with "At no time" in 23% (Item 3: Lack of energy and strength) to 94% (Item 6: Life not worth living) of the cohort. Signs of depression were associated with female gender, younger age, and a more severe LBP profile (Table 1).

Associations between the MDI sum score and outcome

The categorised MDI had statistically significant associations with LBP intensity and activity limitation at 3-months and 12-months follow-up (all $p < .05$). However, the effects, especially regarding pain outcomes, were small, and the amount of variance in the outcome explained by MDI was very low (Table 2).

Associations between the MDI total score and single items

Correlation coefficients between single items and the full MDI and the variance explained in total MDI by each item appear from Table 3. Items 2 (Have you lost interest in your daily activities?), 3 (Have you felt lacking energy and strength?), and 8 (Have you felt restless/Have you felt subdued or slowed down?) were considered candidates for brief screening questions based on the

Table 1 Baseline characteristics of the cohort separated according to signs of depression

	Total cohort n = 925	No depression n = 843	Mild to severe depression n = 82	p-value*
Females	45%	43%	61%	<0.01
Age, mean (sd)	43 (12)	44 (12)	40 (12)	<0.01
Duration of LBP				<0.01
0-2 weeks	62%	65%	39%	
2-4 weeks	13%	13%	21%	
1-3 months	11%	11%	10%	
>3 months	14%	12%	30%	
>3 previous LBP episodes	49%	48%	57%	0.10
LBP intensity, median (IQR)	7 (5–8)	7 (5–8)	8 (6–8)	<0.01
Leg pain >0	56%	54%	72%	<0.01
RMDQ, mean (sd)	51 (24)	50 (24)	65 (20)	<0.01

*p-value for test of no difference between 'no depression' and 'mild to severe depression' the duration of LBP categories for non-depressed sum to 101% due to rounding of figures.

Table 2 Associations between the total MDI scale and outcomes and between five candidate items and outcomes

	β coefficients (95% CI)			
	LBP 3-months	LBP 12-months	RMDQ 3-months	RMDQ 12-months
Total MDI scale				
MDI categorised	Adj. $R^2 = 0.03$	Adj. $R^2 = 0.01$	Adj. $R^2 = 0.03$	Adj. $R^2 = 0.02$
No depression (reference)				
Mild depression	1.59 (.91; 2.27)	.96 (.17; 1.74)	13.14 (5.59;20.68)	6.94 (−.36;14.24)
Moderate depression	.89 (.01; 1.78)	1.08 (.08; 2.08)	18.19 (8.64;27.74)	13.26 (4.13;22–38)
Severe depression	.78 (−.45; 2.02)	1.24 (−.21; 2.69)	18.45 (4.67; 32.23)	15.11 (1.90;28.32)
Single candidate items				
Item 1: Low in spirits or sad	Adj. $R^2 = 0.03$	Adj. $R^2 = 0.04$	Adj. $R^2 = 0.06$	Adj. $R^2 = 0.03$
At no time (reference)				
Some of the time	0.53 (0.24; 0.82)	0.52 (0.19; 0.84)	7.15 (3.99; 10.31)	4.88 (1.89; 7.86)
Slightly less than half the time	0.26 (−0.55; 1.08)	0.44 (−0.44; 1.33)	7.41 (−1.48; 16.31)	5.42 (−2.86; 13.71)
Slightly more than half the time	0.80 (0.08; 1.51)	0.32 (−0.52; 1.15)	16.05 (8.35; 23.75)	6.45 (−1.19; 14.09)
Most or all of the time	1.61 (0.71; 2.41)	2.32 (1.39; 3.24)	25.13 (15.81; 34.45)	19.45 (10.98; 27.93)
Item 2: Lost interest	Adj. $R^2 = 0.02$	Adj. $R^2 = 0.03$	Adj. $R^2 = 0.05$	Adj. $R^2 = 0.02$
At no time (reference)				
Some of the time	0.16 (−0.14; 0.47)	0.55 (0.21; 0.90)	5.25 (1.90; 8.60)	4.76 (1.63; 7.89)
Slightly less than half the time	0.98 (0.40; 1.56)	1.00 (0.36; 1.65)	16.58 (10.23; 22.93)	6.15 (0.25; 12.06)
Slightly more than half the time	0.34 (−0.23; 0.91)	0.67 (0.01; 1.33)	9.18 (3.00; 15.36)	8.81 (2.79; 14.84)
Most or all of the time	0.86 (0.17; 1.55)	0.76 (−0.01; 1.54)	13.85 (6.30; 21.40)	7.60 (0.51; 14.70)
Item 3: Lacking energy	Adj. $R^2 = 0.04$	Adj. $R^2 = 0.05$	Adj. $R^2 = 0.09$	Adj. $R^2 = 0.05$
At no time (reference)				
Some of the time	0.15 (−0.20; 0.49)	0.46 (0.07; 0.84)	3.92 (0.18; 7.65)	1.72 (−1.80; 5.23
Slightly less than half the time	0.67 (0.15; 1.19)	1.07 (0.49; 1.65)	12.26 (6.65; 17.88)	7.73 (2.46; 13.00)
Slightly more than half the time	0.76 (0.24; 1.28)	0.78 (0.17; 1.38)	14.34 (8.75; 19.93)	10.91 (5.37; 16.46)
Most or all of the time	1.33 (0.83; 1.82)	1.50 (0.93; 2.06)	20.71 (15.37; 26.05)	13.79 (8.64; 18.93)
Item 4: Felt less self-confident	Adj. $R^2 = 0.01$	Adj. $R^2 = 0.02$	Adj. $R^2 = 0.04$	Adj. $R^2 = 0.02$
At no time (reference)				
Some of the time	0.41 (0.07; 0.75)	0.38 (0.00; 0.76)	4.64 (0.92; 8.36)	4.02 (0.54; 7.50)
Slightly less than half the time	0.54 (−0.21; 1.29)	0.85 (−0.10; 1.79)	9.99 (1.88; 18.11)	9.10 (0.66; 17.54)
Slightly more than half the time	0.70 (−0.06; 1.47)	0.54 (−0.35; 1.42)	15.67 (7.41; 23.93)	7.72 (−0.35; 15.78)
Most or all of the time	1.12 (0.23; 2.02)	1.88 (0.88; 2.88)	16.83 (6.98; 26.69)	16.05 (6.91; 25.18)
Item 8: Restless or slowed down	Adj. $R^2 = 0.02$	Adj. $R^2 = 0.005$	Adj. $R^2 = 0.04$	Adj. $R^2 = 0.01$
At no time (reference)		*		
Some of the time	−0.03 (−0.35; 0.29)	0.27 (−0.10; 0.63)	3.76 (0.23; 7.28)	3.26 (−0.07; 6.60)
Slightly less than half the time	0.13 (−0.42; 0.69)	0.35 (−0.26; 0.95)	6.41 (0.29; 12.53)	5.42 (−0.09; 10.94)
Slightly more than half the time	0.09 (−0.45; 0.62)	0.40 (−0.21; 1.02)	5.98 (0.10; 11.86)	4.94 (−0.73; 10.60)
Most or all of the time	1.25 (0.66; 1.84)	0.86 (0.18; 1.54)	19.13 (12.67; 25.60)	8.27 (2.02; 14.53)

*All associations between items and outcomes and total MDI and outcomes were statistically significant ($p < .05$) except for the association between item 8 and LBP at 12-months. Confidence intervals that span across zero indicate that this particular category was not significantly different from the reference.

correlation coefficients, and in addition item 1 (Have you felt low in spirits or sad?) and item 4 (Have you felt less self-confident) were included in the analyses of prognostic capacity because they had R-squared values equal to that of item 8.

Associations between single candidate items and outcome

All candidate items were significantly associated with the outcome measures except for item 8 in relation to LBP intensity at 12-months (Table 2). Effect sizes were

Table 3 Correlations between the total MDI score and single items and amount of variance in the MDI score explained by each item

	Spearman's rho	R-squared
Item 1	.66	.56
Item 2	.72	.59
Item 3	.77	.62
Item 4	.63	.56
Item 5	.61	.48
Item 6	.34	.25
Item 7	.59	.42
Item 8	.74	.56
Item 9	.62	.35
Item 10	.56	.36

All correlations and regression models were statistically significant ($p < .001$).

comparable to those of the categorised total MDI, and, as for the total scale, little of the variance in the outcomes was explained. For all outcome measures items 1 and 3 explained the most variance and were considered the best choices as brief screening questions although not performing pronouncedly better than other candidate questions.

Prediction of outcomes by the brief screening questions as compared to the total MDI

Patients with signs of depression had more frequently persistent pain at 3-months follow-up regardless of whether the definition of depression was based on the total MDI, item 1, item 3, or items 1 and 3 combined (Figure 1). However, the predictive accuracy of depression was low with all definitions (AUC: 0.52 to 0.57). A slight increase in the predictive accuracy was gained by combining items 1 and 3 as compared to using only one of them. The positive likelihood ratio, i.e. the increase in risk of a poor prognosis associated with depression, was higher for the total MDI scale than for single items, whereas a combination of items 1 and 3 performed best regarding the negative likelihood ratio, i.e. identification of those with reduced risk of a poor prognosis.

Depression predicted activity limitation more accurately than it predicted pain (Figure 2), but the accuracies were low, also regarding activity limitation (AUC: 0.54 to 0.62). Item 3 performed somewhat better than the total MDI score due to a lower negative likelihood ratio. Very little was achieved by combining items 1 and 3.

Predictions of 12-months outcomes were very similar to those of 3-months outcome and are not reported.

Discussion

Our main finding was that item 1 (feeling low in spirits or sad) and item 3 (lacking energy and strength) of the MDI were reasonable alternatives to the total scale when ultra-brief screening questions are needed. In addition we found that depression measured by the MDI was associated with prognosis in patients with LBP, but prediction of outcome had low accuracy.

As in previous studies [11-13] depression was not frequent in this cohort of patients seeking chiropractic care for LBP. Therefore it was not surprising that depression on its own did not predict outcome with any certainty given that a high number of factors appear to influence

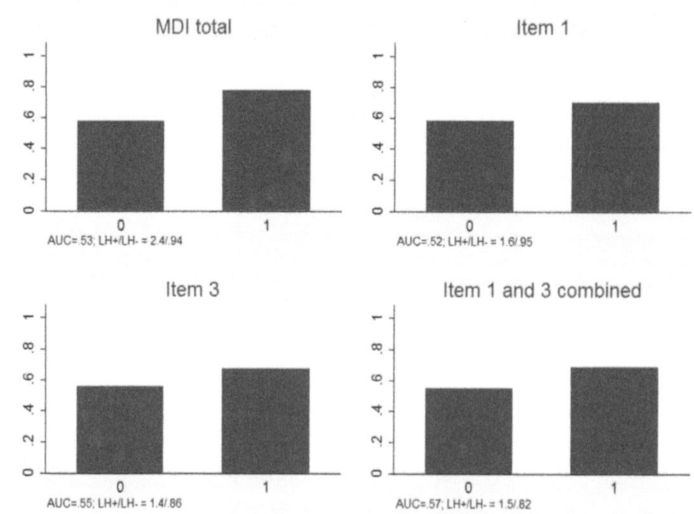

Figure 1 Proportion of patients with persistent pain at 3-months follow-up in depressed (1) and non-depressed (0) according to four ways of screening. AUC = Area under the curve. LH + = Positive likelihood ratio. LH- = Negative likelihood ratio.

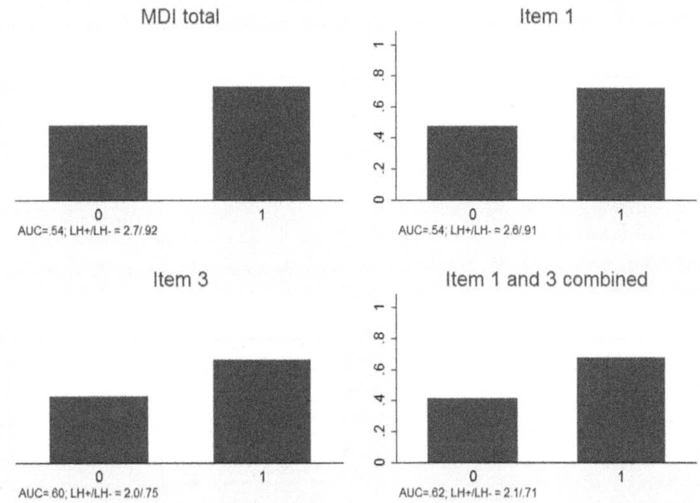

Figure 2 Proportion of patients with persistent activity limitations at 3-months follow-up in depressed (1) and non-depressed (0) according to four ways of screening. AUC = Area under the curve. LH + = Positive likelihood ratio. LH- = Negative likelihood ratio.

the course of LBP [8]. One previous study investigating depression as a prognostic factor in chiropractic patients with LBP used the Hospital Anxiety and Depression Scale and found that depression was associated with outcome but not an independent predictor [12]. It was not within the scope of this paper to investigate whether MDI scores were independently associated with outcome. Moreover, it was not investigated if cognitive elements were included in treatment for patients with signs of depression which may reduce the predictive value of depression.

A recent study demonstrated substantial overlap between depression and pain-related psychological factors such as anxiety, self-efficacy, and kinesiophobia, and the combined construct of pain-related emotional distress was an important indicator of risk of poor prognosis in patients from general practice [31]. To examine complex psychological constructs in large clinical cohorts, simple ways of collecting information on each element are essential.

We suggest that items 1 and 3 from the MDI or the two in combination can be used as reasonable substitutes for the MDI scale, although we recognise that items 2 and 4 performed almost correspondingly. With the applied categorisation of MDI, the recommended items predicted activity limitation as well as the total MDI did and were only slightly less accurate in the prediction of pain. The accuracy in terms of AUC and the negative likelihood ratio favoured item 3 slightly over item 1, whereas item 1 should be preferred if positive predictive value is the main priority.

A 2-item screening test for depression taken from the Primary Care Evaluation of Mental Disorders Procedure (PRIME-MD) has previously been recommended for physical therapist treating LBP [15]. The PRIME-MD questions "During the past month, have you often been bothered by feeling down, depressed, or hopeless?" and "During the past month, have you often been bothered by little interest or pleasure in doing things?" reflects the same aspects of depression as MDI items 1 and 2. However, our results indicated that in the investigated setting, item 3 should be preferred to item 2. This was likely due to item 3 having high scores considerably more frequently than item 2 in our cohort. Also 1-item questions simply asking if patients feel depressed [22], or to what extent they have felt depressed during the last month [23], appear useful for diagnostic screening. However, none of these questions were tested as prognostic factors and future research in this area should provide direct comparisons of existing brief screening questions.

This study was based on a large sample from ordinary clinical practice with rather complete data available. Drop-out rates of 21% and 26% at follow-up was a limitation, and slightly higher MDI scores at baseline in those who dropped out may have resulted in underestimation of the effect of depression on outcome. However, there is no reason to believe that single items would be affected differently by drop-outs than the total scale, and we do not consider drop-out a major issue in relation to the aim of this study.

Another limitation was the categorisation of the MDI which reduced the available information but was performed since the continuous measure did not fit a linear model. We used a previously validated categorisation as this was believed to best mirror the general use of the MDI, but it is possible that other cut-points would be preferable in this population. Smoothened linear plots of outcomes as a function of the MDI sum score gave no obvious reason to alter the categorisation. It was deemed necessary to combine mild to severe depression for the calculations of the predictive capacity of the MDI which may have lowered the accuracy. However, this did not affect the choice of questions to be used for a brief screening tool.

We presented results on combining items 1 and 3 with *or* (i.e. any of the two should be positive) which increased the accuracy of prediction activity limitation slightly. In order to increase the specificity of the screening questions it would appear logical to combine the two items by *and* (i.e. both should be positive), but with the applied cut-point nothing was achieved by that.

We chose to prioritise sensitivity when dichotomising the items since we consider an increased attention on potential psychological issues in patients for whom it is irrelevant less problematic than not being aware of depressive symptoms in those for whom it matters. The cut-point had no implications for the identification of the best screening items and could be altered if wanting a lower number of false positives.

In conclusion, signs of depression were infrequent in this LBP cohort seeking chiropractic care. Depression was associated with outcome but not a major explanation of poor prognosis. Single items of the MDI performed almost as good as prognostic factors as did the entire scale and items 1 or 3 can be used as alternatives to the total scale when a brief screening tool is needed. Head-to-head comparisons with other screening questions for depression are needed in order to recommend one rather than another. In short, depression is of importance in LBP when present but not prevalent in chiropractic practice. Therefore we recommend screening for depression with a very brief tool. This could be item 1 or item 3 from the MDI.

Additional file

Additional file 1: Major (ICD-10) depression inventory.

Competing interests
The authors have no financial or non-financial competing interests to declare. The Foundation for Chiropractic Research and Post Graduate Education, Denmark funded the study and is continuously financing the Nordic Institute of Chiropractic and Clinical Biomechanics.

Authors' contributions
AK formed the study idea. All authors were involved in the design of the study, interpretation of data, revision of the manuscript, and all gave final approval of the manuscript. AK performed the data analysis and wrote the initial draft of the manuscript.

Acknowledgements
The authors want to thank participating patients, clinicians in the research network of the Nordic Institute for Chiropractic and Clinical Biomechanics, and the Foundation for Chiropractic Research and Post Graduate Education.

References
1. Bener A, Verjee M, Dafeeah EE, Falah O, Al-Juhaishi T, Schlogl J, Sedeeq A, Khan S: **Psychological factors: anxiety, depression, and somatization symptoms in low back pain patients.** *J Pain Res* 2013, **6**:95–101.
2. Bair MJ, Robinson RL, Katon W, Kroenke K: **Depression and pain comorbidity: a literature review.** *Arch Intern Med* 2003, **163**(20):2433–2445.
3. Schneider E, Linden M, Weigmann H, Wagner T, Quail D, Hundemer HP, Hegerl U: **Early reduction in painful physical symptoms is associated with improvements in long-term depression outcomes in patients treated with duloxetine.** *BMC Psychiatry* 2011, **11**:150.
4. Fishbain DA, Cutler R, Rosomoff HL, Rosomoff RS: **Chronic pain-associated depression: antecedent or consequence of chronic pain? A review.** *Clin J Pain* 1997, **13**(2):116–137.
5. Gambassi G: **Pain and depression: the egg and the chicken story revisited.** *Arch Gerontol Geriatr* 2009, **49**(Suppl 1):103–112.
6. Kroenke K, Wu J, Bair MJ, Krebs EE, Damush TM, Tu W: **Reciprocal relationship between pain and depression: a 12-month longitudinal analysis in primary care.** *J Pain* 2011, **12**(9):964–973.
7. Vos T, Flaxman AD, Naghavi M, Lozano R, Michaud C, Ezzati M, Shibuya K, Salomon JA, Abdalla S, Aboyans V, *et al*: **Years lived with disability (YLDs) for 1160 sequelae of 289 diseases and injuries 1990–2010: a systematic analysis for the Global Burden of Disease Study 2010.** *Lancet* 2012, **380**(9859):2163–2196.
8. Kent PM, Keating JL: **Can we predict poor recovery from recent-onset non-specific low back pain? A systematic review.** *Man Ther* 2008, **13**(1):12–28.
9. Melloh M, Elfering A, Kaser A, Salathe CR, Barz T, Aghayev E, Roder C, Theis JC: **Depression impacts the course of recovery in patients with acute low-back pain.** *Behav Med* 2013, **39**(3):80–89.
10. Hill JC, Whitehurst DG, Lewis M, Bryan S, Dunn KM, Foster NE, Konstantinou K, Main CJ, Mason E, Somerville S, *et al*: **Comparison of stratified primary care management for low back pain with current best practice (STarT Back): a randomised controlled trial.** *Lancet* 2011, **378**(9802):1560–1571.
11. Langworthy JM, Breen AC: **Psychosocial factors and their predictive value in chiropractic patients with low back pain: a prospective inception cohort study.** *Chiropr Osteopath* 2007, **15**:5.
12. Leboeuf-Yde C, Rosenbaum A, Axen I, Lovgren PW, Jorgensen K, Halasz L, Eklund A, Wedderkopp N: **The Nordic subpopulation research programme: prediction of treatment outcome in patients with low back pain treated by chiropractors–does the psychological profile matter?** *Chiropr Osteopath* 2009, **17**:14.
13. Kongsted A, Johannesen E, Leboeuf-Yde C: **Feasibility of the STarT back screening tool in chiropractic clinics: a cross-sectional study of patients with low back pain.** *Chiropr Man Ther* 2011, **19**:10.
14. Schade CP, Jones ER Jr, Wittlin BJ: **A ten-year review of the validity and clinical utility of depression screening.** *Psychiatr Serv* 1998, **49**(1):55–61.
15. Haggman S, Maher CG, Refshauge KM: **Screening for symptoms of depression by physical therapists managing low back pain.** *Phys Ther* 2004, **84**(12):1157–1166.
16. Smarr KL, Keefer AL: **Measures of depression and depressive symptoms: beck depression inventory-II (BDI-II), center for epidemiologic studies depression scale (CES-D), geriatric depression scale (GDS), hospital anxiety and depression scale (HADS), and patient health questionnaire-9 (PHQ-9).** *Arthritis Care Res (Hoboken)* 2011, **63**(Suppl 11):S454–466.
17. Bech P, Rasmussen NA, Olsen LR, Noerholm V, Abildgaard W: **The sensitivity and specificity of the major depression inventory, using the present state examination as the index of diagnostic validity.** *J Affect Disord* 2001, **66**(2–3):159–164.
18. Olsen LR, Jensen DV, Noerholm V, Martiny K, Bech P: **The internal and external validity of the major depression inventory in measuring severity of depressive states.** *Psychol Med* 2003, **33**(2):351–356.
19. Kent PM, Keating JL, Taylor NF: **Primary care clinicians use variable methods to assess acute nonspecific low back pain and usually focus on impairments.** *Man Ther* 2009, **14**(1):88–100.
20. Shaw EJ, Sutcliffe D, Lacey T, Stokes T: **Assessing depression severity using the UK quality and outcomes framework depression indicators: a systematic review.** *Br J Gen Pract* 2013, **63**(610):e309–317.

21. Mirkhil S, Kent PM: **The diagnostic accuracy of brief screening questions for psychosocial risk factors of poor outcome from an episode of pain: a systematic review.** *Clin J Pain* 2009, **25**(4):340–348.
22. Ayalon L, Goldfracht M, Bech P: **'Do you think you suffer from depression?' Reevaluating the use of a single item question for the screening of depression in older primary care patients.** *Int J Geriatr Psychiatry* 2010, **25**(5):497–502.
23. Reme SE, Eriksen HR: **Is one question enough to screen for depression?** *Scand J Public Health* 2010, **38**(6):618–624.
24. Eirikstoft H, Kongsted A: **Patient characteristics in low back pain subgroups based on an existing classification system. A descriptive cohort study in chiropractic practice.** *Man Ther* 2014, **19**(1):65–71.
25. Danish National Commitee on Biomedical Research Ethics: **Guidelines about Notification.** http://www.cvk.sum.dk/English/guidelinesaboutnotification.aspx.
26. Jensen MP, Karoly P, O'Riordan EF, Bland F Jr, Burns RS: **The subjective experience of acute pain. An assessment of the utility of 10 indices.** *Clin J Pain* 1989, **5**(2):153–159.
27. Kent P, Lauridsen HH: **Managing missing scores on the Roland Morris disability questionnaire.** *Spine (Phila Pa 1976)* 2011, **36**(22):1878–1884.
28. Albert HB, Jensen AM, Dahl D, Rasmussen MN: **Criteria validation of the roland morris questionnaire. A danish translation of the international scale for the assessment of functional level in patients with low back pain and sciatica.** *Ugeskr Laeger* 2003, **165**(18):1875–1880.
29. Lauritsen JM: *EpiData data entry. Data management and basic statistical analysis system.* Odense, Denmark: The EpiData Association; 2008.
30. Kamper SJ, Maher CG, Herbert RD, Hancock MJ, Hush JM, Smeets RJ: **How little pain and disability do patients with low back pain have to experience to feel that they have recovered?** *Eur Spine J* 2010, **19**(9):1495–1501.
31. Campbell P, Bishop A, Dunn KM, Main CJ, Thomas E, Foster NE: **Conceptual overlap of psychological constructs in low back pain.** *Pain* 2013, **154**(9):1783–1791.

13

Do MRI findings identify patients with chronic low back pain and Modic changes who respond best to rest or exercise: a subgroup analysis of a randomised controlled trial

Rikke K. Jensen[1*], Peter Kent[1,2] and Mark Hancock[3]

Abstract

Background: No previous clinical trials have investigated MRI findings as effect modifiers for conservative treatment of low back pain. This hypothesis-setting study investigated if MRI findings modified response to rest compared with exercise in patients with chronic low back pain and Modic changes.

Methods: This study is a secondary analysis of a randomised controlled trial comparing rest with exercise. Patients were recruited from a specialised outpatient spine clinic and included in a clinical trial if they had chronic low back pain and an MRI showing Modic changes. All patients received conservative treatment while participating in the trial. Five baseline MRI findings were investigated as effect modifiers: Modic changes Type 1 (any size), large Modic changes (any type), large Modic changes Type 1, severe disc degeneration and large disc herniation. The outcome measure was change in low back pain intensity measured on a 0–10 point numerical rating scale at 14-month follow-up ($n = 96$). An interaction ≥ 1.0 point (0–10 scale) between treatment group and MRI findings in linear regression was considered clinically important.

Results: The interactions for Modic Type 1, with large Modic changes or with large Modic changes Type 1 were all potentially important in size (−0.99 (95 % CI −3.28 to 1.29), −1.49 (−3.73 to 0.75), −1.49 (−3.57 to 0.58), respectively) but the direction of the effect was the opposite to what we had hypothesized—that people with these findings would benefit more from rest than from exercise. The interactions for severe disc degeneration (0.74 (−1.40 to 2.88)) and large disc herniation (−0.92 (3.15 to 1.31)) were less than the 1.0-point threshold for clinical importance. As expected, because of the lack of statistical power, no interaction term for any of the MRI findings was statistically significant.

Conclusions: Three of the five MRI predictors showed potentially important effect modification, although the direction of the effect was surprising and confidence intervals were wide so very cautious interpretation is required. Further studies with adequate power are warranted to study these and additional MRI findings as potential effect modifiers for common interventions.

Background

In most patients with low back pain (LBP), the cause of pain cannot be definitively attributed to a specific pathology and patients are therefore labelled as having 'non-specific LBP'. Non-specific LBP is estimated to be approximately 85 % of LBP in primary care [1]; however, most clinicians believe that it is not one condition but consists instead of several different subgroups. They also treat non-specific LBP differently depending on patterns of signs and symptoms [2] and preliminary results suggest that targeting treatment to LBP subgroups might be more effective than generic 'one-size-fits all' approaches [3].

There are many ways to potentially classify non-specific LBP into treatment-relevant subgroups, one of which is to use pathoanatomic findings seen on Magnetic Resonance Imaging (MRI). Although there is little evidence for the clinical relevance of most MRI findings, some, such as

* Correspondence: rikke.kruger.jensen@rsyd.dk
[1]Research Department, Spine Centre of Southern Denmark, Hospital Lillebaelt, Institute of Regional Health Research, University of Southern Denmark, Oestre Hougvej 55, 5500 Middelfart, Denmark
Full list of author information is available at the end of the article

Modic changes, have been shown to be associated with LBP. A systematic review in 2008 [4] that investigated this relationship found positive associations between the presence of Modic changes and LBP in seven of 10 studies, with odds ratios ranging from 2 to 20. In addition, a stronger association with pain for Modic changes Type 1 than for other types was shown by Thompson et al. [5], who reported a higher positive predictive value for pain generation during discography for Modic changes Type 1 (0.81) than for Type 2 (0.64) or Type 3 (0.57).

Exercise therapy is a management strategy for non-specific LBP that is guideline-recommended and widely used [6]. As patients' pathoanatomical source of pain is most likely diverse, it may be that MRI findings can identify subgroups of patients with chronic non-specific LBP who benefit more from exercise therapy than others. For example, on theoretical grounds, patients with chronic LBP and Modic changes could be a subgroup of patients that would be less likely to benefit from exercise, as the histology of Modic changes has shown fissured and disrupted endplates [7] that might indicate less tolerance of additional, exercise-induced, loading of the spine.

Based on the hypothesis that rest and reduction of spinal load would lead to better healing of the bone and subsequent reduction in pain, a two-group randomised controlled trial (RCT) investigated if rest was more effective than exercise [8] for people with Modic changes. The results showed no difference between the two treatment outcomes on pain, disability, quality of life or any other outcome measures immediately post-treatment (10 weeks) and at 14-month follow-up. A limitation of those results was that all patients had some type of Modic change, so it was not possible to determine if the presence of any Modic change acted as an effect modifier. However, we also collected information on the type and size of Modic changes as well as the presence or absence of other MRI findings such as disc herniation and disc degeneration. These data now provide the unique opportunity to investigate if the type or size of Modic changes, or the presence or absence of other MRI findings, acted as effect modifiers. To our knowledge, MRI findings have not previously been tested as effect modifiers for response to conservative interventions in an RCT, which seems a major gap in our knowledge.

Therefore, the purpose of this hypothesis-setting, secondary analysis was to investigate if MRI findings modified the treatment response to rest or exercise in patients with chronic LBP and Modic changes.

Method

Study design

This secondary analysis was performed using data from a (two-group) RCT that investigated the effect of rest compared with exercise in patients with chronic LBP and Modic changes. To increase the validity of this subgroup analysis, it was performed using the approach recommended by Sun et al. [9] which included pre-specification of both the direction of subgroup effects and the hypotheses underlying them, and the investigation of only a limited number of subgroups.

Study population

Patients were recruited from a specialised outpatient spine clinic, the Spine Centre of Southern Denmark, where they had been referred by medical practitioners and chiropractors in primary care for investigation of non-response to conservative care. From August 2007 to December 2008, MRI was routinely performed on all patients meeting the following criteria: (i) no contraindications for MRI, (ii) LBP or leg pain of at least 3 on a 0–10 point Numerical Rating Scale (NRS), (iii) duration of current symptoms from 2 to 12 months, and (iv) age above 18 years.

Patients with an MRI showing Modic changes (Type 1, 2 or 3) that extended beyond the endplate into the vertebral body underwent a clinical examination and were invited to participate in the study unless they met any of the following exclusion criteria: (i) unable to participate in the project because of other physical or mental conditions, (ii) had symptoms and clinical signs of lumbar nerve root compression (e.g. leg pain dominating over back pain, positive straight-leg-raise test or neurological deficit), or (iii) had undergone previous spinal surgery with no pain relief after the operation.

Randomisation and intervention

Patients were allocated to one of the two intervention groups (rest or exercise) by means of computerised minimisation software [10]. In total, 100 patients were included and of those, 49 were randomised to the rest group and 51 to the exercise group.

The rest group was instructed to avoid physically demanding activity and to rest twice daily for 1 h, by lying down. The patients participated in a group meeting once every second week to imitate the treatment session structure of the exercise group and thereby, the potential non-specific effect of being in a group. The exercise group received exercises for the stabilising muscles in the low back and abdomen together with dynamic exercises, exercises for postural instability and light physical fitness training. The patients exercised in a group once a week and were instructed to do additional home exercises three times a week. The duration of the interventions was 10 weeks and follow-up data were obtained at the end of this period (post-treatment at 10 weeks) and at 14 months after baseline. At 14 months, follow-up data on 96 participants were available (96 %). For the flow of the trial, see

Fig. 1. Full details of the recruiting procedure and interventions have previously been reported [8].

Outcomes

Current back pain measured on a 0–10 point NRS [11] was the primary outcome in the original trial, collected via self-reported questionnaire. For this secondary analysis, the change in current back pain between baseline and 14-month follow-up was chosen a priori as the treatment outcome, as this enabled the marginal means to be calculated for each subgroup.

Variables of interest

MRIs were obtained at baseline. The MRI system was a 0.2 T (Magnetom Open Viva; Siemens AG, Erlangen, Germany) and a body spine surface coil was used with the patient in the supine position. The imaging protocol consisted of sagittal and axial T1- and T2-weighted sequences. The evaluation of the MRI changes (L1 to S1) was performed by an experienced musculoskeletal radiologist using standardised evaluation protocols [12, 13]. Previous evaluation of the use of these protocols by the same radiologist had shown substantial to almost perfect reproducibility with Kappa values from 0.73 to 1.0 for the Modic change variables [12] and from moderate to almost perfect with values from 0.59 to 0.97 for the disc-related changes [13]. The radiologist was blinded to any patient information except for name, age and sex.

Five potential effect modifiers for treatment with either rest or exercise were chosen from the baseline MRI variables and limited to that number to reduce the risk of type I error. The potential effect modifiers of interest were (i) type of Modic changes (Type 1 compared with not having Type 1 changes), (ii) size of Modic changes (large Modic changes compared with small), (iii) large Modic Type 1 changes (large Modic changes Type 1 compared with not having this finding), (iv) disc degeneration (severe disc degeneration compared with not having this finding) and (v) disc herniation (large disc herniations compared with not having this finding). The rationales for these variables are reported in Table 1.

The definition of a patient being positive for *Modic changes Type 1* was the presence of a Type 1 finding on at least one of the 11 lumbar endplates and regardless of other types present on the same or other segmental levels. A patient was classified as being positive for *large Modic changes* if they had any type of Modic change, of ≥25 % of vertebral height on at least one of the 11 lumbar endplates regardless of other Modic changes present on other segmental levels. *Large Modic changes Type 1* was defined as having at least one Modic change which was both Type 1 and ≥25 % of vertebral height. In the MRI protocol [13], 'disc height' was graded from 0 to 3 and 'disc signal intensity' was graded from 0 to 3 (with higher numbers indicating more severe changes). For the purpose of this study, *severe disc degeneration* was defined as one or more discs with either (i) 'disc height' = grade 3, or (ii) the combination of 'disc height' = grade 2 and 'disc signal intensity' = grade 3 within the same disc. Disc herniations was evaluated according to the same MRI protocol [13], and for the purpose of this study, patients were classified as being positive for *large disc herniation* if they had one or more disc herniations categorised as broad-based protrusion, extrusion or a sequestration independent of the status of the other discs.

Analysis

Data were analysed by linear regression models performed separately for each of the five potential effect modifiers. The dependent variable was change score in pain on a 0–10 point NRS (baseline score minus 14-month follow-up score). Each model included the treatment group variable, the potential effect modifier and the

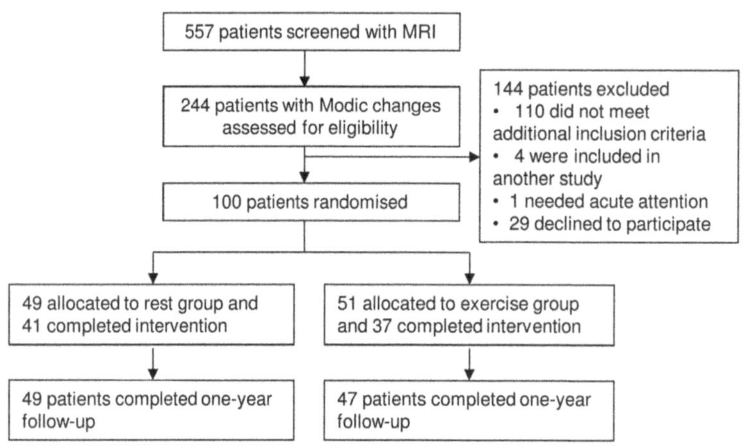

Fig. 1 Flow of patients within the study

Table 1 Rationale for variables

Modic changes Type 1 (compared with not having Type 1)

The histology of Type 1 shows fissured endplates and vascular granulation tissue adjacent to the endplate [7] and could potentially be an early state of bone healing. Therefore, we hypothesised that patients with Modic changes Type 1 would benefit more from rest than from exercise, as rest would facilitate bone healing compared with the compression forces added from exercise.

Large modic changes (compared with small ones)

Kuisma et al. [26] found that extensive Modic changes (≥25 % of vertebral height) were associated with a higher pain score in a working population. Large Modic changes could represent larger disruptions of the endplate and vertebral body and might therefore signal a better outcome from rest than from exercise.

Large modic changes Type 1 (compared with not having this finding)

Based on the hypotheses mentioned above for Modic type and size, we expected that people with large Modic changes Type 1 would benefit more from rest than from exercise.

Severe disc degeneration (compared with not having this finding)

Hancock et al. [27] reported that disc degeneration grade of ≥3 (Pfirrmann grade 1–5) was more than 5 times more likely to be present in patients with acute LBP than in controls without current LBP. Severe disc degeneration and mild disc degeneration could respond differently to conservative treatment. However, the available evidence does not clearly indicate a direction of a potential subgroup effect. Patients with severe disc degeneration could benefit from exercise due to the overall positive effects of physical activity. On the other hand, exercise could lead to increased load on a degenerated joint which could potentially result in a negative outcome.

Large disc herniation (compared with not having this finding)

Patients with LBP and sciatica receiving active conservative treatment [28] who also had broad-based protrusions and extrusions ('large' herniations) had a better outcome in leg pain and physical function than patients with disc bulges or focal protrusions. However, the evidence is sparse and it is possible that 'large' herniations could benefit either from the general effects of exercise or from less load with rest.

interaction term between the two. The interaction term was used to quantify size of the effect modification.

It has been estimated that the detection of a statistically significant subgroup interaction effect in an RCT requires a sample size approximately four times that required to detect a main effect of the same size [14]. Previous authors have suggested secondary analysis of RCTs as an approach to develop hypotheses for potentially important effect modifiers that can then be tested in suitably large trials [15]. As the current hypothesis-setting study was clearly underpowered, our focus was on the estimated effect size rather than statistical significance. If the interaction was greater than the threshold for MCID of 1.0 NRS points identified by Lauridsen et al. [16], we further explored the clinical interpretation by assessing the effect of intervention (rest compared with exercise) separately for those positive for the subgroup and negative for the subgroup, by calculating the marginal means for the subgroups. In addition, the number of patients achieving a MCID >1.0 point on a 0–10 NRS was calculated for those patients who were subgroup negative or positive.

Ethics

This analysis was based on existing data collected for an RCT [8] approved by the Ethics Committee for the Region of Southern Denmark (approval # S-VF-20060111), registered in ClinicalTrials.gov (Identifier # NCT00454792) and performed following the Declaration of Helsinki principles. For all participants in the original RCT signed informed consent was obtained as required by the Ethics Committee for the Region of Southern Denmark. In Denmark, such secondary analysis does not require additional ethics approval (The Act on Processing of Personal Data, December 2012, Section 5.2; Act on Research Ethics Review of Health Research Projects, October 2013, Section 14.2).

Results

Data from 49 patients in the rest group and 47 in the exercise group were available from the original RCT and were used for these analyses. The mean age was 46 years (range 21–60) and 69 % were women.

Participants in both treatment groups had similar sociodemographic and clinical characteristics at baseline, including age, sex, body mass index, type of occupation, sick leave, pain, activity limitation, general health, depression and expectations of treatment effect. Also, the distributions of the MRI variables of interest were similar between the two groups (Table 2). Distribution of the MRI variables per disc level is shown in Additional file 1.

In the regression analyses, the interaction terms for type of Modic changes (Modic Type 1 compared with not having Type 1), size of Modic changes (large changes compared with small ones) and large Modic changes Type 1 (compared with not having this finding) were all greater than or approximated the 1.0-point threshold for clinical importance (Table 3). However, although we hypothesized that patients with these characteristics would benefit more from rest than from exercise, the direction of the effect was the opposite for all three variables. For example, the effect of rest versus exercise was less in participants with

Table 2 Distribution of MRI variables in the treatment groups

		Rest	Exercise	*p*-value
Modic changes Type 1	Yes	38	36	0.91
	No	11	11	
Large Modic changes (any type)	Yes	34	33	0.93
	No	15	14	
Large Modic changes Type 1	Yes	28	28	0.81
	No	21	19	
Severe disc degeneration	Yes	18	18	0.88
	No	31	29	
Large disc herniation	Yes	13	19	0.15
	No	36	28	

Table 3 Results of linear regression models for change score in pain at 14-month follow-up

	Beta coefficient	*p*-value	95 % confidence interval
Modic changes Type 1			
Treatment[a]	0.82	0.42	−1.19;2.82
Modic changes Type 1	−1.79	0.03	−3.41; −0.17
Interaction: Modic Type 1 & treatment	*−0.99*	*0.39*	*−3.28;1.29*
Constant	2.09	0.004	0.67;3.51
Large Modic changes (any type)			
Large Modic changes	1.23	0.13	−0.37;2.84
Treatment	1.08	0.26	−0.80;2.95
Interaction: large Modic changes & treatment	*−1.49*	*0.19*	*−3.73;0.75*
Constant	−0.14	0.83	−1.49;1.20
Large Modic changes Type 1			
Large Modic changes Type 1	0.07	0.93	−1.42;1.55
Treatment	0.89	0.27	−0.70;2.47
Interaction: large Modic changes Type 1 & treatment	*−1.49*	*0.16*	*−3.57;0.58*
Constant	0.68	0.24	−0.46;1.83
Severe disc degeneration			
Severe disc degeneration	−0.002	0.998	−1.53;1.52
Treatment	−0.24	0.78	−1.55;1.07
Interaction: severe disc degeneration & treatment	*0.74*	*0.50*	*−1.40;2.88*
Constant	0.72	0.13	−0.22;1.67
Large disc herniation			
Large disc herniation	0.73	0.34	−0.78;2.24
Treatment	0.38	0.56	−0.90;1.66
Interaction: large disc herniation & treatment	*−0.92*	*0.42*	*−3.15;1.31*
Constant	0.43	0.38	−0.53;1.39

[a]Rest compared with exercise

large Modic changes than in those with small Modic changes; the point estimate and 95 % CI for the interaction was −1.49 (−3.73 to 0.75). The interaction terms for disc degeneration and disc herniation did not meet the threshold for clinical importance (Table 3). As expected, none of the interaction terms for any of the MRI findings was statistically significant, most likely due to the small sample size.

As the interaction terms for type of Modic changes, size of Modic changes and large Modic changes Type 1 were larger than or approximated the 1.0-point threshold for clinical importance, therefore we further explored treatment effects for those in the subgroup compared with those not in the subgroup (Table 4). Patients with Modic changes Type 1 were 0.17 points (95 % CI −1.28 to 0.93) worse with rest than exercise, while those without Modic changes Type 1 were 0.82 points (−1.23 to 2.86) better with rest (Table 4). Patients with large Modic changes were 0.41 (−1.62 to 0.79) points worse with rest, while those without large Modic changes were 1.08 points better with rest (−0.97 to 3.12). Similar findings were identified for patients with large Modic changes Type 1 compared with those without this finding (Table 4). We also present the findings as the number of patients achieving an MCID in the subgroups in Table 5. As an example, of those with Modic changes Type 1, 7 % fewer patients reached the MCID if they received rest compared with exercise, while in those without Modic Type 1 changes, 9 % more reached the MCID if they received rest compared with exercise.

A graphical display of the comparison of outcome in pain for the two treatment groups for the three potential effect modifiers reaching the threshold of 1.0 point, together with treatment effect for those in the subgroup or not in the subgroup (i.e. MRI finding positive vs. MRI finding negative) and interaction effect is shown in Figs. 2, 3 and 4.

Discussion

Statement of principal findings

To our knowledge, this is the first study investigating MRI findings as effect modifiers for response to conservative interventions in a LBP RCT. Although none of the interaction terms for any of the MRI findings tested were statistically significant, Modic changes Type 1, large Modic changes and large Modic changes Type 1 showed tentative evidence of effect modification that was potentially important in size (point estimates ranging from −0.99 to −1.49 on the NRS). Surprisingly, the direction of the effect modification was opposite to those specified in our hypothesis and this is further reason for caution when interpreting the findings. That all three results were consistently in the direction opposite to our hypothesis suggests the notion, that exercise would aggravate physically larger or early stage Modic changes, may have been biologically plausible but overly simplistic. Although this study was underpowered, thereby increasing the risk of the results being due to chance, it suggests which of these potential effect modifiers might be analysed in subsequent studies and provides data suitable for calculating sample sizes for such studies.

Strengths and weaknesses of the study

A strength of the current study is that it was based on data from an RCT, which is the definitive type of data in which to quantify effect modification [17]. In addition, the MRIs were reported using a standardised protocol by a radiologist who had previously demonstrated consistency in evaluating spinal pathologies and was blinded to both the treatment group and the clinical outcome, however, in

Table 4 Change in pain at 14-month follow-up in the two treatment groups

	Rest (mean (95% CI))	Exercise (mean (95% CI))	Treatment effect[a] (mean (95% CI))
Modic changes Type 1	0.13 (−0.62;0.88)	0.31 (−0.47;1.08)	−0.17 (−1.28;0.93)
No Modic changes Type 1	2.91 (1.51;4.31)	2.09 (0.69;3.49)	0.82 (−1.23;2.86)
Modic changes large (≥25 %)	0.68 (−0.18;1.53)	1.09 (0.22;1.96)	−0.41 (−1.62;0.79)
Modic changes small (<25 %)	0.93 (−0.35;2.22)	−0.14 (−1.47;1.19)	1.08 (−0.97;3.12)
Large Modic changes Type 1 (≥25 %)	0.14 (−0.79;1.08)	0.75 (−0.18;1.68)	−0.61 (−1.82;0.61)
No large Modic changes Type 1	1.57 (0.49;2.65)	0.68 (−0.45;1.82)	0.89 (−0.93;2.70)

Change in pain (95 % CI) at 14-month follow-up on a 0–10 point NRS in the two treatment groups for type of Modic changes, size of Modic changes and large Modic changes Type 1
[a]Rest compared with exercise

other settings and with other MRI variables the reliability could vary. Our choice of MRI variables as potential effect modifiers was not exhaustive and other variables could have been potentially important. However, as recommended by Sun et al. [9], we limited the number of variables to cautiously selected potential effect modifiers with, whenever possible, pre-specified assumptions about the direction of the effect. The hypotheses were built on the literature but, as this was often sparse, the likely direction of the effect was not always obvious a priori and we took the pragmatic view that an effect modifier might have potential importance regardless of the direction of the effect. A limitation to the generalisability of the results is that patients in the study population all had some type of Modic changes.

In a study by Bendix et al. [18] investigating Modic changes using low-field MRI (0.3 T) compared with high-field MRI (1.5 T), the authors found a difference in the prevalence rate, with Modic changes Type 1 being detected three times more often using low field MRI, whereas Type 2 was detected two times more often when using high field MRI. As the MRI system used in the current study was low-field (0.2 T), this may have affected the observed prevalence of Type 1 and 2, but it is unknown whether one MRI approach is more accurate than the other or simply more sensitive and less specific. In addition, using only T1- and T2-weighted sequences to identify the type of Modic change may add to the uncertainty of identifying Modic changes Type 1, as this is optimally visualised using a fluid sensitive (STIR) sequence which was not used in the current study.

Table 5 Number of patients achieving a Minimal Clinical Important Difference

Subgroup	Rest	Exercise	Treatment effect
Modic changes Type 1	24 % ($n = 9$)	31 % ($n = 11$)	7 % fewer patients in the rest group achieved MCID
No Modic changes Type 1	64 % ($n = 7$)	55 % ($n = 6$)	9 % more patients in the rest group achieved MCID
Modic changes large (≥25 %)	32 % ($n = 11$)	39 % ($n = 13$)	7 % fewer patients in the rest group achieved MCID
Modic changes small (<25 %)	33 % ($n = 5$)	29 % ($n = 4$)	4 % more patients in the rest group achieved MCID
Large Modic changes Type 1 ((≥25 %)	25 % ($n = 7$)	36 % ($n = 10$)	11 % fewer patients in the rest group achieved MCID
No large Modic changes Type 1	43 % ($n = 9$)	37 % ($n = 7$)	6 % more patients in the rest group achieved MCID

Number of patients (in percentage) achieving a Minimal Clinical Important Difference (MCID >1.0-point on a 0–10 point NRS) at 14-month follow-up in the two subgroups

The MCID was set to 1 point, which is a small difference that is at the lower end of reported estimates for MCIDs. However, the MCID we used was based on the value estimated from a previous chronic LBP sample from the same hospital department and therefore is likely to be the most appropriate for our study sample [16]. Similarly, the RCT from which the data is used in the current study showed that these patients' pain scores, on average, changed very little over 1 year (0.8 (95 % CI 0.3 to 1.3)) suggesting that their MCID would also likely be low [8].

Meaning of the study and comparison with other studies

To our knowledge, there have been very few RCTs that have formally investigated treatment effect modifiers for exercise therapy [19] and previous attempts to identify subgroups of responders to exercise have used aspects of the clinical presentation. For example, Long et al. [20] found that short-term activity and short-term pain limitation were improved in people with a directional preference, if that exercise was matched to their directional preference rather than being unrelated to that preference. In the current study, we have taken a different approach by focusing on MRI findings rather than aspects of the clinical presentation. Both approaches may yield useful evidence but clearly there is a need to improve the effects of exercise by better targeting [19].

There have also been few previous studies of MRI findings as effect modifiers for LBP or sciatica treatments and, to our knowledge, all have investigated invasive interventions, such as injections and various types of surgery. Two of these studies found evidence of significant treatment

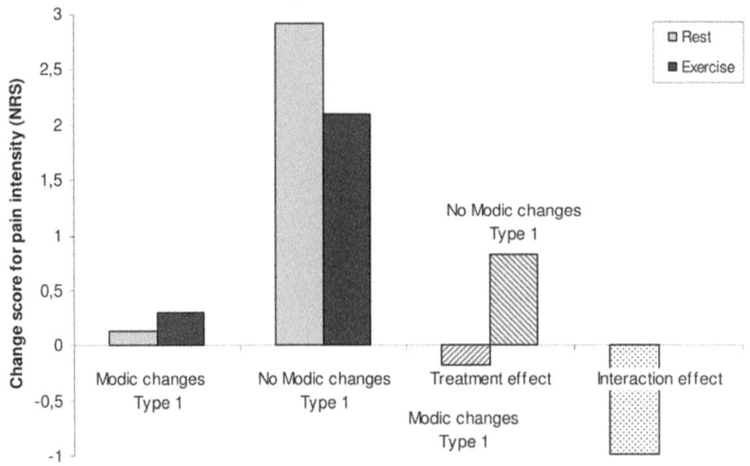

Fig. 2 Treatment effect in patients with and without Modic changes Type 1. Comparison of changes in pain and the treatment effect (rest compared with exercise) in patients receiving rest or exercise subgrouped into those with and without Modic changes Type 1

effect modification (calculations based on data presented in manuscripts) [21, 22]. One study found that people with LBP and Modic changes Type 1 (compared with Modic changes Type 2) had less activity limitation following Disprosan (steroid) injections than if they had saline injections [21]. The other found that sciatica patients with central disc herniation (compared with those without central disc herniation) had less pain following surgery than if they had rehabilitation instead [22]. As early activation and exercise are the most widely recommended treatment for LBP [6], it seems an oversight to not investigate pathoanatomic findings as potential effect modifiers for response to exercise.

Investigation into MRI findings as effect modifiers is complex for a number of reasons. A spinal MRI contains a large amount of anatomical information that requires a detailed protocol to be comprehensively described. When working with a dataset of small sample size, testing for effect modification inevitably leads to data reduction being required and this risks overlooking potentially important information such as location of disc herniation, signal intensity in herniation, location of Modic changes or irregular endplates. Also, numerous MRI findings are present at the same time at a segmental vertebral level and also across all five lumbar segments. For example, vertebral endplate signal changes (Modic changes) and vertebral disc herniation almost always co-exist with other degenerative disc findings, such as reduction of height and signal intensity of the disc [23, 24]. One approach to integrating this multiplicity would be to adjust for the co-existence of other MRI findings in the statistical modelling, but in this study that was not possible due to the lack of power. Alternatively,

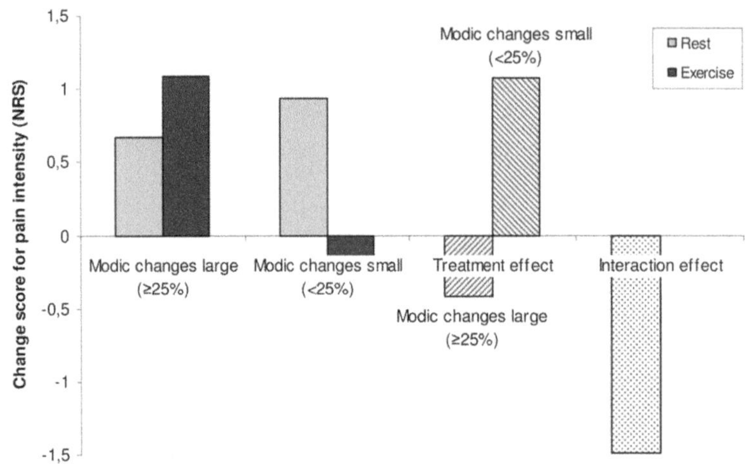

Fig. 3 Treatment effect in patients with and without large Modic changes. Comparison of changes in pain and the treatment effect (rest compared with exercise) in patients receiving rest or exercise subgrouped into those with and without large Modic changes

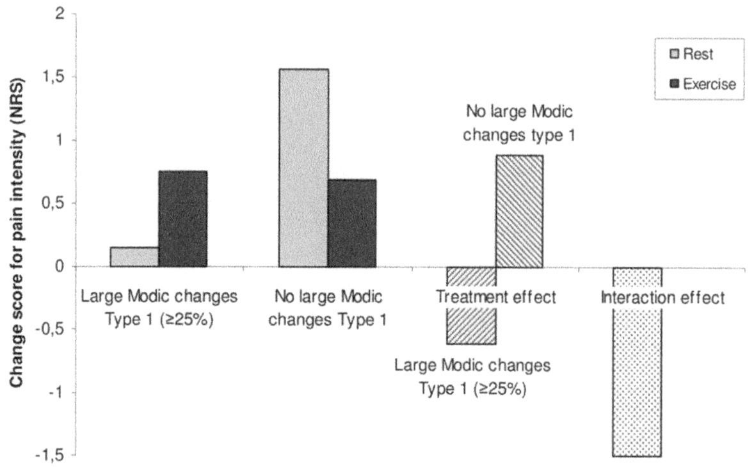

Fig. 4 Treatment effect in patients with and without large Modic changes Type 1. Comparison of changes in pain and the treatment effect (rest compared with exercise) in patients receiving rest or exercise subgrouped into those with and without large Modic changes Type 1

other statistical methods such as Latent Class Analyses could be used to define clusters of MRI findings and those clusters could then be tested as potential effect modifiers, instead of solitary MRI findings [25]. However, those types of analyses using MRI findings are still very novel and require further validation.

Conclusion

In this study, Modic changes Type 1, large Modic changes and large Modic changes Type 1 showed potentially important treatment modification effects by meeting or exceeding our threshold of a 1.0-point difference in pain intensity (0–10 NRS) at 14-month follow-up. Severe disc degeneration and large disc herniations did not reach that threshold. The results need to be interpreted very cautiously as this was a hypothesis-setting study with a relatively small sample, none of the potential effect modifications reached statistical significance, and the effects were in the direction opposite to our hypothesis. Despite this, the findings can be used to indicate some MRI effect modifiers suitable for investigation in subsequent studies of LBP treatment effect and these estimates of effect could be used to adequately power those studies.

Additional file

Additional file 1: Distribution of MRI variables per disc level. Distribution of type and size of Modic changes per disc level (one disc level = 2 endplates) in 96 patients (1056 endplates) with low back pain and Modic changes. Table B. Distribution of severe disc degeneration and type of herniation per disc level in 96 patients (480 discs) with low back pain and Modic changes. (PDF 35 kb)

Abbreviations

LBP: Low back pain; MRI: Magnetic resonance imaging; RCT: Randomised controlled trial; NRS: Numerical rating scale; MCID: Minimal clinically important difference; CI: Confidence interval; STIR: Short tau inversion recovery.

Competing interests

The authors declare that they have no competing interests.

Authors' contributions

RKJ, PK and MH all participated in conception and design of the project and in interpretation of the data. RKJ performed the analyses and wrote the draft manuscript. PK and MH made substantial contributions to the analyses and revising the manuscript. All authors have given their final approval of the version to be published.

Acknowledgement

RKJ and PMK are partially funded by The Foundation for Chiropractic Research and Postgraduate Education. The authors thank Suzanne Capell, professional English language editor, for editing the manuscript and Joan Solgaard Sorensen, radiologist, for coding the MRI protocols.

Author details

[1]Research Department, Spine Centre of Southern Denmark, Hospital Lillebaelt, Institute of Regional Health Research, University of Southern Denmark, Oestre Hougvej 55, 5500 Middelfart, Denmark. [2]Department of Sports Science and Clinical Biomechanics, University of Southern Denmark, Campusvej 55, 5230 Odense M, Denmark. [3]Faculty of Human Sciences, Macquarie University, Balaclava Rd, North Ryde 2113NSW, Australia.

References

1. Deyo RA, Rainville J, Kent DL. What can the history and physical examination tell us about low back pain? JAMA. 1992;268:760–5. doi:10.1001/jama.1992.03490060092030.
2. Kent P, Keating J. Do primary-care clinicians think that nonspecific low back pain is one condition? Spine (Phila Pa 1976). 2004;29:1022–31.
3. Fersum KV, Dankaerts W, O'Sullivan PB, Maes J, Skouen JS, Bjordal JM, et al. Integration of subclassification strategies in randomised controlled clinical trials evaluating manual therapy treatment and exercise therapy for non-specific chronic low back pain: a systematic review. Br J Sports Med. 2010;44:1054–62. doi:10.1136/bjsm.2009.063289.
4. Jensen TS, Karppinen J, Sorensen JS, Niinimaki J, Leboeuf-Yde C. Vertebral endplate signal changes (Modic change): a systematic literature review of prevalence and association with non-specific low back pain. Eur Spine J. 2008;17:1407–22. doi:10.1007/s00586-008-0770-2.
5. Thompson KJ, Dagher AP, Eckel TS, Clark M, Reinig JW. Modic changes on MR images as studied with provocative diskography: clinical relevance–a retrospective study of 2457 disks. Radiology. 2009;250:849–55.

6. Koes BW, van Tulder M, Lin CW, Macedo LG, McAuley J, Maher C. An updated overview of clinical guidelines for the management of non-specific low back pain in primary care. Eur Spine J. 2010;19:2075–94.
7. Modic MT, Steinberg PM, Ross JS, Masaryk TJ, Carter JR. Degenerative disk disease: assessment of changes in vertebral body marrow with MR imaging. Radiology. 1988;166:193–9.
8. Jensen RK, Leboeuf-Yde C, Wedderkopp N, Sorensen JS, Manniche C. Rest versus exercise as treatment for patients with low back pain and Modic changes. A randomized controlled clinical trial. BMC Med. 2012;10:22. doi:10.1186/1741-7015-10-22.
9. Sun X, Briel M, Walter SD, Guyatt GH. Is a subgroup effect believable? Updating criteria to evaluate the credibility of subgroup analyses. BMJ. 2010;340:c117. doi:10.1136/bmj.c117.
10. 'Minim', an MS-DOS program by Stephen Evans, Patrick Royston and Simon Day. [http://www-users.york.ac.uk/~mb55/guide/minim.htm]. Accessed 8 July 2015.
11. Childs JD, Piva SR, Fritz JM. Responsiveness of the numeric pain rating scale in patients with low back pain. Spine (Phila Pa 1976). 2005;30:1331–4.
12. Jensen TS, Sorensen JS, Kjaer P. Intra- and interobserver reproducibility of vertebral endplate signal (modic) changes in the lumbar spine: the Nordic Modic Consensus Group classification. Acta Radiol. 2007;48:748–54.
13. Solgaard SJ, Kjaer P, Jensen ST, Andersen P. Low-field magnetic resonance imaging of the lumbar spine: reliability of qualitative evaluation of disc and muscle parameters. Acta Radiol. 2006;47:947–53.
14. Brookes ST, Whitely E, Egger M, Smith GD, Mulheran PA, Peters TJ. Subgroup analyses in randomized trials: risks of subgroup-specific analyses; power and sample size for the interaction test. J Clin Epidemiol. 2004;57:229–36.
15. Kamper SJ, Maher CG, Hancock MJ, Koes BW, Croft PR, Hay E. Treatment-based subgroups of low back pain: a guide to appraisal of research studies and a summary of current evidence. Best Pract Res Clin Rheumatol. 2010;24:181–91. doi:10.1016/j.berh.2009.11.003.
16. Lauridsen HH, Hartvigsen J, Manniche C, Korsholm L, Grunnet-Nilsson N. Responsiveness and minimal clinically important difference for pain and disability instruments in low back pain patients. BMC Musculoskelet Disord. 2006;7:82.
17. Kent P, Hancock M, Petersen DH, Mjosund HL. Clinimetrics corner: choosing appropriate study designs for particular questions about treatment subgroups. J Man Manip Ther. 2010;18:147–52. doi:10.1179/106698110X12640740712419.
18. Bendix T, Sorensen JS, Henriksson GA, Bolstad JE, Narvestad EK, Jensen TS. Lumbar modic changes-a comparison between findings at low- and high-field magnetic resonance imaging. Spine (Phila Pa 1976). 2012;37:1756–62.
19. Kent P, Mjosund HL, Petersen DH. Does targeting manual therapy and/or exercise improve patient outcomes in nonspecific low back pain? A systematic review. BMC Med. 2010;8:22. doi:10.1186/1741-7015-8-22.
20. Long A, Donelson R, Fung T. Does it matter which exercise? A randomized control trial of exercise for low back pain. Spine (Phila Pa 1976). 2004;29:2593–602.
21. Cao P, Jiang L, Zhuang C, Yang Y, Zhang Z, Chen W, et al. Intradiscal injection therapy for degenerative chronic discogenic low back pain with end plate Modic changes. Spine J. 2011;11:100–6. doi:10.1016/j.spinee.2010.07.001.
22. Pearson AM, Blood EA, Frymoyer JW, Herkowitz H, Abdu WA, Woodward R, et al. SPORT lumbar intervertebral disk herniation and back pain: does treatment, location, or morphology matter? Spine (Phila Pa 1976). 2008;33:428–35. doi:10.1097/BRS.0b013e31816469de.
23. Schmid G, Witteler A, Willburger R, Kuhnen C, Jergas M, Koester O. Lumbar disk herniation: correlation of histologic findings with marrow signal intensity changes in vertebral endplates at MR imaging. Radiology. 2004;231:352–8.
24. Wang Y, Videman T, Battie MC. ISSLS prize winner: lumbar vertebral endplate lesions: associations with disc degeneration and back pain history. Spine (Phila Pa 1976). 2012;37:1490–6. doi:10.1097/BRS.0b013e3182608ac4.
25. Jensen RK, Jensen TS, Kjaer P, Kent P. Can pathoanatomical pathways of degeneration in lumbar motion segments be identified by clustering MRI findings. BMC Musculoskelet Disord. 2013;14:198. doi:10.1186/1471-2474-14-198.
26. Kuisma M, Karppinen J, Niinimaki J, Ojala R, Haapea M, Heliovaara M, et al. Modic changes in endplates of lumbar vertebral bodies: prevalence and association with low back and sciatic pain among middle-aged male workers. Spine (Phila Pa 1976). 2007;32:1116–22.
27. Hancock M, Maher C, Macaskill P, Latimer J, Kos W, Pik J. MRI findings are more common in selected patients with acute low back pain than controls? Eur Spine J. 2012;21:240–6. doi:10.1007/s00586-011-1955-7.
28. Jensen TS, Albert HB, Sorensen JS, Manniche C, Leboeuf-Yde C. Magnetic resonance imaging findings as predictors of clinical outcome in patients with sciatica receiving active conservative treatment. J Manipulative Physiol Ther. 2007;30:98–108.

A literature review of clinical tests for lumbar instability in low back pain: validity and applicability in clinical practice

Silvano Ferrari[1*], Tiziana Manni[2], Francesca Bonetti[3], Jorge Hugo Villafañe[4] and Carla Vanti[1]

Abstract

Background: Several clinical tests have been proposed on low back pain (LBP), but their usefulness in detecting lumbar instability is not yet clear. The objective of this literature review was to investigate the clinical validity of the main clinical tests used for the diagnosis of lumbar instability in individuals with LBP and to verify their applicability in everyday clinical practice.

Methods: We searched studies of the accuracy and/or reliability of Prone Instability Test (PIT), Passive Lumbar Extension Test (PLE), Aberrant Movements Pattern (AMP), Posterior Shear Test (PST), Active Straight Leg Raise Test (ASLR) and Prone and Supine Bridge Tests (PB and SB) in Medline, Embase, Cinahl, PubMed, and Scopus databases. Only the studies in which each test was investigated by at least one study concerning both the accuracy and the reliability were considered eligible. The quality of the studies was evaluated by QUADAS and QAREL scales.

Results: Six papers considering 333 LBP patients were included. The PLE was the most accurate and informative clinical test, with high sensitivity (0.84, 95% CI: 0.69 - 0.91) and high specificity (0.90, 95% CI: 0.85 -0.97).
The diagnostic accuracy of AMP depends on each singular test. The PIT and the PST demonstrated by fair to moderate sensitivity and specificity [PIT sensitivity = 0.71 (95% CI: 0.51 - 0.83), PIT specificity = 0.57 (95% CI: 039 - 0.78); PST sensitivity = 0.50 (95% CI: 0.41 - 0.76), PST specificity = 0.48 (95% CI: 0.22 - 0.58)].
The PLE showed a good reliability (k = 0.76), but this result comes from a single study. The inter-rater reliability of the PIT ranged by slight (k = 0.10 and 0.04), to good (k = 0.87).
The inter-rater reliability of the AMP ranged by slight (k = −0.07) to moderate (k = 0.64), whereas the inter-rater reliability of the PST was fair (k = 0.27).

Conclusions: The data from the studies provided information on the methods used and suggest that PLE is the most appropriate tests to detect lumbar instability in specific LBP. However, due to the lack of available papers on other lumbar conditions, these findings should be confirmed with studies on non-specific LBP patients.

Keywords: Joint instability, Lumbar instability, Low back pain, Physical examination, Reproducibility of results, Prone instability test, Passive lumbar extension test, Aberrant movements pattern, Posterior shear test

Background

Low back pain (LBP) is a growing health problem in the industrialized world. Despite the high medical expenses required for its management, the prevalence of LBP is increasing [1]. LBP is a heterogeneous condition, and the identification of different sub-groups could help the management decisions [2,3]. One of these sub-groups is lumbar segmental instability [4,5].

The radiologically determined instability is characterized by a loss of passive integrity, causing excessive vertebral translation or rotation. The maximum lumbar flexion-extension radiographs in standing position are considered to be a reference standard to detect the function of the passive stabilization system [6,7]. This imaging method is commonly used to evaluate lumbar segmental mobility in isthmic and degenerative spondylolisthesis and degenerative

* Correspondence: silvano.ferrari@fastwebnet.it
[1]Master of Manual Therapy and Musculoskeletal Rehabilitation, Department of Molecular Medicine, University of Padova, Padova, Italy
Full list of author information is available at the end of the article

disc dysfunctions. The radiographic diagnosis of spondylolisthesis is considered to be one of the most efficient methods of identifying lumbar instability [8].

Some authors refer to the concept of instability also considering the so-called "clinical" or "functional" instability, in which no defect of the body architecture of the lumbar spine, and no excessive detectable translation or rotation are shown. However, a poor trunk muscle function and/or an insufficient motor control is believed to be a factor in abnormal inter-segmental movement and LBP [9-11]. Despite this type of instability has not been demonstrated enough as a clinical entity and is not really measureable by any gold standard, it is one of the most frequent fields of interest for chiropractors and manual therapists.

Clinicians have used several clinical tests to detect the spinal instability and/or the ability of the muscles to stabilize the lumbar spine [12]. Recently, some of these tests have been suggested in the "Clinical Practice Guidelines linked to the International Classification of Functioning, Disability and Health from the Orthopaedic Section of the American Physical Therapy Association", to assess the impairments of body functions in LBP [5]. The most commonly used tests are the Prone Instability Test (PIT), the Passive Lumbar Extension (PLE) test, the Aberrant Movements Pattern (AMP), the Posterior Shear Test (PST), the Prone Bridge Test (PBT), the Supine Bridge Test (SBT), and the Active Straight Leg Raise Test.

Previous reviews separately investigated the diagnostic accuracy [13] or the reliability [14] of the instability tests, but a complete vision about their diagnostic validity to detect lumbar instability is lacking. A single literature review on both the diagnostic accuracy (sensitivity, specificity and likelihood ratios) and the inter-rater reliability of these clinical tests does not exist. More specifically, a researcher could be interested in investigating the reliability of the tests that previously demonstrated sufficient face validity.

The objective of this literature review was to assess the methods used for diagnosis (primarily the accuracy with additional reporting of reliability of these tests) of the clinical tests for lumbar instability in individuals with LBP and investigate their applicability in daily practice.

Methods

This is a literature review of all the studies presenting a diagnosis of the clinical tests for lumbar instability in individuals with LBP in literature. PRISMA Guidelines [15] were followed during the design, search and reporting stages of this review on diagnostic test studies.

Literature search

A literature search of relevant literature was performed from July 2012 to December 2013. A comprehensive search, limited to articles in English, Italian and Spanish, was conducted in the following databases: Medline, Embase, Cinahl, PubMed, Scopus. Diagnostic test studies regarding humans published between 1972 and December 2013 were included. Narrative or systematic reviews, guidelines and meta-analyses were excluded.

Two authors (SF and TM) independently performed two different and parallel searches to avoid leaving out relevant articles. The search strategies are shown in Figure 1.

The results of these seven searches were unified into a single item set. From the results of the initial search, double citations were removed and then the titles, abstracts and full texts of retrieved articles were independently evaluated for definitive inclusion. When the two reviewers were unable to reach a consensus, a third reviewer (CV) was consulted. In addition to the Internet-assisted search, references were pulled from a textbook on diagnostic accuracy of orthopedic clinical tests [16], and from reference lists of included studies. Finally, an independent hand search including scanning of reference lists from other systematic reviews [13,14] was performed.

Study selection

Several criteria were used to select eligible studies. Articles examining clinical tests for lumbar instability were included if they met the following criteria:

1) Diagnostic accuracy studies on adult population with sub-acute or chronic LBP were considered if clinical instability tests were employed as index tests. Dynamic radiographs were the reference test to diagnose lumbar instability. The subject articles had to report data which would allow computation of parametric statistical tests of diagnostic accuracy [sensitivity, specificity, or positive and negative likelihood ratios (+LR and -LR)].
2) Reliability studies on healthy or LBP adult population were considered if they concerned the use of clinical tests to diagnose lumbar instability by one or more clinicians. Articles had to report the parametric statistical tests of relationship or agreement.
3) Finally, only the studies in which each test was investigated by at least one study concerning both the accuracy and the reliability were considered eligible.

Data extraction and quality assessment

One author (TM) gathered data regarding clinical tests, with its description and score, study population (e.g. age, gender, setting, clinical characteristics), inclusion and exclusion criteria, diagnostic reference standard, differences in operationalizing the index tests, study raters.

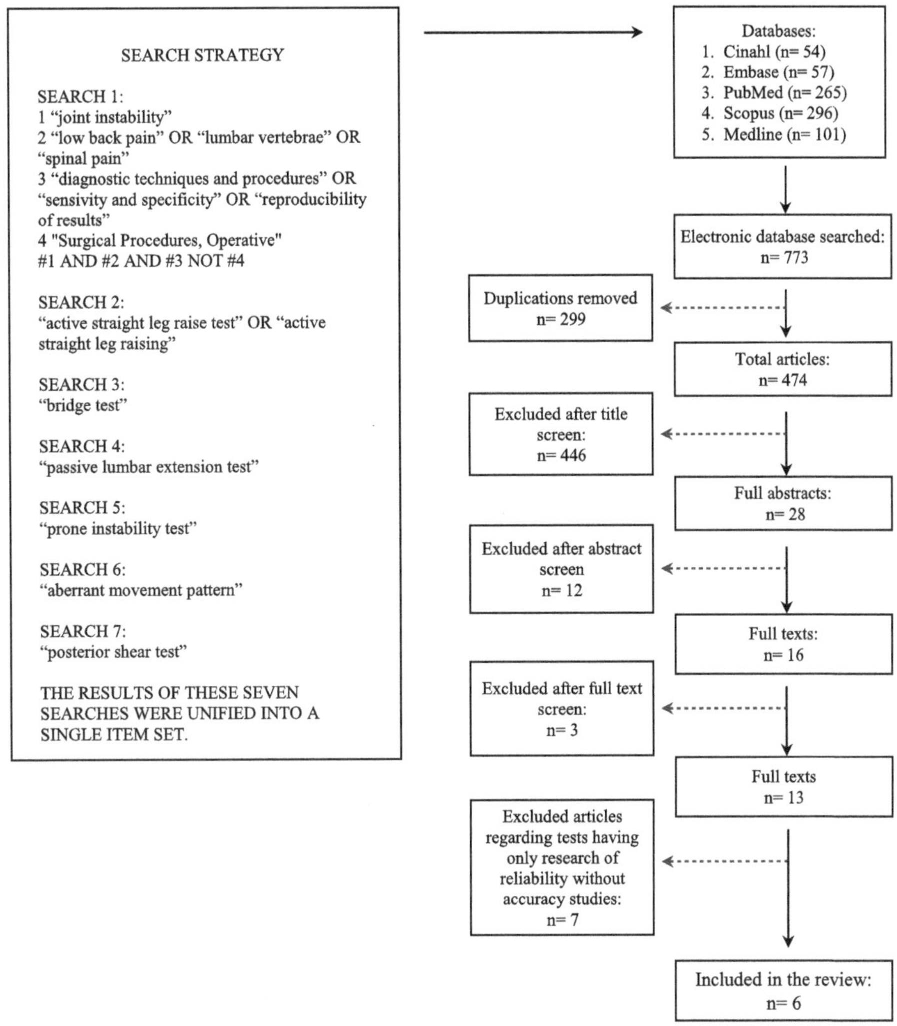

Figure 1 Flow chart.

Study results about sensitivity, specificity, LR+, LR-, and reliability were collected (or calculated, if included articles did not provide these data). Other authors (SF and FB) verified data extraction once completed. The methodological quality of included articles was independently assessed by 2 reviewers (TM and FB), using different tools for the 2 types of studies: the Quality Assessment of Diagnostic Accuracy Studies (QUADAS) tool for diagnostic accuracy articles [17] and the Quality Appraisal of Reliability Studies (QAREL) checklist for diagnostic reliability articles [18].

Data synthesis and analysis

Kappa statistics were used to assess agreement between the 2 raters on article selection and QUADAS and QAREL ratings [19]. The QUADAS and QAREL statement delineates essential items to be reported in diagnostic test studies (Table 1 and Table 2).

Concerning sensitivity and specificity, the acceptable levels were set between 50% (unacceptable test) and 100% (perfect test) [20]. The diagnostic accuracy was considered satisfactory, thus affecting the probability of lumbar instability, with + LR $\geq$ 2.0 or - LR $\leq$0.50 [21].

Concerning reliability, the following criteria has been used to determine the strength of the coefficients: $\leq$ 0.25 = little or no relationship; 0.26 – 0.50 = fair degree of relationship; 0.51 – 0.75 = moderate to good relationship; 0.76 – 1.00 = good to excellent relationship [22].

Results

Figure 1 shows the process of study selection. Initial searching identified 773 citations. Following the first screening, 299 articles were excluded and 474 citations were retained for the second screening; after reviewing the titles, 446 were excluded and 28 considered of interest, looking at the abstracts 16 were maintained and 13 retrieved in full text.

Table 1 QUADAS (Quality Assessment of Diagnostic Accuracy Study) tool results

Item		*Fritz* et al. [24]	*Kasai* et al. [25]
1.	Was the spectrum of patients representative of the patients who will receive the test in practice?	Y	U
2.	Were selection criteria clearly described?	Y	N
3.	Is the reference standard likely to correctly classify the target condition?	Y	Y
4.	Is the time period between reference standard and index test short enough to the reasonably sure that the target condition did not change between the two tests?	Y	U
5.	Did the whole sample or a random selection of the sample, receive verification using a reference standard of diagnosis?	Y	Y
6.	Did patients receive the same reference standard regardless of the index result?	Y	Y
7.	Was the reference standard independent of the index (i.e. The index test did not form part of the reference standard)?	Y	Y
8.	Was the execution of the index described in sufficient detail to permit replication of the test?	Y	Y
9.	Was the execution of the reference standard described in sufficient detail to permit its replication?	Y	U
10.	Were the index test results interpreted without knowledge of the result of the reference standard?	Y	Y
11.	Were the reference standard results interpreted without knowledge of the results of the index test?	Y	Y
12.	Were the same clinical data available when test results were interpreted as would be available when the test is used in practice?	Y	Y
13.	Were uninterpretable/intermediate test results reported?	Y	Y
14.	Were withdrawals from the study explained?	Y	Y

Legend: Y = yes, N = no, U = unclear.

Table 2 QAREL application results

Item		*Hicks* et al. [23]	*Fritz* et al. [24]	*Schneider* et al. [27]	*Ravenna* et al. [26]	*Rabin* et al. [12]
1.	Was the test evaluated in a sample of subjects who were representative of those to whom the authors intended the results to be applied?	Y	Y	Y	Y	Y
2.	Was the test performed by raters who were representative of those to whom the authors intended the results to be applied?	Y	U	Y	Y	Y
3.	Were raters blinded to the findings of the other raters during the study?	Y	Y	Y	Y	Y
4.	Were raters blinded to their own prior findings of the test under evaluation?	*N/A*	*N/A*	*N/A*	*N/A*	*N/A*
5.	Were raters blinded to the results of the accepted reference standard or disease status for the target disorder (or variable) being evaluated?	*N/A*	Y	*N/A*	*N/A*	U
6.	Were raters blinded to clinical information that was not intended to be provided as part of the testing procedures or study design?	U	U	Y	N	N
7.	Were raters blinded to additional cues that were not part of the test?	U	U	U	U	U
8.	Was the order of examination varied?	N	Y	Y	Y	N
9.	Was the stability (or theoretical stability) of the variable being measured taken into account when determining the suitability of the time-interval between repeated measures?	(PIT) N	(AMP) Y	N	N	N
10.	Was the test applied correctly and interpreted appropriately?	Y	Y	Y	N	Y
11.	Were appropriate statistical measures of agreement used?	Y	Y	Y	N	U

Y = yes, N = no, U = unclear, N/A = not applicable; PIT = Prone Instability Test, AMP = Aberrant Movement Pattern.

Using the inclusion and exclusion criteria a further 7 articles were excluded. This study finally included 6 papers, considering 333 LBP patients, for the review [12,23-27].

Quality scores

Two articles of the 6 studies (33%) were identified as having high methodological rigor according to the QUADAS tool (Table 1). Table 2 shows the distribution of studies according to the scores obtained from the assessment of their methodological quality, following the QAREL tool.

Diagnostic accuracy of the tests

The diagnostic accuracy was investigated by 2 authors only: Fritz et al. [24] and Kasai et al. [25] Four lumbar instability tests were considered: the PLE test, the PIT, the AMP, and the PST. The main characteristics of the studies on diagnostic accuracy are shown in Table 3, whereas Table 4 shows the results.

Kasai et al. [25] found that the PLE test was the most accurate clinical test, with high sensitivity (0.84, 95% CI: 0.7 - 0.93) and specificity (0.90, 95% CI: 0.82 - 0.95), in a sample of subjects diagnosed with spinal stenosis or lumbar spondylolisthesis or lumbar degenerative scoliosis. The positive and negative LR's were informative.

The diagnostic accuracy of AMP depends on each singular test. Low sensitivity (0.26, 95% CI: 0.15 - 0.42) and good specificity (0.86, 95% CI: 0.77 - 0.92) were found by Kasai et al. [25] for the Instability Catch Signs. The Painful Catch Sign and the Apprehension Sign showed the same trend, low sensitivity (0.37, 95% CI: 0.24 - 0.54 and 0.18, 95% CI: 0.22 - 0.64 respectively) and good specificity (0.73, 95% CI: 0.61 - 0.8 and 0.88, 95% CI: 0.61 - 0.78 respectively). These tests are included in the AMP, also studied by Fritz et al. [24], who reported low sensitivity (0.18, 95% CI: 0.08 - 0.36) and high specificity (0.95, 95% CI: 0.77 - 0.99) for the AMP test in a cohort of patients with chronic LBP.

The article by Fritz et al. [24] is the only one that studied the diagnostic accuracy of the PIT and the PST. Both tests demonstrated by fair to moderate diagnostic test accuracy. PIT sensitivity = 0.71 (95% CI: 0.53 - 0.85); specificity = 0.57 (95% CI: 0.37 - 0.76); PST sensitivity = 0.50 (95% CI: 0.34 - 0.66); specificity = 0.48 (95% CI: 0.28 - 0.68).

Reliability of the tests

The reliability of the four clinical tests was studied in 5 papers [12,23,24,26,27]. The main characteristics of the studies on reliability and their results are shown in Table 5, whereas Table 6 shows the results in terms of inter-rater reliability.

The PLE test showed a better reliability, but this result comes from a single study [12]. The inter-rater reliability of this test resulted good (k = 0.76).

Five studies investigated the inter-rater reliability of the PIT. This reliability was considered fair by Schneider et al. [27] (k = 0.46) and Ravenna et al. [26] (k = 0.10 and 0.04), moderate by Fritz et al. [24] and Rabin et al. [12] (k = 0.69 and k = 0.67, respectively), and good by Hicks et al. [23] (k = 0.87).

The inter-rater reliability of the AMP was studied by Hicks et al. [23] Fritz et al. [24] and Rabin et al. [12]. Whereas Fritz et al. [24] found poor reproducibility (k = –0.07), Hicks et al. [23] (k = 0.60) and Rabin et al. [12] (k = 0.64) calculated moderate reliability. The inter-rater reliability of the Posterior Shear Test was only studied by Fritz et al. [24] showing poor reliability (k = 0.27).

Implications for clinical practice

The data from the studies provided information on the tests and methods used, the error of measurement and also the validity of the tests. However, only 5 studies (83.3%) provided information concerning the setting and the years of raters clinical experience, whereas all studies identified the person performing the assessment and his/her professional competence.

Discussion

This literature review was aimed to identify the most reliable findings concerning the assessment of methods for diagnosis of the clinical tests for lumbar instability in LBP subjects.

The lumbar instability is traditionally a field of debate. Lumbar segmental instability in the absence of defects of the bony architecture of the lumbar spine has also been cited as a significant cause of chronic low back pain [5,28]. The differences between surgical instability criteria and "functional instability" criteria were defined by Panjabi [29] decades ago. Chiropractics and Manual Therapists are more interested in the lost of motor control than in hypermobility detectable with flexion/extension radiological imaging, which is more useful to spine surgeons. However, the difficulty to clinically detect abnormal or excessive inter-segmental motion makes these tests often insensitive and unreliable and it becomes a limit for the clinical diagnosis of lumbar segmental instability [30,31]. The lack of studies in this field emerges also by our research, which found many studies about reliability of tests used by clinicians but few about their accuracy. Being aware that this criterion is too rigorous for manual therapists we have chosen to be rigorous and we have been forced to do our research having as reference the best reference (gold standard) to instability, that is dynamic X-rays. The result is that many other tests used in the manual clinical practice to detect lumbar clinical instability (i.e. active hip abduction test or hip extension test) have not been considered because no study had investigated their accuracy. These tests are

Table 3 Summary of the studies on diagnostic accuracy

Article	Clinical tests, scores	Inclusion (I) and exclusion (E) criteria	Population	Reference standard and positive criteria	Rater/s
Fritz et al. [24]	- **Aberrant Movement Pattern** (Painful arc on flexion, painful arc on return, instability catch, Gower sign, reverse lumbopelvic rhythm). *Positive test: at least 1 of the 5 signs was present.* - **Prone instability test** *Positive test: pain provoked during the first part of the test decreases when the test is repeated with the legs off the floor.* - **Posterior Shear Test** *Positive test: familiar symptoms are provoked.*	I: LBP with or without referred pain on the lower extremities, < 60 yrs E: contraindications to radiographic assessment (e.g., current pregnancy), previous lumbar fusion surgery, inability (e.g., pain or muscle spasm) to actively flex and extend the spine adequately to permit an assessment of segmental motion	N.49 - Age: 39.2 ± 11.3 yrs - Duration of symptoms (median days) 78 - Distribution of symptoms: back/buttock only 63.3%, symptoms distal to the knee 30.6% - Previous history of LBP: 83.7% - LBP episodes becoming more frequent: 30.6%	Dynamic X-ray: the patient stands at the edge of a tall stool with feet flat on the floor and arms folded across the chest. The patient is instructed to flex forward as far as possible for the flexion X-Ray. For the extension X-ray, the patient stands with arms folded, and is asked to extend as far as possible. Criteria for instability: sagittal plane translation greater than 4.5 mm or greater than 15% of the vertebral body width, or sagittal plane rotation greater than 15° at L1/L2, L2/L3, L3/L4 levels, greater than 20° at L4/L5, or greater than 25° at L5/S1. *Instability diagnosis: 2 segments with either rotational or translational instability OR 1 segment with both translational and rotational instability*	1 Physical Therapist
Kasai et al. [25]	- **Passive lumbar extension test:** The subject was in the prone position; both lower extremities the were elevated concurrently to a height of about 30 cm from the bed while maintaining the knees extended and gently pulling the legs. Positive test when the subject complained of strong pain in the lumbar region ("low back pain", "very heavy feeling on the low back", "feeling as if the low back was coming off") during elevation of both lower legs, and such pain disappeared when they returned to the initial position. In contrast, when the subject complained of an abonrmal sensation (mild numbness or prickling sensation) the test was negative. - **Instability catch sign:** The subject was asked to bend his body forward as much as possible and then return to the erect position; subject who was not able to return to erect position because of sudden low back pain was judged positive to the test.	I: lumbar degenerative diseases E: /	N. 122 subjects with lumbar degenerative diseases: 89 lumbar spinal canal stenosis; 21 lumbar spondylolisthesis; 12 lumbar degenerative scoliosis. - 39 ± 8.8 yrs; - mean illenss duration 11.2 months; - Complain of pain: 70.5% lumbago, 60.7% intermittent claudicatio, 42.6% neurological symptoms in the lower legs	Dynamic x-ray: flexion-extension films of the lumbar spine, lateral vision. 3 criteria to asses radiological instability: angular motion > 20°; transactional motion > 5 mm; cutoff value of - 5° for the intervertebral endplate angle on the flexion film. *Radiograph instability: positive for 1 o more of the 3 criteria.*	n°3 Orthopedics n°2 for testing PLE test (who had 12 and 15 yrs of clinical experience) n°1 for testing Instability catch sign (with 20 yrs of clinical experience). *For RX evaluation:* *n°2 Orthopedics who had 8 and 14 yrs of clinical experience.*

Legend: / = data no present in the article.

Table 4 Results of diagnostic accuracy studies

Test	2x2 table		Sensitivity	Specificity	PPV	NPV	+LR (95% CI)	-LR (95% CI)
	TP	FP						
	FN	TN						
PIT [23]	20	9	71.4	57.1	69.0	60.0	1.67	0.50
	8	12					(0.97-2.88)	(0.97-2.88)
PLE [24]	32	8	84.2	90.5	80.0	92.7	8.84	0.18
	6	76					(4.51-17.34)	(0.08-0.37)
AMP [23]	5	1	17.9	95.2	83.3	46.5	3.75	0.86
	23	20					(0.47-29.75)	(0.71-1.05)
ICS [24]	10	12	26.3	85.7	45.5	72.0	1.84	0.86
	28	72					(0.87-3.89)	(0.87-1.06)
PCS [24]	14	23	36.8	72.6	37.8	71.8	1.35	0.87
	24	61					(0.78-2.32)	(0.66-1.15)
AS [24]	7	10	18.4	88.1	41.2	70.5	1.55	0.93
	31	74					(0.64-3.76)	(0.78-1.1)
PST [23]	16	11	50.0	47.6	59.3	36.5	0.96	1.05
	16	10					(0.56-1.63)	(0.60-1.85)

T: True, F: False, P: Positive, N: Negative; PPV = Positive Predictive Value; NPV = Negative Predictive Value; +LR = Positive Likelihood Ratio; −LR = Negative Likelihood Ratio; PIT = Prone Instability Test; PLE = Passive Lumbar Extension Test; AMP = Aberrant Movements Sign; ICS: Instability Catch Sign; PCS: Painful Catch Sign; AS: Apprehension Sign; PST = Posterior Shear Test.

not present in this review, so that, in latest analysis, our study could be considered as a literature review of accuracy of lumbar clinical tests with additional reporting of reliability information.

Six high-quality studies were selected and four lumbar clinical instability tests (PLE test, PIT, AMP and PST) satisfied the inclusion criteria.

Accuracy

The characteristics of the samples of the 2 subject studies [24,25] cannot be considered accurate. Fritz et al. [24] studied a population whose majority had a prior history of LBP, and in which only 30.6% (n = 15) of people complained about distal knee symptoms. Kasai et al. [25], however, investigated a population with specific lumbar conditions (lumbar spinal canal stenosis, lumbar spondylolisthesis or lumbar scoliosis), most of whom had intermittent claudication, and 42.6% (n = 52) had neurological leg symptoms.

The PLE test was the most accurate and informative test, even though it was measured by only one study, in patients affected by lumbar degenerative diseases. Despite the PLE test appears to be a potentially effective clinical test to detect lumbar instability, the characteristics of the investigated sample and the presence of only one study on its diagnostic accuracy may suggest the necessity of studies on non-specific LBP patients.

The PIT demonstrated low to moderate sensitivity and specificity [24] indicating that this test has limited accuracy in diagnosing lumbar instability in patients with LBP.

The PST showed relatively poor sensitivity and specificity [24], indicating that this test is less accurate than the PLE test and the PIT to detect lumbar instability.

The Instability Catch Sign, the Painful Catch Sign and the Apprehension Sign are three of the five signs included in the AMP investigated by Fritz et al. [24]. The relatively low sensitivity and high specificity resulting from the study of Kasai et al. [25] suggest caution in the use of these tests to diagnose lumbar instability. According to Hicks et al. [23], these 5 tests should be used together, as a complete observation of the trunk movement and the 5 signs could be considered as only one comprehensive test. However, positive results on AMP and PIT, which demonstrated moderate sensitivity and specificity, were considered predictive for a favorable response to stabilization exercises [32].

Reliability

The characteristics of the samples were not always well explained or were not reliable. The PLE test [12] and the PIT [12,23,24] demonstrated good inter-rater reliability. The reliability of PLE test is evident in younger subjects referred to outpatient physical therapy [12]. Five studies on PIT demonstrated very different inter-rater reliability scores. Nevertheless, the 2 studies showing fair reliability [26,27] are affected by possible bias; in the first case [27] due to a very limited sample size and in the second case

Table 5 Summary of the articles on reliability

Article	Clinical test and scores	Inclusion (I) and exclusion (E) criteria	Population	Reliability	Rater/s
Hicks et al. [23]	- **Painful arc in flexion** - **Painful arc on return** - **Instability catch** - **Gower sign ("thigh climbing")** - **Reversal of lumbopelvic rhythm** - **Aberrant Movement Pattern:** positive if at least one of the five previously cited signs is present. - **Prone Instability Test:** *Positive test: pain provoked during the first part of the test disappears when the test is repeated with the legs off the floor.*	I: current complaints of LBP. E: symptoms referred below the knee, LBP which may be attributed to current pregnancy, fractures in acute phase, tumor, infection, previous lumbar surgical fusion.	N 63 20-66 yrs - Gender: 38♀, 25♂ - Previous LBP episodes, 51/63. - Age 36.0 ± 10.3	Inter-rater reliability. For each pair of raters, the first rater performs all clinical examination measures on each subject; the second rater, who is blinded to the results of the first evaluation, then performs the same examination procedures, after a minimum of 15- minutes.	N. 4 PT1: PT and chiropractor with 3 yrs of experience as a chiropractor and 2 yrs as an OMT PT2: PT with 6 yrs of experience in orthopedic setting PT3: OMT with 8 yrs of experience PT4: PT with 4 yrs of experience on orthopedic environment. *3 pair of raters: PT1 + PT2, PT2 + PT3, PT1 + PT4*
Fritz et al. [24]	- **Aberrant Movement Pattern:** Painful arc on flexion; Painful arc on return; Instability catch; Gower sign ("thigh climbing"); Reverse lumbopelvic rhythm. *Positive test when at least 1 of the previous 5 signs was present.* - **Prone Instability Test:** *Positive test when pain provoked during the first part of the test decreases when the test is repeated with the legs off the floor.* - **Posterior Shear Test:** *Positive test if familiar symptoms are provoked.*	I: complaint of LBP with or without radiation into the lower extremities, < 60 yrs E: contraindications to radiographic assessment (e.g., current pregnancy), previous lumbar fusion surgery, inability (e.g. pain or muscle spasm) to actively flex and extend the spine adequately to permit an assessment of segmental motion.	N. 38 patients taken by a sample of 49 patients with these characteristics: - Age: 39.2 ± 11.3 yrs; - Duration of symptoms (median days) 78; - Distribution of symptoms: back/buttock only 63.3%, symptoms distal to the knee 30.6%; - Previous history of LBP: 83.7% - LBP episodes becoming more frequent: 30.6%	Inter-rater reliability. The second rater repeats the assessment 5 minutes after the first rater's assessment	N. 2 physical therapists
Schneider et al. [27]	- **Prone instability test:** *Positive test when pain provoked during the first part of the test disappears when the test is repeated with the legs off the floor.*	I: History of LBP, age between 18 and 65 years, ability to tolerate lying prone E: History of prior lumbar surgery, stenosis, scoliosis greater than 20°, unstable spondylolisthesis, positive nerve root tension or radiculopathy, any red flags suggestive of spinal pathology.	N. 39 volunteer patients with history of LBP and undergoing chiropractic treatment at the time of their enrollment in the study	Inter-rater reliability.	N. 2 experienced doctors of chiropractic (25 and 10 years of clinical experience, respectively).

Table 5 Summary of the articles on reliability *(Continued)*

Ravenna et al. [26]	- **Prone Instability Test with additional guidelines:** → A trunk stabilizing belt is placed around the subject and the table at shoulder level, → A stool may be placed under the subject's feet if the feet do not comfortably reach the floor. *Positive and negative criteria:* ● *Positive level if the subject reports a decrease of pain with the second P/A, lifting the legs in the second part of the test* ● *Negative test if the subject reports superficial bone-on-bone pressure;* ● *Negative test if the subject reports an increase in symptoms lifting the legs during the second part of the test;* ● *Negative level if the subject reports an increase or same with the second P/A, compared with the first.*	I: chronic or recurrent LBP; age 18 to 60 years; current symptoms of LBP, but not acute phase. E: BMI > 30 kg/m^2, disk herniation, symptoms referred below the knee, lower extremity weakness or loss of reflexes, history of spinal surgery or fracture, spinal deformity, systemic inflammatory condition, neurologic disease or other serious medical conditions. LBP attributable to pregnancy or a primary hip problem.	- N. 30 - Age 36.1 ± 11.8 yrs - Men: 56.7% - Diagnosis: degenerative disk disease 16.6%, disk problem 10%, LBP 73.4% - Previous LBP episodes: 83.0% - Current VAS (0–10): 2.8 ± 1.6	● Inter-rater reliability for PIT examined under 2 conditions: ● PIT test with additional guidelines ● PIT test without additional guidelines.	N. 2 examiners: Second-year physical therapy student Licensed physical therapist with 2 years of clinical experience in outpatient orthopedic physical therapy
Rabin et al. [12]	- **Aberrant Movement Pattern.** Painful arc on flexion; Painful arc on return; Instability catch; Gower sign ("thigh climbing"); Reverse lumbopelvic rhythm. *Positive test when at least one of the cited five signs is present.* - **Prone Instability Test:** *Positive when pain elicited during the first part of the test is relieved or abolished during the second part.* - **Passive Lumbar Extension Test:** *Positive if LBP is elicited.*	I: age between 18 and 60 years, main complaint of LBP and/or related leg symptoms (i.e., pain, paresthesia) E: pregnancy; history suggesting a non-mechanical origin of symptoms (e.g., malignancy, inflammatory conditions), LBP due to a fracture, osteoporosis, regular use of corticosteroids, rheumatoid arthritis, presence of 2 or more signs suggesting lumbar nerve root compression.	N. 30 consecutive patients with LBP of any duration, with or without associated leg symptoms. - Age: 33.5 ± 8.0 yrs - Gender: 15♀, 15♂ - Duration of symptoms: 164.4 ± 321.8 days - Previous LBP episodes: 20 subjects	Interrater reliability AMP was assessed by the two raters simultaneously; PIT and PLE are assessed by the two raters separately (second assessment 5 minutes after the first one).	N. 4 raters physical therapists, with experience ranging from 13 to 25 yrs. One rater with postprofessional master's degree (contributes to rating all subjects). Other raters with bachelor degree in physical therapy contribute to rating in 23, 4, and 3 subjects, respectively.

Table 6 Summary of results on reliability

Article	Test	Reliability	Results
Hicks et al. [23]	Aberrant Movement Pattern	Inter-rater reliability	k = 0.60 (95% CI: 0.44; 0.73)
	Prone Instability Test		k = 0.87 (95% CI: 0.80; 0.94)
Fritz et al. [24]	Aberrant Movement Pattern	Inter-rater reliability	k = −0.07 (95% CI: −0.45; 0.31)
	Prone Instability Test		k = 0.69 (95% CI: 0.59; 0.79)
	Posterior Shear Test		k = 0.27 (95% CI: 0.14; 0.41)
Schneider et al. [27]	Prone Instability Test	Inter-rater reliability	k = 0.46 (95% CI: 0.15, 0.77)
			k weighed = 0.58
Ravenna et al. [26]	Prone Instability Test with additional guidelines	Inter-rater reliability	(With*) k = 0.10 (95% IC: −0.27; 0.47)
			k weighed = 0.27 (95% IC: −0.08; 0.61)
			(Without*) k = 0.04 (95% IC: −0.34; 0.42)
			k weighed = 0.47 (95% IC: 0.15; 0.78)
Rabin et al. [12]	Aberrant Movement Pattern	Inter-rater reliability	k = 0.64 (95% IC 0.32; 0.90)
	Prone Instability Test		k = 0.67 (95% IC 0.29; 1.00)
	Passive Lumbar Extension test		k = 0.76 (95% IC 0.46; 1.00)
	Active Straight Leg Raising		k = 0.53 (95% IC 0.2; 0.84)

* = Additional guidelines.

[26] due to procedures and methodological weaknesses as the involvement of novel raters and the use of a modified test. The main statistical problem was the presence of few samples that could invalidate the k score. Despite all the other 4 studies adopting the PIT closely followed its original description, some differences in the positivity criteria were found. Hicks et al. [23] and Schneider et al. [27] judged the test positive when the pain disappeared in the second part of the test; Fritz et al. [24] when the pain decreased, whilst for Rabin et al. [12] the pain had to be both relieved or abolished.

After having excluded the two studies with the main methodological weaknesses, the reliability of the PIT appeared from moderate to good.

The AMP reliability was investigated in three studies [12,23,24] but their results were not similar and ranged from insufficient reliability [24] to moderate reliability [12,23]. The PST was investigated by only one study and scored the lowest reliability [24], which is insufficient to recommend its use.

Implications for clinical practice

After an initial inspection of the articles it appears that the information derived from the studies could provide a useful picture of the items that contribute to the definition of "applicability in rehabilitation practice". Sufficient information was provided on the execution of the tests, whereas little information regarded the duration, and the time needed to process data. Considering that in clinical practice a standard manual therapy session normally lasts 30 minutes, it may be the case that a series of tests proposed in the literature cannot be repeated by the clinicians due to lack of time. The attempt to identify methods for the evaluation of lumbar instability in patients with LBP allowed us to select some tests that are suitable for clinicians in everyday clinical practice. The time needed to test and process data are compatible with clinical practice and research purposes. Starting from the same key-words used for the search of the articles of the literature review, 4 clinical tests (PIT, PLE, AMP and PST) investigated by 2 studies [24,25] met the criteria of applicability in clinical practice.

Limits

The main limitation of this review is the small number of articles found on any single test. Only 2 studies concerned the diagnostic accuracy, while for the studies investigating the reliability, the results are limited by statistical or methodological weaknesses. For example, the Ravenna's [26] conclusions should be cautiously interpreted also for some significant modifications made to standardize the PIT, such as the different hip and knee positions, the use of a stabilization scapular belt and a stool for foot placement.

The average age and the characteristics of the spinal dysfunctions of the samples were not homogeneous in the different studies, thus reducing the external validity of the results. Another limitation of this review concerns the insufficient homogeneity regarding the execution and interpretation of the tests. As already mentioned, a lack of standardization of a test affects comparative analyses among different studies and the implementation of that test in clinical practice.

Conclusions

The actual state of the art of clinical tests for lumbar instability include 6 studies of almost 333 patients and 4 clinical tests. Our data suggest that the PLE test is the most suitable test for detecting lumbar instability, thanks to its excellent diagnostic accuracy, and good reliability. Further studies on the diagnostic properties of the PLE test to detect lumbar instability among different populations with LBP are suggested.

After more than 20 years from the definition of the importance of diagnostic clinical tests for lumbar instability in individuals with LBP, clinicians can use some tests showing encouraging results in terms of accuracy and reliability. Nevertheless, their application in daily practice might be affected by insufficient research and evidence on their performances. Future research should be oriented to compare in the same study different assessment methods on the same sample size, in order to evaluate their reliability and validity.

Competing interests

The authors declare that they have no competing interests. The authors disclose any financial and personal relationships with other people or organizations that could inappropriately influence this work.

Authors' contributions

SF was the main supervisor on location and overlooked every step of the process. SF and CV conceived the study and were responsible for drafting the manuscript. All authors were responsible for the study design. TM and FB performed the data collection. JUV undertook the analyses. All authors read and approved the final manuscript.

Acknowledgements

We would like to thank Anna Trevisan for assisting with the literature search, Giovanni Gobitti for helping us in the statistical analysis, Fabio Cassola and Paola D'Ovidio for their help in the language review.

Author details

[1]Master of Manual Therapy and Musculoskeletal Rehabilitation, Department of Molecular Medicine, University of Padova, Padova, Italy. [2]Physical Therapy Private Practice, Treviso, Italy. [3]Physioup Physical Therapy Private Practice, Rome, Italy. [4]IRCCS Don Gnocchi Foundation, Milan, Italy.

References

1. Martin BI, Deyo RA, Mirza SK, Turner JA, Comstock BA, Hollingworth W, et al. Expenditures and health status among adults with back and neck problems. JAMA. 2008;299(6):656–64. doi:10.1001/jama.299.6.656.
2. Childs JD, Fritz JM, Piva SR, Erhard RE. Clinical decision making in the identification of patients likely to benefit from spinal manipulation: a traditional versus an evidence-based approach. J Orthop Sports Phys Ther. 2003;33(5):259–72.
3. Hall H, McIntosh G, Boyle C. Effectiveness of a low back pain classification system. Spine J. 2009;9(8):648–57. doi:10.1016/j.spinee.2009.04.017.
4. Abbott JH, McCane B, Herbison P, Moginie G, Chapple C, Hogarty T. Lumbar segmental instability: a criterion-related validity study of manual therapy assessment. BMC Musculoskelet Disord. 2005;6:56.
5. Delitto A, George SZ, Van Dillen LR, Whitman JM, Sowa G, Shekelle P, et al. Low back pain. J Orthop Sports Phys Ther. 2012;42(4):A1–57. doi:10.2519/jospt.2012.0301.
6. Dupuis PR, Yong-Hing K, Cassidy JD, Kirkaldy-Willis WH. Radiologic diagnosis of degenerative lumbar spinal instability. Spine. 1985;10(3):262–76.
7. Nizard RS, Wybier M, Laredo JD. Radiologic assessment of lumbar intervertebral instability and degenerative spondylolisthesis. Radiol Clin North Am. 2001;39(1):55–71. 1.
8. O'Sullivan PB, Phyty GD, Twomey LT, Allison GT. Evaluation of specific stabilizing exercise in the treatment of chronic low back pain with radiologic diagnosis of spondylolysis or spondylolisthesis. Spine. 1997;22(24):2959–67.
9. Hodges PW, Moseley GL. Pain and motor control of the lumbopelvic region: effect and possible mechanisms. J Electromyogr Kinesiol. 2003;13(4):361–70.
10. Lee P, Helewa A, Goldsmith CH, Smythe HA, Stitt LW. Low back pain: prevalence and risk factors in an industrial setting. J Rheumatol. 2001;28(2):346–51.
11. Macedo LG, Latimer J, Maher CG, Hodges PW, Nicholas M, Tonkin L, et al. Motor control or graded activity exercises for chronic low back pain? A randomised controlled trial. BMC Musculoskelet Disord. 2008;9:65. doi:10.1186/1471-2474-9-65.
12. Rabin A, Shashua A, Pizem K, Dar G. The interrater reliability of physical examination tests that may predict the outcome or suggest the need for lumbar stabilization exercises. J Orthop Sports Phys Ther. 2013;43(2):83–90. doi:10.2519/jospt.2013.4310.
13. Alqarni AM, Schneiders AG, Hendrick PA. Clinical tests to diagnose lumbar segmental instability: a systematic review. J Orthop Sports Phys Ther. 2011;41(3):130–40. doi:10.2519/jospt.2011.3457.
14. May S, Littlewood C, Bishop A. Reliability of procedures used in the physical examination of non-specific low back pain: a systematic review. Aust J Physiother. 2006;52(2):91–102.
15. Moher D, Liberati A, Tetzlaff J, Altman DG, Group P. Preferred reporting items for systematic reviews and meta-analyses: the PRISMA statement. Int J Surg. 2010;8(5):336–41. doi:10.1016/j.ijsu.2010.02.007.
16. Cleland JA. Orthopaedic Clinical Examination: An Evidence-Based Approach for Physical Therapists. Carlstadt, NJ: Icon Learning Systems; 2005. p. 516. ISBN 1-929007-87-6.
17. Whiting P, Rutjes AW, Reitsma JB, Bossuyt PM, Kleijnen J. The development of QUADAS: a tool for the quality assessment of studies of diagnostic accuracy included in systematic reviews. BMC Med Res Methodol. 2003;3:25.
18. Lucas NP, Macaskill P, Irwig L, Bogduk N. The development of a quality appraisal tool for studies of diagnostic reliability (QAREL). J Clin Epidemiol. 2010;63(8):854–61. doi:10.1016/j.jclinepi.2009.10.002.
19. Villafañe JH, Zanetti L, Isgrò M, Cleland JA, Bertozzi L, Gobbo M, et al. Methods for the assessment of neuromotor capacity in non-specific low back pain: Validity and applicability in everyday clinical practice. J Back Musculoskelet Rehabil. 2014. In Press.
20. van der Wurff P, Meyne W, Hagmeijer RH. Clinical tests of the sacroiliac joint. Man Ther. 2000;5(2):89–96.
21. Vanti C, Bonfiglioli R, Calabrese M, Marinelli F, Guccione A, Violante FS, et al. Upper Limb Neurodynamic Test 1 and symptoms reproduction in carpal tunnel syndrome. A validity study. Man Ther. 2011;16(3):258–63. doi:10.1016/j.math.2010.11.003.
22. Jewell D. Guide to Evidence-Based Physical Therapist Practice. 2nd ed. Sudbury MA: Jones & Bartlett Learning; 2011. p. 230.
23. Hicks GE, Fritz JM, Delitto A, Mishock J. Interrater reliability of clinical examination measures for identification of lumbar segmental instability. Arch Phys Med Rehabil. 2003;84(12):1858–64.
24. Fritz JM, Whitman JM, Childs JD. Lumbar spine segmental mobility assessment: an examination of validity for determining intervention strategies in patients with low back pain. Arch Phys Med Rehabil. 2005;86(9):1745–52.
25. Kasai Y, Morishita K, Kawakita E, Kondo T, Uchida A. A new evaluation method for lumbar spinal instability: passive lumbar extension test. Phys Ther. 2006;86(12):1661–7.
26. Ravenna MM, Hoffman SL, Van Dillen LR. Low interrater reliability of examiners performing the prone instability test: a clinical test for lumbar shear instability. Arch Phys Med Rehabil. 2011;92(6):913–9.
27. Schneider M, Erhard R, Brach J, Tellin W, Imbarlina F, Delitto A. Spinal palpation for lumbar segmental mobility and pain provocation: an interexaminer reliability study. J Manipulative Physiol Ther. 2008;31(6):465–73. doi:10.1016/j.jmpt.2008.06.004.
28. Long DM, BenDebba M, Torgerson WS, Boyd RJ, Dawson EG, Hardy RW, et al. Persistent back pain and sciatica in the United States: patient characteristics. J Spinal Disord. 1996;9(1):40–58.
29. Panjabi MM. The stabilizing system of the spine. Part II. Neutral zone and instability hypothesis. J Spinal Disord. 1992;5(4):390–6. discussion 7.

30. Dvorak J, Panjabi MM, Novotny JE, Chang DG, Grob D. Clinical validation of functional flexion-extension roentgenograms of the lumbar spine. Spine. 1991;16(8):943–50.
31. Pope MH, Frymoyer JW, Krag MH. Diagnosing instability. Clin Orthop Relat Res. 1992;279:60–7.
32. Hicks GE, Fritz JM, Delitto A, McGill SM. Preliminary development of a clinical prediction rule for determining which patients with low back pain will respond to a stabilization exercise program. Arch Phys Med Rehabil. 2005;86(9):1753–62.

Reliability of diagnostic ultrasound in measuring the multifidus muscle

Eirik Johan Skeie[1*], Jan Arve Borge[2], Charlotte Leboeuf-Yde[3], Jenni Bolton[4] and Niels Wedderkopp[5]

Abstract

Background: Ultrasound is frequently used to measure activity in the lumbar multifidus muscle (LMM). However previous reliability studies on diagnostic ultrasound and LMM have included a limited number of subjects and few have used Bland-Altman's Limits of Agreement (LOA). Further one does not know if activity affects the subjects' ability to contract the LMM.

Methods: From January 2012 to December 2012 an inter- and intra-examiner reliability study was carried out in a clinical setting. It consisted of a total of four experiments with 30 subjects in each study. Two experienced examiners performed all measurements. Ultrasound measurements were made of: 1. the LMM in the resting state, 2. during a contracted state, 3. on subsequent days, and, before and after walking. Reliability and agreement was tested for 1. resting LMM, 2. contracted LMM, and 3. thickness change in the LMM. Mean values of three measurements were used for statistical analysis for each spinal level. The intra-class correlation coefficient (ICC) 3.1 and 3.2 was used to test for reliability, and Bland-Altman's LOA method to test for agreement.

Results: All of the studies indicate high levels of reliability, but as the LMM thickness increased (increasing contraction) the agreement between examiners was poorer than for low levels of contraction.

Conclusions: The use of diagnostic ultrasound to measure the LMM seems to be reliable in subjects who have little or no change in thickness of the LMM with contraction.

Keywords: Diagnostic ultrasound, Measurement, Lumbar multifidus, Agreement, Reliability, Limits of agreement, Intraclass correlation coefficient

Introduction

The lumbar multifidus muscle and low back pain

It is well known that non-specific low back pain (LBP) is a prevalent disorder often with numerous recurring episodes [1]. Currently there is no objective clinical test that is able to differentiate subjects with nonspecific LBP from pain free subjects, nor is there any clinical test than can predict the occurrence or recurrence of LBP. Even though the exact cause of LBP remains unknown, some studies indicate that fat infiltrations in the multifidus musculature (LMM) are associated with back pain [2]. Numerous studies have been carried out on the LMM in relation to the presence of LBP with and without radiculopathy [3-9], as well as LMM size and function as a prognostic factor for LBP [10,11], predictive effects of changes in the LMM in LBP patients [12,13] and LMM changes in relation to treatment of LBP [14-16]. Changes of the LMM function have also been noted in people who previously had LBP [17] and even in those with experimentally induced LBP [18]. Therefore it seems possible that there may be a link between the function and/or morphology of the LMM and LBP. Hence function of the LMM may be easily altered by pain and slow to recover.

Evaluating the LMM with diagnostic ultrasound

When evaluating the LMM with ultrasound, this is done by comparing the thickness of resting muscle with that of activated muscle. The reason for this is findings in prior studies that have demonstrated reduced ability to contract the LMM in low back pain patients [7,9] as well as in patients who have previously suffered from LBP [17]. Hodges et al. [19] investigated the use of ultrasound to measure muscle contraction on several muscles

* Correspondence: eirikjs@online.no
[1]MChiro, MSc, Ulriksdal 2, 5009 Bergen, Norway
Full list of author information is available at the end of the article

other than the LMM. The study found the architectural parameters measured by ultrasound and EMG showed a nonlinear relationship, and the majority of muscle thickness change took place in the range up to 30% of maximal voluntary contraction [19]. For the LMM a close correlation was found between values measured by ultrasound and activity measured by EMG when the contractions were in the range of 19 to 34% of maximum contraction [20].

Earlier studies on diagnostic ultrasound and the LMM differed greatly on methodology, procedures, equipment, muscles tested, sample size, LBP presentation, and levels of physical fitness of participants. A systematic review by Hebert et al. [21] reported poor methodological quality of previous studies on diagnostic ultrasound and LMM, only 6 of the 24 studies included in the systematic review were considered high quality studies.

When measuring the thickness of the LMM, earlier studies have shown that averaging the thickness of three measurements optimizes reproducibility [22,23]. Very good inter-rater agreements between novice and experienced examiners have been found when measuring LMM thickness [24]. Good inter- and intra-rater reliability has also been reported between experienced examiners [25] and novice examiners [23,26,27]. In order to activate the LMM one can lift either the contralateral arm or leg. An earlier study found only marginal difference in contraction when lifting the contralateral arm or leg: The same study also noted that transducer position has little effect on intra and inter-rater reliability of diagnostic ultrasound and the LMM [23]. The systematic review by Hebert et al. [21] highlights that reliability increases with more experienced examiners, and that only a minority of studies have reported low levels of reliability.

Need for further studies on diagnostic ultrasound

Criticism has been raised against several of the studies on inter- and intra-rater reliability of the LMM when measured with diagnostic ultrasound. Hebert et al. [21] highlighted different methods in measuring the LMM in previous studies, and several of these had small sample sizes (<15), asymptomatic subjects, and only some of the studies looked at the measurement of contraction. None of the previous studies investigated how general activity, such as gait might affect measurements of the LMM using diagnostic ultrasound. The reason for investigating gait, is the suggestion that the spine is the key to locomotion of the lower limbs [28]. More recent studies have shown increased electromyographic activity in the LMM during walking [29].

Methodological considerations

Previous studies that investigated reproducibility of measurements of LMM with diagnostic ultrasound have done so by examining reliability of measurements. To test this statistically, the intra-class correlation coefficient (ICC) is commonly used. However, the concept of reproducibility consists also of agreement. Agreement is best illustrated with Bland-Altman's Limits of Agreement (LOA) method [30-33] because it helps detect any systematic differences between the individual measurements (i.e., fixed bias) and is able to identify possible outliers. However only rarely in previous studies on diagnostic ultrasound and the LMM have both these methods been used [26].

Aim and objectives of the present study

In order to bring forth a coherent picture on the issue of the potential usefulness of ultrasound diagnosis on the LMM in people with LBP, a number of projects were carried out. We started with the most basic aspects, moving towards the more advanced ones, using both the ICC and LOA methods for our statistical analyses. Specifically, the study had the four following objectives in relation to the ultrasound diagnostic procedure on the LMM:

1. To study the inter-examiner reliability of diagnostic ultrasound when measuring LMM thickness on one still image.
2. To study the inter-examiner reliability of diagnostic ultrasound when measuring LMM contraction on two sets of still images.
3. To study the intra-examiner reliability of diagnostic ultrasound when measuring LMM contraction on two different occasions.
4. To study the stability of measurements of LMM contraction with diagnostic ultrasound by comparing these before and after the subjects exercised.

Methods

Examiners

Inter and intra-examiner reliability was tested between two chiropractors who were both experienced in diagnostic ultrasound for the musculoskeletal system. Examiner 1 had four years of experience in diagnostic ultrasound and examiner 2 had eight years of experience. At the time of the study both the examiners held a postgraduate diploma in diagnostic ultrasound. Before the study, both examiners agreed upon and developed the protocol of diagnostic ultrasound that was applied in this study.

Study subjects

An a priori decision was made to include 30 study subjects to test each of the four study objectives. These subjects were recruited consecutively from a chiropractic practice from January 2012 to December 2012. The sample size was considered a convenience sample as the study was conducted in a routine clinical practice setting. The majority of these subjects were LBP patients although patients with other spinal complaints such as mid back pain, neck pain, and/or extremity pain were also included. In addition some pain-free subjects were recruited from outside the clinic. This case mix was to include subjects with the potential ability to produce a contraction of the LMM as well as those with the potential not to. Subjects were recruited during the clinic's opening hours, normally around the end of the day and during lunch hours when both examiners were available. Each of the total 120 subjects took part in only one of the projects outlined above. All subjects gave verbal and written consent to inclusion in the study. Application for ethics approval was sent to the Regional Committees for Medical and Health Research Ethics (REC) in Norway. REC considered the project a quality assurance project and therefore no special permission from REC was needed to complete the project.

Procedures

Ultrasound measurements

In this study all the measurements of the LMM were taken with the subjects in a prone position with a pillow placed under the abdomen to flatten the lumbar lordosis as this provides better contact for the transducer. A Medison Accuvix V10 ultrasound scanner with a 3–7 MHz curvilinear probe was used. To identify the level of the LMM in the lumbar spine, the transducer was placed longitudinally along the spine with the midpoint over the spinous processes of interest. The sacrum was recognized as a longitudinal structure in contrast to the shorter curved spinous processes. The probe was then moved laterally and angled slightly medially until the facet joint in question could be visualized as described by Kiesel [20]. At this point the probe was directly overlying the LMM, and a measurement was taken from the apex of the facet joint to the plane between the thoracolumbar fascia and the subcutaneous fat. The reason for utilizing the on-screen callipers was to make the study as clinically relevant as possible. Previous studies have analysed the images offline. However, this is not common in a clinical setting. Care was taken not to move too far laterally as this would lead to imaging of the erector spinae muscles and not the LMM. Figure 1 illustrates placement of the calipers.

Objective 1: Inter-examiner reliability of LMM thickness on the same still image

For all study subjects in objective 1, a single image was generated of the LMM by one of the examiners. The first examiner then placed a marker on the image on the mammillary process of the level to be measured. Examiner 1 subsequently measured the distance three times with the calliper software on the ultrasound machine, saving each image onto the ultrasound machine's hard drive. The callipers and saved images were removed before examiner 2 entered the room, leaving only the still image with the marker in place on the screen. Examiner 2 then performed the same measurement procedure. Thereafter the data were transferred to a separate paper by examiner 1 who calculated mean values.

Objective 2: Inter-examiner reliability of LMM contraction on separate still images

For all subjects, images of the LMM in the resting and contracted states were generated independently by each of the examiners. The spinal level to be measured was chosen from predetermined criteria (a total of thirty average measurements, fifteen from the left and fifteen from the right, and evenly distributed between L3-L5). Examiner 1 generated an image of the LMM in the resting state with the subject in prone position (Figure 1). Thereafter a split screen was utilized and the subject performed the contralateral arm lifting task as described by Kiesel [20] but with no hand held load. Then a second image (Figure 1: Image 2) was captured of the contracted LMM with the arm in the elevated position, and the thickness of the LMM was measured on screen of the two images (Figure 1: Image 1: resting thickness, Figure 1: Image 2: contracted thickness). This procedure was performed three times by both examiners for each subject, giving three sets of measurements of the LMM in the resting and contracted states for each level for each examiner. The three sets of images with the measurements in place were saved onto the ultrasound machine's hard drive. Examiner 1 removed the saved images from the screen before examiner 2 entered the room. Examiner 2 then repeated the same procedure. After examiner 2 left the room, the data were then transferred to two separate sheets of paper by examiner 1. Examiner 1 calculated mean measurements for the individual measurements by both examiners (mean resting and contraction values). In addition contraction of the LMM was expressed as raw change in thickness (contracted LMM minus resting LMM). Contraction was expressed as an exact change in thickness and not in a relative percentage because there is missing evidence to support that the LMM contracts as a unit.

Objective 3: Intra-examiner reliability of LMM contraction using two sets of still images on two different days

For all subjects, three sets of measurements were generated on two different days giving a total of six sets of measurements per subject. Examiner 1 performed all measurements. To reduce the risk of recall, a minimum of five days

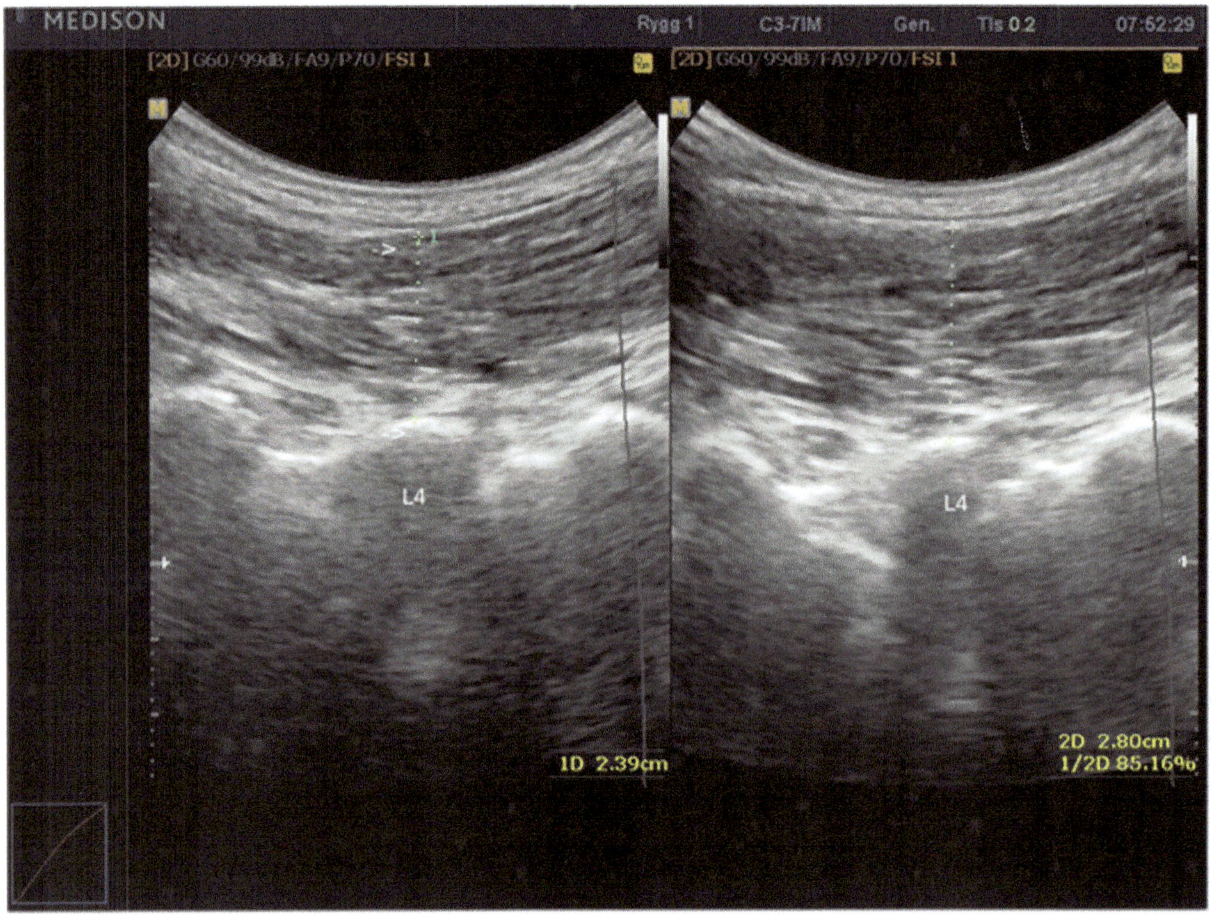

Figure 1 Ultrasound image of resting LMM (left image) contracted LMM (right image). Calipers placed on the apex of facet joint of L4, and on the interface between the thoracolumbar fascia and subcutaneous fat.

elapsed between measurements during which a large number of patients had been examined, making recall of previous measurements unlikely. The procedure for obtaining the images was the same as for objective 2. The measurements obtained by the examiner were saved onto the ultrasound machine, and recorded on two different sets of paper that were kept separate until all measurements had been obtained. The first sets of measurements were deleted off the ultrasound machines hard drive on the same day as they were generated. This was done to avoid examiner 1 being able to read the first set of measurements when performing measurements on the second day. Examiner 2 then calculated the mean of resting and contracting LMM values for day 1 and day 2.

Objective 4: Repeatability of measurements of LMM contraction with diagnostic ultrasound before and after the subjects walked around the table

For all subjects examiner 1 generated two sets of images. Again, examiner 1 performed all measurements. The procedure for obtaining resting and contraction measurements of LMM were the same as in objectives 2 and 3. For each subject three sets of measurements were taken both before and after the subject walked around the table (exercised). When recording the measurements, examiner 1 first saved the first three sets of measurements on the ultrasound machine's hard drive, after which the subject exercised. During the exercise the first sets of measurements had been cleared from the screen. The second three sets of measurements taken were saved on the same subject file but annotated as "after". The reason for clearing the images from the screen was to prevent examiner 1 from reading the measurements from the "before" measurements when recording the second sets of measurements. After the measurements were completed, examiner 2 transferred the data onto a separate sheet of paper and calculated mean values for the individual measurements by examiner 1 (mean resting thickness and contraction thickness before the patient had walked, and mean resting and contraction values after the subject had walked around the table). The contraction was expressed as raw change in thickness (contracted LMM – resting LMM).

Statistical analyses

Correlation between examiners was measured in three ways:

1. For study objectives 1 to 4, ICC were determined in two ways, both as two way mixed single measures (3.1) and as two way mixed average measures (3.2) in order to evaluate inter- and intra-rater reliability. ICC 3.1 and 3.2 are the correct forms of ICC to use when the subjects are randomly selected but the examiners are not [34]. In this analysis, both subjects and examiners are seen as potential sources of systematic variability.

There is no consensus of what constitutes a good ICC value [35]. According to the guidelines by Kottner et al. [33] the ICC values should be at least 0.90 or 0.95 if individual and important decisions should be made based on ICC statistics. A systematic review by Hebert et al. [21] on the reliability of diagnostic ultrasound on the abdominal and lumbar trunk muscles used ICC values above 0.75 to indicate good reliability and below 0.75 to indicate poor reliability.

2. LOA were also calculated for study objectives 1, 2 and 4 and shown in order to determine differences between the means of the measurements. The LOA is shown as a graph in which the individual measurements are plotted making it possible to observe if the results vary as a function of the size of the measurements.

3. In addition to the ICC values for study objective 3, a linear plot was constructed in order to evaluate the level of LMM contraction in the subjects on two different days.

The analyses were carried out by an independent person (NW) using STATA version 12.1.

Results

Descriptive data

A detailed description of the study subjects is shown in Table 1. Each experiment consisted of a different sample of 30 subjects.

Objective 1. To study the inter-examiner reliability of diagnostic ultrasound when measuring LMM thickness on one still image

Good inter-examiner reliability was found between examiners (Table 2). The mean difference between examiners was low and the LOA narrow in range (Figure 2, Table 3). The greatest difference on an individual measurement between the two examiners, gave a measurement difference of approximately 2% when applied to the average LMM thickness.

Objective 2. To study the inter-examiner reliability of diagnostic ultrasound when measuring LMM contraction on two sets of still images

Good inter-examiner reliability was also found between examiners when measuring resting and contracted LMM (Table 2). The LOA plots (Figures 3 and 4, and Table 3) for resting and contracted LMM showed a small average difference between examiner 1 and 2. However the LOA plots (Figures 3 and 4, and Table 3) were substantially wider than in study 1. The average difference between examiners measuring resting LMM was very low (Table 3), but the greatest difference on an individual measurement equated to a difference of as much as 21% between examiners (Figure 3). For the contracted LMM the average difference between examiners measuring resting LMM was very low (Table 3). But the greatest difference on an individual measurement of the LMM resulted in a 19% difference between examiners (Figure 4).

When LMM contraction was expressed as contracted LMM minus relaxed LMM good inter-examiner reliability was found (Table 2). The LOA plot (Figure 5, Table 3) demonstrated a low average difference between the examiners. But compared with the LOA plots (Figures 3 and 4) for measurements of contracted and relaxed LMM, the average difference between examiners increased when expressing contraction as LMM

Table 1 Descriptive data on subjects

Subjects, total.									
Total (N)	**Male (N)**	**Female (N)**	**Mean age (Yrs.)**	**Age range (Yrs.)**	**SD (Yrs.)**	**LBP (N)**	**Neck/Midback pain (N)**	**Extremity pain (N)**	**Pain free (N)**
120	64	56	38	20-69	±12	88	23	4	5
Study objective 1									
30	18	12	38	20-69	±13	25	5	0	0
Study objective 2									
30	14	16	37	20-65	±12	20	5	1	4
Study objective 3									
30	15	15	38	20-59	±11	23	7	0	0
Study objective 4									
30	17	13	40	20-68	±11	20	6	3	1

Table 2 Mean measurements for LMM and ICC values for study objective 1–4

Objective 1 Interexaminer reliability of measuring LMM thickness using one still image			
Mean LLM thickness examiner 1	Mean LLM thickness examiner 2	ICC average	ICC individual
27.9 mm ± 3.2 mm	27.9 mm ± 3.2 mm	0.999 (0.997-0.999)	0.997 (0.994-0.999)
Objective 2 Interexaminer reliability of measuring LMM contraction using two sets of still images.			
Mean relaxed LLM thickness examiner 1 (distance 1)	Mean relaxed LLM thickness examiner 2 (distance 1)	ICC average	ICC individual
28.9 mm ± 6.4 mm	29.0 mm ± 6.1 mm	0.97 (0.94-0.99)	0.95 (0.89-0.98)
Mean contracted LLM thickness examiner 1 (distance 2)	Mean contracted LLM thickness examiner 2 (distance 2)	ICC average	ICC individual
32.1 mm ± 7.0 mm	32.0 mm ± 6.7 mm	0.97 (0.94-0.99)	0.95 (0.90-0.98)
Distance 2–1 examiner 1	Distance 2–1 examiner 1	ICC average	ICC individual
3.1 mm ± 2.2 mm	3.0 mm ± 2.0 mm	0.98 (0.96-0.99)	0.97 (0.92-0.98)
Objective 3 Intraexaminer reliabilty of measuring LMM contraction using 2 sets of still images taken on 2 different days.			
Mean relaxed LLM thickness (distance 1 day 1)	Mean relaxed LLM thickness (distance 1 day 2)	ICC average	ICC individual
28.4 mm ± 5.3 mm	28.4 mm ± 4.8 mm	0.99 (0.97-0.99)	0.97 (0.94-0-99)
Mean contracted LLM thickness (distance 2 day 1)	Mean contracted LLM thickness (distance 2 day 2)	ICC average	ICC individual
29.7 mm ± 6.0 mm	29.6 mm ± 5.5 mm	0.97 (0.93-0.99)	0.94 (0.88-0.97)
Distance 2–1 day 1	Distance 2–1 day 2	ICC average	ICC individual
1.4 mm ± 1.7 mm	1.3 mm ± 1.7 mm	0.97 (0.93-0.99)	0.94 (0.88-0.97)
Objective 4 Measuring LMM contraction before and after a motor task on two sets of still images.			
Mean relaxed LLM thickness (distance 1 before task)	Mean contracted LLM thickness (distance 2 before task)	Mean relaxed LLM thickness (distance 1 after task)	Mean contracted LLM thickness (distance 2 after task)
30.6 mm ± 5.5 mm	34.1 mm ± 6.6 mm	29.9 mm ± 5.3 mm	34.6 mm ± 6.4 mm
Distance 2–1 before	Distance 2–1 after	ICC average	ICC individual
3.5 mm ± 2.6 mm	3.5 mm ± 2.5 mm	0.98 (0.97-0.99)	0.97 (0.94-0.99)

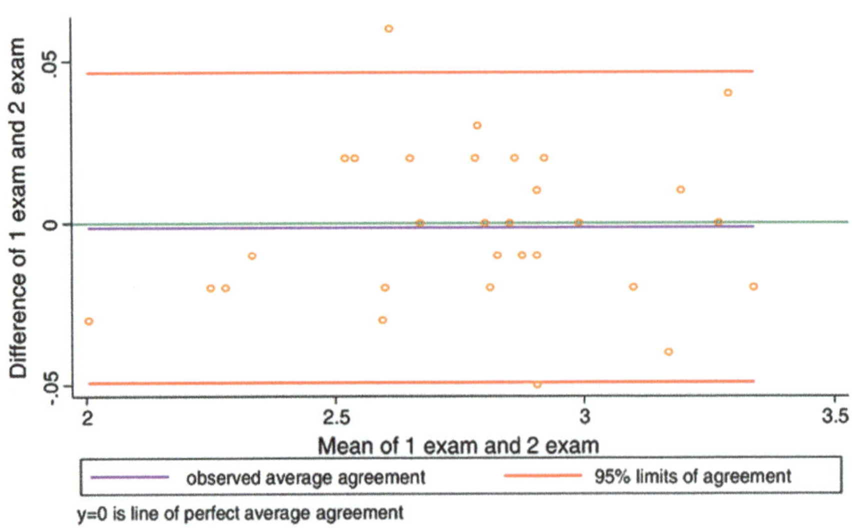

Figure 2 LOA plot showing agreement between examiner 1 and examiner 2. Study objective 1, measurement of LMM thickness on one still image (N = 30).

Table 3 Mean difference and LOA range study 1, 2, and 4

Objective 1		
	Mean difference	**LOA range**
Relaxed LMM	0.01 mm ± 0.24 mm	[−0.48; 0.47 mm]
Objective 2		
Relaxed LMM	0.08 mm ± 2.0 mm	[−4.07; 3.92 mm]
Contracted LMM	0.06 mm ±2.0 mm	[−3.93; 4.06 mm]
Contracted-Relaxed LMM	0.14 mm ±0.55 mm	[−0.94; 1.22 mm]
Objective 4		
Relaxed LMM	0.7 mm ± 0.9 mm	[−1.09; 2.49 mm]
Contracted LMM	0.7 mm ± 0.9 mm	[−1.18; 2.51 mm]
Contracted-Relaxed LMM	0.04 mm ± 0.65 mm	[−1.32; 1.25 mm]

minus relaxed LMM. The greatest difference on an individual measurement equated to a 45% difference in measurements between the two examiners. The LOA (Figure 5) demonstrated a funnel shape with the opening to the right. On the x-axis the volume increased towards the right suggesting poorer agreement with increasing muscle thickness.

It is also possible to express contraction as a relative percentage change and not as a raw measurement. This was performed as a separate analysis to see if it changed the LOA plot. Figure 6 shows contraction expressed this way. This resulted in a change in the funnel shape of the LOA plot into a more linear increase indicating that the examiners agreed less as the muscle thickness increased.

Objective 3. To study the intra-examiner reliability of diagnostic ultrasound when measuring LMM contraction on two different days

Again, there was good intra-examiner reliability both for relaxed and contracted LMM (Table 2). ICC values for contraction expressed as contracted LMM minus relaxed LMM (Table 2) also demonstrated excellent intra-examiner reliability.

The linear plot in Figure 7 shows little change in measurements from day to day, and that the vast majority of the subjects had little or no ability to contract their LMM. Only five subjects are seen on the right end of the scale demonstrating a volume change representing contraction. Four of the subjects had around 4 mm volume increase of the LMM and one subject had around 6 mm volume change. On average this equates to a relative thickness change between 14 and 20%. This study did not attempt to correlate the level of pain with contraction, so it is not possible to determine whether these subjects suffered from LBP.

Objective 4. To study the repeatability of measurements of LMM contraction with diagnostic ultrasound before and after the subjects walked around the table

There was good intra-examiner reliability for relaxed and contracted LMM on days 1 and 2 (Table 2). Good intra-examiner agreement was also seen for contraction expressed as contracted minus relaxed LMM (Table 2). The LOA plots for relaxed and contracted LMM (Figures 8 and 9) were very similar to those in study objective 2

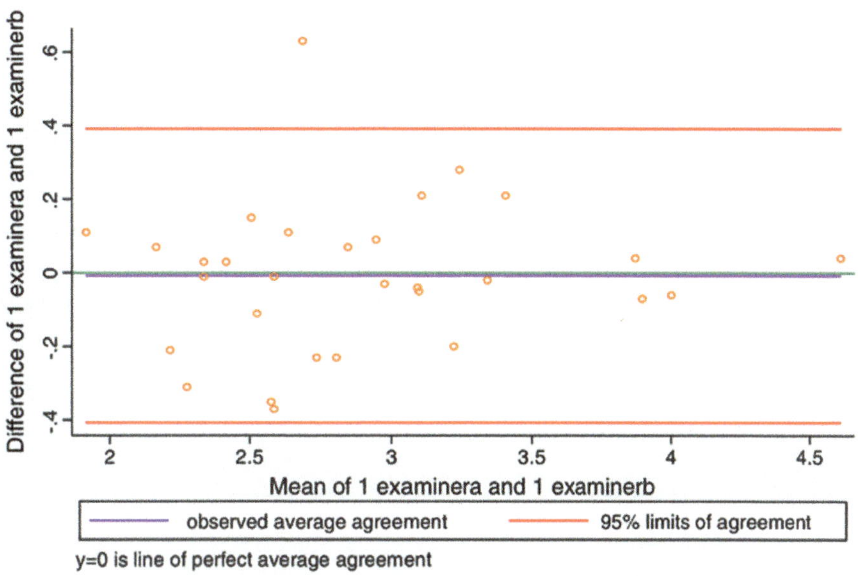

Figure 3 LOA plot showing agreement between examiner 1 and examiner 2. Study objective 2, measurement of resting LMM on two sets of images (N = 30).

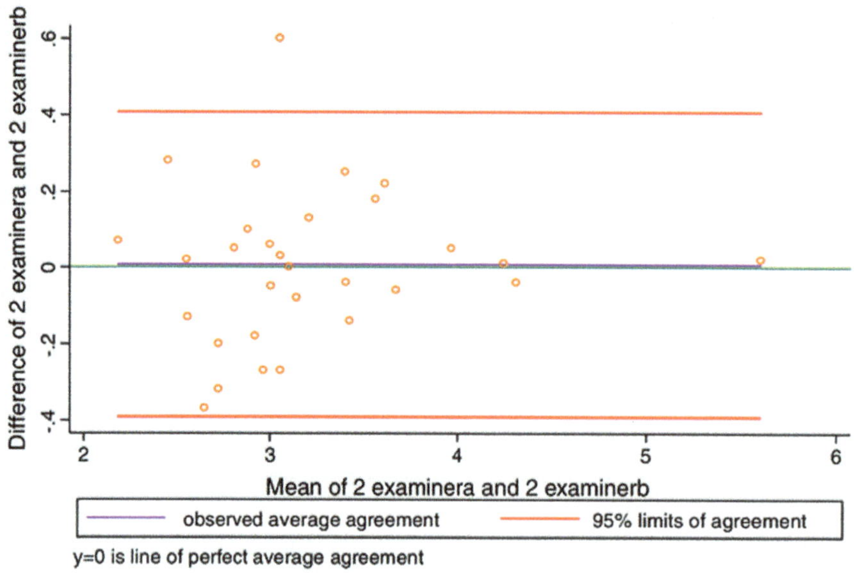

Figure 4 LOA plot showing agreement between examiner 1 and examiner 2. Study objective 2, measurement of contracted LMM on two sets of images (N = 30).

(Figures 3 and 4). The average difference for relaxed and contracted LMM was still low although greater than those found in study 2 (Table 3). Nonetheless the standard deviation for resting and contracted LMM is lower than that seen in study objective 2. The greatest difference for an individual measurement was equal to 6% measurement difference before and after the subject exercised. For contracted LMM the greatest difference on an individual measurement was equal to 5% measurement difference. When expressing contraction as (contracted LMM minus relaxed LMM) a similar plot to Figure 5 is seen in Figure 10. Again a moderate funnel shape can be seen, indicating less agreement as the LMM thickness increases. The average difference is also very low (Table 3). The greatest difference in LMM contraction on an individual measurement gave a measurement difference in muscle thickness as high as 7% before and after the subject exercised.

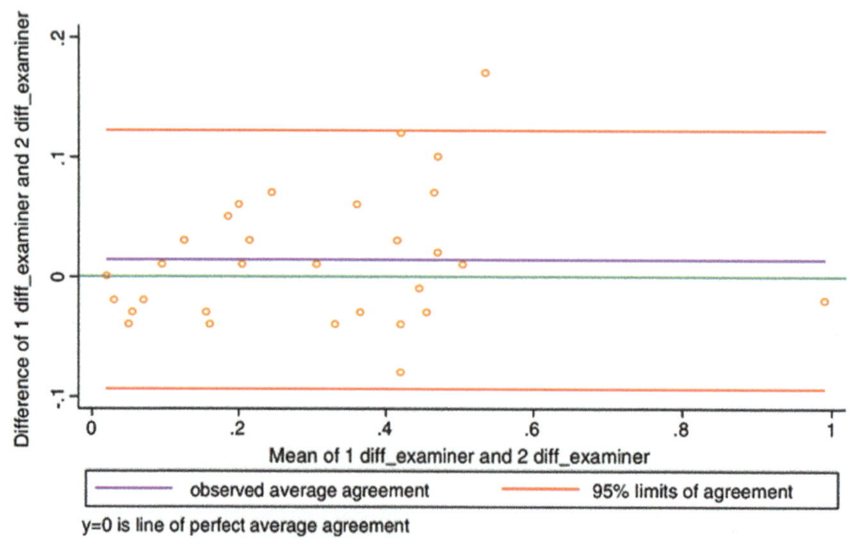

Figure 5 LOA plot showing agreement between examiner 1 and examiner 2. Study objective 2, measurement of contraction (distance 2 – distance 1) LMM on two sets of images (N = 30).

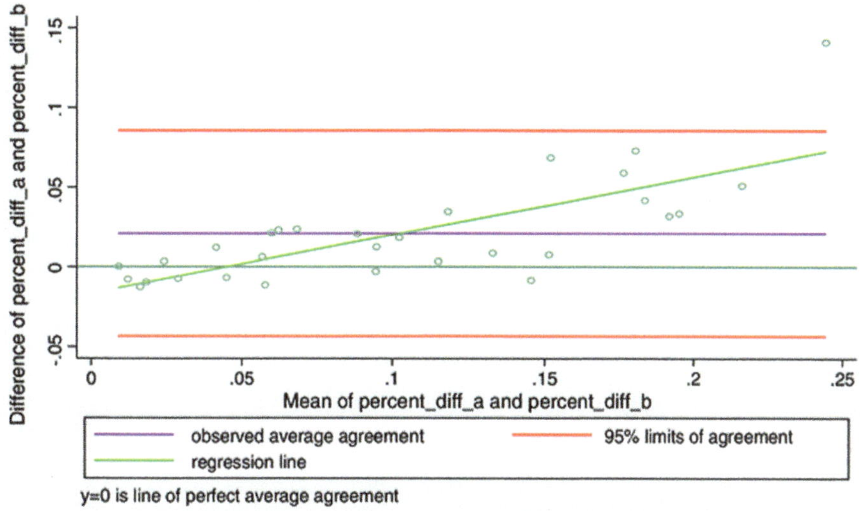

Figure 6 LOA plot showing agreement between examiner 1 and examiner 2. Study objective 2, measurement of LMM contraction expressed as relative % (distance 2 – distance 1)/distance 1) on two sets of images (N = 30).

Discussion

We performed four independent studies to test if diagnostic ultrasound can be used to reliably examine the thickness of the LMM in situations that relate to the various stages of examination. To analyse our data, we used both ICC and LOA. Our results were encouraging. Average measurements were used for analysis. The reliability of the measurements of LMM thickness was good in all four studies. This was the case when two examiners used the same still image, when they used two sets of still images, when one examiner measured the same person on two different days, and before/after the study-subject had walked around for a while.

However, it was noted that good agreement was mainly present in subjects who had little or no change in muscle thickness (contraction), probably making this method less reliable to measure thickness change as seen with contraction. Because this study sample consisted mainly of people with chronic back problems, it was not possible to study further the cut-points for good and less good reliability.

Limitations and weaknesses

Another weakness was that the examiners in these four experiments were clinicians in the clinic where the study subjects were treated. This meant that they would have met and/or treated several of these subjects. Nevertheless, many patients come through this clinic over time, a large proportion of which would be examined with diagnostic ultrasound. It would be impossible for the clinicians to remember individual values to a larger extent, and none

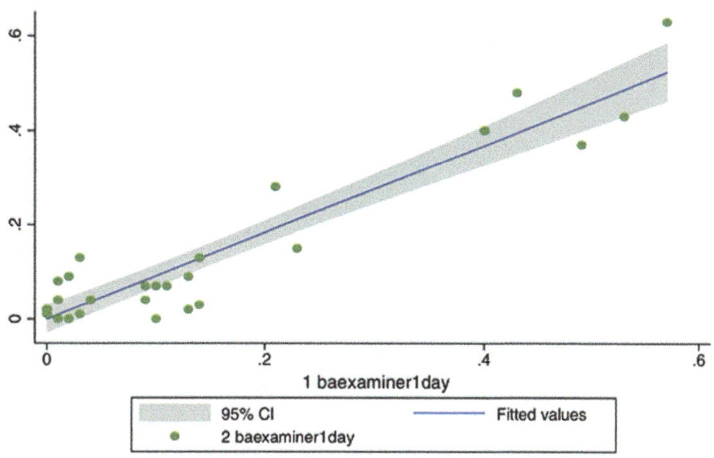

Figure 7 Scatter plot of subjects in study objective 3. Day to day scatter, x-axis shows day 1, y axis day 2.

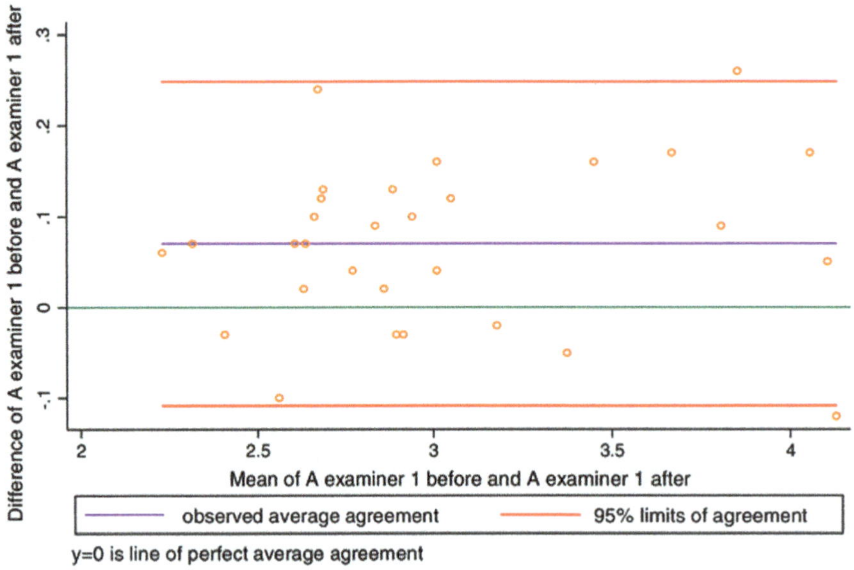

Figure 8 LOA plot showing agreement between examiner 1 before and after the subject performed a motor task. Study objective 4, measuring resting LMM before and after a simple motor task on two sets of images (N = 30).

of them had a special need to "prove" anything, but performed this study with an open and curious mind. It is unlikely that the results would be biased for this reason.

The subjects in this study were recruited from a clinical setting, the majority of which had LBP. This can be seen as both a strength and a weakness. It would have been preferable with a more mixed study sample, but the presence of people with LBP made it possible to study the usefulness of diagnostic ultrasound in a typical setting. The negative aspect is that the results cannot necessarily be generalized to other populations.

Comparison with other studies

When comparing our results to others one can only look at the ICC values. Our results, are all similar to previous

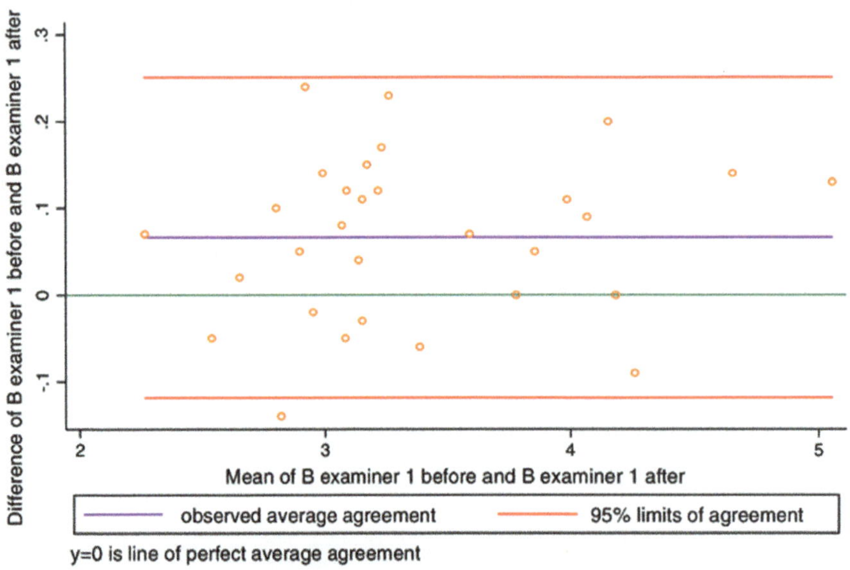

Figure 9 LOA plot showing agreement between examiner 1 before and after the subject performed a motor task. Study objective 4, measuring contracted LMM before and after a simple motor task on two sets of images (N = 30).

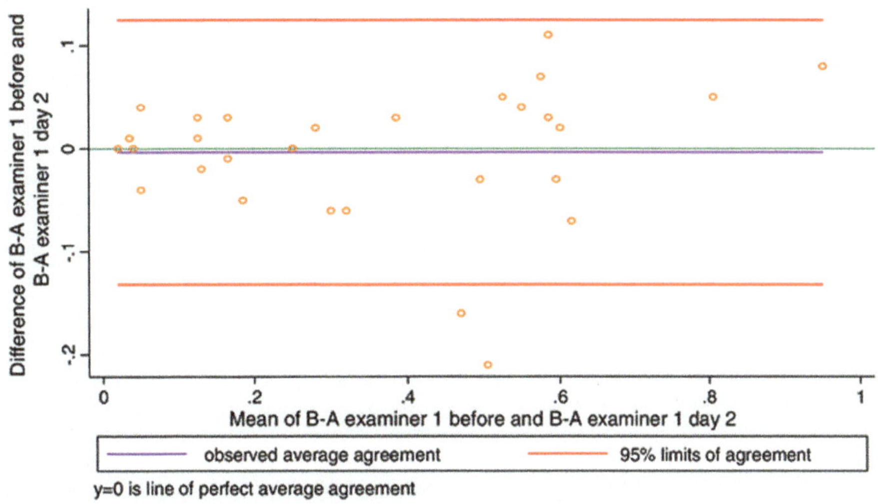

Figure 10 LOA plot showing agreement between examiner 1 before and after the subject performed a motor task. Study objective 4, measurement of contraction (distance 2 – distance 1) LMM on two sets of images (N = 30).

studies [21-23,26,27]. The main difference from our study to others is that we have demonstrated through the LOA analysis, a poorer agreement between two examiners who measure LMM thickness on two different sets of images. We also found less agreement between two examiners who measure contraction of the LMM. The agreement does seem to diminish when the thickness of the LMM is increasing more than 4 mm (relative increase of approximately 14%).

It has previously been shown that it is difficult for subjects with LBP to contract the LMM [18]. Our study did not aim to correlate LBP and ability to contract the LMM, however the majority of the subjects were LBP sufferers and this might be the reason why the majority of subjects had little or no ability to contract the LMM. We also included subjects without LBP, which may be reflected in the measurements that indicate a thickness increase in the LMM. As we only wanted to investigate the measurements this needs to be explored further in other studies.

Recommendations for further studies

Further exploration of utilization of diagnostic ultrasound on the LMM is needed. The examiners showed a low level of agreement when measuring LMM thickness change in the subjects who were able to contract of the LMM, but a good level of agreement when measuring LMM thickness change in the subjects who were not capable of contracting the LMM. It could be possible to categorize the contraction in groups to see if this increases the agreement. However this would be easier if one could use relative contraction measured in % as a scale. But if one were to use relative contraction as a measurement, further studies need to be conducted to see if different parts of the LMM contracts as a unit. From a more clinical perspective correlation between pain and LMM contraction measured with diagnostic ultrasound needs to be performed, as well as studies that examine subjects who never had low back pain to obtain more knowledge of how the LMM normally would contract. The clinical utilization of diagnostic ultrasound in measuring the muscle contraction of the LMM is not clear, as normal ranges are not fully established [36]. However, diagnostic ultrasound could possibly be used for identifying subjects who are not capable of contracting the LMM.

Conclusion

Our results indicate that ultrasound examination of the lumbar multifidus muscle is a reliable method when used by experienced examiners in people with chronic LBP, with poor contracting ability of their multifidus muscles and the average of three measurements is utilized.

Competing interests

The authors have no financial or non-financial competing interests to declare. The foundation Et Liv i Bevegelse (ELIB) partly funded the study.

Authors' contributions

EJS, JAB, and CLY formed the study idea. All authors were involved in the design of the study, interpretation of data, revision of the manuscript, and all gave final approval of the manuscript. NW performed the data analysis. JB revised the manuscript and was also supervisor for the projects part of the MSc at the Anglo European College of Chiropractic and Bournemouth University. Parts of this study was used for an MSc degree in diagnostic ultrasound at the Anglo- European College of Chiropractic. EJS, JAB, CLY and JB set up the study. EJS and JAB conducted all intra and inter-rater measurements. NW performed the statistical analysis. EJS drafted the manuscript. CLY, JB and NW reviewed the manuscript. All authors reviewed and approved the manuscript in its final form.

Acknowledgements
The authors want to thank participating subjects, and especially Jeffrey Hebert for his input on reviewing this article. The authors would also thank the Norwegian Chiropractic Association for financial support towards the MSc degree in musculoskeletal ultrasound for EJS and JAB.

Funding
This study recieved funding from the Norwegian independant research foundation Et liv i bevegelse (ELIB).

Author details
[1]MChiro, MSc, Ulriksdal 2, 5009 Bergen, Norway. [2]DC, MSc, Ulriksdal 2, 5009 Bergen, Norway. [3]Department Spincenter of Southern Denmark Hospital Lillebælt, Østre Hougvej 55, DK-5500 Middelfart, Denmark. [4]Anglo European College of Chiropractic. Research Department, 13-15 Parkwood Road, Bournemouth BH5 2DF England, UK. [5]Orthopaedic Department, Center for Spine Surgery, Hospital of Lillebaelt, Institute of Regional Health Service Research and Center for Research in Childhood Health, University of Southern Denmark, Østre Hougvej 55, DK5500 Middelfart, Denmark.

References

1. Donelson R, McIntosh G, Hall H. Is it time to rethink the typical course of low back pain? PMR. 2012;4(6):394–401.
2. Kjaer P, Bendix T, Sorensen JS, Korsholm L, Leboeuf-Yde C. Are MRI-defined fat infiltrations in the multifidus muscles associated with low back pain? BMC Med. 2007;5:2. doi:10.1186/1741-7015-5-2.
3. Zhao WP, Kawaguchi Y, Matsui H, Kanamori M, Kimura T. Histochemistry and morphology of the multifidus muscle in lumbar disc herniation: comparative study between diseased and normal sides. Spine. 2000;25 (17):2191–9.
4. Yoshihara K, Nakayama Y, Fujii N, Aoki T, Ito H. Atrophy of the multifidus muscle in patients with lumbar disk herniation: histochemical and electromyographic study. Orthopedics. 2003;26(5):493–5.
5. Kader DF, Wardlaw D, Smith FW. Correlation between the MRI changes in the lumbar multifidus muscles and leg pain. Clin Radiol. 2000;55(2):145–9.
6. Hides J, Gilmore C, Stanton W, Bohlscheid E. Multifidus size and symmetry among chronic LBP and healthy asymptomatic subjects. Man Ther. 2008;13(1):43–9.
7. Danneels L, Coorevits P, Cools A, Vanderstraeten G, Cambier D, Witvrouw E, et al. Differences in electromyographic activity in the multifidus muscle and the iliocostalis lumborum between healthy subjects and patients with sub-acute and chronic low back pain. Eur Spine J. 2002;11(1):13–9.
8. Parkkola RR, Rytökoski UU, Kormano MM. Magnetic resonance imaging of the discs and trunk muscles in patients with chronic low back pain and healthy control subjects. Spine. 1993;18(7):830–6.
9. Wallwork TL, Stanton WR, Freke M, Hides JA. The effect of chronic low back pain on size and contraction of the lumbar multifidus muscle. Man Ther. 2008;14(5):496–500.
10. Lee HI, Song J, Lee HS, Kang JY, Kim M, Ryu JS. Association between cross-sectional areas of lumbar muscles on magnetic resonance imaging and chronicity of low back pain. Ann Rehabil Med. 2011;35(6):852–9.
11. Heydari A, Nargol AVF, Jones APC, Humphrey AR, Greenough CG. EMG analysis of lumbar paraspinal muscles as a predictor of the risk of low-back pain. Eur Spine J. 2010;19(7):1145–52.
12. Wong AYL, Parent EC, Funabashi M, Stanton TR, Kawchuk GN. Do various baseline characteristics of transversus abdominis and lumbar multifidus predict clinical outcomes in non-specific low back pain? A systematic review. Pain. 2013;154(12):2589–602.
13. Zielinski KA, Henry SM, Ouellette-Morton RH, DeSarno MJ. Lumbar multifidus muscle thickness does not predict patients with low back pain who improve with trunk stabilization exercises. Arch Phys Med Rehabil. 2013;94(6):1132–8.
14. Danneels L, Vanderstraeten G, Cambier D, Witvrouw E, Bourgois J, Dankaerts W, et al. Effects of three different training modalities on the cross sectional area of the lumbar multifidus muscle in patients with chronic low back pain. Br J Sports Med. 2001;35(3):186–91.
15. Weber BRB, Grob DD, Dvorák JJ, Müntener MM. Posterior surgical approach to the lumbar spine and its effect on the multifidus muscle. Spine. 1997;22(15):1765–72.
16. Hides JA, Jull GA, Richardson CA. Long-term effects of specific stabilizing exercises for first-episode low back pain. Spine. 2001;26(11):E243–8.
17. Macdonald D, Moseley GL, Hodges PW. Why do some patients keep hurting their back? Evidence of ongoing back muscle dysfunction during remission from recurrent back pain. Pain. 2009;142(3):183–8.
18. Kiesel KB, Uhl T, Underwood FB, Nitz AJ. Rehabilitative ultrasound measurement of select trunk muscle activation during induced pain. Man Ther. 2008;13(2):132–8.
19. Hodges PW, Pengel LHM, Herbert RD, Gandevia SC. Measurement of muscle contraction with ultrasound imaging. Muscle Nerve. 2003;27(6):682–92.
20. Kiesel KB, Uhl TL, Underwood FB, Rodd DW, Nitz AJ. Measurement of lumbar multifidus muscle contraction with rehabilitative ultrasound imaging. Man Ther. 2007;12(2):161–6.
21. Hebert JJ, Koppenhaver SL, Parent EC, Fritz JM. A systematic review of the reliability of rehabilitative ultrasound imaging for the quantitative assessment of the abdominal and lumbar trunk muscles. Spine. 2009;34 (23):E848–56.
22. Koppenhaver SL, Parent EC, Teyhen DS, Hebert JJ, Fritz JM. The effect of averaging multiple trials on measurement error during ultrasound imaging of transversus abdominis and lumbar multifidus muscles in individuals with low back pain. J Orthop Sports Phys Ther. 2009;39(8):604–11.
23. Larivière C, Gagnon D, De Oliveira E, Henry SM, Mecheri H, Dumas J-P. Ultrasound measures of the lumbar multifidus: effect of task and transducer position on reliability. PMR. 2013;5(8):678–87.
24. Wallwork TL, Hides JA, Stanton WR. Intrarater and interrater reliability of assessment of lumbar multifidus muscle thickness using rehabilitative ultrasound imaging. J Orthop Sports Phys Ther. 2007;37(10):608–12.
25. Van K, Hides JA, Richardson CA. The use of real-time ultrasound imaging for biofeedback of lumbar multifidus muscle contraction in healthy subjects. J Orthop Sports Phys Ther. 2006;36(12):920–5.
26. Koppenhaver SL, Hebert JJ, Fritz JM, Parent EC, Teyhen DS, Magel JS. Reliability of rehabilitative ultrasound imaging of the transversus abdominis and lumbar multifidus muscles. Arch Phys Med Rehabil. 2009;90(1):87–94.
27. Wong AYL, Parent EC, Kawchuk GN. Reliability of two ultrasonic imaging analysis methods in quantifying lumbar multifidus thickness. J Orthop Sports Phys Ther. 2012;43(4):251–62.
28. Gracovetsky S. An hypothesis for the role of the spine in human locomotion: a challenge to current thinking. J Biomed Eng. 1985;7(3):205–16.
29. Saunders SW, Schache A, Rath D, Hodges PW. Changes in three dimensional lumbo-pelvic kinematics and trunk muscle activity with speed and mode of locomotion. Clin Biomech. 2005;20(8):784–93.
30. Zaki R, Bulgiba A, Ismail R, Ismail NA. Statistical methods used to test for agreement of medical instruments measuring continuous variables in method comparison studies: a systematic review. PLoS One. 2011;7(5): e37908. doi:10.1371/journal.pone.0037908.
31. Hanneman SK. Design, analysis, and interpretation of method-comparison studies. Adv Crit Care. 2008;19(2):223–34.
32. Bland JMJ, Altman DGD. Statistical methods for assessing agreement between two methods of clinical measurement. Lancet. 1986;1(8476):307–10.
33. Kottner JJ, Audige LL, Brorson SS, Donner AA, Gajewski BJB, Hróbjartsson AA, et al. Guidelines for reporting reliability and agreement studies (GRRAS) were proposed. Int J Nurs Stud. 2011;48(6):661–71.
34. Rankin G, Stokes M. Reliability of assessment tools in rehabilitation: an illustration of appropriate statistical analyses. Clin Rehabil. 1998;12(3):187–99.
35. Shrout PE. Measurement reliability and agreement in psychiatry. Stat Methods Med Res. 1998;7(3):301–17.
36. Teyhen DS, Childs JD, Stokes MJ, Wright AC, Dugan JL, George SZ. Abdominal and lumbar multifidus muscle size and symmetry at rest and during contracted states normative reference ranges. J Ultrasound Med. 2012;31(7):1099–110.

Use of the measure your medical outcome profile (MYMOP2) and W-BQ12 (Well-Being) outcomes measures to evaluate chiropractic treatment: an observational study

Barbara I Polus[†], Amanda J Kimpton[†], Max J Walsh[*†]

Abstract

Background: The objective was to assess the use of the Measure Yourself Medical Outcome Profile (MYMOP2) and W-BQ12 well-being questionnaire for measuring clinical change associated with a course of chiropractic treatment.

Methods: Chiropractic care of the patients involved spinal manipulative therapy (SMT), mechanically assisted techniques, soft tissue therapy, and physiological therapeutic devices.
Outcome measures used were MYMOP2 and the Well-Being Questionnaire 12 (W-BQ12).

Results: Statistical and clinical significant changes were demonstrated with W-BQ12 and MYMOP2.

Conclusions: The study demonstrated that MYMOP2 was responsive to change and may be a useful instrument for assessing clinical changes among chiropractic patients who present with a variety of symptoms and clinical conditions.

Background

In an era of accountability, health care providers are increasingly required to use reliable and valid outcome measures to assess changes in patient characteristics, including function and activities of daily living, following intervention. A review of outcome measures for primary care illustrates the evolution of instruments that acknowledge the importance of subjective perceptions of health and which focus on the measurement of function and quality of life [1].

Subjective outcome measures provide another dimension in the clinician's understanding of the patient's complaint when compared to standard objective measures (such as range of motion, palpation). Common subjective outcome measures include condition-specific tools such as the Revised Oswestry Disability Index and Neck Disability Index for assessing functional disability due to low back and neck pain respectively. Standardised questionnaires such as the Short form 36 (SF36) and the Well-being Questionnaire (W-BQ12) are used to assess general health status or quality of life - especially changes in self-concept over time following therapeutic intervention.

A recent approach is to assess change over time for specific symptoms or complaints identified by patients to be most important to them [1-3]. The Measure Yourself Medical Outcome Profile (MYMOP) has been recently developed to evaluate such patient-generated measures over time following therapeutic intervention [1]. The MYMOP is a brief patient generated, problem specific questionnaire which requires the respondent to specify one or two symptoms which are concerning them most and which they are seeking treatment for. A daily activity that is being restricted or prevented by these symptoms is also documented [4].

The MYMOP was initially published in 1996 [1] and was revised to MYMOP2 after a second validation in 1999 and included another section relating to medication [3]. It is a sensitive measure of within-person change over time; is capable of measuring the effects of a wide

* Correspondence: max.walsh@rmit.edu.au
† Contributed equally
Division of Chiropractic, School of Health Sciences, RMIT University, Plenty Rd Bundoora, Melbourne, Australia

variety of care; and is a brief and simple questionnaire that can be completed during a consultation [1].

It has been used successfully to evaluate patient outcomes in a number of clinical settings including acupuncture [2,5], massage therapy in an Aboriginal community [6], acute exacerbations of chronic bronchitis [7], and more recently chiropractic management of patellar tendinopathy [8].

In the past the Short Form 36 (SF-36) has been the principal outcome measure for overall health in primary care. There are a number of studies that have evaluated the effectiveness of chiropractic care on patient's health and general health status as measured by the Short-Form 36 [9,10]. The MYMOP provides health practitioners with an alternative that is more easily incorporated into the practice setting because of its brevity. A comparative study of MYMOP and the SF-36 has been conducted [1]. MYMOP concurrent validity was supported by its ability to detect different degrees of change in relation to scores in acute and chronic conditions, and by its correlations with SF-36 scores. MYMOP correlated more closely with the subjective clinical findings than the SF 36. Paterson's study also showed that the MYMOP measure was capable of being responsive to changes in symptoms despite being brief.

The 12-item Well-being Questionnaire (W-BQ12) is another patient-centred subjective outcome measure that is geared towards people with long-term illness and has been found to be reliable and valid [11,12]. The W-BQ12 and MyMOP2 are two patient-centred outcome measures that are part of a set of five questionnaires that have been recently assembled to assess a range of outcomes experienced by people having acupuncture for long-term health problems [13].

Two of these five patient-centred survey instruments have recently been used to evaluate outcomes experienced by patients in response to body wall therapies such as massage [6] and chiropractic [8]. It was considered a significant step forwards to assess the utility of these questionnaires in another practice setting.

Therefore the aim of this observational study was to assess the utility of the MYMOP2 and W-BQ12 health outcomes measures for measuring clinical change associated with a course of chiropractic treatment delivered by student chiropractors in a clinical teaching facility. The W-BQ12 was also used as a tool to assess the validity of the well being component of the MyMOP2 against the validated W-BQ12 instrument in this clinical practice setting.

Methods

A prospective, multicentre, practice based, observational study was conducted using patients presenting with spinal complaints to the RMIT University (Melbourne, Australia) chiropractic teaching clinics. For this observational study the patient's presenting complaint was not limited to a specific condition. Any patient who fulfilled the inclusion criteria was invited to participate in the study and were reviewed after 6 weekly treatments. The RMIT Human Research Ethics Committee approved all protocols and forms utilised for the study.

Patients were invited to participate in the study if they were: over the age of 18 years; had no treatment from any health professional for their complaint in the preceding four weeks; and suffered from a condition amenable to treatment by one or more chiropractic therapies. Patients were excluded if the following criteria were met: a requirement for immediate referral for medical treatment or where chiropractic intervention was contraindicated such as fracture, infection e.g. septic arthritis or malignancy; any additional physical treatment for their complaint during the course of the study; inability to complete or understand the required informed consent or outcome measures and inability to comply with the treatment schedule.

Under supervision of qualified chiropractic clinicians, treatment was provided by final year student chiropractors. Assessment prior to treatment included a full clinical history, physical, orthopaedic, neurological, palpatory and radiological examination. All participants received one or more chiropractic techniques taught and applied in the RMIT University chiropractic teaching clinics. These treatment protocols included: manual manipulative procedures such as spinal manipulative technique of high-velocity and low-amplitude thrust (SMT); soft tissue therapy; Logan Basic technique; and mechanical-force manually-assisted manipulation such as biomechanical blocking, drop-piece and activator. Segmental spinal dysfunction (subluxation) was assessed as described by Gatterman [14]. Patient management also included advice on nutrition, exercise and static stretching regimens as required.

Outcome Measures

Two health and well-being questionnaires were used with consenting patients prior to and after completion of 6 treatments delivered over a minimum of one month and a maximum of three months. The questionnaires were either self-completed or administered by a student chiropractor if the patient requested this. The questionnaires were:

- 12 Item Well-being Questionnaire (W-BQ12)
- Measure Yourself Medical Outcome Profile v2 (MYMOP2 - see Figure 1)

A description of the MYMOP2 subcategories is given in Table 1.

The W-BQ12 is a 12-item scale measuring four components: positive well-being (PWB), energy (E), negative

*** MYMOP2 ***

Full name .... Date of birth ....

Address and postcode...

....

Today's date .... Practitioner seen ....

Choose one or two symptoms (physical or mental) which bother you the most. Write them on the lines.

Now consider how bad each symptom is, over the last week, and score it by circling your chosen number.

SYMPTOM 1:	0	1	2	3	4	5	6
....	As good as it could be						As bad as it could be
SYMPTOM 2:	0	1	2	3	4	5	6
....	As good as it could be						As bad as it could be

Now choose one activity (physical, social or mental) that is important to you, and that your problem makes difficult or prevents you doing. Score how bad it has been in the last week.

ACTIVITY:	0	1	2	3	4	5	6
....	As good as it could be						As bad as it could be

Lastly how would you rate your general feeling of wellbeing during the last week?

0	1	2	3	4	5	6
As good as it could be						As bad as it could be

How long have you had Symptom 1, either all the time or on and off? Please circle:

0 - 4 weeks   4 - 12 weeks   3 months - 1 year   1 - 5 years   over 5 years

Are you taking any medication FOR THIS PROBLEM ? Please circle: YES/NO

IF YES:

1. Please write in name of medication, and how much a day/week

....

2. Is cutting down this medication: Please circle:

Not important   a bit important   very important   not applicable

IF NO:

Is avoiding medication for this problem:

Not important   a bit important   very important   not applicable

MYMOP. Measure Yourself Medical Outcome Profile

Figure 1 MYMOP2 questionnaire.

well-being (NWB) and general well-being (GWB). Items 1-4 are summed to produce the negative well-being score; Items 5-8 produce a total energy score; and Items 9-12 produce the positive well-being score. The negative well-being score is reversed and then added with the energy and positive well-being scores to produce a general well-being score (range: 0-36). The higher the score on this reliable and valid instrument, the greater sense of general well-being [15].

The Measure Yourself Medical Outcome Profile [3] is a 'patient-centred' outcome scale where patients are asked to nominate one or two symptoms (physical or

Table 1 Description of MYMOP2 subcategories

Category	Code	Description
Symptom 1	S1	The symptom which is most important to the patient described in the patient's own words.
Symptom 2	S2	Optional and is second symptom which is **part of the same problem** as symptom 1
Activity	A	An activity of daily living of importance to the patient in which Symptoms 1 and 2 interfere with. Written in patient's own words
Well-being	W	Patient asked how they would rate their general feeling of well-being over the last 7 days on a scale of 0 to 6, with 6 being as bad as it could be
Profile	P	Equals the mean of the scores recorded.

mental) of a specific problem they need assistance with and consider the severity of these symptoms over the last week. The third item asks the patient to list an activity (such as walking) that they have had difficulty completing due to their problem. The fourth item asks patients to rate their general well-being over the last week. Student chiropractors inserted the previously chosen symptoms and activity onto the follow-up form prior to this being given to the patient to score. Therefore, the patient was aware of the symptoms they had previously nominated, but not the previous score. Each of the four items is rated on a seven point scale where 0 is *'as good as it could be'* and 6 *'as bad as it could be'.* Hence, a decrease in the MYMOP2 score represents an improvement in health outcome. A mean of the four item scores is calculated and is referred to as the MYMOP2 "profile score".

The latest version of the MYMOP2 questionnaire (MYMOP2) was used in the present study and comprises another section relating to medication [3].

Data analysis

All data were coded and entered into an Excel spreadsheet and then imported into SPSS v16.0 to perform statistical analysis.

The Wilcoxon signed rank test was used to compare baseline and post-treatment values for the outcome measures to investigate the responsiveness or sensitivity to change of both instruments.

Unpaired t-tests were used to compare the baseline (pre-treatment) characteristics of the group of patients who completed both initial and follow-up outcome measures and the initial total group. This test was completed to ensure that there was no difference in characteristics between the two groups (no follow-up and follow-up groups).

Chi-squared calculations were used to assess differences in pre-treatment categorical data.

Correlations between MYMOP2 and W-BQ12 scales were analysed using Spearman's correlation coefficients (r_s) as a measure of the responsiveness, validity, in terms of well-being, and clinical usefulness of the instruments in a chiropractic student clinic setting.

All significance levels were set at $p < .05$.

Results

Fifty-two (52) patients agreed to participate in the study, with each patient completing the MYMOP2 and W-BQ12 questionnaires prior to initial treatment.

Of the initial 52 subjects, 33 completed the full treatment schedule and were re-assessed after six treatments. There were no significant differences between the baseline (pre-treatment) characteristics of the total initial group (N = 52) compared to the group who completed the base-line and follow-up surveys (N = 33).

Region of chief complaint

Back and/or neck pain was the most common presenting complaint, experienced by 71.2% of the initial sample of patients, with no significant differences between males and females in presenting region.

There was no significant difference in the distribution of region of main symptom between the total initial sample and the treatment group.

Pre-treatment MYMOP2 scores

The MYMOP2 scores from the initial consultation are documented in Table 1. A MYMOP2 score of 6 represents 'as bad as it could be' and a score of 0 represents 'as good as it could be'.

While scores for females tended to be higher than for males for all sub-scores of the MYMOP2, there were no statistically significant differences except for profile scores where females had a statistically significantly higher score ($p = .004$).

Age groups

The distribution of presenting (pre-treatment) MYMOP2 scores according to age groups is shown in Figure 2.

The 52 subjects were broken down into the following age groups: <20yo (n = 5), 20-39 (n = 25), 40-59 (n = 15) and >60 (n = 7).

The older age groups tended to have higher scores across each sub-score but there were no significant differences between the various age groups.

Treatment effects on MYMOP2 and W-BQ12 scores

The effect of treatment on MYMOP2 and W-BQ12 scores is shown in Table 2 and Figures 3 and 4 respectively. Large significant changes occurred in all MYMOP2 categories following treatment ($p < .0001$), with improvements over baseline from 40 to 65 percent.

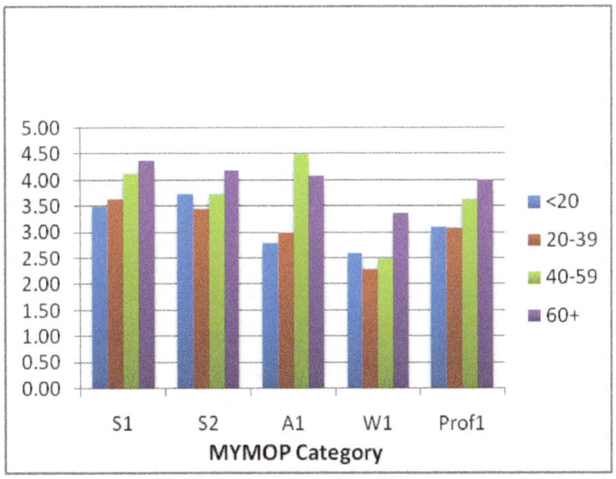

Figure 2 **Presenting mean MYMOP2 scores according to age group.**

The W-BQ-12 scores were negative well-being (NWB), Energy (E), Positive Well-being (PWB) and General Well-being (GWB). Figure 4 compares the pre treatment and post treatment scores. All W-BQ12 scores showed a significant improvement in scores following treatment ($p < .05$), noting that a decrease in negative well-being corresponds to a positive effect of treatment.

Correlation between MYMOP2 and W-BQ12 scores

Correlations between MYMOP2 scales and W-BQ12 scales were assessed using Spearman's correlation coefficients (r_s) as shown in Table 3.

The MYMOP2 scales of Symptom 1 and Profile showed a moderate negative correlation with the General Wellbeing (GWB) and Energy scales of the W-BQ12. The Wellbeing scale of the MYMOP2 had a strong negative correlation with the GWB, a moderate negative correlation with the PWB and Energy scales and a positive moderate correlation with the Negative wellbeing scale.

The Activity scale of the MYMOP2 had no significant correlations with any of the W-BQ12 scales.

Correlations between MYMOP2 scales and W-BQ12 scales were assessed using Spearman's correlation coefficients (r_s) as shown in Table 3.

Discussion

This observational study had two objectives. The first objective was to assess the effectiveness of the MYMOP2 and W-BQ12 questionnaires in measuring clinical changes following chiropractic care on patients attending the RMIT University chiropractic teaching clinics. The second objective was to investigate the validity of the MyMOP2 instrument to detect a change in well-being of patients attending the RMIT chiropractic teaching clinic.

The mean baseline MYMOP2 profile score was 3.4 (+/- 1.0) for the 52 presenting chiropractic patients as demonstrated in this study which is similar to that obtained in a study of massage therapy for subjects with chronic musculoskeletal complaints [6]. It is lower than those of patients attending for acupuncture in medical practices (4.7) [2], and for those patients attending general practice in the UK (4.6) [1]. The presenting MYMOP2 scores were not dependent on age or gender except for the Profile sub score where females had a significantly higher score. Given there is no difference in other sub scores there is no apparent reason why females should have a higher Profile score.

There was a statistically significant improvement in all MYMOP2 sub-scales following chiropractic treatment indicating a positive effect of the therapy. These changes were similar to changes found in the other studies referred to above.

The improvements were also of clinical significance defined as a change in score that is of importance to the individual patient involved. The MYMOP2 uses a 7-point score for which the minimum clinically important change in score after intervention should be between 0.5-1.0: any change greater than 1.0 can be considered clinically significant [16].

The changes in all MYMOP2 scores were equal to or greater than 1.0 (for Symptom 1 and Symptom 2 changes were greater than 2.0), suggesting that, in general, the effect of therapy was clinically significant to patients.

There were also significant improvements in the W-BQ12 scores, once again suggesting a positive effect of the treatment. According to Pouwer et al [15], the W-BQ12 is a reliable and valid measure of well-being and has been used in a number of studies to measure clinical changes following treatment [6,17,18]. It is of interest to compare the changes observed in the W-BQ12 in our study with that of another recent large study that measured a range of treatment effects of traditional acupuncture - including changes in self concept - the target of the W-BQ12 [19]. In this latter setting, the W-BQ12 was not found to be responsive. The authors of this latter study attributed the lack of responsiveness of the W-QB12 to two possible causes: either the socioeconomically diverse population or the preponderance of musculoskeletal problems present in their sample. While our study is unable to comment on the first possibility, all participants in our study presented with musculoskeletal pain of spinal origin. Therefore, in contrast to the Paterson *et al* study [19], our study suggests that the W-BQ12 may be a useful outcome measure for use within a chiropractic clinical practice setting.

Table 2 Patient characteristics

	Total group (n = 52) Pre-Tx data	Tx group (n = 33) Pre-Tx data	Tx group (n = 33) Post-Tx data
Gender			
Male	24 (46.1%)	16 (48.5%	
Female	28 (53.9%)	17 (51.5%)	
Age Mean -yrs (SD)	39.4 (17.3)	40.9 (18.4)	
Range yrs	18 - 82	18-82	
Age categories -yrs			
<20	5 (9.6%)	3 (9.1%)	
20-39	24 (46.1%)	14 (42.4%)	
40-59	15 (28.8%)	10 (30.3%)	
<60	8 (15.4%)	6 (18.2%)	
Mean MYMOP2 scores (SD)[a]			
Symptom 1 S1 (SD)	3.9 (1.1)	3.9 (1.1)	**1.5 (1.2)**
Symptom 2 S2 (SD)	3.6 (1.2)	3.5 (1.2)	**1.5 (1.1)**
Activity A (SD)	3.9 (1.4)	3.9 (1.5)	**1.4 (1.1)**
Well-being W (SD)	2.5 (1.3)	2.6 (1.3)	**1.6 (1.3)**
Profile P (SD)	3.4 (1.0)	3.5 (0.9)	**1.6 (1.0)**
Mean W-BQ12 scores (SD) [b]	**1.4 (1.5)**	**1.4 (1.3)**	**1.0 (1.3)**
Negative well-being NWB Energy E	**7.1 (2.5)**	**6.9 (2.5)**	**7.7 (2.5)**
Positive well-being PWB	**8.6 (2.5)**	**8.5 (4.4)**	**10.0 (4.4)**
General well-being GWB	**26.1 (5.4)**	**25.8 (5.8)**	**28.6 ()**

SD = standard deviation.

[a] MYMOP2, 6 is "as bad as it can be" and 0 is "as good as it can be".

[b] W-BQ 12,each subscale has a maximum score of 12 except total well-being score which has a maximum of 36.

The correlation between MYMOP2 and W-BQ12 scores was moderate to strong for most scales other than the Activity scale of the MYMOP2 which had no significant correlations with any of the W-BQ12 scales (see Table 3).

MYMOP2 has been shown to be highly responsive to changes in symptoms whether acute or chronic, as well as correlating with the findings of the SF-36 [1].

Based on this and the observational findings of this study, the MYMOP2 has potential as a clinically useful tool to assess chiropractic care in terms of health status and general well-being. The official MYMOP website [16] lists the strengths and weaknesses of the MYMOP2 questionnaire. The major strengths are considered as: patient-centred, applicable to any problem, quick and easy to complete and score, and very responsive to change. The main weakness is that it is problem specific which makes it unsuitable for patients who cannot identify their problem.

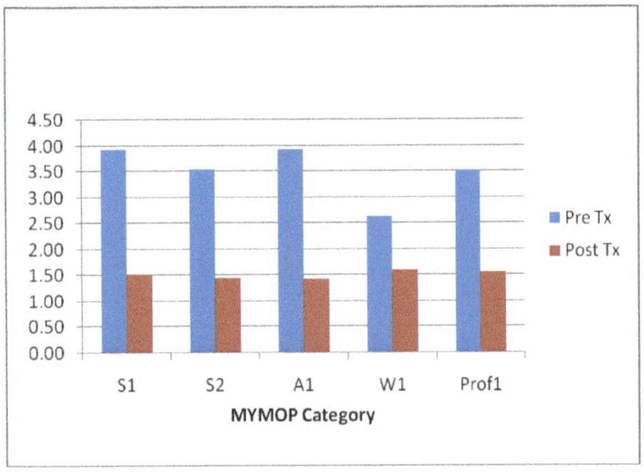

Figure 3 Comparison of pre and post treatment MYMOP2 scores.

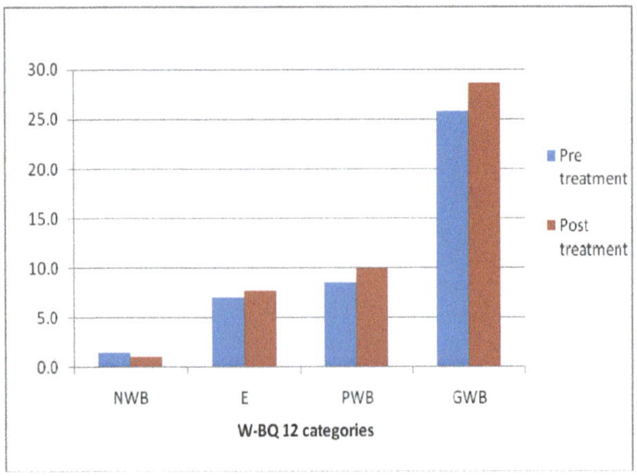

Figure 4 Comparison of pre and post treatment WBQ-12 scores.

Table 3 Correlation coefficients for MYMOP2 vs W-BQ12 scales

	W-BQ12 scales	General Well-Being	Positive Well-Being	Energy	Negative Well-being
MYMOP2 Scales					
Symptom 1 (S1)	r_s p (2-tailed)	- .330 .015	-.221* .107	.320 .018	**.058*** **.675**
Activity (A)	r_s p (2-tailed)	-.229* .103	-.037* .792	-.268* .058	**.058*** **.682**
Wellbeing (WB)	r_s p (2-tailed)	- .512 < .001	-.311 .022	-.445 .001	**.358** **.008**
Profile (P)	$\mathbf{r_s}$ **p (2-tailed)**	**-.372** **.006**	**-.172*** **.212**	**-.370** **.006**	**.201*** **.144**

* = no statistical significance.

The use of a non-experimental (observational) study design has well-established limitations. First, it is not possible to attribute any change to the intervention itself as other confounding effects (notably natural history and regression to the mean), could be responsible for the change observed. However, as the changes observed were both statistically and clinically significant, such an interpretation is less likely. Further, the purpose of the study was to document how these patient-centred outcome measures performed in a chiropractic clinical practice setting. A non-experimental, observational research design was considered appropriate for such an investigation and minimised disruption to the provision of the chiropractic service.

Another limitation of this observational study was that the practitioners were student chiropractors with minimal clinical experience. This may have had some impact on the observed findings as well as influencing the external validity of the study.

Conclusions

This study assesses the use of the MYMOP2 and W-BQ12 questionnaires as outcome measures to monitor changes following chiropractic therapy. Within the limitations of this study, it was shown that both questionnaires were responsive to change. The MYMOP2 also correlated well with the W-BQ12 questionnaire. It thus appears to be a useful instrument for assessing change among chiropractic patients and in the assessment of patient perceived well-being for chiropractic patients who present with a variety of symptoms and clinical conditions.

Acknowledgements

We are grateful to Clare Bradley for permission to use the W-BQ12 questionnaire and to Charlotte Paterson for use of the MyMOP2 and her continued support and encouragement in the use of patient-centred questionnaires.

This study was undertaken by RMIT chiropractic students as part of the requirements for the Master of Chiropractic degree. The authors wish to thank the following students who participated in this study and did such an excellent job in completing the study.

Catherine Langford, Conor Sexton, Luke Nichols, Marcus Kennedy, Paije Cox, Samuel Floreani, Simon Vannapraseuth, Adam Sherriff

Brett S. Jarosz, Shane W. Lincoln, Lauren Lupone, Catherine Andrews, Andrew B. Lincoln, Karen E. Phillips, Terrence D. Brown, Michael Melling-Williams, Jennifer Johnson, Sally Oborne.

Bolkunowicz DC, Buda RA, Grorud R, Kitsou NJ, McKenzie BJ, Mibus JA, Mond A, Ronning TW, Shambrook JG.

Authors' contributions

BP conceived the study, participated in its design and its coordination. BP, AK and MW supervised the student chiropractors in the collection and analysis of data. MJW undertook a further overall statistical analysis of data and drafted the manuscript. All authors read and approved the final manuscript.

Competing interests

The authors declare that they have no competing interests.

References

1. Paterson C: **Measuring outcomes in primary care: a patient generated measure, MYMOP2, compared with SF-36 health survey.** *BMJ* 1996, **312**:1016-20.
2. Hull SK, Page CP, Skinner BD, Linville JC, Coeytaux RR: **Exploring outcomes associated with acupuncture.** *J Altern Complement Med* 2006, **12(3)**:247-254.
3. Paterson C, Britten N: **In pursuit of patient-centred outcomes: a qualitative evaluation of MYMOP2, measure yourself medical outcome profile.** *J Health Serv Res Policy* 2000, **5**:27-36.
4. Paterson C: **Seeking the patients perspective: A qualitative assessment of EuroQol, COOP-WONCA charts and MYMOP2.** *Quality of Life Research* 2004, **13**:871-81.
5. Paterson C: **Complementary practitioners as part of the primary health care team: consulting patterns, patient characteristics and patient outcomes.** *Family Practice* 1997, **14**:347-54.
6. Paterson C, Vindigni D, Polus B, Browell T, Edgecombe G: **Evaluating a massage therapy training and treatment programme in a remote aboriginal community.** *Complementary therapies in clinical practice* 2008, **14**:158-67.
7. Paterson C, Langan CE, Anderson P, Maclaine G, Rose L, Walker S, Campbell M: **Assessing patient outcomes in acute exacerbations of choric bronchitis: the measure you medical outcome (MYMOP2), medical outcomes study 6-item general health survey (MOS 6A) and EuroQol (EQ-5D).** *Quality of Life Research* 2000, **9**:521-27.
8. Jarosz BS: **Chiropractic treatment of chronic patellar tendinopathy in a professional basketball player: a case report.** *Chiropr J Aust* 2010, **40(1)**:3-8.
9. Walsh MJ, Reece J, Donnoli F: **General health status in a sample of chiropractic patients with uncomplicated biomechanical neck or low back pain.** *Chiropr J Aust* 2008, **38**:75-80.
10. Bronfort G, Goldsmith CH, Nelson CF, Boline PD, Anderson AV: **Trunk exercise combined with spinal manipulative or NSAID therapy for**

chronic low back pain: a randomized, observer-blinded clinical trial. *J Manipulative Physiol Ther* 1996, **19**:570-82.

11. Bradley C: **The 12-Item Well-Being Questionnaire: origins, current state of development, and availability.** *Diabetes care* 2000, **23**:875.
12. Mitchell J, Bradley C: **Psychometric evaluation of the 12-Item Well-Being Questionnaire for use with people with macular disease.** *Qual Life Res* 2001, **10**:465-73.
13. Paterson C: **Patient-centred outcome measurement.** In *Acupuncture research: strategies for establishing an evidence base.* Edited by: MacPherson H, Hammerschlag R, Lewith G, Schnyer RN. London: Churchill Livingstone; 2007.
14. Gatterman M: **Chiropractic management of spine related disorders.** Philadelphia: Lippincott Williams & Wilkins;, 2 2004.
15. Pouwer F, van der Ploeg HM, Adèr HJ, Heine RJ, Snoek FJ: **The 12-item well-being questionnaire. An evaluation of its validity and reliability in Dutch people with diabetes.** *Diabetes Care* 1999, **22(12)**:2004-10.
16. **MYMOP.** [http://sites.pcmd.ac.uk/mymop/], Accessed July 2010.
17. DAFNE study group: **Training in flexible, intensive insulin management to enable dietary freedom in people with type 1 diabetes: dose adjustment for normal eating (DAFNE) randomised control trial.** *BMJ* 2002, **325**:746-52.
18. Riazi A, Bradley C, Barendse S, Ishii H: **Development of the well-being questionnaire short form in Japanese: the W-BQ12.** *Health Qual Life Outcomes* 2006, **4**:40.
19. Paterson C, Unwin J, Joire D: **Outcomes of traditional Chinese medicine (traditional acupuncture) treatment for people with long-term conditions.** *Complement Ther Clin Pract* 2010, **16**:3-9.

Peroneal neuropathy misdiagnosed as L5 radiculopathy: a case report

Michael D Reife[1,2*] and Christopher M Coulis[3,4,5]

Abstract

Objective: The purpose of this case report is to describe a patient who presented with a case of peroneal neuropathy that was originally diagnosed and treated as a L5 radiculopathy.

Clinical features: A 53-year old female registered nurse presented to a private chiropractic practice with complaints of left lateral leg pain. Three months earlier she underwent elective left L5 decompression surgery without relief of symptoms.

Intervention and outcome: Lumbar spine MRI seven months prior to lumbar decompression surgery revealed left neural foraminal stenosis at L5-S1. The patient symptoms resolved after she stopped crossing her legs.

Conclusion: This report discusses a case of undiagnosed peroneal neuropathy that underwent lumbar decompression surgery for a L5 radiculopathy. This case study demonstrates the importance of a thorough clinical examination and decision making that ensures proper patient diagnosis and management.

Keywords: Peroneal neuropathy, Lumbar radiculopathy, Chiropractic

Background

The most common entrapment neuropathy in the lower extremity is common peroneal mononeuropathy, accounting for approximately 15% of all mononeuropathies in adults [1]. Most injuries occur at the fibular head and can be the result of many factors including chronic low grade infection [2], varicose veins [3], schwannoma [4], nerve herniation through a fascial defect [5], giant plexiform neurofibromatosis [6], pneumatic compression [7], total knee arthroplasty, proximal tibial osteotomy [8], ganglion cysts [9], weight loss [10], associated endocrine or metabolic disorders including diabetes mellitus, alcoholism, thyrotoxicosis or Vitamin B depletion [11], high ankle sprain and leg crossing/squatting [12,13]; the most common cause of which is habitual leg crossing [14]. In this paper, we present a case of peroneal neuropathy that was originally misdiagnosed as a lumbar radiculopathy.

* Correspondence: mdrdc@snet.net
[1]Private Practice, 8 Independence Drive, Marlborough, CT 06447, USA
[2]Basic and Clinical Sciences, University of Bridgeport College of Chiropractic, 75 Linden Ave, Bridgeport, CT 06604, USA
Full list of author information is available at the end of the article

Case presentation

The patient is a 53-year-old registered nurse who was referred to the author's office in August 2003 by her primary care physician with a chief complaint of left leg pain. Her symptoms began in October 2002 after she fell off an ambulance landing on her left hip. Plain x-rays of her hip revealed mild osteoarthritis. Two months later lumbar spine magnetic resonance imaging (MRI) revealed degenerative disc disease, posterior disc bulging and facet arthropathy at L5-S1 resulting in moderate left foraminal stenosis. Subsequently, she was treated with physical therapy which included exercises, trans-cutaneous electrical nerve stimulation (TENS), lumbar traction and anti-inflammatory medications. Due to persistent symptoms, she followed-up with a neurosurgeon in January 2003. He ordered a lumbar spine CT scan which revealed mild spondylosis at L3-S1. The neurosurgeon diagnosed her with left L5 radiculopathy. She continued with physical therapy and anti-inflammatory medications and received three epidural injections which provided mild intermittent relief. Her symptoms persisted and in May 2003 she underwent elective left L5-S1 hemilaminectomy with diskectomy. She did not improve after the surgery and developed increased pain in her left lateral leg. A second

MRI June 2003 revealed a large fluid collection that extended from the spinal canal through the laminectomy defect and into the subcutaneous tissue. This was thought to be a CSF fistula. She underwent a second surgery three weeks after the first surgery to repair a cerebral spinal fluid leak and recurrent extruded disk at L5-S1. She improved somewhat after the second surgery and was referred for a physical therapy strengthening program. Her symptoms however, persisted and she was unable to work.

The patient presented for chiropractic evaluation and treatment two and a half months after her second surgery. Her complaints were left lateral leg pain, described as a deep bone ache as if her leg was on fire. She stated her pain felt like a screwdriver being driven into her left lateral ankle. Her pain was rated as a constant but of variable intensity, level 2-8 out of 10 with an average pain of 4. She also presented with a new onset of right lumbosacral junction pain described as an ache rated as level 3 out of 10. She stated her low back pain was provoked when she leaned forward. She denied weakness, paresthesias, bowel or bladder loss or retention or thigh pain. Her left lower extremity complaint was aggravated with inversion of her left foot, internal rotation of her left hip, sitting, lying down and sleeping. Her symptoms were mildly relieved with walking, eversion of her left foot and if she performed a "figure four" of her left thigh.

Physical examination revealed an ectomorph body type standing 174 centimeters (68.5 inches) and weighing 57 kilograms (125 pounds). During the interview she sat the entire time with her right leg crossed over her left with her right foot wrapped behind her left ankle. Postural exam revealed decreased lumbar lordosis and thoracic kyphosis. Palpation reproduced tenderness over the left lateral leg inferior to the head of the fibula across the peroneal muscles. There was considered to be paraspinal tenderness and spasm at L2-L5 levels and over the posterior superior iliac spines, worse on the right side. Lumbosacral ranges of motion appeared normal. Deep tendon reflexes were 2+ patellas and 2+ achilles bilaterally. Plantar reflexes were down going. Hypesthesia was found over the left lateral leg and dorsum of her left foot. Motor examination found grade 4 weakness with dorsiflexion of the left foot and toes and eversion of the left foot. The remainder of the lower extremities muscles were graded 5/5. Her gait was normal. Straight leg raise was negative. Subjective tightness was found with the gastrocnemius and hip external rotator muscles. Passive inversion of the left foot reproduced leg pain.

She was instructed to stop crossing her legs and six days later she reported less pain along her left lateral leg and was sleeping better. She was followed for two months and discharged at that time symptom-free.

Discussion

In the thigh, the peroneal division of the sciatic nerve supplies the short head of the biceps femoris muscle. Near the distal thigh, just above or in the popliteal fossa, the sciatic nerve divides into the tibial and common peroneal nerve (CPN). The CPN extends around the neck of the fibula where it is superficial and susceptible to direct trauma [14]. At the level of the fibular neck, the nerve passes beneath the peroneus longus tendon to enter the peroneal tunnel [15]. The CPN gives off the lateral cutaneous nerve of the calf proximal to the head of the fibula, which supplies sensation to the upper third of the anterolateral leg. After entering the lateral leg compartment deep to the peroneus longus tendon, the CPN divides into deep (DPN) and superficial peroneal (SPN) branches [16]. The DPN innervates the anterior compartment muscles, including tibialis anterior and extensor digitorum brevis, extensor hallucis, peroneus tertius, and extensor digitorum longus in addition to supplying the sensory branch between the first and second toes. Conversely, the SPN innervates the lateral compartment muscles of the leg including the peroneus longus and brevis muscles and supplies sensation to the lower 2/3 of the anterolateral leg and dorsum of the foot [17-19]. The CPN is most vulnerable as it becomes superficial over the fibular neck just distal to the head of the fibula [20], whereas the DPN and SPN are more vulnerable distally in the leg, ankle and foot [21]. Plantar flexion and inversion motions of the foot can stretch or compress the CPN in the peroneal tunnel [15,22].

Injury to the common peroneal nerve results in a foot drop described as slapping or tripping [20]. Pain may occur at the site of compression as well as distally into the lateral leg. At times there may be a radiation of pain into the thigh [15]. Numbness and tingling can occur along the lateral leg and dorsum of the foot [14]. Peroneal neuropathies occurring at the fibular neck affect the DPN more commonly than the SPN. Also with common peroneal neuropathies, weakness can be more prominent in muscles supplied by the DPN [22]. Neuropathy of both the DPN and the SPN will cause weakness with dorsiflexion of the foot and toes and eversion of the foot. If only the DPN is affected, there will be weakness with foot and toe dorsiflexion and sensory deficit to the web of skin between the first and second toes [22]. In severe cases of peroneal neuropathy there will be obvious foot drop. Milder cases of foot dorsiflexion weakness are assessed with heel walking and manual muscle testing. Sensory loss is typically found over the lateral leg and dorsum of the foot sparing the fifth toe [14]. Palpation or pressure over the peroneal tunnel region can reproduce the patient symptoms. Resisted inversion of the foot can also reproduce pain [15].

The history and exam may be the most helpful at arriving at a diagnosis for suspected peroneal neuropathy. Neurodiagnostic testing (EMG/NCV) may be required to provide a more complete understanding and can allow for localization of the lesion. Misidentification of the lesion can result in unnecessary surgery or delay in surgery. Electrodiagnostic testing can also establish that a physiologically relevant nerve injury is present and may also provide insight into the timing of injury and underlying pathophysiology of injury (demylination vs. axonal disruption). EMG should be used if the patient does not improve with time or treatment, is considered a surgical candidate secondary due to intractable pain or the presence of progressive weakness, or there are equivocal MRI findings [23].

MRI has utility in the evaluation for peroneal neuropathy as it can detect the proximal portion of the CPN at the knee for space occupying lesions, edema and change in nerve size. However, in most cases of peroneal neuropathy these findings are not evident. [21]. High-resolution Sonography may be used to detect structural lesions such as an intramural ganglion or inflammatory changes and color duplex ultrasonography and angiography may be used for assessment of vascular compromise including popliteal pseudo-aneurysm of the popliteal artery [24].

Clinical findings can aid in determining the etiology of a patient's condition. L5 radiculopathy and peroneal neuropathy can both present with weakness of the foot dorsiflexors and toe extensors, however, L5 radiculopathy may present with weakness during foot inversion versus weakness with foot eversion associated with peroneal neuropathy [14]. Additionally, reflex changes at the patella, medial hamstring and Achilles tendon can distinguish a L4, L5 or S1 radiculopathy from a common peroneal neuropathy [25]. Sensory changes to light touch or pinprick may not improve the clinical picture as dermatomal patterns and peripheral nerve distributions can have much overlap and sensory evaluation may be prone to subjective bias [26]. Finally, adverse nerve root tension, including femoral nerve stress test and straight leg raise can indicate a lumbar nerve root involvement which is absent during peroneal neuropathy. On the other hand, passive or forceful ankle inversion tensions the peroneal nerve which may reproduce symptoms of a peroneal neuropathy [15].

Injury to the sciatic nerve, especially when the peroneal portion is affected, can mimic a common peroneal neuropathy at the fibular head. Partial sciatic nerve injuries usually affect the lateral division (common peroneal nerve) more commonly than the medial division (tibial nerve); this is believed to be due to limited supportive tissue surrounding the peroneal nerve and the fact the peroneal nerve is taut and secured at both its proximal and distal ends. These high sciatic nerve lesions can be caused by static notch injections, hip trauma, hip surgery and gluteal compartment hemorrhage. High sciatic nerve lesions are differentially diagnosed from common peroneal nerve lesions through needle EMG of the short head of the biceps femoris which receives innervation from the peroneal division of the sciatic nerve [27].

One must also consider the presence of other neuropathies, such as a diabetic neuropathy, which can present with foot drop and dysesthesias. Diabetic polyneuropathy generally occurs bilaterally versus unilaterally for a mononeuropathy or peripheral entrapment syndrome [11]. Diabetic symmetric distal polyneuropathy includes tingling, buzzing or a prickling sensation in a stocking distribution. Absent Achilles reflexes are a frequently encountered sign in diabetic polyneuropathy. Weakness generally involves the extensor hallucis longus muscles rather than dorsiflexion of the feet. Loss of vibration at the toes is also common with diabetic polyneuropathy [28]. Diabetic mononeuropathy or Mononeuritis multiplex can involve one nerve or multiple nerves. The cause is thought to be vasculitis, ischemia or infarction of the nerve. The onset is acute and self-limiting, generally resolving over six weeks. Entrapment syndromes begin slowly and continually progress until intervention [29]. Other conditions can produce peripheral neuropathies including human immuno-deficiency virus (HIV), nutritional deficits, polyarteritis nodosa, sarcoidosis, SLE, toxemia and uremia [14]. The patient in our case study did not exhibit signs or symptoms of a systemic condition.

Conclusion

This case represents a patient who underwent L5-S1 hemilaminectomy and discectomy for the diagnosis of a L5 radiculopathy. After two surgeries and over a year of physical therapy the patient presented to the authors office. In this instance the authors had the foresight of the failed low back surgery leading to the diagnosis of a peroneal neuropathy. The importance of this case study is the differential diagnosis between a L5 radiculopathy and peroneal neuropathy. The patient's sensory complaints, exam findings and imaging studies mimicked a L5 radiculopathy. There are indications however, pointing to a peroneal neuropathy, which included weakness with foot eversion along with dorsiflexion and toe extension, tenderness over the fibular neck and peroneal tunnel and a history of increased pain with ankle inversion and relief upon ankle eversion. Ideally, electrodiagnostic testing would have been performed prior to the second surgery and would have essentially ruled out lumbar spine involvement. Additionally, an EMG/NCV may have provided a more conclusive diagnosis of peroneal neuropathy, however, in this particular case, following a trial of treatment targeting the common peroneal nerve, the patient reported resolution of her symptoms thus eliminating the need for further diagnostic testing or clarification.

We presented a case of undiagnosed peroneal neuropathy in a female who presented to a chiropractic office that was non-responsive to two lumbar decompression surgeries and interventional pain procedures that responded to a simple direction to not sit cross legged. This adds to the existing literature of previously-reported cases and concludes that clinicians managing such patients must exhibit careful diagnostic acumen and clinical decision making to ensure proper patient treatment and management.

Consent

Written informed consent was obtained from the patient for publication of this case report and any accompanying images. A copy of the written consent is available for review by the Editor-in-Chief of this journal.

Competing interests

The authors declare that they have no competing interests.

Authors' contributions

Both authors wrote, reviewed and made editorial changes in the manuscript. Both authors read and approved the final manuscript.

Author details

[1]Private Practice, 8 Independence Drive, Marlborough, CT 06447, USA. [2]Basic and Clinical Sciences, University of Bridgeport College of Chiropractic, 75 Linden Ave, Bridgeport, CT 06604, USA. [3]Department of Veterans Affairs Connecticut Healthcare System, West Haven, CT 06516, USA. [4]Shoreline Spine & Pain Associates, PC, 2415 Boston Post Rd., Guilford, CT 06437, USA. [5]Clinical Sciences, University of Bridgeport College of Chiropractic, 75 Linden Ave., Bridgeport, CT 06604, USA.

References

1. Cruz-Martinez A: **Peroneal neuropathy after weight loss.** *J Peripher Nerv Syst* 2000, **5**:101–105.
2. Schulze J, Troeger H: **Fibular nerve compression due to an unusual cause. A case report.** *Handchir Mikrochi Plast Chir* 2004, **36**(1):25–28.
3. Yamamoto N, Koyano K: **Neurovascular compression of the common peroneal nerve by varicose veins.** *Eur J Vasc Endovasc Surg* 2004, **28**(3):335–338.
4. Mahitchi E, Van Linthoudt D: **Schwannoma of the deep peroneal nerve. An unusual presentation in rheumatology.** *Praxis* 2007, **96**(3):69–72.
5. Yang LJ, Gala VC, McGillicuddy JE: **Superficial peroneal nerve syndrome: an unusual nerve entrapment. Case report.** *J Neurosurg* 2006, **104**(5):820–823.
6. Cebesoy O, Tutar E, Isik M, Arpacioglu O: **A case of isolated giant plexiform neurofibroma involving all branches of the common peroneal nerve.** *Arch Orthop Trauma Surg* 2007, **127**(8):709–712.
7. Fukuda H: **Bilateral peroneal nerve palsy caused by intermittent pneumatic compression.** *Intern Med* 2006, **45**(2):93–94.
8. Mont MA, Dellon AL, Chen F, Hungerford MW, Krackow KA, Hungerford DS: **The operative treatment of peroneal nerve palsy.** *J Bone Joint Surg Am* 1996, **78**(6):863–869.
9. Greer-Bayramoglu RJ, Nimigan AS, Gan BS: **Compression neuropathy of the peroneal nerve secondary to a ganglion cyst.** *Can J Plast Surg* 2008, **16**(3):181–183.
10. Shahar E, Landau E, Genizi J: **Adolescence peroneal neuropathy associated with rapid marked weight reduction: case report and literature review.** *Eur J Paediatr Neurol* 2007, **11**(1):50–54.
11. Stewart JD: *Focal Peripheral Neuropathies.* New York: Elsevier; 1987:290–305.
12. Yilmaz E, Karakurt L, Serin E, Güzel H: **Peroneal nerve palsy due to rare reasons: a report of three cases.** *Acta Orthop Traumatol Turc* 2004, **38**(1):75–78.
13. Sangwan SS, Marya KM, Kundu ZS, Yadav V, Devgan A, Siwach RC: **Compressive peroneal neuropathy during harvesting season in Indian farmers.** *Trop Doct* 2004, **34**(4):244–246.
14. Agarwal P, Griffith A: **Peroneal mononeuropathy.** *Emedicine* 2012. http://emedicine.medscape.com/article/1141734-overview.
15. Pecina M, Krmpotic-Nemantic J, Markiewitz A: **Peroneal Tunnel Syndromes.** In *Tunnel Syndromes.* 2nd edition. Boca Raton, Fl: CRC Press; 1997:207–211.
16. Rosse C, Gaddum-Rosse P: *Hollinshead's textbook of anatomy.* 5th edition. Philadelphia: Lippincott-Raven publishers; 1997.
17. Kosinski C: **The course, mutual relations and distribution of the cutaneous nerves of the metazonal region of leg and foot.** *J Anat* 1926, **60**(3):274–297.
18. Hethfield KW, Williams JR: **Peripheral neuropathy and myopathy associated with bronchogenic carcinoma.** *Brain* 1954, **77**(1):122–137.
19. Huelke DF: **The origin of the peroneal communicating nerve in adult man.** *Anat Rec* 1958, **132**(1):81–92.
20. Fabre T, Piton C, Andre D, Lasseur E, Durandeau A: **Peroneal nerve entrapment.** *J Bone Joint Surg Am* 1998, **80**:47–53.
21. Donovan A, Rosenberg ZS, Cavalcanti CF: **MR imaging of entrapment neuropathies of the lower extremity. Part 2. The knee, leg, ankle, and foot.** *Radiographics* 2010, **30**(4):1001–1019.
22. Brazis P, Masdeu J, Biller J: **Peripheral Nerves.** In *Localization in Clinical Neurology.* 4th edition. Philadelphia, PA: Lippincott Williams and Wilkins; 2001:60–65.
23. Fridman V, David WS: **Electrodiagnostic evaluation of lower extremity Mononeuropathies.** *Neuro Clin May* 2012, **30**(2):505–528.
24. Nodera H, Sato K, Terasawa Y, Takamatsu N, Kaji R: **High-resolution sonography detects inflammatory changes in vasculitic neuropathy.** *Muscle Nerve* 2006, **34**(3):380–381.
25. Berry H, Richardson PM: **Common peroneal nerve palsy: a clinical and electrophysiological review.** *J Neurol Neurosurg Psychiatry* 1976, **39**(12):1162–1171.
26. Hage JJ, van der Steen LP, de Groot PJ: **Difference in sensibility between the dominant and nondominant index finger as tested using the Semmes-Weinstein monofilaments pressure aesthesiometer.** *J Hand Surg Am* 1995, **20**(2):227–229.
27. Katirji B, Wilbourn AJ: **High sciatic lesion mimicking peroneal neuropathy at the fibular head.** *J Neurol Sci* 1994, **121**(2):172–175.
28. Llewelyn JG: **The diabetic neuropathies: types, diagnosis & management.** *J Neurosurg Psychiatry* 2003, **74**(10):ii15–ii19.
29. Viniti A, Mehrabyan A, Colen L, Boulton A: **Focal entrapment neuropathy in diabetes.** *Diabetes Care July* 2004, **27**(7):1783–1788.

18

Research on placebo analgesia is relevant to clinical practice

Charles W Gay[1*] and Mark D Bishop[2,3]

Abstract

Over the decades, research into placebo responses has shed light onto several endogenous (i.e. produced from within) mechanisms underlying modulation of pain perception initiated after the administration of inert substances (i.e. placebos). Chiropractors and manual therapists should embrace analgesic-placebo-research in an attempt to maximize clinical benefit. Historical views that placebo responses are fake, passive, undesirable, and require deception and therefore should be minimized and avoided in clinical practice are outdated. Further, statements that contend the placebo response represents a single mechanism are overly simplistic. This commentary will discuss research that shows that there are several active biological processes underlying modulation of pain perception involved in placebo analgesia and its counterpart nocebo hyperalgesia. We contend that it is highly likely that, to some extent, all of these biological processes are engaged, in varying degrees, following all interventions and represent endogenous pain modulating processes. Failure, of chiropractors and manual therapists, to embrace a more contemporary view of analgesic-placebo-research serves as a barrier to transferring knowledge into clinical practice and represents a missed opportunity to improve the delivery of current treatments.

Keywords: Placebo, Endogenous pain modulation, Placebo response

Background

Evidence-based medicine deals with the use of current best evidence in clinical decision-making and other aspects of patient care. The assumption that simply having the evidence available or providing authoritative clinical practice guidelines will result in practice change and improved patient outcomes is incorrect [1,2]. A number of physician behaviors have been identified that act as barriers to translating evidence into clinical practice [3]. Two domains of those barriers are physician's knowledge and attitudes. This commentary addresses knowledge awareness and outdated attitudes surrounding the clinical improvement seen following the administration of a placebo. By addressing these potential barriers chiropractors and manual therapists may be more open to analgesic-placebo-research and its counterpart hyperalgesia-nocebo-research. In turn, clinical practice may be influenced by knowledge gained from this field, applying evidence to decision-making and the context in which interventions are delivered with a goal of improving patient outcomes.

Main text

Misconceptions about placebo responses continue in the general public and among healthcare professionals [4,5]. There has been a push for healthcare professionals to re-think what a placebo response represents and the applicability of knowledge gained from placebo-analgesia-research that can be applied ethically in clinical practice [6-12]. Rethinking placebo and nocebo responses as endogenous modulatory mechanisms broadens the focus of care beyond just the intervention to include the context in which interventions are delivered. Historical views that placebo responses represent fake, passive, and undesirable results; require deception; and should be minimized and avoided in clinical practice continue today among healthcare providers. Further, the placebo response has been described as a single mechanism through which an intervention may induce a positive therapeutic outcome [9]. Harboring such views may bias manual therapy practitioners away from valuable clinical evidence that may

* Correspondence: chaz.gay@ufl.edu
[1]Rehabilitation Science Doctoral Student, University of Florida, Gainesville, Florida, USA
Full list of author information is available at the end of the article

influence their clinical decision making. This commentary presents research that opposes these views.

Changes in the perceived intensity of pain are often attributed to a variety of factors lumped into three board categories: (1) condition related factors, (2) the specific effects of treatment, and/or (3) treatment contextual effects [13]. Condition related factors include the natural course of the condition and regression to the mean. Specific treatment effects are the unique effects associated with the 'active' ingredient of the treatment. Treatment context includes a host of signs, symbols and physician interactions that convey information to the individual. In recent years, researchers have used placebo-analgesia and its negative equivalent, nocebo-hyperalgesia to investigate the neuronal underpinnings of treatment contextual effects. Although, these three categories are practical and useful, they can create a misconception that there are unique biological pathways that do not overlap or interact underlying the categories. This misconception is highlighted by the notion that a predictable estimate of change in pain perception can be determined simply by a treatment's active biological properties.

For example, findings from one study significantly challenge the convention that an active biological agent produces a consistent therapeutic effect within an individual. By convention, researchers acknowledge that the active biological agent in a drug will vary across people, depending on a multitude of personal factors. However, what is not acknowledged so frequently is that within one individual, the therapeutic effect can significantly vary. By experimentally manipulating an individual's expectation through instructional sets, it was shown that the therapeutic effect of the active ingredient of remifentanil, a potent synthetic μ-opioid agonist, can be significantly modulated [14]. The study manipulated subjects' expectations by instructing them that remifentanil is a widely used opioid that relieves pain when infused intravenously, but can worsen pain when the infusion ceases [14]. Hidden administration of the drug produced less perceived pain than baseline, open administration of the drug produced significantly more hypoalgesia than hidden administration and when the drug was continuously administered but the subjects were told it had stopped, the perception of pain retuned to baseline values [14]. The estimated therapeutic effect size of the active ingredient in remifentanil spanned from no effect to a moderate effect, depending on the expectancy created by the instructional set.

Embedded in every pain-relieving treatment are contextual effects. Physician interactions, signs and symbols convey information to the individual with the potential for producing therapeutic and counter-therapeutic responses (ie placebo and nocebo responses respectively) [15]. The estimated therapeutic effect of treatment context following the administration of an inert substance has been shown to be substantial, albeit variable [15-21]. One factor that is not causing the therapeutic effect is the inert substance (ie placebo). Therefore, placebo-analgesia-research provides valuable information about the context in which interventions are delivered. Research into principle mediators of the contextual effects suggest expectancy, desire for a positive outcome and classical conditioning account for a significant portion of the variance in contextual effects [22-24]. Chiropractors and manual therapists should be aware that the context in which they deliver their interventions is as important as the intervention they are giving. Further evidence suggesting the effectiveness of a manual therapy intervention is influenced by patient's expectation comes from a study published by Bialosky et al. [25]. The study showed that by using different instructional sets to positively, negatively and neutrally influence the subjects expectation, the effect of spinal manipulation on a dynamic pain sensitivity measure (temporal summation of second pain) varied [25].

Placebo-analgesia-research has also shown that deception is not integral to inducing a placebo response. One study administered open labeled placebos with patient education that described an active biological pathway for symptom improvement [26]. In this study, the investigators told irritable bowel syndrome (IBS) subjects, that they would be randomized to receive either a placebo sugar pill or no treatment. Subjects receiving the placebo pill were told placebos have been found to produce clinically effective results though a mind-body connection and that by taking the pill, the subjects would be harnessing their own recuperative powers. Greater clinical improvement was found in the placebo group compared to the no-treatment group [26]. Another study examined the repeatability of contextual effects after subjects were told they received an inert substance. In this study, individuals, who received inert pain-relieving cream and experienced pain reductions, were then told they had received a placebo cream. On a subsequent visit those same individuals were again able to experience pain relief a second time using an inert cream [27]. Both of these studies challenge deception's role as a necessary component of the context in which an inert treatment is delivered that produces a positive therapeutic effect.

Finally, placebo-analgesia-research has shed light onto neural mechanisms underlying endogenous pain modulation. Cortical networks involved in processing and modulating the pain experience have been identified and continue to be reinvestigated, redefined and undergo reconceptualization. Activity in these cortical networks influence the perception of pain and modulation can be inhibitory or facilitatory. Research has identified various neurotransmitters including opioids, cannabinoids, dopamines and cholecystokinins, that are used within these cortical networks [28-31]. Attributing clinical benefit following the administration of an inert substance to a single mechanism, or terming it a placebo mechanism fails to account for the numerous neural and other biological pathways involved in producing and influencing the perception of pain [32,33].

Conclusion

Over the decades, research into placebo responses has shed light onto several endogenous (i.e. produced from within) mechanisms underlying modulation of pain perception initiated by the administration of inert substances (i.e. placebos/nocebos). In addition, this growing body of work emphasizes the need for chiropractors' and manual therapists' to be more alert to, and embrace, 'psychologically informed practice'; that is, practice in which recognition of neural mechanisms is equally as important as identification of structural pathology. Chiropractors and manual therapists should embrace analgesic-placebo-research in an attempt to maximize endogenous pain relieving mechanisms to produce maximum clinical benefit. Historical views that placebo responses are fake, passive, undesirable, and require deception and therefore should be minimized and avoided in clinical practice are outdated. Further, statements that contend the placebo response represents a single mechanism are too simplistic. Instead, in this commentary the authors discussed how several active biological processes underlie analgesic-placebo responses. We contend that it is highly likely that to some extent all of these biological processes, which represent endogenous pain relieving processes, are engaged to various degrees following all interventions that produce a positive clinical outcome.

Failure to embrace a more contemporary view of analgesic-placebo-research may negatively bias chiropractors' and manual therapists' opinions about the potential clinical value of results emerging from this field. These biases serve as a barrier to successfully translating potential benefits for patients into clinical practice in an ethical manner. Analgesic-placebo-research provides insight on how to improve the delivery of current treatments by optimizing clinical benefit and matching the right treatment to the right spinal pain patient at the right time.

Competing interests

The authors of this manuscript attest there are no conflicts of interest to report.

Authors' contributions

CWG and MDB contributed equally to the concept, the drafting, and critical revision of the manuscript. All authors read and approved the final manuscript.

Acknowledgements

This manuscript was written while CWG received support from the University of Florida Alumni Fellowship, NCMIC Foundation and the National Center of Complementary and Alternative Medicine (F32 AT007729-01A1), MDB received support from the National Center of Complementary and Alternative Medicine (R01AT006334).

Author details

[1]Rehabilitation Science Doctoral Student, University of Florida, Gainesville, Florida, USA. [2]Associate Professor, Department of Physical Therapy, University of Florida, Gainesville, Florida, USA. [3]Center for Pain Research & Behavioral Health, University of Florida, Gainesville, Florida, USA.

References

1. Mafi JN, McCarthy EP, Davis RB, Landon BE: **Worsening trends in the management and treatment of back pain.** *JAMA Intern Med* 2013, **173**(17):1573–81.
2. National Research Council: *Relieving Pain in America: Blueprint for Transofrming Prevention, Care, Education, and Research.* Washington, DC: The National Academies Press; 2011.
3. Pierson DJ: **Translating evidence into practice.** *Respiratory care* 2009, **54**:1386–1401.
4. Bishop FL, Jacobson EE, Shaw JR, Kaptchuk TJ: **Scientific tools, fake treatments, or triggers for psychological healing: How clinical trial participants conceptualise placebos.** *Soc Sci Med* 2012, **74**(5):767–74.
5. Kisaalita NR, Robinson ME: **Analgesic placebo treatment perceptions: acceptability, efficacy, and knowledge.** *J Pain* 2012, **13**:891–900.
6. Miller FG, Kaptchuk TJ: **The power of context: reconceptualizing the placebo effect.** *J R Soc Med* 2008, **101**:222–225.
7. Brody H, Colloca L, Miller FG: **The placebo phenomenon: implications for the ethics of shared decision-making.** *J Gen Intern Med* 2012, **27**:739–742.
8. Kisaalita NR, Roditi D, Robinson ME: **Factors affecting placebo acceptability: deception, outcome, and disease severity.** *J Pain* 2011, **12**:920–928.
9. Bialosky JE, Bishop MD, George SZ, Robinson ME: **Placebo response to manual therapy: something out of nothing?** *J Man Manip Ther* 2011, **19**:11–19.
10. Linde K, Fassler M, Meissner K: **Placebo interventions, placebo effects and clinical practice.** *Philos Trans R Soc Lond B Biol Sci* 2011, **366**:1905–1912.
11. Benz LN, Flynn TW: **Placebo, nocebo, and expectations: leveraging positive outcomes.** *J Orthop Sports Phys Ther* 2013, **43**:439–441.
12. Benedetti F, Amanzio M: **Mechanisms of the placebo response.** *Pulm Pharmacol Ther* 2013.
13. Fillingim RB, Price DD: **What is controlled for in placebo-controlled trials?** *Mayo Clin Proc* 2005, **80**:1119–1121.
14. Bingel U, Wanigasekera V, Wiech K, Ni Mhuircheartaigh R, Lee MC, Ploner M, Tracey I: **The effect of treatment expectation on drug efficacy: imaging the analgesic benefit of the opioid remifentanil.** *Sci Transl Med* 2011, **3**:70ra14.
15. Miller FG, Colloca L: **Semiotics and the placebo effect.** *Perspect Biol Med* 2010, **53**:509–516.
16. Price DD, Finniss DG, Benedetti F: **A comprehensive review of the placebo effect: recent advances and current thought.** *Annu Rev Psychol* 2008, **59**:565–590.
17. Hrobjartsson A: **The uncontrollable placebo effect.** *Eur J Clin Pharmacol* 1996, **50**:345–348.
18. Hrobjartsson A, Gotzsche PC: **Is the placebo powerless? An analysis of clinical trials comparing placebo with no treatment.** *N Engl J Med* 2001, **344**:1594–1602.
19. Hrobjartsson A, Gotzsche PC: **Is the placebo powerless? Update of a systematic review with 52 new randomized trials comparing placebo with no treatment.** *J Intern Med* 2004, **256**:91–100.
20. Hrobjartsson A, Gotzsche PC: **Unsubstantiated claims of large effects of placebo on pain: serious errors in meta-analysis of placebo analgesia mechanism studies.** *J Clin Epidemiol* 2006, **59**:336–338. discussion 339–341.
21. Benedetti F, Carlino E, Pollo A: **How Placebos Change the Patient's Brain.** *Neuropsychopharmacology* 2011, **36**:339–354.
22. Vase L, Petersen GL, Riley JL 3rd, Price DD: **Factors contributing to large analgesic effects in placebo mechanism studies conducted between 2002 and 2007.** *Pain* 2009, **145**:36–44.
23. Finniss DG, Kaptchuk TJ, Miller F, Benedetti F: **Biological, clinical, and ethical advances of placebo effects.** *Lancet* 2010, **375**:686–695.

24. George SZ, Robinson ME: **Dynamic nature of the placebo response.** *J Orthop Sports Phys Ther* 2010, **40:**452–454.
25. Bialosky JE, Bishop MD, Robinson ME, Barabas JA, George SZ: **The influence of expectation on spinal manipulation induced hypoalgesia: an experimental study in normal subjects.** *BMC Musculoskelet Disord* 2008, **9:**19.
26. Kaptchuk TJ, Friedlander E, Kelley JM, Sanchez MN, Kokkotou E, Singer JP, Kowalczykowski M, Miller FG, Kirsch I, Lembo AJ: **Placebos without deception: a randomized controlled trial in irritable bowel syndrome.** *PLoS One* 2011, **5:**e15591.
27. Chung SK, Price DD, Verne GN, Robinson ME: **Revelation of a personal placebo response: its effects on mood, attitudes and future placebo responding.** *Pain* 2007, **132:**281–288.
28. Colloca L, Benedetti F: **Nocebo hyperalgesia: how anxiety is turned into pain.** *Curr Opin Anaesthesiol* 2007, **20:**435–439.
29. Benedetti F: **Placebo-induced improvements: how therapeutic rituals affect the patient's brain.** *J Acupunct Meridian Stud* 2012, **5:**97–103.
30. Benedetti F, Thoen W, Blanchard C, Vighetti S, Arduino C: **Pain as a reward: changing the meaning of pain from negative to positive co-activates opioid and cannabinoid systems.** *Pain* 2013, **154:**361–367.
31. Zubieta JK, Stohler CS: **Neurobiological mechanisms of placebo responses.** *Ann N Y Acad Sci* 2009, **1156:**198–210.
32. Tracey I: **Getting the pain you expect: mechanisms of placebo, nocebo and reappraisal effects in humans.** *Nat Med* 2010, **16:**1277–1283.
33. Benedetti F: **What do you expect from this treatment? Changing our mind about clinical trials.** *Pain* 2007, **128:**193–194.

Accuracy of clinical tests in the diagnosis of anterior cruciate ligament injury: a systematic review

Michael S Swain[1,2*], Nicholas Henschke[1,3], Steven J Kamper[1,4], Aron S Downie[1,2], Bart W Koes[5] and Chris G Maher[1]

Abstract

Background: Numerous clinical tests are used in the diagnosis of anterior cruciate ligament (ACL) injury but their accuracy is unclear. The purpose of this study is to evaluate the diagnostic accuracy of clinical tests for the diagnosis of ACL injury.

Methods: Study Design: Systematic review. The review protocol was registered through PROSPERO (CRD42012002069).
Electronic databases (PubMed, MEDLINE, EMBASE, CINAHL) were searched up to 19th of June 2013 to identify diagnostic studies comparing the accuracy of clinical tests for ACL injury to an acceptable reference standard (arthroscopy, arthrotomy, or MRI). Risk of bias was appraised using the QUADAS-2 checklist. Index test accuracy was evaluated using a descriptive analysis of paired likelihood ratios and displayed as forest plots.

Results: A total of 285 full-text articles were assessed for eligibility, from which 14 studies were included in this review. Included studies were deemed to be clinically and statistically heterogeneous, so a meta-analysis was not performed. Nine clinical tests from the history (popping sound at time of injury, giving way, effusion, pain, ability to continue activity) and four from physical examination (anterior draw test, Lachman's test, prone Lachman's test and pivot shift test) were investigated for diagnostic accuracy. Inspection of positive and negative likelihood ratios indicated that none of the individual tests provide useful diagnostic information in a clinical setting. Most studies were at risk of bias and reported imprecise estimates of diagnostic accuracy.

Conclusion: Despite being widely used and accepted in clinical practice, the results of individual history items or physical tests do not meaningfully change the probability of ACL injury. In contrast combinations of tests have higher diagnostic accuracy; however the most accurate combination of clinical tests remains an area for future research.

Clinical relevance: Clinicians should be aware of the limitations associated with the use of clinical tests for diagnosis of ACL injury.

Keywords: Anterior cruciate ligament, Diagnosis, Medical history taking, Physical examination, Diagnostic test accuracy

* Correspondence: mswain@georgeinstitute.org.au
[1]The George Institute for Global Health, Sydney Medical School, University of Sydney, Missenden Rd, PO Box M201, 2050 Sydney, Australia
[2]Department of Chiropractic, Faculty of Science, Macquarie University, 2109 Sydney, Australia
Full list of author information is available at the end of the article

Background

The anterior cruciate ligament (ACL) is an important stabilising structure of the knee and its disruption is associated with pain and activity limitation [1]. The annual incidence of ACL injury ranges from 0.01% to 0.05% [2], however it is higher in sporting groups and most frequently affects individuals during late adolescence and early adulthood [3–5]. The prevalence of ACL injury in adults presenting to primary care with acute knee pain is estimated to be 4% [6]. Many cases are initially missed [7] in primary care and these undiagnosed ACL injuries are of concern because of the risk of cartilage tear and premature knee osteoarthritis [8].

Clinical diagnosis of ACL injury is based upon history and physical examination findings with suspected cases confirmed by MRI or arthroscopy [9]. Numerous clinical tests and findings have been proposed to aid the diagnosis of ACL injury. A popping sound, swelling and instability following high impact sport trauma along with a positive Lachman's, anterior draw or pivot shift test is the most common method of clinical diagnosis [9]. However, there are over 25 specific physical tests and numerous features from the clinical history that have been proposed for detection of ACL injury [10]. At present the diagnostic accuracy of these tests is unclear.

Most existing reviews evaluating the accuracy of tests to diagnose ACL injury [6,11–14] are now over a decade old and contain methodological limitations such as inclusion of inappropriate studies and pooling of estimates from heterogeneous studies. Since these reviews were published there has been much progress in the diagnostic field with regard to study appraisal and synthesis [15]. There is now a greater appreciation of how design features may lead to biased estimates of diagnostic test accuracy and when meta-analysis is justified. In addition it is likely that more recent primary research studies have been conducted in the area of ACL diagnosis.

The objective of this systematic review was to report the diagnostic accuracy of clinical tests for the diagnosis of ACL injury and describe the quality of research evaluating these tests.

Methods

A systematic review protocol [16] was registered at the International Prospective Register of Systematic Reviews - PROSPERO 2012:CRD42012002069.

Identification of selected studies

Electronic databases (PubMed, MEDLINE, EMBASE, and CINAHL) were searched for eligible diagnostic studies from the earliest year possible up to 19th of June 2013. The search strategy was developed for PubMed and modified for use in other databases (Additional file 1: Table S1). The reference lists of all included publications and relevant systematic reviews were checked and forward citation searches performed.

Eligibility criteria

Diagnostic studies were eligible if they compared the accuracy of history taking or physical examination to an acceptable reference standard (arthroscopy, arthrotomy, or MRI) in the identification of ACL injury. Both prospective and retrospective studies were eligible for inclusion. We did not include case control studies as they substantially overestimate diagnostic accuracy compared with studies that use a clinical population [17].

The focus of this review was on studies that evaluated patients presenting to a care provider for diagnosis of knee pain or dysfunction, where the diagnostic accuracy of individual, or combinations of, history features or physical assessment procedures was evaluated. Studies in which a substantial proportion of recruited patients had already been diagnosed with ACL injury were excluded to minimise verification bias [17].

Included studies had to report sufficient data on diagnostic tests to enable construction of a 2 × 2 table so estimates of diagnostic accuracy (such as sensitivity and specificity) could be calculated. Studies that evaluated the accuracy of an unspecified combination of history and physical examination, such as clinical diagnosis or global clinician judgment were excluded as they do not allow for replication, validation and generalization of the study results [18].

If studies had been reported in abstracts or conference proceedings, the related full publications were retrieved if available, but only full articles published in peer-reviewed journals were included. Studies published in all languages were considered eligible and translations were sought where necessary.

Study selection

Two authors (MS and NH) independently screened all titles and abstracts identified in the searches with respect to the inclusion and exclusion criteria. Full text copies of potentially relevant articles were retrieved and final inclusion or exclusion was determined. Disagreements regarding inclusion were resolved by consensus, including a third review author (SK) where necessary.

Data extraction

Three review authors (MS, NH, SK) independently extracted information from the included studies. Data were extracted into a specifically designed spreadsheet and included details on the study design, setting, enrolment procedures, number of participants, patient demographics, and time since initial ACL injury. Details of the type of index test and the type of reference standard were also extracted and the proportion of participants with ACL injuries was calculated for each included study.

Diagnostic two-by-two tables (true positive, false positive, true negative and false negative) were either extracted from the publications or reconstructed using information from other reported parameters (sensitivity, specificity, or predictive values). Uninterpretable index test outcomes, such as an equivocal finding were dealt with as a negative index test finding. The authors of one study [19] were contacted and provided additional information.

Quality assessment

The quality of each included study was assessed by two review authors (MS, NH) using the QUality Assessment of Diagnostic Accuracy Studies (QUADAS-2) checklist [20]. The QUADAS-2 checklist consists of four domains relating to patient selection, index test, reference standard, and flow and timing. Each domain is assessed in terms of risk of bias, and the first 3 domains are also assessed in terms of applicability. The review authors classified each item as "yes" (adequately addressed), "no" (inadequately addressed), or "unclear" (inadequate detail presented to allow a judgment to be made). Disagreements were resolved by consensus and consulting with a third (SK) review author where necessary.

Synthesis of results

The two-by-two tables were used to calculate index test summary statistics: sensitivity, specificity, likelihood ratios along with their 95% confidence intervals using MetaDiSc 1.4. Index test accuracy was presented as forest plots of likelihood ratios, as likelihood ratios provide the best way for clinicians to use diagnostic data to establish clinical diagnoses in patient care [21]. Categorisation of likelihood ratios was adopted from Jaeschke et al. [18] where positive likelihood ratios (+LR) <5 and a negative likelihood ratios (–LR) >0.2 were considered small, +LR 5–10 and –LR 0.1-0.2 were moderate, and + LR>10 and –LR <0.1 were considered large, with respect to changing the pre to post-test probability.

Both clinical and statistical heterogeneity as well as methodological quality were evaluated to determine the appropriateness of meta-analysis. Assessment of clinical heterogeneity involved comparison of the study populations, settings, performance of index tests and reference standards among included studies. Assessment of statistical heterogeneity involved visual inspection of forest plots and performance of the chi-square (χ^2) test and calculation of the inconsistency index (I^2) which quantifies the proportion of variation across the included studies that is due to heterogeneity rather than chance [22].

Results

Study selection

The initial database searches retrieved 21,691 citations of which 10,796 citations remained after duplicates were removed (Figure 1). Screening of the titles and abstracts identified 285 potentially relevant articles that were retrieved in full text format. Forwards and backwards citation tracking identified 12 potentially relevant articles which were also retrieved. Fourteen articles were finally included, of which 11 were published in English [19,23–32] and three in German [33–35]. Additional file 2: Table S2 lists the reasons for excluding 28 articles that were included in one or more of the previous five systematic reviews.

Description of included studies

Of the 14 included articles, 10 had a prospective study design [19,23,24,28–30,32–35], two used a retrospective design [26,27] and for two studies [25,31] the design was unclear (Table 1).

Only one study [19] evaluated the diagnostic accuracy of clinical tests in primary care. The other 13 studies evaluated the accuracy of clinical tests in secondary contact settings, defined here as either a referral to an orthopaedic department or presentation to an accident and emergency department. In three studies the reference standard was MRI [19,24,27], eight studies applied arthroscopy [23,26,29–32,34,35] and three studies applied either arthroscopy or arthrotomy [25,28,33]. Only five studies [25–27,29,30] reported in detail the method of index test application with slight variations between them in the way the index tests was performed.

Nine studies [19,23,26,28,30–32,34,35] assessed diagnostic accuracy for partial or complete ACL injuries, however only four of these [19,23,30,32] provided sufficient information to determine if the index test result pertained to a partial or complete disruption of the ACL. Injury severity (partial or complete ACL disruption) was unclear and treated as partial *and* complete injuries in the remaining studies. Nine studies [19,24–26,28,30,31,33,35] described ACL injuries with concomitant injury to other knee structures, while comorbid knee injuries were unclear or not reported in the remaining five studies [23,27,29,32,34].

There was variability between participants in the included studies with respect to sample size (50–350), average age (25–40 years), proportion of males (52%-100%) and time since ACL injury (one day to longer than one year). The prevalence of verified partial *and* complete ACL injury ranged from 21%-81%.

Quality assessment

The QUADAS-2 ratings of risk of bias and study applicability are shown in Table 2. Only one study [19] adequately addressed all risk of bias domains. For the 14 studies, risk of bias was high or unclear with regard to patient selection for 10 studies, for the index text four studies, for the reference standard nine studies and for flow and timing eight studies.

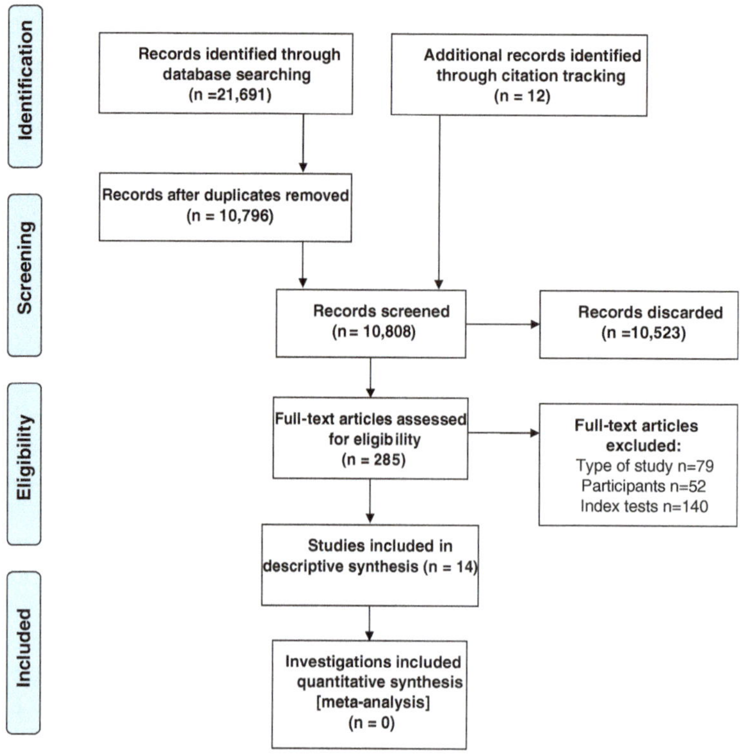

Figure 1 PRISMA flow diagram of studies through the review.

Only one study [19] clearly stated that the reference standard was assessed without knowledge of the results of the index test, while in 12 studies this was unclear [23–26,28–35]. In one study the reference standard was not applied independently of clinical tests [27]. Six studies [24,27,28,32,34,35] included all enrolled participants in the analysis. Across the remaining eight studies [19,23,25,26,29–31,33] the number of participants left out of the analyses ranged from 1%-71% of those originally included.

Diagnostic accuracy of clinical tests

A total of nine clinical index tests were identified by this review. Five tests were items from the clinical history (popping sound at time of injury, giving way, effusion, pain, ability to continue activity) and four index tests were applied as part of physical assessment (the anterior draw test, Lachman's test, prone Lachman's test, the pivot shift). Three of the tests were also performed under anaesthesia (anterior draw test, Lachman's test, pivot shift test). Diagnostic accuracy statistics for all index tests are presented as supplemental material (Additional file 3: Table S3). The anterior draw, Lachman and pivot shift tests were each evaluated in subgroups where the tests were applied in secondary contact settings to identified partial *and* complete ACL injury. The chi-square test ranged from $\chi^2 = 50.66$, 6df, $P < 0.001$ to $\chi^2 = 6.55$, 4df, $P = 0.16$ and the inconsistency indexes were typically high (>75%) ranging from 99.2% to 38.9%. The three physical tests plotted on the ROC plane as well the subgroups sensitivity and specificity forest plots are presented as supplementary information (Additional file 4: Figure S1, Additional file 5: Figure S2). The variability in patient spectrum and performance of index tests among the included studies resulted in important clinical and statistical heterogeneity. In addition, only a small number of studies evaluate specific clinical tests, with all but one study at high risk of bias, so a decision was made not to perform a meta-analysis. The diagnostic accuracy of individual clinical tests for ACL injury along with thresholds for defining clinical usefulness (i.e. small, moderate and large change in post-test probability) are illustrated in Figure 2. The number of studies that evaluated each individual test ranged from two studies for clinical history items to nine studies for Lachman's test.

Only two studies [19,30], from different settings (primary and secondary care), investigated test accuracy for clinical history items. Clinical history items had low value in correctly diagnosing ACL injury (+LR range 0.93-2.54, −LR range 0.15-1.18) (Figure 2).

Six studies [19,23,24,27,31,34] reported the accuracy of the anterior draw test in diagnosing ACL injury. Small, moderate and large +LR (range 1.94-87.88) were observed for the anterior draw test across studies. The

Table 1 Characteristics of included studies

First author, year	Design	Setting	Participants	Partial *and* complete ACL tear prevalence % (n)	Complete ACL tear prevalence % (n)	Reference standard(s)
Beldame, 2011 [23]	Prospective	University hospital, France.	*112 patient/knees with an indication for knee arthroscopy.	37.5% (42)	28.5% (32)	Arthroscopy
Boeree, 1991 [24]	Prospective	Orthopaedic clinic, UK.	203 patient/knees referred from GPs or the A&E.	29.1% (51)	nr	MRI
Decker, 1988 [33]	Prospective	Hospital, Germany.	†108 patient/knees suspected to have knee ligament injury.	61.1% (66)	nr	Arthroscopy/ Surgery
Harilainen, 1987 [25]	Unclear	Emergency department, Finland.	†350 patient/knees with acute knee injury.	41.7% (146)	nr	Arthroscopy/ Arthrotomy
Katz, 1986 [26]	Retrospective	Community hospital, USA.	85 participant/knees with knee injuries presenting for arthroscopy.	25.9% (22)	nr	Arthroscopy
Lee, 1988 [27]	Retrospective	Orthopaedic department of a hospital, USA.	79 magnetic resonance studies of the knee were reviewed.	29.1% (22)	nr	MRI
Lucie, 1984 [28]	Prospective	Orthopaedic clinic, USA.	50 patient/knees with acute traumatic knee haemarthrosis.	76.0% (38)	nr	Arthroscopy/ Arthrotomy
Mulligan, 2011 [29]	Prospective	Orthopaedic surgery and sports medicine service, USA.	*†52 patient/knees with a complaint of knee pain referred from emergency department.	44.2% (23)	nr	Arthroscopy
Noyes, 1980 [30]	Prospective	Orthopaedic/Sports medicine knee clinic, USA.	*85 injured knees (83 patients) that had traumatic haemarthrosis.	71.8% (61)	43.5% (37)	Arthroscopy
Richter, 1996 [34]	Prospective	Hospital, Germany.	74 patient/knees with effusion of the knee following trauma.	78.4% (58)	64.9% (48)	Arthroscopy
Schwartz, 1997 [35]	Prospective	Hospital, Germany.	58 patient/knees with acute knee injury.	81.0% (47)	65.5% (38)	Arthroscopy
Tonino, 1986 [31]	Unclear	Hospital, Netherlands.	*66 patient/knees with acute symptoms of a ligamentous lesion of the knee after trauma.	45.5% (30)	nr	Arthroscopy
Wagemakers, 2010 [19]	Prospective	GP clinics, Netherlands.	*134 patient/knees with new knee symptoms.	20.9% (28)	12.7% (17)	MRI
Wong, 1999 [32]	Prospective	Orthopaedic department of a hospital, Hong Kong.	91 patient/knees with an acute knee haemarthrosis.	nr	56.0% (51)	Arthroscopy

nr: not reported.
*Not all participants evaluated by index test(s).
†Not all participants evaluated by reference standard.

large +LR estimates all had wide confidence intervals and were reported in studies with high risk of bias. All −LRs (range 0.23-0.74) for the anterior draw test were within the small threshold.

Nine studies [19,23–25,27,31,32,34,35] investigated the accuracy of Lachman's test in diagnosing ACL injury. Small, moderate and large LRs (+LR range 1.39-40.81, −LR range 0.02-0.52) were reported for Lachman's test across the studies. Studies that report moderate or large LRs tended to be at risk of bias and had wide confidence intervals. One study [29] investigated the prone Lachman's test and reported small and imprecise LRs (+LR 3.50, −LR 0.38).

Five studies [23,24,30,31,34], all at risk of bias, evaluated the accuracy of the pivot shift test. Small, moderate and large +LRs (range 4.37-16.42) and small −LRs (range 0.38-0.84) were reported for the pivot shift test in all studies. Accuracy estimates with moderate and large +LRs tended to lack precision.

Five studies at high risk of bias [26,28,30,31,33] investigated physical tests when examination was performed under anaesthesia (EUA) (Additional file 6: Figure S3). The anterior draw test, Lachman's test and pivot shift test appear to provide improved diagnostic accuracy when examination is performed under anaesthesia. While LRs are moderate-large the confidence intervals around the +LR estimates are wide.

Only one study, from the primary care setting with low risk of bias, provided data on the effect of combining clinical tests [19]. Specifically, this included two or three positive history tests (from a list of popping sensation, giving way, effusion, immediate pain at trauma and continuation of activity impossible) as well as a positive anterior draw or Lachman's test (Figure 3). The addition of a positive anterior draw test to the combinations of two positive history tests increase the +LR (4.81) close to moderate diagnostic threshold. The addition of a third

Table 2 Risk of bias and applicability concerns summary based on the QUADAS-2 checklist

	Risk of bias				Applicability concerns concerns		
First author, year	Patient selection	Index test	Reference standard	Flow and timing	Patient selection	Index test	Reference standard
Beldame, 2011 [23]	?	+	+	-	+	+	+
Boeree, 1991 [24]	-	?	+	+	+	+	+
Decker, 1988 [33]	?	+	?	-	+	+	+
Harilainen, 1987 [25]	+	?	?	-	+	+	+
Katz, 1986 [26]	-	+	?	+	+	+	+
Lee, 1988 [27]	-	+	?	-	+	+	+
Lucie, 1984 [28]	-	+	?	-	+	+	+
Mulligan, 2011 [29]	+	+	?	?	+	+	+
Noyes, 1980 [30]	-	?	+	-	?	+	+
Richter, 1996 [34]	-	+	?	+	+	+	+
Schwartz, 1997 [35]	-	+	+	+	+	+	+
Tonino, 1986 [31]	-	+	?	?	+	+	+
Wagemakers, 2010 [19]	+	+	+	+	+	+	+
Wong, 1999 [32]	+	?	?	+	+	+	+

Judgements on risk of bias and applicability concerns: – = high risk; ? = unclear risk; + = low risk.

history test produced a large but imprecise +LR (35.64) but reduced the –LR (0.82).

Discussion

This systematic review included 14 studies that evaluated the diagnostic accuracy of clinical tests for ACL injury. Just one study, which was the only study performed in primary care, had a low risk of bias and showed that results of individual tests produce only small changes in the probability of ACL injury. The same study investigated the diagnostic accuracy of combining history items with physical tests and reported improved accuracy when doing so. The other studies, performed in secondary contact settings, had moderate to high risk of bias and reported quite diverse and imprecise estimates of diagnostic accuracy. Based upon these findings, clinical tests in combination, but not individually, may assist the diagnosis of ACL injury.

The key strengths of the review include a pre-specified and registered review protocol, the use of inclusion criteria to ensure that the study settings reflected clinical practice and the evaluation of study quality using the QUADAS-2 checklist. This review also reported likelihood ratios as they are the preferred approach to report estimates of diagnostic accuracy [21]. The limitations of the study were that sparse data were available on most clinical tests and that we were unable to perform a meta-analysis due to heterogeneity in the estimates of diagnostic accuracy, risk of bias and clinical characteristics. The heterogeneity among studies is well illustrated by the results for Lachman's test, where reported +LRs ranged from 1.5 to 102, risk of bias varied and ACL injury prevalence in the included studies ranged from 21% to 81%.

The clinical tests reviewed are those most commonly used for the diagnosis of ACL injury in clinical practice. Our findings suggest that a clinician cannot rely on a single clinical test in isolation, particularly one from the clinical history, to identify patients with ACL injury. Due to the fact that diagnostic decisions regarding ACL injury are not made on the basis of a single test, studies should ideally focus on test performance in combination. The best estimates of diagnostic accuracy come from Wagemakers et al. [19] whose data suggest that there may be some potential in combining clinical tests, specifically the anterior draw test with two or three of the following five history findings: popping sensation, giving way, effusion, immediate pain at trauma and inability to continue activity. Notwithstanding, these findings must be interpreted with caution as a major drawback of Wagemakers et al's study was its low power to sufficiently analyse multiple combined tests. An important direction for future research is identification of the optimal combination of currently available clinical tests to accurately diagnose ACL injury. While the literature regarding the accuracy of currently used tests is of variable quality, those identified in this body of literature (and included in this review) are the logical candidates to investigate using more robust methods. Such studies are well suited to primary care settings (limiting referral bias), but sample sizes will need to be substantially larger than studies to date in order to investigate multiple sequencing of index tests.

In contrast to our findings, previous systematic reviews have concluded that individual clinical tests can be used to accurately diagnose ACL injury [11,14]. The

Index test / First Author	Risk of Bias 1	2	3	4	Likelihood ratio - LR	+ LR
Popping						
Wagemakers, 2010	+	+	+	+	0.51 (0.31 - 0.85)	2.3 (1.5 - 3.6)
Wagemakers, 2010	+	+	+	+	0.51 (0.26 - 0.98)	2.1 (1.4 - 3.4)
Noyes, 1980	-	?	+	-	0.95 (0.65 - 1.40)	1.1 (0.5 - 2.3)
Giving way						
Wagemakers, 2010	+	+	+	+	0.63 (0.39 - 1.02)	1.6 (1.1 - 2.4)
Wagemakers, 2010	+	+	+	+	0.58 (0.30 - 1.12)	1.7 (1.1 - 2.5)
Noyes, 1980	-	?	+	-	0.29 (0.10 - 0.83)	1.4 (1 - 1.9)
Effusion						
Wagemakers, 2010	+	+	+	+	0.78 (0.56 - 1.10)	1.6 (0.9 - 2.7)
Wagemakers, 2010	+	+	+	+	0.65 (0.39 - 1.08)	2.0 (1.1 - 3.4)
Noyes, 1980*	-	?	+	-	0.59 (0.33 - 1.04)	1.5 (0.9 - 2.6)
Noyes, 1980†	-	?	+	-	0.28 (0.14 - 0.57)	2.1 (1.2 - 3.9)
Pain						
Wagemakers, 2010‡	+	+	+	+	0.15 (0.02 - 1.08)	1.3 (1.1 - 1.4)
Wagemakers, 2010‡	+	+	+	+	0.28 (0.04 - 1.93)	1.2 (1.0 - 1.4)
Noyes, 1980§	-	?	+	-	0.93 (0.66 - 1.31)	1.2 (0.5 - 2.7)
Noyes, 1980‖	-	?	+	-	1.18 (0.51 - 2.73)	0.9 (0.7 - 1.3)
Noyes, 1980¶	-	?	+	-	0.52 (0.09 - 2.86)	1.1 (0.9 - 1.3)
Continue activity						
Wagemakers, 2010	+	+	+	+	0.45 (0.23 - 0.88)	1.7 (1.2 - 2.3)
Wagemakers, 2010	+	+	+	+	0.45 (0.19 - 1.07)	1.6 (1.2 - 2.3)
Noyes, 1980	-	?	+	-	0.23 (0.11 - 0.47)	2.5 (1.3 - 4.9)
Anterior draw						
Wagemakers, 2010	+	+	+	+	0.29 (0.12 - 0.72)	2.0 (1.5 - 2.6)
Wagemakers, 2010	+	+	+	+	0.23 (0.06 - 0.84)	1.9 (1.5 - 2.6)
Beldame, 2011	?	+	+	-	0.35 (0.24 - 0.52)	4.4 (1.9 - 9.9)
Beldame, 2011	?	+	+	-	0.27 (0.17 - 0.44)	4.8 (2.1 - 10.8)
Richter, 1996	-	+	?	+	0.37 (0.25 - 0.57)	5.4 (1.5 - 19.9)
Boeree, 1991	-	?	+	+	0.48 (0.36 - 0.64)	6.7 (3.7 - 12.1)
Tonino, 1986	-	+	?	?	0.74 (0.59 - 0.93)	12.6 (0.8 - 207.6)
Lee, 1988	-	+	?	-	0.23 (0.11 - 0.48)	87.9 (5.5 - 1400)
Lachman						
Wagemakers, 2010	+	+	+	+	0.42 (0.19 - 0.95)	1.5 (1.2 - 2.0)
Wagemakers, 2010	+	+	+	+	0.52 (0.22 - 1.26)	1.4 (1 - 1.9)
Schwarz, 1997	-	+	+	+	0.16 (0.05 - 0.46)	2.0 (1.1 - 3.9)
Beldame, 2011	?	+	+	-	0.24 (0.15 - 0.40)	3.7 (1.9 - 7.2)
Beldame, 2011	?	+	+	-	0.15 (0.08 - 0.29)	4.0 (2.1 - 7.8)
Boeree, 1991	-	?	+	+	0.41 (0.30 - 0.58)	6.5 (3.8 - 11)
Richter, 1996	-	+	?	+	0.08 (0.03 - 0.21)	7.5 (2 - 27.3)
Wong, 1999	+	?	?	+	0.43 (0.29 - 0.62)	5.0 (2.2 - 11.7)
Harilainen, 1987	+	?	?	-	0.02 (0.01 - 0.07)	35.7 (15 - 84.7)
Tonino, 1986	-	+	?	?	0.12 (0.04 - 0.31)	40.8 (2.6 - 634.8)
Lee, 1988	-	+	?	-	0.11 (0.03 - 0.34)	102.0 (6.4 - 1618)
Prone Lachman						
Mulligan, 2011	+	+	?	?	0.38 (0.13 - 1.06)	3.5 (0.6 - 21.2)
Pivot shift						
Beldame, 2011	?	+	+	-	0.47 (0.32 - 0.68)	4.4 (1.5 - 12.8)
Beldame, 2011	?	+	+	-	0.38 (0.24 - 0.60)	5.0 (1.7 - 14.5)
Noyes, 1980	-	?	+	-	0.77 (0.65 - 0.91)	6.3 (0.9 - 44.9)
Noyes, 1980	-	?	+	-	0.65 (0.50 - 0.85)	9.1 (1.3 - 64.6)
Tonino, 1986	-	+	?	?	0.84 (0.71 - 1.00)	8.2 (0.5 - 140.3)
Boeree, 1991	-	?	+	+	0.72 (0.61 - 0.86)	8.8 (3.4 - 22.6)
Richter, 1996	-	+	?	+	0.53 (0.41 - 0.69)	16.4 (1.1 - 255)

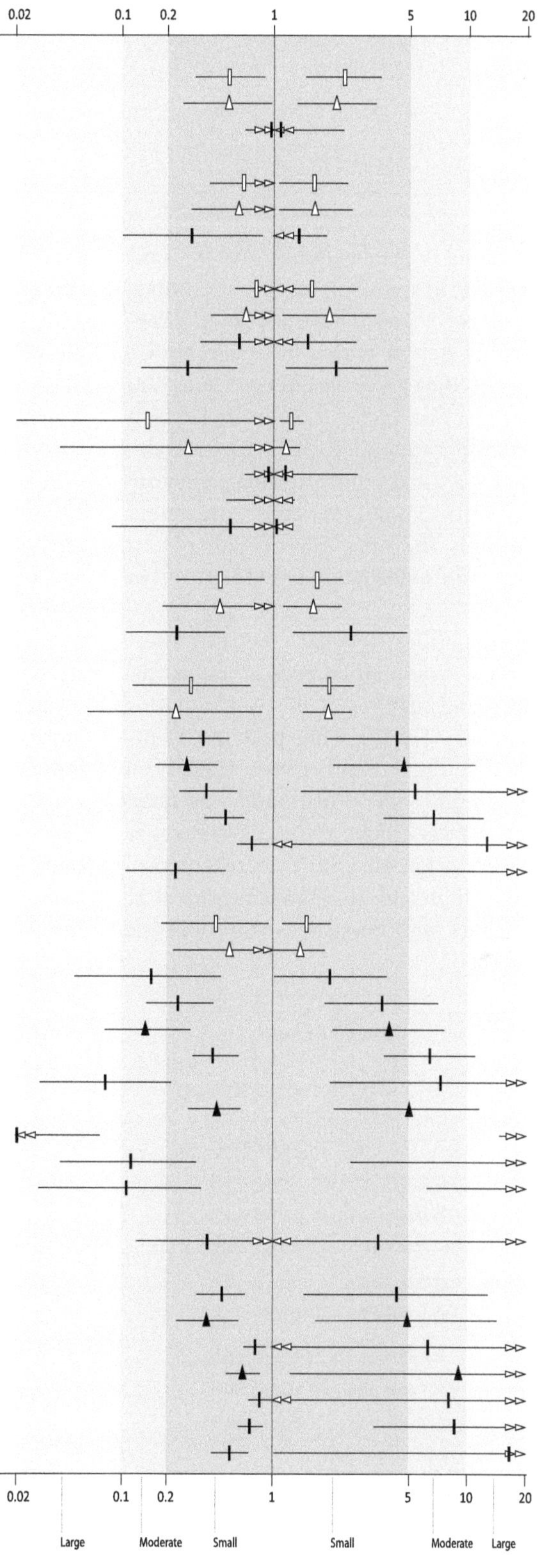

Risk of Bias
1. Patient selection
2. Index test
3. Reference test
4. Flow and timing

Partial *and* Complete / Complete
Primary care
Secondary contact

Figure 2 (See legend on next page.)

(See figure on previous page.)

Figure 2 Diagnostic accuracy of clinical examination for ACL injury. Legend: Risk of bias judgements: (–) = high risk; (?) = unclear risk; (+) = low risk. LR thresholds: +LR <5 and -LR >0.2 = small; +LR 5–10 and; –LR 0.1–0.2 = moderate and +LR >10 and –LR <1 = large. Studies that reported estimates for complete ACL injury as well as partial *and* complete ACL injury estimates have been plotted together to provide a comparison of test performance. Different symbols are used for the estimates for complete versus partial and complete ACL injury and for primary care versus secondary contact settings. *joint effusion 2 hours; †joint effusion 12 hours; ‡immediate pain at trauma; §pain none to slight; ||pain moderate to severe; ¶guarded or painful ROM 24 hours after injury. Guide for interpretation: Greater distance between the –LR and +LR symbols for the test indicates better diagnostic performance.

difference in conclusions is primarily because we only included studies evaluating a clinical sample with diagnostic uncertainty. Other reviews have included case–control studies, a study design which has been shown to inflate estimates of diagnostic accuracy [36]. Our decision to interpret test accuracy via clinically usefully thresholds of likelihood ratios also distinguishes this from previous reviews. A final point of difference concerns our decision not to pool accuracy estimates, which we believe this is the only appropriate course given the risk of bias and heterogeneity evident in the included studies.

Although we applied a critical approach to study selection we still identified several methodological issues that affect internal validity and may result in overestimation of diagnostic test accuracy [17,37]. The spectrum of patients in the included studies varied because of different methods in patient sampling. Most obviously, the characteristics of the samples varied due to the differences in study inclusion and exclusion criteria. Two recent prospective cohort studies illustrate this: Wagemakers et al. [19] included participants with new knee symptoms and excluded participants who were suspected of knee fracture; whereas Beldame et al. [23] included participants with indication for knee arthroscopy, meaning the sample was subject to referral filter bias [37]. The paucity of diagnostic studies for ACL injury conducted in primary care also suggests caution should be taken when generalising these findings to this setting.

In some instances the index tests were not applied to all participants prior to the application of the reference test, or the reference test was performed without a clinical test. There was under reporting of reasons for patient exclusion and withdrawals. Reporting was deficient in most primary studies which limited our appraisal of study quality. This is perhaps most evident with respect to risk of bias domains associated with blinding of the index tests and reference standards. Where multiple index tests were applied concurrently it is unclear the extent to which knowledge of prior testing (test review bias) overestimated the accuracy of index tests. Similarly, there was concern that the invasive nature of knee arthroscopy or surgery as a reference test may have affected the flow of participants through some studies. In these

First Author / Combined test	Likelihood ratio - LR	Likelihood ratio + LR
Wagemakers, 2010		
1 History	0.21 (0.05 to 0.81)	1.4 (1.2 to 1.7)
1 History + Anterior draw	0.29 (0.13 to 0.64)	2.9 (1.9 to 4.1)
1 History + Lachman	0.35 (0.16 to 0.78)	1.9 (1.4 to 2.5)
2 History	0.57 (0.37 to 0.89)	2.3 (1.5 to 3.7)
2 History + Anterior draw	0.63 (0.45 to 0.87)	4.8 (2.3 to 10.2)
2 History + Lachman	0.45 (0.27 to 0.76)	3.8 (2.2 to 6.5)
3 History	0.87 (0.74 to 1.01)	14.3 (1.7 to 122.8)
3 History + Anterior draw	0.82 (0.69 to 0.99)	35.6 (2.0 to 640.4)
3 History + Lachman	0.80 (0.65 to 0.98)	20.0 (2.5 to 163.3)

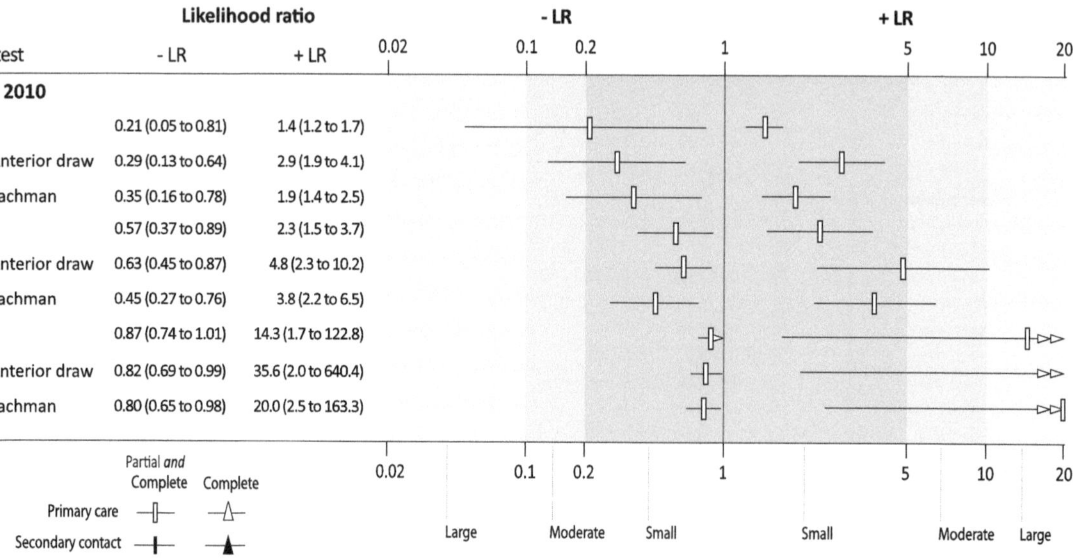

Figure 3 Diagnostic accuracy of composite index tests for partial *and* complete ACL injury in primary care. Legend: Thresholds: +LR <5 and -LR >0.2 = small; +LR 5–10 and; –LR 0.1–0.2 = moderate and +LR >10 and -LR <1 = large. Guide for interpretation: Greater distance between the –LR and +LR symbols for the test indicates better diagnostic performance.

instances a patient with a negative index test may not have received a reference test creating partial verification bias.

Conclusion

This systematic review of clinical tests for ACL injury incorporates the most recent knowledge of diagnostic test accuracy methods. The findings highlight the lack of clinical test accuracy data to support the use of history and physical examination to diagnose ACL injury. Most diagnostic studies on this topic contain methodological flaws which can overestimate the diagnostic accuracy of clinical tests. The available high quality evidence suggests that tests are not useful on their own but combinations may prove to be more useful.

Additional files

Additional file 1: Table S1. PubMed search strategy.

Additional file 2: Table S2. Excluded articles from previous systematic reviews.

Additional file 3: Table S3. Summary statistics for Index tests in the diagnosis of ACL injury.

Additional file 4: Figure S1. Anterior draw, Lachman and pivot shift tests plotted on the ROC plane. Legend: Green: Primary care study setting. Red: Secondary contact study setting.

Additional file 5: Figure S2. Subgroup sensitivity and specificity forest plots. Legend: Anterior draw, Lachman and pivot shift test sensitivity and specificity for partial *and* complete ACL injury in secondary contact settings.

Additional file 6: Figure S3. Diagnostic accuracy of index test EUA in the diagnosis of partial and complete ACL injury. Legend: Risk of bias judgements: (–) = high risk; (?) = unclear risk; (+) = low risk. LR thresholds: +LR <5 and –LR >0.2 = small; +LR 5–10 and; –LR 0.1–0.2 = moderate and +LR>10 and -LR <1 = large. Studies that reported estimates for complete ACL injury as well as partial and complete ACL injury estimates have been plotted together to provide a comparison of test performance. Different symbols are used for the estimates for complete versus partial and complete ACL injury and for primary care versus secondary contact settings. Guide for interpretation: Greater distance between the –LR and +LR symbols for the test indicates better diagnostic performance.

Abbreviations

ACL: Anterior cruciate ligament; QUADAS: QUality assessment of diagnostic accuracy studies; +LR: Positive likelihood ratio; -LR: Negative likelihood ratio; EUA: Examination under anaesthesia.

Competing interests

The authors declare that they have no competing interests.

Authors' contributions

Conception and design: MSS, NH, SJK, BWK, CGM. Analysis and interpretation of the data: MSS, NH, SJK, ASD, BWK, CGM. Drafting of the article: MSS, NH, SJK, ASD, CGM. Critical revision of the article for important intellectual content: MSS, NH, SJK, ASD, BWK, CGM. Final approval of the article: MSS, NH, SJK, ASD, BWK, CGM. Statistical expertise: NH, SJK, CGM. Administrative, technical, or logistic support: MSS, NH, SJK, CGM. Collection and assembly of data: MSS, NH, SJK, ASD. All authors read and approved the final manuscript.

Author details

[1]The George Institute for Global Health, Sydney Medical School, University of Sydney, Missenden Rd, PO Box M201, 2050 Sydney, Australia. [2]Department of Chiropractic, Faculty of Science, Macquarie University, 2109 Sydney, Australia. [3]Institute of Public Health, University of Heidelberg, 69120 Heidelberg, Germany. [4]Department of Epidemiology and Biostatistics, EMGO + Institute, VU University Medical Center, 1081BT Amsterdam, Netherlands. [5]Department of General Practice, Erasmus MC, University Medical Centre, 50 3015 GE Rotterdam, Netherlands.

References

1. Lerat JL, Moyen BL, Cladiere F, Besse JL, Abidi H: **Knee instability after injury to the anterior cruciate ligament. Quantification of the Lachman test.** *J Bone Joint Surg Br* 2000, **82**:42–47.
2. Moses B, Orchard J, Orchard J: **Systematic review: annual incidence of ACL injury and surgery in various populations.** *Res Sports Med* 2012, **20**:157–179.
3. Gianotti SM, Marshall SW, Hume PA, Bunt L: **Incidence of anterior cruciate ligament injury and other knee ligament injuries: a national population-based study.** *J Sci Med Sport* 2009, **12**:622–627.
4. Janssen KW, Orchard JW, Driscoll TR, van Mechelen W: **High incidence and costs for anterior cruciate ligament reconstructions performed in Australia from 2003–2004 to 2007–2008: time for an anterior cruciate ligament register by Scandinavian model?** *Scand J Med Sci Sports* 2012, **22**:495–501.
5. Shea KG, Grimm NL, Ewing CK, Aoki SK: **Youth sports anterior cruciate ligament and knee injury epidemiology: who is getting injured? In what sports? When?** *Clin Sports Med* 2011, **30**:691–706.
6. Jackson JL, O'Malley PG, Kroenke K: **Evaluation of acute knee pain in primary care.** *Ann Intern Med* 2003, **139**:575–588.
7. Bollen SR, Scott BW: **Rupture of the anterior cruciate ligament–a quiet epidemic?** *Injury* 1996, **27**:407–409.
8. Louboutin H, Debarge R, Richou J, Selmi TA, Donell ST, Neyret P, Dubrana F: **Osteoarthritis in patients with anterior cruciate ligament rupture: a review of risk factors.** *Knee* 2009, **16**:239–244.
9. Cimino F, Volk BS, Setter D: **Anterior cruciate ligament injury: diagnosis, management, and prevention.** *Am Fam Physician* 2010, **82**:917–922.
10. Magee DJ: *Orthopedic physical assessment 5th ed.* Saunders Elsevier: St. Louis, Mo; 2008.
11. Benjaminse A, Gokeler A, van der Schans CP: **Clinical diagnosis of an anterior cruciate ligament rupture: a meta-analysis.** *J Orthop Sports Phys Ther* 2006, **36**:267–288.
12. Scholten RJ, Opstelten W, van der Plas CG, Bijl D, Deville WL, Bouter LM: **Accuracy of physical diagnostic tests for assessing ruptures of the anterior cruciate ligament: a meta-analysis.** *J Fam Pract* 2003, **52**:689–694.
13. Solomon DH, Simel DL, Bates DW, Katz JN, Schaffer JL: **Does this patient have a torn meniscus or ligament of the knee? Value of the physical examination.** *JAMA* 2001, **286**:1610–1620.
14. van Eck CF, van den Bekerom MPJ, Fu FH, Poolman RW, Kerkhoffs GMMJ: **Methods to diagnose acute anterior cruciate ligament rupture: a meta-analysis of physical examinations with and without anaesthesia.** *Knee Surg Sports Traumatol Arthrosc* 2013, **21**:1898–1903.
15. Leeflang MM, Deeks JJ, Gatsonis C, Bossuyt PM: **Cochrane Diagnostic Test Accuracy Working G: Systematic reviews of diagnostic test accuracy.** *Ann Intern Med* 2008, **149**:889–897.
16. Swain M, Henschke N, Maher C, Keuerleber J: Diagnostic accuracy of history and physical examination to diagnose knee anterior cruciate ligament injury. PROSPERO 2012:CRD42012002069 Available from http://www.crd.york.ac.uk/PROSPERO/display_record.asp?ID=CRD42012002069 (accessed 20th August 2013).
17. Lijmer JG, Mol BW, Heisterkamp S, Bonsel GJ, Prins MH, van der Meulen JHP, Bossuyt PMM: **Epmerical evidence of design-related bias in studies of diagostic tests.** *JAMA* 1999, **282**:1061–1066.
18. Jaeschke R, Guyatt GH, Sackett DL: **Users' guides to the medical literature. III. How to use an article about a diagnostic test B. What are the results and will they help me in caring for my patients?** *JAMA* 1994, **271**:703–707.
19. Wagemakers HP, Luijsterburg PA, Boks SS, Heintjes EM, Berger MY, Verhaar JA, Koes BW, Bierma-Zeinstra SM: **Diagnostic accuracy of history taking and physical examination for assessing anterior cruciate ligament lesions of the knee in primary care.** *Arch Phys Med Rehabil* 2010, **91**:1452–1459.
20. Whiting PF, Rutjes AW, Westwood ME, Mallett S, Deeks JJ, Reitsma JB, Leeflang MM, Sterne JA, Bossuyt PM, Group Q: **QUADAS-2: a revised tool**

for the quality assessment of diagnostic accuracy studies. *Ann Intern Med* 2011, **155:**529–536.

21. Grimes DA, Schulz KF: Refining clinical diagnosis with likelihood ratios. *Lancet* 2005, **365:**1500–1505.
22. Higgins JP, Thompson SG, Deeks JJ, Altman DG: Measuring inconsistency in meta-analyses. *BMJ* 2003, **327:**557–560.
23. Beldame J, Bertiaux S, Roussignol X, Lefebvre B, Adam JM, Mouilhade F, Dujardin F: Laxity measurements using stress radiography to assess anterior cruciate ligament tears. *Orthop Traumatol Surg Res* 2011, **97:**34–43.
24. Boeree NR, Ackroyd CE: Assessment of the menisci and cruciate ligaments: an audit of clinical practice. *Injury* 1991, **22:**291–294.
25. Harilainen A: Evaluation of knee instability in acute ligamentous injuries. *Ann Chir Gynaecol* 1987, **76:**269–273.
26. Katz JW, Fingeroth RJ: The diagnostic accuracy of ruptures of the anterior cruciate ligament comparing the Lachman test, the anterior drawer sign, and the pivot shift test in acute and chronic knee injuries. *Am J Sports Med* 1986, **14:**88–91.
27. Lee JK, Yao L, Phelps CT, Wirth CR, Czajka J, Lozman J: Anterior cruciate ligament tears: MR imaging compared with arthroscopy and clinical tests. *Radiology* 1988, **166:**861–864.
28. Lucie RS, Wiedel JD, Messner DG: The acute pivot shift: clinical correlation. *Am J Sports Med* 1984, **12:**189–191.
29. Mulligan EP, Harwell JL, Robertson WJ: Reliability and diagnostic accuracy of the lachman test performed in a prone position. *J Orthop Sports Phys Ther* 2011, **41:**749–757.
30. Noyes FR, Bassett RW, Grood ES, Butler DL: Arthroscopy in acute traumatic hemarthrosis of the knee. Incidence of anterior cruciate tears and other injuries. *J Bone Joint Surg Am* 1980, **62:**687–695.
31. Tonino AJ, Huy J, Schaafsma J: The diagnostic accuracy of knee testing in the acutely injured knee. Initial examination versus examination under anaesthesia with arthroscopy. *Acta Orthop Belg* 1986, **52:**479–487.
32. Wong JWK, Chien EP, Yip DKH, Tang WM, Chin ACW, Peh WCG: Is MRI necessary to confirm an acute ACL rupture? *Hong Kong J Sports Med Sports Sci* 1999, **8:**1–5.
33. Decker R, Ruf W: [The diagnostic certainty of various methods of evaluating recent trauma to knee ligaments]. *Unfallchirurgie* 1988, **14:**204–210. German.
34. Richter J, David A, Pape HG, Ostermann PA, Muhr G: [Diagnosis of acute rupture of the anterior cruciate ligament. Value of ultrasonic in addition to clinical examination]. *Unfallchirurg* 1996, **99:**124–129. German.
35. Schwarz W, Hagelstein J, Minholz R, Schierlinger M, Danz B, Gerngross H: [Manual ultrasound of the knee joint. A general practice method for diagnosis of fresh rupture of the anterior cruciate ligament]. *Unfallchirurg* 1997, **100:**280–285. German.
36. Rutjes AWS, Reitsma JB, Vandenbroucke JP, Glas AS, Bossuyt PMM: Case–control and two-gate designs in diagnostic accuracy studies. *Clin Chem* 2005, **51:**1335–1341.
37. Leeflang MMG, Bossuyt PMM, Irwig L: Diagnostic test accuracy may vary with prevalence: implications for evidence-based diagnosis. *J Clin Epidemiol* 2009, **62:**5–12.

20

Chiropractor interaction and treatment equivalence in a pilot randomized controlled trial: an observational analysis of clinical encounter video-recordings

Stacie A Salsbury[1*], James W DeVocht[1], Maria A Hondras[2], Michael B Seidman[1], Clark M Stanford[3] and Christine M Goertz[1]

Abstract

Background: Chiropractic care is a complex health intervention composed of both treatment effects and non-specific, or placebo, effects. While doctor-patient interactions are a component of the non-specific effects of chiropractic, these effects are not evaluated in most clinical trials. This study aimed to: 1) develop an instrument to assess practitioner-patient interactions; 2) determine the equivalence of a chiropractor's verbal interactions and treatment delivery for participants allocated to active or sham chiropractic groups; and 3) describe the perceptions of a treatment-masked evaluator and study participants regarding treatment group assignment.

Methods: We conducted an observational analysis of digital video-recordings derived from study visits conducted during a pilot randomized trial of conservative therapies for temporomandibular pain. A theory-based, iterative process developed the 13-item *Chiropractor Interaction and Treatment Equivalence Instrument*. A trained evaluator masked to treatment assignment coded video-recordings of clinical encounters between one chiropractor and multiple visits of 26 participants allocated to active or sham chiropractic treatment groups. Non-parametric statistics were calculated.

Results: The trial ran from January 2010 to October 2011. We analyzed 111 complete video-recordings (54 active, 57 sham). Chiropractor interactions differed between the treatment groups in 7 categories. Active participants received more interactions with clinical information (8 vs. 4) or explanations (3.5 vs. 1) than sham participants within the therapeutic domain. Active participants received more directions (63 vs. 58) and adjusting instrument thrusts (41.5 vs. 23) in the procedural domain and more optimistic (2.5 vs. 0) or neutral (7.5 vs. 5) outcome statements in the treatment effectiveness domain. Active participants recorded longer visit durations (13.5 vs. 10 minutes). The evaluator correctly identified 61% of active care video-recordings as active treatments but categorized only 31% of the sham treatments correctly. Following the first treatment, 82% of active and 11% of sham participants correctly identified their treatment group. At 2-months, 93% of active and 42% of sham participants correctly identified their group assignment.

Conclusions: Our findings show the feasibility of evaluating doctor-patient interactions in chiropractic clinical trials using video-recordings and standardized instrumentation. Clinical trial design and clinician training protocols should improve and assess the equivalence of doctor-patient interactions between treatment groups.
(Continued on next page)

* Correspondence: stacie.salsbury@palmer.edu
[1]Palmer College of Chiropractic, Palmer Center for Chiropractic Research, 741 Brady Street, Davenport, IA 52803, USA
Full list of author information is available at the end of the article

(Continued from previous page)

Trial registration: This trial was registered in ClinicalTrials.gov as NCT01021306 on 24 November 2009.

Keywords: Chiropractic, Musculoskeletal manipulations, Observational study, Physician-patient relations, Placebo effect, Randomized controlled trials, Sham treatment, Verbal behavior, Video recording

Background

Chiropractic care is a complex health intervention. Complex health interventions are those healthcare therapies constructed from multiple independent and interacting components rather than composed of a single active ingredient, such as a medication [1-3]. With chiropractic care, these interacting components may include the biomechanical characteristics of spinal or joint manipulation, the therapeutic components of chiropractic care, and the non-specific effects of health interventions in general. The biomechanical characteristics of spinal manipulation [4-8] are commonly described in terms of force-time profile (e.g., loading rates, peak and pre-load forces) [8-10] or the thrust characteristics of location, direction and duration [9,11]. Therapeutic components of chiropractic care may include the underlying theoretical paradigm (i.e., subluxation, biomechanical, or somatic dysfunction) [12-15], specific techniques applied [16-19], and treatment frequency or dose [20]. The non-specific or contextual effects of health interventions are often termed 'placebo effects' [3,21,22]. Placebo effects are physiological responses to an intervention that vary by individual and in extent due to the nature of an intervention, its invasiveness, and the patient's expectations for cure or relief and which may have an impact on patient-reported outcomes, such as pain [23-26]. Placebo effects of a health intervention may include such diverse facets as treatment credibility [3,27], therapeutic ritual [28-30], patient response to clinical observation [28], patient and provider expectations [21,27,31-34], classical conditioning [32,34], the biological pathways involved in pain perception [22,31,32], and patient-practitioner interactions [21,27,31,35].

In clinical trials of chiropractic, manual therapy, acupuncture, medical or surgical interventions, or complementary and alternative medicine (CAM), the notion of the placebo effect may be conflated with the placebo treatment, that is, the comparative or control group [22,23,28,34]. These placebo treatments often are termed 'sham' treatments [36,37]. An ideal sham intervention is a procedure that mimics the active treatment in every way except for the absence of the therapeutic component under investigation [23]. Thus, when conducting a randomized controlled trial (RCT) that involves a placebo or sham treatment group, it is not sufficient to provide a sham that is both credible and non-therapeutic [3,21,38,39]. In order to accurately determine the effectiveness of an active treatment, investigators must ensure that non-specific treatment effects (e.g., doctor-patient interactions, time demands, touch or other contact) are the same for participants in the sham group as for the therapeutic group [3,21,23,38,39].

While clinical trials of chiropractic care and other complex health interventions may examine the effects of a treatment on patient-centered outcomes, such as pain or disability [40-42], few trials have considered how placebo effects associated with these therapies may impact patient outcomes [3,21,22,27,43]. One reason researchers have not evaluated placebo effects in clinical trials of chiropractic is the lack of research instruments or data collection processes to quantify these effects. The overall purpose of this observational study was to assess the feasibility of quantifying doctor-patient interactions in sham-controlled chiropractic clinical trials. We also compared these findings to participant perceptions of their treatment group assignment from that same trial. Thus, our specific aims were fourfold. First, we developed a theory-derived data collection tool, the *Chiropractor Interactions and Treatment Equivalence Instrument* (CITE-I), to assess video-recordings of clinical encounters between doctors of chiropractic (DCs) and chiropractic patients. Secondly, we evaluated the equivalence of one chiropractor's verbal interactions and treatment delivery for participants randomized to the active treatment and sham-controlled chiropractic care groups in an expertise-based, pilot RCT of Activator Methods Chiropractic Technique (AMCT) for temporomandibular disorder (TMD) [44]. Next, we described the video evaluator's masked assessment of participant treatment assignment with the RCT participants' beliefs about their treatment group assignment. Finally, we described participants' perceptions of their treatment group assignment after the first treatment visit and following 2 months of treatment.

Methods

We conducted an observational analysis of digital video-recordings derived from study visits with participants who received an active or sham chiropractic treatment during a pilot RCT of 4 conservative therapies for TMD-related jaw pain. A theory-based, iterative process developed the 5-domain, 13-variable, *Chiropractor Interaction and Treatment Equivalence Instrument.* In these methods, we describe the design of the pilot RCT, video-recording procedures, the instrument development process, and data collection and analysis procedures.

Pilot RCT design

The institutional review boards of the Palmer College of Chiropractic, Davenport, Iowa (Approval Number 2009D121), and The University of Iowa, Iowa City, Iowa (Approval Number 200808726) approved the study protocol and human research participant protections for the pilot RCT. This trial was registered in ClinicalTrials.gov as NCT01021306 on 24 November 2009. The trial began January 2010, with data collection completed October 2011. The methods and results of the pilot RCT were described elsewhere [44]. Participants had at least a 6-month history of jaw pain consistent with chronic myofascial TMD. Eighty participants were randomly allocated to one of four treatment groups: active AMCT (n = 20), sham AMCT (n = 19), dental reversible interocclusal splint therapy (RIST) (n = 20), or self-care only (n = 21). Participants in all four groups received a basic self-care training module of relaxation, stretching and self-awareness pain modulation therapy. The self-care treatment group received this module, alone. Participants signed a written informed consent. The informed consent document instructed participants that they may be randomized to a "placebo treatment group" with treatments similar in appearance to AMCT and that the investigators did not expect the TMD condition of participants assigned to this group to worsen over the course of the study [23,38]. The consent document informed participants that study visits would be video-recorded to evaluate the doctor's interactions with participants and that these recordings would not be destroyed.

One DC with over 20 years of experience using the AMCT protocol provided the intervention to all participants in both the active and sham AMCT groups. The DC delivered both treatments with a hand-held, spring-loaded device – the Activator Adjusting Instrument (AAI) (Activator IV, Activator Methods International Ltd., Phoenix, AZ) instead of a manual thrust common to many forms of chiropractic spinal manipulation [17,45]. The DC mimicked the active AMCT protocol for the sham group by using a detuned AAI that made just a sound (like the active AAI), but delivered no thrust. The DC delivered the AMCT protocol, including treatment to the full spine, extremities, and temporomandibular joints for participants in both groups [44]. The DC also performed a gentle occipital stretching procedure following delivery of the standard AMCT treatment. Training on the study protocol emphasized the DC should offer the same type of verbal communication and spend a similar amount of time with patients in each treatment group, including in self-care instruction, examination and testing procedures, and treatment delivery [44].

All participants randomized to the AMCT groups were to receive 12 study visits over 2 months [44]. Primary outcomes included an 11-point numerical rating scale for TMD-related pain [46] and the 14-item Oral Health Impact Profile (OHIP-14) [47] to assess quality of life at 2 months and 6 months. Participant ratings of treatment believability were gathered for all 4 treatment groups following the first and twelfth study visits [19]. Participants also answered the following statement on a 5-item scale ('strongly believe' to 'do not know'): "There are two types of treatments in this research study: active and inactive (placebo). Please indicate which type of treatment you believe you are receiving". Participant responses for 'strongly believe' and 'somewhat believe' for active treatment and 'strongly believe' and 'somewhat believe' for inactive (placebo) treatment were combined in this analysis.

Video recording and handling process

The study protocol included video recordings of each chiropractic study visit. Thus, our study sample was the video-recorded observations of participant study visits, and not the participants themselves. A digital video-camera (Panasonic model HDC-H520; Newark, NJ, USA) was set up on a tripod in a corner of the treatment room before the participant entered. A card with the participant identification (ID) number and current date was placed in front of the video-camera and recorded for a few seconds. The video-camera was to be positioned to visualize the participant's entire body lying on the treatment table (from crown of head to feet), as well as the DC as he moved around the table delivering the study treatment. The clinic receptionist used a remote control unit to begin the video-recording process as the participant entered the treatment room and to stop the recording when the participant left the treatment room. The video files were copied from the camera to an external hard drive and named with the participant ID number and recording date. No other identifying information was recorded to maintain participant confidentiality. A study co-leader (JWD) copied the video files from the external hard drive in the chiropractic clinic to a second external hard drive for data transfer to the research center. The HD video-recordings were converted from *.m2ts to *.mp4 files using Roxio Toast Titanium 10 software (Corel Corporation, Ottawa, Ontario, Canada). This version of the video-recordings was stored at the research center on a password-protected computer for long-term back-up and data analysis.

Instrument development process

Four team members developed the assessment instrument and data collection process to codify the doctor-patient interactions during the chiropractic visits (see Author Information for respective contributions). Team members remained blinded to participants' treatment assignment throughout the instrument development, data collection and analysis processes. The instrument development process went through 3 primary stages as described below.

Stage 1: Preliminary video-recordings review and research question

Two researchers (JWD, SAS) jointly reviewed several video-recordings to examine various aspects of the doctor-patient interactions such as verbal communications (i.e., clinician utterances, participant replies), non-verbal behaviors, and contextual effects (e.g., social interactions, humor, or use of touch) as well as factors related to the recording process to identify the initial coding framework and the strengths and limitations of these video-recordings as data sources. For example, most of the video-recordings did not visualize the participant during pre-treatment consultations or post-treatment interactions due to camera position. In addition, the audio-track often did not record the participants' side of these conversations clearly. The treatment table muffled participants' voices when lying prone during much of the AMCT-protocol. Similarly, the camera position for many video-recordings did not allow complete visualization of the non-verbal behaviors (e.g., facial expressions, body position, treatment delivery, AAI positioning) of the DC when his back was to the camera, nor could participants observe these doctor behaviors when they were lying prone. Further, the participants' ideal body position (i.e., from the crown of the head to the feet) was captured in only about 25% of the videos recorded.

Based on such contextual factors, the investigators (SAS, JWD, MAH) concluded that an analysis of doctor-patient interactions could neither focus on the non-verbal communications of the DC nor emphasize participants' verbal responses. However, we noted the recordings captured most of the chiropractor's verbal utterances as well as the "clicking" sounds produced by the thrust of the active and detuned AAIs. A previous study using AAI as a placebo treatment noted this clicking sound supported patients' assessments of treatment credibility [37]. The team then focused the research question and instrument development process on quantification of the equivalence of the DC's verbal communications and AAI delivery between the active and sham AMCT groups.

Stage 2: Construct identification and instrument development

Literature reviews identified published instruments available for the assessment of doctor-patient interactions in medical encounters [48-50]. Among these, the Roter Interaction Analysis System (RIAS) was identified as the most widely used method of analyzing patient-provider interactions during healthcare encounters [49], and served as the theoretical framework from which our instrument was derived. The RIAS classifies medical communications into two conceptual categories - the socioemotional and task dimensions [49]. While the RIAS has excellent psychometric properties [49], a major limitation of this instrument for an analysis of patient-provider communications within the context of clinical research is that conversational styles of communication in RCTs differ from those in naturally-occurring medical encounters in important ways [30,35,51]. In routine clinical practice, physicians may tailor patient education, advice and support to the individual needs of the patient [27]. In contrast, the communications from the research clinician to the research participant within an RCT is a protocol-driven, or scripted, conversation to minimize its influence on treatment outcomes [28,35,43]. In addition, while research participants are masked to their treatment assignment at the start of a RCT, clinician behavior may lead them to identify whether they are receiving an active or placebo/sham treatment [27,30,35,37,43,51,52]. Thus, the clinician's verbal communications and treatment delivery should not unmask participants to treatment assignment [43]. Finally, the research clinicians' verbal interactions may directly impact outcomes assessments in an RCT should the doctor communicate any observed or perceived changes in health status, such as an improvement or decline, to participants [43,51,53].

At this stage, the team first focused instrument development on two theoretical categories of the RIAS: socio-emotional, or 'care-oriented', communications and instrumental, or 'cure-oriented', communications [49,54] to assure these key features of doctor-patient interactions were identified. Video-recordings were viewed over several team meetings to identify how these thematic constructs were expressed by the clinician during treatment. Each member coded the video-recordings using a paper copy of the current assessment form. Video reviewers placed a hash mark in the appropriate cell for each utterance from the clinician and any clicks from the AAI thrust. An utterance was defined as any verbalization that expressed a single idea to a participant. Thus, a sentence in which the DC directed the participant to "turn your head to the right, and to the center, and to the left" would equate 3 unique utterances. Team members stopped the video-recording frequently to discuss how each had categorized the various utterances, the rationale for such categorization, and sought consensus on each classification.

The team reviewed 2–4 video-recordings per session, determined categorical or definitional revisions, and identified form changes. For instance, clinician utterances on participants' health status (i.e., need for more or fewer adjustments since the last visit) required an added domain for "treatment effectiveness" with optimistic, pessimistic and neutral statements on patient outcomes constituting key variables. This category was of particular importance within a sham-controlled trial where verbal indications of treatment effectiveness may increase participant expectancies for future response [31], serve as a conditioning protocol [31], and impact patient outcome measures [31]. We included a variable for the duration of the study visit to assess whether the clinician spent an equivalent amount time with participants in each group. We also added a tally of AAI clicks (an auditory stimulus that may condition the participant and increase the placebo response [31]) as a rough indicator of the 'dose' delivered of active or sham AMCT.

Stage 3: Process pre-testing, evaluator training and instrument refinement

SAS and JWD evaluated video-recordings until the team members achieved consensus on the instrument domains, variables, examples and data collection format as no new categories were identified with additional video-recording reviews. MAH confirmed the completeness of initial data collection form. While the team did not assess inter-rater agreement using formal statistics, comparison of categorical totals at the end of each data collection session revealed a high level of agreement between reviewers, with most categories tallying within 1 [for categories with low tallies (0–8 hash marks), such as treatment effectiveness] to 3 points [for categories with high tallies (30–50 hash marks) such as directions or AAI clicks] for each evaluator.

During pre-testing, the team also identified treatment duration differences, with the first treatment visit (T1) lasting 10–20 minutes longer than subsequent study visits (T2-T12). During the T1 visit, the DC spent considerable time discussing the participants' past medical history, the study protocol, and follow-up activities. As these visits appeared tailored to the individual participant, and differed considerably in duration and content from the other treatment visits, we decided not to include these visits in the analysis for this study.

The team member (MBS) who served as the video evaluator was trained on the video analysis instrument. As in previous coding rounds, team members coded the recordings as a group and discussed unclear utterances, variable definitions and examples. Early in the training, the video evaluator had categorical inconsistencies (primarily with therapeutic domain variables) that were resolved through these discussions. The instrument was reorganized so the most used variables (*clinical information, directions, Activator clicks)* were placed at the top of the grid. Categorical tallies after each coding round noted few differences between the team members.

The team members reviewed and accepted the Chiropractor Interaction and Treatment Equivalence Instrument (CITE-I) for use in the interaction equivalence study. This version of the CITE-I included 5 domains with 13 variables. The affective domain consisted of 2 socio-emotional variables [49,54] categorizing the clinician's verbal interactions as *social/humor* or *name use*. The therapeutic domain included 3 instrumental variables [49,54]: *clinical information*, *explanations*, and *logistics*. The procedural domain consisted of 3 variables addressing treatment implementation and fidelity [55] including adherence, delivery, and dose: *directions, cautions,* and *Activator clicks,* or the sound produced by the adjusting instrument. The treatment effectiveness domain categorized *optimistic, pessimistic* and *neutral* statements about health or treatment outcomes [31]. Lastly, the encounter context domain tabulated the *duration* of the treatment encounter as an additional measure of dose, as well as any *unclear statements* made by the clinician that the video evaluator could not definitively place into another category. The CITE-I also included a field to denote how much of the participant's *body position* was on the video and a *notes field* to record additional details of the interaction context, blinding issues, etc. The final item on the CITE-I asks the video evaluator to denote which study treatment he believed the participant to have received (active, placebo/sham or not sure). Figure 1 presents the CITE-I instrument including variable definitions and examples.

Data collection

One team member (MBS) evaluated the video-recordings of the chiropractic visits using the CITE-I. A flash drive of video-recordings included mixed participants from discontinuous study visits to assure the evaluator did not view an entire treatment series sequentially. The evaluator viewed the recordings while wearing headphones to minimize external distractions. When necessary, portions of the video-recordings were replayed to enhance the accuracy of data collection. This process was repeated until all video recordings were evaluated.

Data management and data analysis

Completed CITE-I forms were submitted to the Office of Data Management for double key entry into an electronic spreadsheet once all video-recordings in an analytic set were evaluated. Tally marks were counted twice and entered as a total for each category by the evaluator, with these sums double checked by data entry personnel. Data were organized by participant ID number, treatment date, and treatment visit number. Participant treatment believability items were data entered at the time of the pilot RCT. Data were analyzed using the SAS statistical analysis software package (Version 9.2, SAS Institute Inc., Cary, North Carolina, USA). We report simple descriptive statistics (median, interquartile ranges [IQR], and/or number and percentage) to characterize our sample of video-recordings. Formal statistical tests of significance were not appropriate at this stage of instrument development as our primary aim was to assess whether video-recordings were a feasible means of evaluating

PTID:_________ Tx Date (mm/dd/yy):___/___/___ Tx Duration: __ :__ __:__ __ **Chiropractor Interaction and Treatment Equivalence Instrument (CITE-I)**

Variable	Definition	Examples	5	10	15	20	25	30	35	40	45	50	Total
Clinical Info Seeking	Questions/comments to obtain clinical or health information	How are you feeling?											
		How are you feeling?											
Directions or Instructions	Instructions given to participant related to treatment protocol	Place your arm... Lift your head. Relax.											
	**If two or move body movements are instructed in one sentence, count each movement separately.*	Place your arm... Lift your head. Relax.											
		Place your arm... Lift your head. Relax.											
Activator Clicks	Sounds produced by Activator Adjusting Instrument	Click!											
		Click!											
Optimistic Health Statement	Positive statement on health improvement / treatment success	Leg check is even. Good. Very nice.											
Pessimistic Health Statement	Negative statements on health decline / treatment nonsuccess	Much worse... Need adjustments											
Neutral Statement	Neutral statements about health or noncommittal sounds	Hmmm... I see... OK.											
Social / Humor	Statements or questions about everyday life / attempt at humor	Family, work, hobby, jokes, weather, laugh											
Cannot Make Out	Statement unclear or soft volume	(whispers)											
Explanation or Recommendation	Info given on protocol or actions pt should take to improve health	I do this to... You should do this...											
Cautions	Statements on uncomfortable or startling touch or treatments	This touch might hurt. I am lowering table.											
Study Logistics	Statements on study or schedule	Appointments, call-ins											

Number of times participant's name spoken:

Participant body position (upper- and lowermost body sections visible, such as head to knee, shoulder to feet, etc):

NOTES (Interaction context, blinding issues, etc.):

In your opinion, which study treatment did this participant receive? ❑$_1$ Active (Activator) Treatment ❑$_2$ Placebo/Sham ❑$_3$ Not sure

Evaluator ID: __ __ __ Evaluation Date (mm/dd/yy):___/___/___

Figure 1 Chiropractor Interaction and Treatment Equivalence Instrument (CITE-I).

doctor-patient interactions and not to test hypotheses based on those interactions.

Results

Video-recording evaluation flowchart

Figure 2 presents a flowchart of the video-recordings evaluated for this study. Each participant allocated to a chiropractic group (n = 39) was to receive 12 visits to the chiropractor per study protocol (n = 468). An equal number of participants from each group (n = 13) had at least 1 video-recording reviewed for this study. Four participants (3 in active AMCT, 1 in sham AMCT) withdrew from the trial before the first treatment, while 9 participants (5 in active AMCT, 4 in sham AMCT) did not have any video-recordings made during the trial. The mean number of video-recordings completed for all participants was 4.4 (range from 0–11).

For this analysis, we excluded all T1 visits from this analysis due to their longer durations and the more personalized nature of the encounters as compared to the T2-T12 visits. Other video-recordings were either not available or incomplete and not included. Of these, the number of missed appointments (n = 59), missed video-recordings (n = 172), and video-recordings excluded due to incomplete recordings (n = 43), either from video-recordings that began after the visit was in progress or that ended before the visit concluded, were equivalent between groups. In total, we analyzed 24% (111/468) of the planned active and sham AMCT study visits in this pilot RCT. The video evaluator coded 54 video-recordings from 13 active AMCT participants and 57 video-recordings from 13 sham AMCT participants for this analysis.

Chiropractor interactions and treatment equivalence

Table 1 presents results for the video analysis of clinician interaction and treatment equivalence between active and sham AMCT groups. Five categories, *clinical information, explanations, directions, optimistic statements,* and *neutral statements* revealed notable differences in the DC's verbal interactions, while two categories, *Activator clicks* and *encounter duration,* denoted disparities in treatment equivalence between the active and sham AMCT groups.

Within the therapeutic domain, the participants in active AMCT had twice as many verbal interactions where

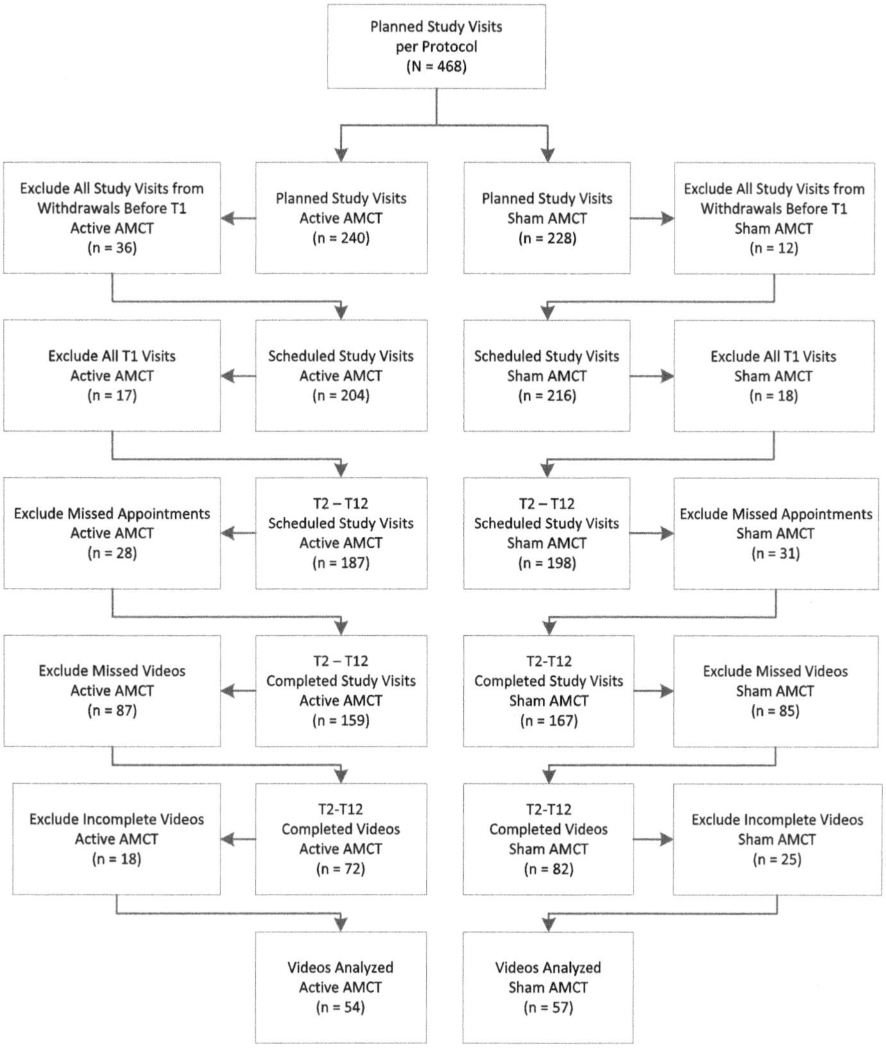

Figure 2 Video-recording flowchart.

the clinician sought *clinical information* than did sham AMCT participants (median 8.0 vs. 4.0 per visit). Active AMCT participants also received more *explanations* on the study protocol or recommendations on actions to take to improve health compared to sham AMCT participants (median 3.5 vs. 1.0 per visit). Statements about study *logistics* favored sham ACMT participants over active AMCT participants (median 2.0 vs. 1.0 per visit).

Within the procedural domain, active AMCT participants received more *directions* from the clinician than did sham AMCT participants (median 63 vs. 58 per visit). Active AMCT participants also received more *Activator clicks* than did sham AMCT participants (median 41.5 clicks vs. 23 clicks per visit). *Cautions* were similar between groups.

Within the treatment effectiveness domain, the DC offered active AMCT participants more *optimistic statements* about health improvements or treatment success than participants in the sham AMCT group (median 2.5 comments vs. 0 comments per visit). Active AMCT participants also received more *neutral statements* about their treatments than did sham AMCT participants (median 7.5 comments vs. 5 comments per visit), while few *pessimistic statements* were offered to participants in either treatment group.

Within the encounter context domain, the mean *encounter duration* was somewhat longer for the active AMCT group than the sham AMCT group (13.5 minutes vs. 10.0 minutes per treatment). More *unclear statements* were recorded for the active AMCT group (median 2.0 versus 1.0). Neither of the affective domain variables (*social/humor* or *name use*) differed appreciably between the treatment groups.

Treatment group assignment evaluation

Table 2 presents the results of the masked assessment of treatment assignment by the video evaluator and compares

Table 1 Video-analysis of chiropractor interaction equivalence between active and sham Activator Methods Chiropractic Technique (AMCT) treatment groups

			Active AMCT (n =54)		Sham AMCT (n =57)	
Domain	**Variable**	**Definition**	**Median (SD)**	**IQR**	**Median (SD)**	**IQR**
Affective	**Social/Humor**	Statements or questions about everyday life or attempts at humor	9.0 (14.9)	14	8.0 (11.2)	13
	Name Use	Number of times the name of the participant was spoken	2.0 (1.3)	2	2.0 (1.5)	1
Therapeutic	**Clinical Information**	Questions or comments to obtain clinical or health information	8.0 (5.3)	7	4.0 (3.1)	4
	Explanations	Information on protocol or actions to take to improve health	3.5 (9.2)	8	1.0 (3.6)	3
	Logistics	Statements on study procedures or treatment schedule	1.0 (1.4)	2	2.0 (2.5)	1
Procedural	**Directions**	Instructions given related to treatment protocol	63.0 (11.6)	15	58.0 (6.7)	8
	Cautions	Statements on uncomfortable or startling touch or treatments	3.0 (1.5)	2	3.0 (1.2)	1
	Activator Clicks	Sounds produced by Activator Adjusting Instrument	41.5 (30.1)	44	23.0 (10.1)	13
Treatment Effectiveness	**Optimistic**	Positive statement on health improvement or treatment success	2.5 (4.0)	6	0 (1.6)	0
	Pessimistic	Negative statement on health improvement or treatment success	0 (1.1)	1	0 (0.7)	0
	Neutral	Neutral statement about health or noncommittal sounds	7.5 (4.1)	6	5.0 (3.6)	4
Encounter Context	**Encounter Duration**	Duration of treatment in minutes	13.5 (4.1)	5	10.0 (1.8)	2
	Unclear Statement	Statement unclear or spoken at soft volume	2.0 (2.6)	3	1.0 (2.0)	3

Table 2 Video evaluator assessment of treatment assignment compared to participant treatment believability ratings

		Active AMCT Videos (n =54)		Sham AMCT Videos (n =57)	
Variable	**Response**	**n^**	**%**	**n^**	**%**
Video Evaluator Assessment of Treatment Assignment	Active AMCT	33	61	16	28
	Sham AMCT	3	6	18	31
	Not Sure	17	31	22	39
		Active AMCT participants (n =17)		**Sham AMCT participants (n =18)**	
Variable	**Response**	**n**	**%**	**n**	**%**
Participant Believability 1st Treatment Visit	Active Treatment+	14	82	12	66
	Inactive Treatment (Placebo)+	1	6	2	11
	Do Not Know	2	12	4	22
		Active AMCT participants (n =14)		**Sham AMCT participants (n =14)**	
Variable	**Response**	**n**	**%**	**n**	**%**
Participant Believability Month 2	Active Treatment+	13	93	8	58
	Inactive Treatment (Placebo)+	1	7	6	42
	Do Not Know	0	0	0	0

+Strongly believe and somewhat believe were combined for presentation.
^Missing data.

these data to participant's perceptions about their treatment assignment. The video evaluator correctly assigned an assessment of 'active treatment' to 33 (61%) of the active AMCT video-recordings, with most of the remaining (n = 17; 31%) video-recordings receiving a 'not sure' designation. The video evaluator assigned an assessment of 'active treatment' (n = 16; 28%), 'placebo/sham' (n = 18; 31%), and 'not sure' (n = 22; 39%) to the sham AMCT video-recordings.

In contrast to the treatment-masked evaluator, study participants more readily identified their treatment group assignments, particularly those in the active AMCT group. After the first study visit, 82% (n = 14) of active AMCT participants rated their treatment as an 'active treatment', with 6% (n = 1) rating the treatment as inactive or placebo, and 12% (n = 2) stating they did not know which treatment they received. After their first treatment, 66% (n = 12) of sham AMCT participants rated their treatment as active, 11% (n = 2) as inactive or placebo, and 22% (n = 4) as did not know. At the 2-month assessment, participant ratings of 'active treatment' increased to 93% (n = 13) for active AMCT participants. For sham AMCT participants, active treatment ratings dropped to 58% (n = 8), with inactive or placebo ratings increasing to 42% (n = 6). No participant in either group stated they did not know their treatment group at the 2-month evaluation.

Discussion

To our knowledge, this study is the first to assess the equivalence of verbal interactions and treatment delivery for a doctor of chiropractic providing active and sham chiropractic interventions within the context of a randomized controlled trial. Many studies of spinal manipulation or other chiropractic therapies have used sham adjustments as a comparator [36,56], including those using a detuned Activator adjusting instrument as the sham [37,57]. Researchers who conduct sham or placebo-controlled trials of complementary therapies, including chiropractic, have espoused the need for the standardization of the non-specific aspects of treatment, including treatment duration and the interventionists' verbal and non-verbal communications, between study groups [37,52,58]. And yet, most have evaluated only patient perceptions of the believability of the sham or their success in masking treatment assignment [37,52,59-61]. Few studies, if any, of chiropractic interventions have discussed the potential placebo effects derived from the doctor's interpersonal interactions with patients.

This study showed the feasibility of quantifying the verbal interactions and treatment equivalence of chiropractors within a clinical trial using a standardized data collection process. This finding has relevance for future clinical studies. Our data collection tool, the Chiropractor Interaction and Treatment Equivalence Instrument, may be tailored for specific chiropractic techniques, other manual therapies, and complementary and alternative medicine therapies, and perhaps to interventions delivered by other healthcare providers. The CITE-I also may be useful for several stages of the clinical trial development and implementation process [53,55,62,63]. For example, researchers might use the CITE-I to train clinicians in the delivery of the study protocol in an effort to provide participants in each treatment group with equivalent doses of interactions with the treatment provider, and equivalent treatments when more than one clinician delivers the study treatments [63]. This training procedure might be performed via video-recordings that are either reviewed by the investigators or by the clinicians themselves, to identify areas to treatment standardization (e.g., number of adjustments, clinical information queries) before the start of the trial [62]. Once the trial is underway, the same instrument might be used for quality control purposes to minimize drift in treatment delivery over the course of the trial [64]. Finally, once the trial is concluded, the CITE-I might be used to assess treatment fidelity over the course of the study [53,55].

Our study found potentially important discrepancies in the DC's verbal interactions, including in communications related to clinical information, explanations, protocol-related directions, and statements about treatment effectiveness between the active and sham groups. In essence, active AMCT participants may have received an 'augmented interaction' with the DC, similar to that delivered by acupuncturists in an RCT specifically designed to assess various components of the placebo effect in patients with irritable bowel syndrome [28]. In that study, participants allocated to the augmented interaction group received acupuncturists' communications that emphasized 5 behaviors shown to support optimal patient-practitioner relationships: a friendly manner, active listening, empathy, thoughtful silence, and communication of confidence in and positive expectations for treatment [28]. These augmented communication styles were not dissimilar to the added interactions the active AMCT participants received when the DC sought more clinical information, offered treatment explanations or self-care recommendations, or shared optimistic statements about participants' changes in health status. These differences in the practitioner's verbal interactions may explain the higher satisfaction levels of participants in the active AMCT group reported in the pilot RCT, and possibly account for some of the difference in outcomes between the two chiropractic groups [44].

We also reported the video evaluator's perceptions of treatment assignment and the RCT participants' perceptions of treatment believability. The video evaluator correctly attributed 'active treatment' to 61% of the active AMCT videos, while incorrectly ascribing 'placebo/sham' to only 6% of the active AMCT group. This finding suggests a perceptible difference in the DC's interactions between treatment groups that allowed a trained evaluator to correctly identify participants who received active AMCT more often than by chance. Similarly, 82% and 93% of active AMCT participants correctly identified their treatment as an active treatment after the first and final treatments, respectively. In contrast, sham AMCT participants shifted their treatment perceptions as inactive from 11% at first treatment to 42% at the final treatment. The video evaluator's and participants' perceptions of treatment assignment might be based on two notable differences in treatment delivery identified in this analysis: treatment duration and number of audible sounds generated by the adjusting instrument during its thrust. Active AMCT participants received study visits that were three minutes longer in duration and during which almost twice as many instrument-assisted adjustments were delivered. The sounds made by the adjusting instrument were identified in a previous study as evidence of treatment credibility [37]. Future chiropractic trials with sham treatment groups should develop study protocols that maximize equivalence in such components of treatment delivery.

While our analysis focused on the doctor's verbal interactions, the non-verbal communications which were not measured in this study may account for the differences noted in the treatment group assignment perceptions of the video evaluator and study participants. Other researchers have identified the importance of such non-verbal communications as tone of voice, facial expression and eye contact [65], the use of touch [65,66], and provider time spent sitting versus standing during clinical encounters [67] on patient satisfaction and health outcomes. Future studies may more closely examine the contributions of non-verbal communication to the placebo effects of chiropractic care although those may be more difficult to adequately record and quantify than were verbal interactions.

Our study has several strengths. Our method of video-recording doctor-patient interactions during chiropractic care is similar to other studies using video-recordings to assess the clinical or communication skills of health professionals [68]. The advantages of video-recordings for this type of research are numerous [69,70]. First, a video-recording is a permanent account of human interactions that are complex, fleeting, and difficult to detail or verify using standard documentation techniques for observational data (e.g., field notes, memos) [69]. As we did during the instrument development process, observers may view video-recorded interactions repeatedly, at different speeds and directions, and with pauses, allowing for thorough and reliable analyses [69,70]. Multiple reviewers also may analyze the same interaction, which may decrease the subjectivity inherent in observational techniques [69,70]. Another strength was the number of recordings analyzed, recorded from multiple participants at different phases of the treatment protocol. In addition, team members were blinded to the treatment assignment of participants throughout the instrument development process as well as during video-recording analysis. These procedures enhance the validity of the study findings [69].

This study had its limitations, including the challenges inherent in the video-recording process [68-71]. Mechanical limitations, such as camera malfunctions, static camera positions, or muffled audio mechanisms, are known issues in research using video-recordings [69-71]. Future studies might position the video-camera on the ceiling, employ two cameras, or use cameras that automatically follow movement to allow fuller visualization of the doctor-patient interaction, as researchers have done in similar studies conducted in emergency departments, physician consultations, or during surgical procedures [64,71,72].

Another limitation is the potential influence of the video-recoding process on the behaviors of the persons whose interactions are recorded [69,70]. Some studies have shown few differences in camera-related behaviors [73] or doctor-patient interactions during video-recorded clinical encounters [68,74], while others indicate improved performance by physicians whose clinical encounters were video-recorded [75]. The frequency with which such behaviors occurred was not evaluated in this analysis, although some patterns were noted that may suggest clinician discomfort with the video-recording process. For example, the camera often was positioned in such a way that it did not visualize the participants' entire body (most notably the neck and head region) or pick up DC utterances while seated at the head of the treatment table. Future studies should assess clinician comfort with the video-recording process directly.

Another limitation is missing data. We analyzed just 24% of the planned study visits in this pilot RCT. While some missing data-points were from missed appointments, more were from unrecorded treatment visits or incomplete video-recordings. Clinic staff missed or truncated the video-recordings when the office was busy or other clinical demands tasks were prioritized. Similar analyses have reported similar challenges capturing all possible events due to problems with the recording device or human error in initiating the video-recording process [72]. Future studies collecting video-recordings to assess doctor-patient interactions should institute pre-treatment checklists and on-going quality control procedures to assure complete datasets.

In this analysis, we opted not to evaluate the video-recordings for the first treatment visit due to the extended duration and content differences for these visits compared to the T2-T12 study visits. Eight active AMCT participants and 6 sham AMCT participants did not have their T1 study visits video-recorded. Finniss and colleagues note, however, that first treatment encounters may be of critical importance in the "development of subsequent robust placebo responses" (p. 688) through a chain of treatment expectancy, conditioning mechanisms, and the perceived effectiveness of the initial interaction [31]. A future study using this or similar datasets might evaluate the doctor-patient interactions using a more discrete data collection system such as the RIAS to assess group differences in medical history taking, rapport building, self-care instructions, and other socio-emotional relationship components during the initial treatment encounter [49]. Such an evaluation also would allow a comparison of the communication strategies of DCs to other healthcare professionals [76-80].

Lastly, this study was a preliminary investigation of doctor-patient interactions with a pilot clinical trial of chiropractic care. We developed the Chiropractic Interaction and Treatment Equivalence Instrument specifically for this preliminary study. While the conceptual framework for the instrument seems logical and our analysis did identify differences in the doctor's interactions between treatment groups, the CITE-I requires further refinement, including formal instrument testing to establish its reliability and validity. Item analysis may identify different domains than those presented here, as well as individual items that are redundant or that might be omitted. Psychometric evaluations of the CITE-I should occur before its use in other clinical studies of chiropractic care or in other manual therapy trials.

Conclusion

Our findings show the feasibility of evaluating doctor-patient verbal interactions and treatment equivalence in chiropractic clinical trials using video-recordings of doctor-patient encounters and a standardized data collection tool, the Chiropractor Interaction and Treatment Equivalence Instrument. The results of our study indicated that doctor-patient interactions in randomized controlled trials of chiropractic therapies may vary between the active care and sham-controlled treatment groups. It is not known how much effect such variation in doctor-patient interaction has on clinical outcomes. However, to accurately compare the clinical value of one form of treatment to that of another, clinical trial design and training protocols of clinicians who deliver study interventions should include steps to minimize the variation of doctor-patient interactions between treatment groups. Future studies to establish the psychometric properties of the CITE-I are needed.

Abbreviations

AAI: Activator adjusting instrument; AMCT: Activator methods chiropractic technique; CAM: Complementary and alternative medicine; CITE-I: Chiropractor interaction and treatment equivalence instrument; DC: Doctor of chiropractic; ID: Identification number; RCT: Randomized controlled trial; RIAS: Roter interaction analysis system; T: Treatment (number); TMD: Temporomandibular joint disorder.

Competing interests

The authors declare that they have no competing interests.

Authors' contributions

MAH, CMS, JWD, CMG and SAS conceived of this study. SAS, MAH, and JWD designed the study methodology and participated in instrument design. SAS directed instrument development, conducted literature reviews, and coordinated the coder training process. JWD coordinated the video-recording, data management and data analysis processes. MAH was a co-investigator for the pilot RCT and provided oversight throughout this study. MBS participated in instrument refinement and completed data collection. SAS, JWD, and MAH interpreted the data and drafted the manuscript. CMG, CMS and JWD provided leadership on the Center grant and the clinical trial that provided the data used in this study. All authors were involved in manuscript revision and gave final approval of the manuscript.

Acknowledgements

This study was supported by grant U19AT004663 from the National Center for Complementary and Alternative Medicine (NCCAM), National Institutes of Health (NIH), Bethesda, MD, USA. This study was conducted in part in a facility constructed with support of the Research Facilities Improvement Program grant C06 RR15433 from the National Center for Research Resources (NCRR), NIH. The contents of this manuscript are solely the responsibility of the authors and do not necessarily represent the official views of NCCAM, NCRR, or NIH.
The results of this study were presented at the 2012 International Research Congress on Integrative Medicine and Health in Portland, OR, USA.
The authors thank Activator Methods International, Phoenix, AZ, for providing the Activator IV instruments used in the pilot study.
The authors thank the study participants for their important contributions to this research. We thank the doctor of chiropractic and office staff for their involvement in the clinical trial. We acknowledge research staff members for their project and data management contributions. We are grateful to Robert D. Vining, DC for his many valuable and thoughtful insights on the nature of doctor-patient relationships.

Author details

[1]Palmer College of Chiropractic, Palmer Center for Chiropractic Research, 741 Brady Street, Davenport, IA 52803, USA. [2]Institute of Sports Science and Clinical Biomechanics, University of Southern Denmark, Odense, Denmark. [3]The University of Illinois, 801 South Paulina Street, 102c (MC621), Chicago, IL 60612, USA.

References

1. Campbell NC, Murray E, Darbyshire J, Emery J, Farmer A, Griffiths F, Guthrie B, Lester H, Wilson P, Kinmonth AL: **Designing and evaluating complex interventions to improve health care.** *BMJ* 2007, **334**(7591):455–459.
2. Craig P, Dieppe P, Macintyre S, Michie S, Nazareth I, Petticrew M: **Developing and evaluating complex interventions: the new Medical Research Council guidance.** *BMJ* 2008, **337**:a1655.
3. Paterson C, Dieppe P: **Characteristic and incidental (placebo) effects in complex interventions such as acupuncture.** *BMJ* 2005, **330**(7501):1202–1205.
4. Jones CH: **The spectrum of therapeutic influences and integrative health care: classifying health care practices by mode of therapeutic action.** *J Altern Complement Med* 2005, **11**(5):937–944.
5. Herzog W: **The biomechanics of spinal manipulation.** *J Bodywork Mov Ther* 2010, **14**(3):280–286.
6. Graham BA, Clausen P, Bolton PS: **A descriptive study of the force and displacement profiles of the toggle-recoil spinal manipulative procedure (adjustment) as performed by chiropractors.** *Man Ther* 2010, **15**(1):74–79.
7. Bronfort G, Haas M, Evans R, Kawchuk G, Dagenais S: **Evidence-informed management of chronic low back pain with spinal manipulation and mobilization.** *Spine J* 2008, **8**(1):213–225.
8. Downie AS, Vemulpad S, Bull PW: **Quantifying the high-velocity, low-amplitude spinal manipulative thrust: a systematic review.** *J Manipulative Physiol Ther* 2010, **33**(7):542–553.

9. Kawchuk GN, Herzog W: **Biomechanical characterization (fingerprinting) of five novel methods of cervical spine manipulation.** *J Manipulative Physiol Ther* 1992, **16**(9):573–577.
10. DeVocht JW, Owens EF, Gudavalli MR, Strazewski J, Bhogal R, Xia T: **Force-time profile differences in the delivery of simulated toggle-recoil spinal manipulation by students, instructors, and field doctors of chiropractic.** *J Manipulative Physiol Ther* 2013, **36**(6):342–348.
11. Nambi SG, Inbasekaran D, Khuman R, Devi S, Satani K: **Clinical effects of short and long lever spinal thrust manipulation in non-specific chronic low back pain: a biomechanical perspective.** *Int J Health Allied Sci* 2013, **2**(4):230–236.
12. McGregor M, Puhl A, Reinhart C, Injeyan H, Soave D: **Differentiating intraprofessional attitudes toward paradigms in health care delivery among chiropractic factions: results from a randomly sampled survey.** *BMC Complement Altern Med* 2014, **14**(1):51.
13. Smith M, Carber LA: **Survey of US chiropractor attitudes and behaviors about subluxation.** *J Chiropr Human* 2008, **15**:19–26.
14. Murphy DR, Schneider MJ, Seaman DR, Perle SM, Nelson CF: **How can chiropractic become a respected mainstream profession? The example of podiatry.** *Chiropr Osteop* 2008, **16**:10.
15. Gleberzon B, Stuber K: **Frequency of use of diagnostic and manual therapeutic procedures of the spine currently taught at the Canadian Memorial Chiropractic College: a preliminary survey of Ontario chiropractors. Part 2 – procedure usage rates.** *J Can Chiropr Assoc* 2013, **57**(2):165–175.
16. Mykietiuk C, Wambolt M, Pillipow T, Mallay C, Gleberzon BJ: **Technique Systems used by post-1980 graduates of the Canadian Memorial Chiropractic College practicing in five Canadian provinces: a preliminary survey.** *J Can Chiropr Assoc* 2009, **53**(1):32–39.
17. Huggins T, Boras AL, Gleberzon BJ, Popescu M, Bahry LA: **Clinical effectiveness of the activator adjusting instrument in the management of musculoskeletal disorders: a systematic review of the literature.** *J Can Chiropr Assoc* 2012, **56**(1):49–57.
18. Gleberzon BJ: **Chiropractic "name techniques": a review of the literature.** *J Can Chiropr Assoc* 2001, **45**(2):86–99.
19. Christensen MG, Kollasch MW, Hyland JK: *Practice Analysis of Chiropractic 2010: A Project Report, Survey Analysis, and Summary of Chiropractic Practice in the United States.* Greeley, CO: National Board of Chiropractic Examiners; 2010.
20. Haas M, Spegman A, Peterson D, Aickin M, Vavrek D: **Dose response and efficacy of spinal manipulation for chronic cervicogenic headache: a pilot randomized controlled trial.** *Spine J* 2010, **10**(2):117–128.
21. Witt CM, Schützler L: **The gap between results from sham-controlled trials and trials using other controls in acupuncture research: the influence of context.** *Complement Ther Med* 2013, **21**(2):112–114.
22. Gay C, Bishop M: **Research on placebo analgesia is relevant to clinical practice.** *Chiropr Man Therap* 2014, **22**(1):6.
23. Brim RL, Miller FG: **The potential benefit of the placebo effect in sham-controlled trials: implications for risk-benefit assessments and informed consent.** *J Med Ethics* 2013, **39**(11):703–707.
24. Hróbjartsson A, Gøtzsche PC: **Placebo interventions for all clinical conditions.** *Cochrane Database Syst Rev* 2010, **1**:CD003974.
25. Puhl AA, Reinhart CJ, Rok ER, Injeyan HS: **An examination of the observed placebo effect associated with the treatment of low back pain: a systematic review.** *Pain Res Manag* 2011, **16**(1):45–52.
26. Krogsbll LT, Hróbjartsson A, Gøtzsche PC: **Spontaneous improvement in randomised clinical trials: meta-analysis of three-armed trials comparing no treatment, placebo and active intervention.** *BMC Med Res Methodol* 2009, **9**(1):1.
27. Licciardone JC, Russo DP: **Blinding protocols, treatment credibility, and expectancy: methodologic issues in clinical trials of osteopathic manipulative treatment.** *J Am Osteopath Assoc* 2006, **106**(8):457–463.
28. Kaptchuk TJ, Kelley JM, Conboy LA, Davis RB, Kerr CE, Jacobson EE, Kirsch I, Schyner RN, Nam BH, Nguyen LT: **Components of placebo effect: randomised controlled trial in patients with irritable bowel syndrome.** *BMJ* 2008, **336**(7651):999–1003.
29. Kaptchuk TJ: **The placebo effect in alternative medicine: can the performance of a healing ritual have clinical significance?** *Ann Intern Med* 2002, **136**(11):817–825.
30. Kaptchuk TJ, Shaw J, Kerr CE, Conboy LA, Kelley JM, Csordas TJ, Lembo AJ, Jacobson EE: **"Maybe I made up the whole thing": placebos and patients' experiences in a randomized controlled trial.** *Cult Med Psychiatry* 2009, **33**(3):382–411.
31. Finniss DG, Kaptchuk TJ, Miller F, Benedetti F: **Biological, clinical, and ethical advances of placebo effects.** *Lancet* 2010, **375**(9715):686–695.
32. Price DD, Finniss DG, Benedetti F: **A comprehensive review of the placebo effect: recent advances and current thought.** *Annu Rev Psychol* 2008, **59**:565–590.
33. Bialosky JE, Bishop MD, Robinson ME, Barabas JA, George SZ: **The influence of expectation on spinal manipulation induced hypoalgesia: an experimental study in normal subjects.** *BMC Musculoskelet Disord* 2008, **9**:19.
34. Bensing JM, Verheul W: **The silent healer: the role of communication in placebo effects.** *Patient Educ Couns* 2010, **80**(3):293–299.
35. Paterson C, Zheng Z, Xue C, Wang Y: **"Playing their parts": the experiences of participants in a randomized sham-controlled acupuncture trial.** *J Altern Complement Med* 2008, **14**(2):199–208.
36. Ernst E, Harkness E: **Spinal manipulation: a systematic review of sham-controlled, double-blind, randomized clinical trials.** *J Pain Symptom Manag* 2001, **22**(4):879–889.
37. Hawk C, Azad A, Phongphua C, Long CR: **Preliminary study of the effects of a placebo chiropractic treatment with sham adjustments.** *J Manipulative Physiol Ther* 1999, **22**(7):436–443.
38. Miller FG, Emanuel EJ, Rosenstein DL, Straus SE: **Ethical issues concerning research in complementary and alternative medicine.** *JAMA* 2004, **291**(5):599–604.
39. Margolin A, Avants SK, Kleber HD: **Investigating alternative medicine therapies in randomized controlled trials.** *JAMA* 1998, **280**(18):1626–1628.
40. Schulz KF, Altman DG, Moher D, CONSORT Group: **CONSORT 2010 statement: updated guidelines for reporting parallel group randomised trials.** *BMC Med* 2010, **8**(1):18.
41. Goertz CM, Pohlman KA, Vining RD, Brantingham JW, Long CR: **Patient-centered outcomes of high-velocity, low-amplitude spinal manipulation for low back pain: a systematic review.** *J Electromyogr Kinesiol* 2012, **22**(5):670–691.
42. Khorsan R, Coulter ID, Hawk C, Choate CG: **Measures in chiropractic research: choosing patient-based outcome assessments.** *J Manipulative Physiol Ther* 2008, **31**(5):355–375.
43. Sikorskii A, Wyatt G, Victorson D, Faulkner G, Rahbar MH: **Methodological issues in trials of complementary and alternative medicine interventions.** *Nurs Res* 2009, **58**(6):444–451.
44. DeVocht JW, Goertz CM, Hondras MA, Long CR, Schaeffer W, Thomann L, Spector M, Stanford CM: **A pilot study of a chiropractic intervention for management of chronic myofascial temporomandibular disorder.** *J Am Dent Assoc* 2013, **144**(10):1154–1163.
45. Fuhr AW, Menke JM: **Status of activator methods chiropractic technique, theory, and practice.** *J Manipulative Physiol Ther* 2005, **28**(2):e1–e20.
46. Farrar JT, Young JP Jr, LaMoreaux L, Werth JL, Poole RM: **Clinical importance of changes in chronic pain intensity measured on an 11-point numerical pain rating scale.** *Pain* 2001, **94**(2):149–158.
47. Locker D, Allen PF: **Developing short-form measures of oral health-related quality of life.** *J Public Health Dent* 2002, **62**(1):13–20.
48. Epstein RM, Franks P, Fiscella K, Shields CG, Meldrum SC, Kravitz RL, Duberstein PR: **Measuring patient-centered communication in patient–physician consultations: theoretical and practical issues.** *Soc Sci Med* 2005, **61**(7):1516–1528.
49. Roter D, Larson S: **The Roter interaction analysis system (RIAS): utility and flexibility for analysis of medical interactions.** *Patient Educ Couns* 2002, **46**(4):243–251.
50. Ong L, De Haes J, Hoos A, Lammes FB: **Doctor-patient communication: a review of the literature.** *Soc Sci Med* 1995, **40**(7):903–918.
51. Barlow F, Scott C, Coghlan B, Lee P, White P, Lewith GT, Bishop FL: **How the psychosocial context of clinical trials differs from usual care: A qualitative study of acupuncture patients.** *BMC Med Res Methodol* 2011, **11**(1):79.
52. White AR, Filshie J, Cummings TM: **Clinical trials of acupuncture: consensus recommendations for optimal treatment, sham controls and blinding.** *Complement Ther Med* 2001, **9**(4):237–245.
53. Sidani S, Braden CJ: *Evaluating Nursing Interventions: A Theory-Driven Approach.* Thousand Oaks, CA: SAGE Publications; 1998.
54. Desjarlais-deKlerk K, Wallace J: **Instrumental and socioemotional communications in doctor-patient interactions in urban and rural clinics.** *BMC Health Serv Res* 2013, **13**(1):261.

55. Carroll C, Patterson M, Wood S, Booth A, Rick J, Balain S: **A conceptual framework for implementation fidelity.** *Implement Sci* 2007, **2**(40):1–9.
56. Scholten-Peeters GG, Thoomes E, Konings S, Beijer M, Verkerk K, Koes BW, Verhagen AP: **Is manipulative therapy more effective than sham manipulation in adults? A systematic review and meta-analysis.** *Chiropr Man Therap* 2013, **21**(1):34.
57. Reed WR, Beavers S, Reddy SK, Kern G: **Chiropractic management of primary nocturnal enuresis.** *J Manipulative Physiol Ther* 1994, **17**(9):596–600.
58. Sawyer CE, Evans RL, Boline PD, Branson R, Spicer A: **A feasibility study of chiropractic spinal manipulation versus sham spinal manipulation for chronic otitis media with effusion in children.** *J Manipulative Physiol Ther* 1999, **22**(5):292–298.
59. Vernon H, MacAdam K, Marshall V, Pion M, Sadowska M: **Validation of a sham manipulative procedure for the cervical spine for use in clinical trials.** *J Manipulative Physiol Ther* 2005, **28**(9):662–666.
60. Brose SW, Jennings DC, Kwok J, Stuart CL, O'Connell SM, Pauli HA, Liu B: **Sham manual medicine protocol for cervical strain-counterstrain research.** *PM&R* 2013, **5**(5):400–407.
61. Vernon HT, Triano JJ, Ross JK, Tran SK, Soave DM, Dinulos MD: **Validation of a novel sham cervical manipulation procedure.** *Spine J* 2012, **12**(11):1021–1028.
62. Ozcakar N, Mevsim V, Guldal D, Gunvar T, Yildirim E, Sisli Z, Semin I: **Is the use of videotape recording superior to verbal feedback alone in the teaching of clinical skills?** *BMC Public Health* 2009, **9**(1):474.
63. Kihlgren M, Kuremyr D, Norberg A, Brane G, Karlson I, Engstrom B, Melin E: **Nurse-patient interaction after training in integrity promoting care at a long-term ward: analysis of video-recorded morning care sessions.** *Int J Nurs Stud* 1993, **30**(1):1–13.
64. Mackenzie CF, Xiao Y: **Video techniques and data compared with observation in emergency trauma care.** *Qual Saf Health Care* 2003, **12**(suppl 2):ii51–ii57.
65. Marcinowicz L, Konstantynowicz J, Godlewski C: **Patients' perceptions of GP non-verbal communication: a qualitative study.** *Br J Gen Pract* 2010, **60**(571):83–87.
66. Cocksedge S, George B, Renwick S, Chew-Graham CA: **Touch in primary care consultations: qualitative investigation of doctors' and patients' perceptions.** *Br J Gen Pract* 2013, **63**(609):e283–e290.
67. Swayden KJ, Anderson KK, Connelly LM, Moran JS, McMahon JK, Arnold PM: **Effect of sitting vs. standing on perception of provider time at bedside: a pilot study.** *Patient Educ Couns* 2012, **86**(2):166–171.
68. Coleman T: **Using video-recorded consultations for research in primary care: advantages and limitations.** *Fam Pract* 2000, **17**(5):422–427.
69. Latvala E, Vuokila-Oikkonen P, Janhonen S: **Videotaped recording as a method of participant observation in psychiatric nursing research.** *J Adv Nurs* 2000, **31**(5):1252–1257.
70. Caldwell K, Atwal A: **Non-participant observation: using video tapes to collect data in nursing research.** *Nurse Res* 2005, **13**(2):42–54.
71. Ram P, Grol R, Rethans JJ, Schouten B, van der Vleuten C, Kester A: **Assessment of general practitioners by video observation of communicative and medical performance in daily practice: issues of validity, reliability and feasibility.** *Med Educ* 1999, **33**(6):447–454.
72. Oakley E, Stocker S, Staubli G, Young S: **Using video recording to identify management errors in pediatric trauma resuscitation.** *Pediatrics* 2006, **117**(3):658–664.
73. Penner LA, Orom H, Albrecht TL, Franks MM, Foster TS, Ruckdeschel JC: **Camera-related behaviors during video recorded medical interactions.** *J Nonverbal Behav* 2007, **31**(2):99–117.
74. Pringle M, Stewart-Evans C: **Does awareness of being video recorded affect doctors' consultation behaviour?** *Br J Gen Pract* 1990, **40**(340):455–458.
75. Rex DK, Hewett DG, Raghavendra M, Chalasani N: **The impact of videorecording on the quality of colonoscopy performance: a pilot study.** *Am J Gastroenterol* 2010, **105**(11):2312–2317.
76. Innes M, Skelton J, Greenfield S: **A profile of communication in primary care physician telephone consultations: application of the Roter Interaction Analysis System.** *Br J Gen Pract* 2006, **56**(526):363–368.
77. Paasche-Orlow M, Roter D: **The communication patterns of internal medicine and family practice physicians.** *J Am Board Fam Prac* 2003, **16**(6):485–493.
78. Bensing JM, Roter DL, Hulsman RL: **Communication patterns of primary care physicians in the United States and The Netherlands.** *J Gen Internal Med* 2003, **18**(5):335–342.
79. Shaw JR, Adams CL, Bonnett BN, Larson S, Roter DL: **Use of the Roter interaction analysis system to analyze veterinarian-client-patient communication in companion animal practice.** *J Am Vet Med Assoc* 2004, **225**(2):222–229.
80. Ong LM, Visser MR, Kruyver IP, Bensing JM, Brink-Muinen A, Stouthard JM, Lammes FB, de Haes JC: **The Roter Interaction Analysis System (RIAS) in oncological consultations: psychometric properties.** *Psychooncology* 1998, **7**(5):387–401.

21

Gimme that old time religion: the influence of the healthcare belief system of chiropractic's early leaders on the development of x-ray imaging in the profession

Kenneth John Young

Abstract

Background: Chiropractic technique systems have been historically documented to advocate overutilization of radiography. Various rationales for this have been explored in the literature. However, little consideration has been given to the possibility that the healthcare belief system of prominent early chiropractors may have influenced the use of the diagnostic modality through the years. The original rationale was the visualisation of chiropractic subluxations, defined as bones slightly out of place, pressing on nerves, and ultimately causing disease. This paradigm of radiography has survived in parts of the chiropractic profession, despite lacking evidence of clinical validity. The purpose of this paper is to compare the characteristics of the chiropractic technique systems that have utilised radiography for subluxation detection with the characteristics of religion, and to discover potential historical links that may have facilitated the development of those characteristics.

Discussion: Twenty-three currently or previously existing technique systems requiring radiography for subluxation analysis were found using a search of the internet, books and consultation with experts. Evidence of religiosity from the early founders' writings was compared with textbooks, published papers, and websites of subsequently developed systems. Six criteria denoting religious thinking were developed using definitions from various sources. They are: supernatural concepts, claims of supremacy, rules and rituals, sacred artefacts, sacred stories, and special language. All of these were found to a greater or lesser degree in the publicly available documents of all the subluxation-based chiropractic x-ray systems.

Summary: The founders and early pioneers of chiropractic did not benefit from the current understanding of science and research, and therefore substituted deductive and inductive reasoning to arrive at conclusions about health and disease in the human body. Some of this thinking and rationalisation demonstrably followed a religion-like pattern, including BJ Palmer's use of radiography. Although access to scientific methods and research education became much advanced and more accessible during the past few decades, the publicly available documents of technique systems that used radiography for chiropractic subluxation detection examined in this paper employed a historically derived paradigm for radiography that displayed characteristics in common with religion.

Keywords: Chiropractic, X-ray, Subluxation, History, Evidence-based practice, Religion

Correspondence: k.young@murdoch.edu.au
School of Arts; Senior Lecturer, School of Health Professions, Murdoch University, South Street, Murdoch 6150, Australia

Background

In 1910, fifteen years after the invention of chiropractic as well as the discovery of the x-ray, BJ Palmer, son of the founder of the profession, began vigorously promoting radiography to chiropractors [1]. Although there was some initial backlash to this invasive technology in a profession that focussed on manual therapy, [2] eventually it was embraced. In fact, chiropractic treatment systems have historically been documented to overutilise radiography [3-5]. However, overuse of diagnostic imaging is not unique to that profession [6-9]. Ionising radiation, even at the low levels used for diagnostic purposes, must be used judiciously due to the known risk of harm [10-12]. The rationale chiropractors have used to justify radiography has included diagnostic uncertainty, contraindications to manipulation/chiropractic adjusting, financial gain, discovery of occult congenital anomalies, routine screening, and biomechanical considerations [5,13-19]. The last item includes the discovery and/or quantification of tiny misalignments of spinal bones thought to impede the flow of vital energy through nerves, and known as chiropractic subluxations. Little evidence exists in the peer-reviewed literature to support this last use of ionising radiation [20,21]. Therefore, techniques using it for this purpose would seem to be driven by something other than purely rational, evidence-based clinical reasoning. Belief in the absence of evidence is essentially the operating system of religion. This observation raised the question as to whether the technique systems that employ plain radiographs for subluxation detection exhibited any similarities to religion.

There is a historical schism in chiropractic around the issue of radiography [22]. Some practitioners advocate a purely diagnostic approach, using radiography for the detection of pathology such as fracture or tumour, some advocate radiography purely for subluxation detection, and some for both. This debate was acknowledged as early as the 1930s. Waldo Poehner wrote about the advantages of using chiropractic radiographic views for chiropractic purposes and standard radiographic views for the detection of pathology, encouraging each camp to see the merit in each other's arguments [23]. The paradigm that the primary use of radiography is to discover or quantify chiropractic subluxations has survived over a hundred years in parts of the chiropractic profession [1]. Although evidence-based guidelines regarding ionising radiation exist, [14,24-26] the profession does not universally endorse them [27,28].

The belief system around the larger issue of the chiropractic subluxation itself has been addressed in an attempt to help practitioners understand the basic concepts of science and to encourage a profession-wide move toward evidence-based care [29,30]. In addition, although the literature contains a number of papers on the subject of religion and dogma in chiropractic, [29,31-37] little consideration has been given to potential religious connotations specifically regarding the use of radiography for subluxation detection.

A short digression into the concept of the subluxation may be useful to readers not familiar with it. The vertebral subluxation is the traditional basis of the chiropractic profession. DD Palmer, who 'discovered' chiropractic in 1895, used the term to describe a 'bone out of place' that impinged the flow of vital energy, which he called 'Innate' or 'Innate Intelligence', to organs throughout the body, thereby causing dis-ease, and disease. This concept is a variant of the 'one cause' theories of healthcare that were common at that time [38]. The entire spectrum of ill health in mankind was attributed to altered transmission of nerve energy from slightly displaced bones affecting various nerves. According to BJ Palmer:

> 'Chiropractic had long maintained... that a vertebral subluxation produced a pressure upon nerves which interfered with the normal and free transmission of mental impulses between the brain and its body; that this unequal state of balance between generation, transmission and expression produced disease. That the *sunnum bonum* of all life and death, health or disease issues pivoted around a study of the correct or incorrect position of vertebrae' [39].

The idea that maximum expression of life can be obtained only when the bones of the spine (or a portion of the spine) are in the 'correct' place so that life force may flow unimpeded is a form of vitalism. In 1993, Gaucher-Peslherbe described the subluxation concept advanced by DD Palmer as being based on a moral conviction rather than a scientifically testable theory [40]. The credulity shown by chiropractors towards vitalistic ideas was noted by Keating who wrote that most members of the profession, at least in the 1920s, were ill-equipped to differentiate various epistemologies, such as uncritical rationalism versus casual empiricism versus the scientific method [2]. This propensity may not be limited to the early 20th century. Moore described it more comprehensively and charitably: 'Contemporary chiropractic belief systems embrace a blend of experience, conviction, critical thinking, open-mindedness, and appreciation of the natural order of things' [38].

The purpose of this paper is to compare the characteristics of the chiropractic technique systems that have utilised radiography for subluxation detection with the characteristics of religion, and to discover potential historical links that may have facilitated the development of those characteristics.

Methods

A six-part strategy was designed. First, the writings of early chiropractic leaders, including DD Palmer and BJ Palmer were reviewed for their religious content. This was seen as relevant, because it was as indicative of the intellectual environment in which they operated. As the self-titled 'Discoverer' and 'Developer' of chiropractic, respectively, they and their inner circles were influential in the profession [41,42]. Their modes of thinking necessarily affected that of their followers. Second, since BJ Palmer was instrumental in introducing radiography to chiropractic, his paradigm for radiography was used as a starting point. Evidence was gathered from his writings on the topic, specifically, *The Subluxation Specific The Adjustment Specific,* [43] *Answers,* [44] *Chiropractic Clinical Controlled Research,* [45] *The Science of Chiropractic,* [46] and Palmer's Introduction to EA Thompson's *Chiropractic Spinography,* [1] as well as quotes from historically scholarly secondary sources such as Keating's *BJ of Davenport,* [2] Dye's *The Evolution of Chiropractic,* [47] Wardwell's *Chiropractic: History and Evolution of a New Profession,* [48] and Moore's *Chiropractic in America* [38]. Third, a list was created of techniques that used plain radiography for the purpose of finding chiropractic subluxations. This was done by searching the internet, entering into Google the key phrases 'chiropractic x-ray', 'chiropractic radiography', 'chiropractic x-ray line drawing', and 'chiropractic subluxation'. PubMed was searched with the term 'chiropractic and technique and x-ray'. Cooperstein and Gleberzon's *Technique Systems in Chiropractic* [49] was used as a source. In addition, two experts in the fields of chiropractic history and technique systems were consulted. In order to be included in this study, current or previously existing chiropractic technique systems had to be named systems. They also had to have specific diagnostic/analytic protocols that included the visualization of subluxations on plain radiographs. The practices of individual chiropractors or groups that used modifications of the techniques were excluded. Fourth, a definition of religion was developed from works on comparative religion and anthropology. This was then modified to be practically applicable with clearly defined, specific parameters. Fifth, the publicly available documents of the technique systems, including their textbooks, published papers, magazine articles and official websites were examined for evidence of the religious characteristics developed as described above. Finally, the information was collated and examined. A list of the six characteristics was created, and evidence from each technique system entered into it; the list was then divided into the six appendices of this paper. Two tables were developed. One is a list of all the technique systems (see Additional file 1: TableS1), and the second is a chart with six headings, each corresponding to a religious characteristic, and a brief synopsis of the evidence from each technique system was entered under each heading, the technique systems appearing in alphabetical order under each heading (see Additional file 2: Table S2). The characteristics of the radiographic paradigm of chiropractic's early leaders were then compared to that of the subsequently developed technique systems, and historical links demonstrated.

Discussion

Religiosity in early chiropractic leaders

The aetiology for the environment within chiropractic that fostered belief over evidence can be demonstrated in the books and papers left by the founders. DD Palmer wrote about his religious convictions in papers published after his death: 'I believe, in fact know, that the universe consists of Intelligence and Matter. This intelligence is known to the Christian world as God' [50]. Palmer continued with his explanation of the way Intelligence or spirit is expressed through the nervous system, and that all physical and mental functions are modified by the physical condition of the body. He concluded with this: 'a correct understanding of these principles and the practice of them constitute the religion of chiropractic' [50]. DD Palmer felt that he had a sacred duty in relieving people's subluxations: 'Knowing that our physical health and the intellectual progress of Innate depend upon the proper alignment of the skeletal frame, we feel it our bounded duty to replace any displaced bones so that physical and spiritual health, happiness, and the full fruition of earthly life may be fully enjoyed' [51]. DD Palmer even explicitly considered turning chiropractic into a religion, as Mary Baker Eddy had done with Christian Science [52].

After his father's death, BJ Palmer expanded on the religious theme. In 1915, feeling the effects of medical attacks on the profession, he compared himself to Jesus Christ. He wrote a detailed description of the crucifixion scene, finishing with: 'Father, forgive, they know not what they do. It behoves us all to be forgiving. I have tried to be charitable to those who would do otherwise' [2]. He continued this theme over time. John J Nugent's advocacy of improved academic standards earned him expulsion from Palmer's school in June 1922. BJ accused him of disloyalty, disrespect and insult to the President as well as making statements derogatory to the institution [53]. Eventually Nugent was influential in the development of national standards for chiropractic education, and Palmer took to calling him the anti-Christ of chiropractic, [53] which seemed to imply Palmer as the Christ. BJ was even known to repeatedly state: 'The first man that cured by laying on of hands they crucified' [48]. Keating noted religious overtones from the early days of chiropractic, [2] citing an illustration in the magazine *The Chiropractor* in 1910 that depicted BJ Palmer nearly nude and improbably muscular, with a halo emanating light rays, fending off death and giving aid to the ill (Figure 1).

Another overtone of religion appeared on the masthead of Palmer's *Fountainhead News,* a weekly newsletter written 'by BJ himself'. Volume 5 number 19, issued on 24 June

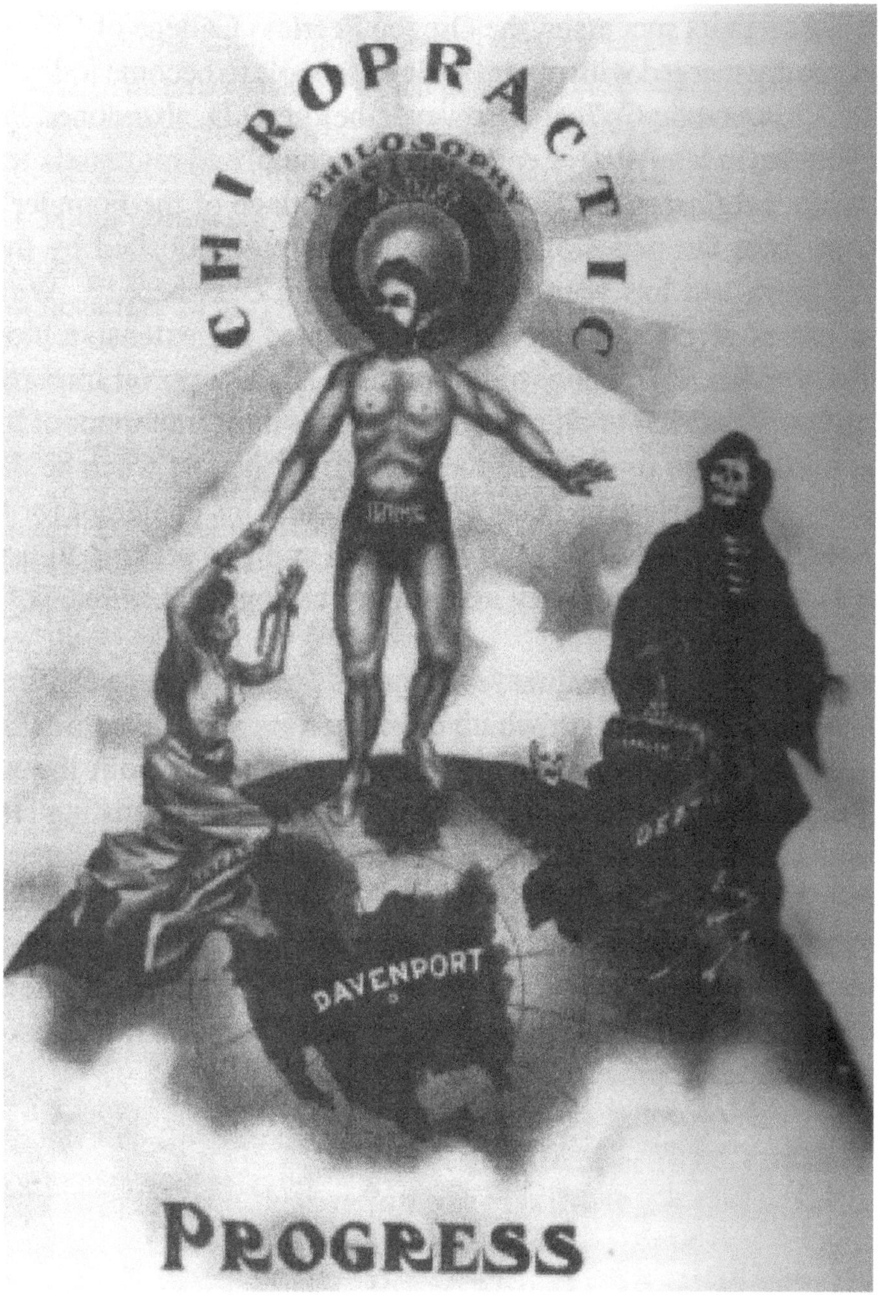

Figure 1 BJ Palmer as healer of the sick, fending off Death, with halo-like emanations from his head, 1910 (with permission from Special Collections and Archives, Palmer College of Chiropractic).

1916 reworked the Gregorian calendar, dating the world (of chiropractic, at least) from 18 September 1895, the supposed date of the first adjustment. The notation for 1916 became AC 21, with AC standing for 'After Chiropractic', a parallel to the Christians' AD, *Anno Domini* [2].

Some of Palmer's 'disciples' held strong convictions, conveying the chiropractic belief with great fervour. In 1927 a Palmer alumnus and teacher in chiropractic philosophy at his alma mater, produced the *Chiropractic Textbook* [54]. In it, author Ralph W Stephenson elucidated his thirty-three principles of chiropractic. He declared explicitly that chiropractic could not be tested by science, but rather came from God and therefore could not be refuted. 'By assuming a major premise, that there is a Universal Intelligence which governs all matter, every inference drawn from that major premise and subjected to specific scrutiny, stands the test' [54]. BJ Palmer was effusive in his praise for this work, writing in its introduction 'Of ALL the books written and compiled on Chiropractic Philosophy, this is by far the best, not excepting my own' [54].

Historian J Stuart Moore also noted a religious thread running through some of the early practitioners of chiropractic. For them, BJ, who was happy to take the role of messiah, provided a focus for an undefined or unfulfilled desire for answers to the mysteries of life and health:

'Chiropractic drew believers with similar yearnings but with at least two clearly distinguishable temperaments that determined how their allegiance to chiropractic would develop. The first type came with deep spiritual longings but no strongly fixed religious faith... chiropractic became a substitute religion, supplying a comprehensive explanation of reality, complete in itself with claims of divine powers, suffering saints and martyrs, and sacred writings and utterances from prophets (the Palmers) who provided the ultimate source of authority – all wrapped in a millennial eschatology' [38].

Another group, Moore noted, were conventional Christians, who made chiropractic fit in with their pre-existing beliefs. He indicated the ease with which chiropractic believers could substitute Palmer's Universal Intelligence as the Christian God and Innate Intelligence as the human manifestation of the divine [38]. Improvements in health due to chiropractic ministrations meant that the chiropractor was, quite literally, the hand of God, revitalising the sick with heaven-sent energy.

BJ began holding an annual homecoming, which he called a lyceum, at the Palmer School starting in the year 1914 [2]. These were part seminar, part spectacle, with celebrities of the day attending as guests and other entertainment. Keating characterised them as the 'traditional opportunity to bedazzle and inspire the faithful to the cause' [2]. Like an old-time tent revival, these gatherings helped renew faith in chiropractic and in Palmer as the leader [2].

These are just a few examples, cited to demonstrate the environment of belief, rather than scepticism, that was disseminated from the highest levels of the early profession. It is reasonable to argue that this situation at least allowed, and even encouraged some subsequent technique originators to accept the basic premises of chiropractic without question.

BJ Palmer and the historical chiropractic paradigm for radiography

BJ Palmer bought the first x-ray machine for the Palmer School of Chiropractic in 1910, theorising that since this new technology allowed the visualisation of bones within the body, subluxations could now be 'proved'. This would legitimise the core theory of chiropractic. 'The advent of the X-Ray [sic] into Chiropractic was to prove that vertebral subluxations did actually exist and could be so proven with the aid of the X-Ray make this visible to the eye' [1]. Palmer then advanced the technology as the critical component of chiropractic practice: 'The spinograph means the difference between failure and success: No results and results. Guess and knowledge. Doubt and positiveness. Theory and fact' [1]. Essentially, BJ Palmer used x-ray to help convince people of the veracity of his claims about subluxation. There is evidence that was effective at this task, because some chiropractors began espousing BJ's rhetoric. For instance, a 1917 Utah newspaper advertisement by chiropractors CB Johnson, IJ McKell and Palmer's former spinographer, EA Thompson, began with the statement that '95% of sickness is caused by slightly misaligned spinal segments' and that 'the X-ray picture is the only absolutely reliable method of securing a correct analysis' [55] (Figure 2). The more recently developed system Chiropractic BioPhysics utilised a credulous approach in their research, gathering evidence for spinal subluxation as visualised on radiographs, an assumption granted prior to commencement of data collection: 'The **PCCRP** [Practicing Chiropractors' Committee on Radiology Protocols] guidelines are the Evidence Based Support for subluxation analysis via x-ray as performed by a large percentage of practicing chiropractors' [27]. Others claimed to refine methods without ever questioning the basic premise of the primary role of the subluxation in the creation of ill health; much in the way theological studies may undertake investigation of a deity without ever questioning its existence. For example, Zimmerman proclaimed that due to his refinements in radiography and treatment methods, '[the chiropractor] is trained to place the tip of the machine so accurately as to do that which has never been done before' [56]. 'The Gonstead Chiropractor goes beyond what many chiropractors consider a spinal assessment by conducting a thorough analysis of your spine using five criteria to detect the presence of the vertebral subluxation complex' [57]. It seemed that in contrast to evidence-based healthcare, the epistemology of 'appeal to authority' was generally found to be highly valued in these systems.

The assertion that vertebral subluxation is the primary cause of ill health is a dogmatic, religious-like position, rather than the basis for a system that responds to changes in evidence in order to provide the best care for a variety of conditions. This belief system extends beyond the use of radiography to the idea of the subluxation in general. However the focus of this paper will be on the elements of the belief as reinforced by radiography. This group by no means represents all of chiropractic, and it should be noted that the American Chiropractic College of Radiology does not endorse this use of ionising radiation, [22] nor do the mainstream radiology guidelines to which many chiropractors adhere [26].

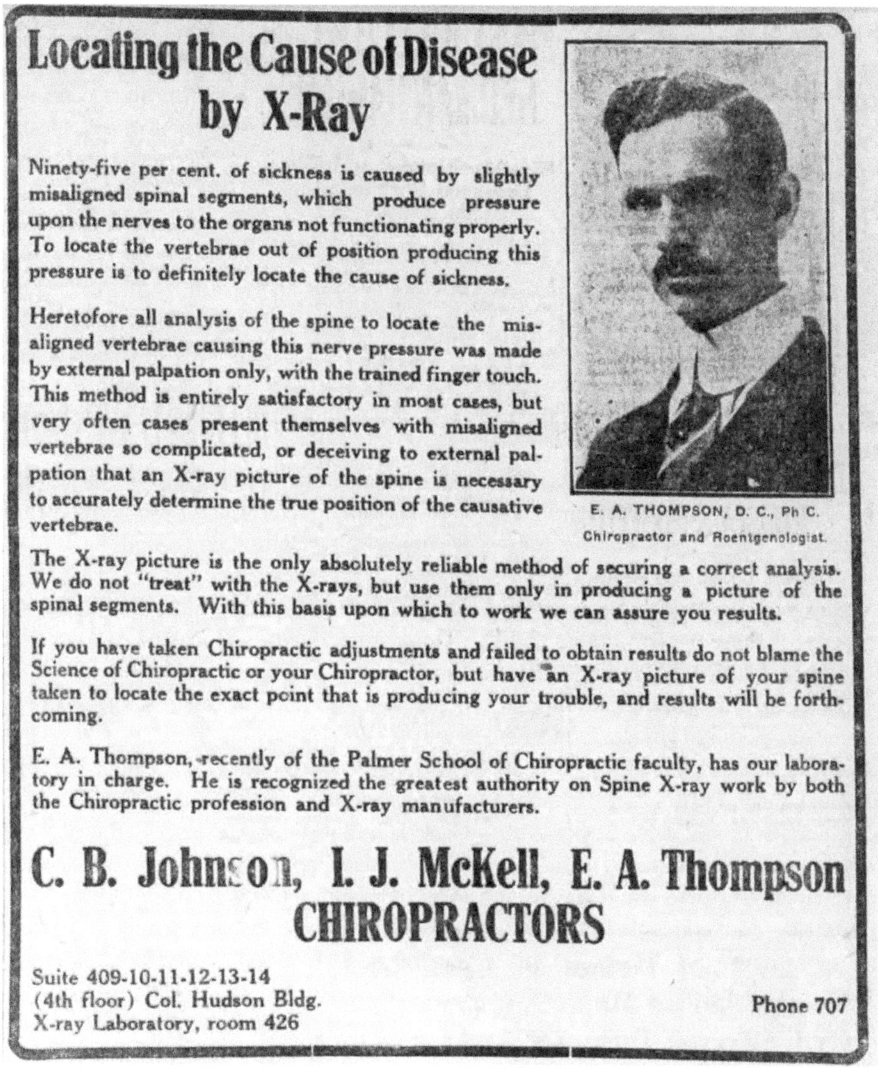

Figure 2 Advertisement in the Ogden (Utah) Standard, 1917.

The techniques that advocate radiography for subluxation analysis

Twenty-three specific, named technique systems were found (see Additional file 1: TableS1), comprised of: Advanced Orthogonal, Applied Spinal Biomechanical Engineering (ASBE), Applied Upper Cervical Biomechanics (AUCB), Atlas Orthogonality, Blair, Chiropractic BioPhysics (CBP), Cowin Upper Cervical Orthogonal, Duff, Gonstead, Grostic, Kale, Knee-Chest Upper Cervical Specific, Logan Basic, Mears, National Upper Cervical Chiropractic Association (NUCCA), Orthospinology, Palmer Upper Cervical Specific (also known as HIO, Hole-in-One or Toggle Recoil), Pettibon, Spinal Orthopedic Neurological Advancement and Research (SONAR), Spinal Stressology, Sutter and Zimmerman. The Palmer original full spine technique was not found to exist as a specific technique today. Pierce-Stillwagon deserves a specific note. Created in 1975, it only briefly required imaging, and then reduced the emphasis on radiography, preferring thermography to locate subluxations [49]. Walter Vernon Pierce subsequently split from Glenn Stillwagon [49] and not enough information on Stillwagon technique was found to meet the inclusion criteria, but the Pierce Results system was found, and will be included below. One paper [58] listed two additional names as techniques, Hildebrandt and Wernsing, but not enough information about their methods or history was found to meet the inclusion criteria. In addition, AA Wernsing's ideas seem largely to have been incorporated into BJ Palmer's Upper Cervical Specific technique [43].

Characteristics of religion

There are a great many definitions of religion, most of which focus solely or primarily on the idea of belief in a deity or guiding hand in life, [59-62] but sociologically based ones exist [63]. As has been noted elsewhere, [64] the variety of perspectives on the topic suggests that religion is difficult to define. Specific characteristics were sought for this paper, in order to have an operational definition. This would allow comparison of the characteristics to the concepts and devices found in the technique systems. Albanese [64] addressed chiropractic specifically, and defined religion as a 'way of organizing reality and relating to it' [65]. When referring to a system of natural healing, that is, non-pharmaceutical and non-surgical, she employed the term 'nature religion' [65]. As will be seen, the chiropractic technique systems examined in this paper did seem to organise reality according to their own standards, eschewing mainstream principles of healthcare, and adopting their own versions of a uniquely chiropractic paradigm for radiography. For the purpose of this paper, an essentially behavioural definition was created, drawing partly from the above references and modified by the author's observations of prominent religions. The definition consisted of six characteristics: 1) supernatural concepts relating to a belief in a supreme power, 2) claims of supremacy to others that are similar, 3) rules that must be followed, including carrying out rituals, 4) sacred artefacts, often utilised in the rituals, 5) sacred stories, and 6) special language. Evidence for each of these characteristics as observed in religions is given as they are individually discussed below. The religious characteristics of these techniques ranged from striking to mild but were not absent from any of the systems.

Evidence-based chiropractic attempts to use diagnostic imaging as well as vocabulary and concepts of health and disease conventional with the medical establishment. However, the above-listed elements of religion were demonstrably present in the publicly available documents of chiropractic technique systems that asserted vertebral subluxation as the primary or sole cause of disease, and that utilised radiographic analysis as their main diagnostic test for this lesion.

Characteristics of religion in the technique systems

Supernatural concepts relating to a belief in a supreme power

Supernatural concepts in religions are usually thought of as the idea of a superior being with some degree of influence on earthly life, or a spirit or life force, something that transcends the laws of nature. For this paper, chiropractic supernatural concepts were vitalism and an ethereal feeling of being 'called' to the profession. Vitalism is the idea of vital energy (life force), called Innate Intelligence or just Innate by the Palmers, the key to health that may be blocked by small misalignments of bones near nerves. Therefore, references to 'nerve interference' preventing full expression of human health were considered vitalism, and therefore supernatural. Some techniques directly referenced BJ Palmer, such as Grostic, where 'misaligned vertebra(e) impinge the flow of innate intelligence and cause illness, or what BJ Palmer later referred to as dis-ease' [66]. Another example was Applied Upper Cervical Biomechanics: 'A chiropractic doctor detects and corrects these spinal misalignments (vertebral subluxation causing nerve interference), restoring normal nerve impulses to the body allowing the body's own innate healing capabilities to function optimally' [67]. Some referenced Palmer's concepts more obliquely, without using the terms 'Innate' or 'Innate Intelligence' but expressing Palmer's ideas nonetheless. For example, Cowin: 'Our procedures are based on the traditional chiropractic concept of vertebral subluxation' [68]. Or Blair: 'The nervous system controls and regulates all parts and functions in the body. When there is nerve interference (subluxation) your body loses the ability to properly self regulate and heal itself. The result can be pain and illness. Blair upper cervical care is often the key to people regaining and maintaining good health' [69]. Some appeared to be peripheral on the topic, but nevertheless expressed the same idea, like Chiropractic BioPhysics, who claimed that their mission was to 'correct human spines and alleviate human suffering' [70].

A calling to the profession was expressed in various ways. Techniques like Spinal Orthopedic Neurological Advancement and Research (SONAR) link the idea for the technique directly to a deity: 'Through the grace of God, Dr. Elliott has developed the SONAR instrument' [71]. Others expressed the idea that their practice was a form of worship, like Advanced Orthogonal: 'we recognize that the human body is fearfully and wonderfully made, and our desire is to honor the Creator of this dynamic body through our approach to health care' [72]. Still others viewed their duty within the profession to include a kind of evangelism: 'Our Mission is to perpetuate the teachings of Dr. Clarence S. Gonstead, fund chiropractic research, and encourage cooperation and camaraderie amongst all who practice the Gonstead technique' [73]. The linkage between profession and religion is expressed outright by a few: 'The Kale Foreign Messenger has been in over 9 countries doing missionary work' [74]. The full evidence from the writings of each technique is found in Appendix 1. All the techniques demonstrated some element of supernatural thinking.

In addition to text referring to the supernatural, a few techniques employed religious imagery in their official publications. Otherworldliness was implied by a picture on the Gonstead website, showing the originator of the technique with hands clasped, wearing a white shirt with high, priestly collar, staring beatifically into the distance, a halo emanating from his upper body [75]. NUCCA had a picture of a sunrise over a road heading off into a heavenly looking horizon [76]. Duff used a chiropractic angel, similar to a medical caduceus, with rays like sunshine emanating from it [77]. It should be noted that there is no evidence that the chiropractic angel was invented with a supernatural implication. Created for a public relations campaign by the American Society of Chiropractors around 1928, many different forms of this symbol have existed over the years, adopted and modified by chiropractic practices and institutions with widely varying approaches to the profession [78].

Other techniques used multimedia that evoked religious comparisons. Orthospinology's website had a video entitled 'Changing the World, one spine at a time', which used music that sounded like a church choir singing over electronic dance music [79]. Whether implied or explicit, these techniques used words, images and sounds often more evocative of religion than mundane and earthly science.

Claims of supremacy

Many religions claim that theirs is the one true path to enlightenment, something Runzo [80] called religious exclusivism [80]. This characteristic was expressed in the writings of the technique systems using radiography for subluxation detection. These were all similar to the attitude BJ and DD Palmer had when they declared chiropractic to be the one cure for the one cause of disease. Assertions of superiority were found for all the techniques, and many claimed it by precision of radiographic analysis or adjustment. This set them apart not just from medical methods, but also from other chiropractic techniques whose methods were similar to their own. In terms of tiniest misalignments discovered, Advanced Orthogonal referred to: 'Digital x-ray analysis to measure misalignments to the 1/100th of a degree' [81]. Cowin averred that their methods would uncover displacements 'as small as 0.75 degrees (or, translated into linear measurements, each as small as 28 thousandths of an inch or 0.7 mm)' [82]. Others claimed superiority due to research, for instance ASBE asserted '12 volumes of A.S.B.E. research discoveries' [83]. AUCB boasted '15 years of unprecedented research' [84]. Many claimed simple, overall superiority: 'the secret of health and longevity has been solved... in Logan Basic Technique more than by all other asserted advances in healing methods since the beginning of time' [85]. SONAR claimed its system as 'far superior to other upper cervical techniques' [71]. Orthospinology declared itself the 'greatest health care procedure in the world' [86]. See Appendix 2 for examples from each technique.

Rules and rituals

Examples of rules followed in religions include such things as the Ten Commandments, Jewish Kosher food restrictions, and Islamic fasting during Ramadan. There are two rules that are common to all these chiropractic techniques: the chiropractic subluxation is the primary basis of disease in humans, and plain film radiographs must be obtained in order to detect or define it. The same set of images was claimed to be necessary, differing according to each technique's rules, regardless of their symptoms. In the upper cervical systems, several views of the neck and lower part of the skull were taken, sometimes with elaborate patient positioning devices (Figure 3). For many of the systems, post treatment radiographs were also required to confirm replacement of the bones. In the full spine systems, radiographs of the entire spine, and often the pelvis were required to search for subluxations. In a best-case scenario for the patient, the images would be examined for pathology in addition to subluxation/postural change. However even this amounted to screening for disease with x-rays. This practice has not been supported in the healthcare literature for over half a century, due to the potential negative consequences of ionising radiation and the low probability of uncovering significant findings [87-93]. Therefore, any of the more recent techniques that advocated radiography for subluxation detection did not follow the evidence for best practice of radiography, but rather their own belief system of healthcare.

Turner [94] defined a religious ritual as 'a stereotyped sequence of activities involving gestures, words, and objects, performed in a sequestered place, and designed to influence preternatural entities or forces on behalf of the actor's goals and interests' [94]. Ritual behaviour has been noted for its rigidity, repetition, and apparent lack of rational motivation [95]. The effect on those that partake of religious rituals has been described as bringing order, comfort, and organization through shared familiar symbols and patterns of behaviour [96]. Religious rituals include baptism, lighting candles at Hanukkah, reciting seven vows while taking seven steps at the Hindu wedding ceremony. The common ritual in all the technique systems was the taking of the radiographs; although the areas imaged and the analytical procedures vary to some degree, they all involved finding a slightly malpositioned vertebra or postural alteration. The images were often used to explain the issues of subluxation or abnormal posture as well as their dire consequences [97,98]. The rules and rituals of the systems indicated a rigidity of methods applied uniformly to all patients, rather than the customized exam and treatment that one would expect from other types of health care practitioners. This may have represented a form of indoctrination. Ritual gives artefacts value and defines the sacred within a community [99].

Many of the techniques also required post-treatment images as routine, with a stated goal of visualising the bone back in the correct place. Post-treatment radiography is a questionable practice, since it is of no benefit to the patient, but does give a dose of ionising radiation.

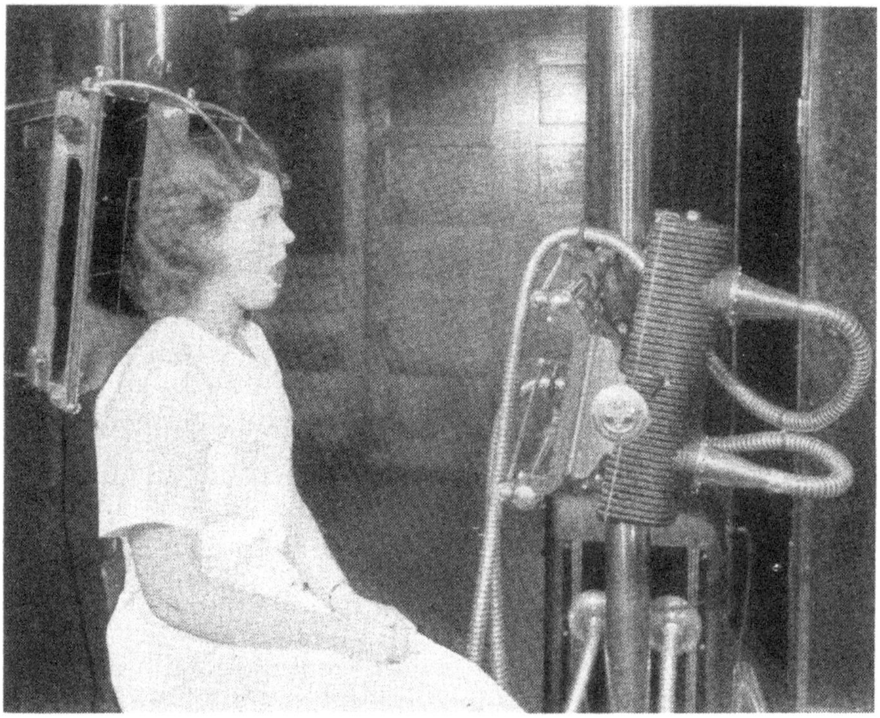

Figure 3 Body positioning devices used in preparation of x-ray for subluxation analysis. (Remier, PA, *Modern X-ray Practice and Chiropractic Spinography*. 1st ed. Davenport, Iowa: Palmer School of Chiropractic, USA, 1938, 260).

However, this practice may be perceived as part of the ritual indoctrination of patients. The entire radiographic procedure could arguably perform the function of creating a stronger bond between practitioner and patient, as well as enhancing belief in the technique system for both. See Appendix 3 for evidence regarding x-ray rules and rituals in all the techniques.

Sacred artefacts

Sacred artefacts varied somewhat from technique to technique, but they all had in common the x-ray machine and the radiographs. These artefacts were used as powerful symbols, around which was woven the story of the technique. Comparison can be made to the crucifix is a symbol upon which the story of Christianity relies, or a turban as an object of strong religious significance for a Sikh. These artefacts help create or augment the ritualistic experience, and thereby indoctrinate new members and perpetuate the system of religion.

In the context of techniques that required radiography for subluxation detection, the x-ray machine allowed the direct visualisation of the health-depleting subluxation (or postural alteration), so its status was elevated to the highest (holy) level. Similarly, the radiographs themselves (whether plain film hard copy or digital images on a screen) demonstrated the visible manifestations of the lesion upon which these practitioners founded their diagnosis and treatment. Their service in reinforcing the reality of the technique systems was likely very strong. People will always be greatly stimulated by the visible. 'Seeing is believing' is a cliché because it is largely accurate. Therefore, to be able to point to a radiographic image and tell a person in pain that his/her problem is 'right here' must be a strong inducement to believing.

In some cases, special head clamps or other body positioning devices specific to the technique may have been used for the radiography. The more elaborate the ritual, the more persuasive it may be, [100] and this precept seemed to have been used by some of these systems. For example, 'Pettibon x-ray analysis may involve over 41 lines and 23 angles to specifically locate the displaced vertebra' [101]. John D Grostic invented a device called a cephalometer that measures the patient's head, and the measurements were then used in conjunction with the radiographs [102]. Blair employed what he called a 'protracto clamp' and special chair to help position the patient for the radiographs [103]. Cowin placed small metal pieces on various anatomical landmarks on the patient's head before x-raying, in order to facilitate subluxation analysis [82]. Some of these techniques used machines to perform the adjustments or employed other tools of questionable diagnostic utility, such as temperature sensing devices to augment the indoctrination process, but only x-ray-related machinery is considered in this paper. These 'sacred artefacts' helped the practitioner rationalise the system and engaged the patients into believing.

Sacred stories

Sacred stories form an important part of religions. They help capture peoples' imaginations. They also take concepts that contravene the majority of human experience and work to elevate either a figure within the religion or the ideas of the religion itself. The idea of Christ walking on water makes him supernatural, inspiring awe and respect; it sets him apart, with abilities above those of mere mortals. It is then not unreasonable to believe that such a superior being should have his words listened to and obeyed. The story of the Buddha's life path of asceticism and respect for all living creatures, as well as his ability to overcome challenges creates a desire to emulate the methods, to become part of the group that enjoys this way of life. Stories create a reality of the author's imagination; they may inspire by showing what happens and why, giving a new perspective on the events in life, and can help listeners/readers understand, evaluate and redirect their lives [104]. The prototypical chiropractic sacred story is that of DD Palmer's first adjustment, which he believed cured deafness in a man. DD then recounted this story as the breakthrough moment when he realised the principle of chiropractic. This would have been a persuasive tale in the days when monistic theories of disease were given serious consideration. In the current context, sacred stories were considered to be the tales of the diagnostic and healing powers of the technique (patient testimonials) or positive statements from practitioners who adopted the technique and believed that their practices flourished because of it (practitioner testimonials).

Typical patient testimonials included the following: '[The chiropractor] took x-rays, and my life was changed in about 2/3 of a second... My spine, which had been 20 degrees to the right, suddenly was realigned. One minute after he actually used the [adjusting] device on me, we took another x-ray ... and it was the first time in twelve years that I was not in pain.' (Atlas Orthogonality) [105] 'He studies x-rays and makes precise and thoughtful recommendations. His pricing is reasonable. I love my body feeling good and highly recommend getting an adjustment if needed. You will be pleased...' (Duff) [106].

Practitioners gave testimonials such as: 'Patients know how long their correction-rehabilitative care will take and how much it will cost, making my pre-pays extraordinary!' (Pettibon) [107]. 'This [Advanced Orthogonal] seminar has been the most influential seminar of my life. It has changed not only the course of my career, but also the life of my family' [108].

Case reports, a weak form of clinical evidence, [109,110] were considered sacred stories as well as case anecdotes. Case anecdotes were stories of patient benefit from the perspective of the practitioner, similar to case reports, but without scholarly rigour in the reporting. These were much more frequently cited in the publicly available documents of the technique systems studied here than higher levels of scientific evidence such as randomised controlled trials. The case reports and anecdotes were usually found in magazines or newsletters, rather than peer-reviewed, scholarly journals.

Unsupported extrapolations and oversimplified analogies of anatomy or physiology were also considered sacred stories. These were interpreted as the equivalents of myths or fables, conveying the morality and correctness of a particular system. The technique systems examined here warned of the detrimental effects of spinal subluxations. Some created analogies to other disease processes, which may become far advanced without the person knowing, until one day it is too late. For instance, the Blair system used several intricate, almost indecipherable analogies, claiming that the body has a momentum like a spinning fan blade [111]. Once a trauma creates a subluxation in the spine, disease begins in one cell then spreads to others geometrically [111]. 'The longer the subluxation exists, the greater becomes the momentum of speed of diseases' [111]. Kale conveyed the danger of spinal misalignment in the most extreme way: 'Mild to moderate malfunction results in sickness and disease, while extreme malfunction results in DEATH!!' [emphasis in original] [97]. These ideas have not been supported by evidence available in peer-reviewed literature [20,21]. They are likely useful to the technique, though, to help hold together its concept of disease, and to gain new believers in patients and practitioners.

Several of the techniques also related the stories of the way in which their founders either came to chiropractic or invented their particular system. William Blair claimed to have been cured of lifelong asthma by upper cervical adjustments [112]. Clarence Gonstead credited being cured of rheumatoid arthritis by a chiropractor when he was a child; receiving regular adjustments so invigorated him that he went on to maintain a superhuman practice schedule for years, apparently seeing 250 patients per day [75]. John F Grostic claimed to be cured of Hodgkin's lymphoma, twice, by BJ Palmer himself [66]. Once healthy, he apparently also kept a gruelling practice schedule [66]. Sharon Freese-Pettibon (wife of technique founder Burl Pettibon) was evidently relieved of several life-threatening conditions, including paralysis, by her future husband's ministrations [113].

Sacred stories also included distorted evidence to support the belief in the use of radiography: 'In CBP® Technique, the use of initial and follow-up spinal x-rays or radiographs is deemed necessary; however, some in chiropractic have condemned the use of follow-radiographs to collect alignment data. Importantly, there is data [sic] to show that the use of medical/chiropractic x-rays constitutes a very minor health risk and in fact has been shown to be of benefit (decreased sickness and cancer mortality rates) in some studies' [114]. Unfortunately, the studies cited either did not actually support the claim of benefit in that they either did not include humans as study subjects, or they did not study diagnostic radiation. The concept of radiation hormesis (beneficial effects) has been discredited [115]. The National Academies of Science have done a long-term, comprehensive review of all known types of radiation, called the Biological Effects of Ionizing Radiation (BEIR) studies. This is the best available evidence, from a consensus of a large majority of scientists, and indicated that there is no such thing as a harmless dose of radiation. Every dose has the potential to cause damage and doses are cumulative: 'The report concludes that the preponderance of information indicates that there will be some risk, even at low doses, although the risk is small' [116]. Given this information, CBP's claims were considered a sacred story, used to support the radiographic paradigm of their system.

These stories may have performed the same function as myths and fables in religion. That is, they elevated the status of the authorities, they inspired awe and a desire to be part of the group, and they formed powerful tools for the recruitment of a flock (patients) and new shepherds (practitioners). See Appendix 4 for examples of the sacred stories of all the techniques.

Special language

Special language is used to describe unique or unusual artefacts, processes or rituals in various religions. It includes words like sacrament, reincarnation, and exorcism. L Ron Hubbard created an extensive vocabulary and copious acronyms for Scientology. For instance, 'thetan' represented a human soul, 'enturbulated' meant troubled, and SP stood for Suppressive Person, that is, someone who disapproved of Scientology [117]. These words seem to reinforce the exceptional nature of the religions and help make them more mysterious and worthy of wonder. In the realm of healthcare, Fuller observed that 'A distinguishing character of these [unorthodox medical] systems is that they utilize vocabularies and techniques designed to induct individuals into a world view predicated upon the "fact" that under certain conditions extramundane forces enter into, and exert sanative influences upon, the human realm. They are, therefore, substantively religious...' [118].

Special language used by the technique systems studied in this paper seemed to be an example of Fuller's idea. The language found in the techniques' descriptions of their radiographic processes included original words or specially derived meanings of ordinary or medical words. For instance, the word 'subluxation' has a meaning in medical literature that is different from the special definition given to it by subluxation-based chiropractors. Since the late 17th century, the term subluxation has denoted a partial dislocation of a joint, and implied severe damage to ligaments, tendons, and the other soft tissue structures that support articulations in the body [119]. However, the writings examined for this paper used the term to indicate a minute misalignment of a joint, sometimes claimed to be less than a degree of angulation or a sub-millimetric displacement [82]. These techniques also included in the definition a component indicating that despite the slightness of the lesion, nerves or the spinal cord were affected to a degree that created manifestations of disease in the organs of the body. Gonstead [120], Duff [121], Zimmerman [56], and others made statements to this effect.

Other special words are names of tools, such as the cephalometer mentioned above [102] and the anatometer, a device by Ralph Gregory of NUCCA, [122] used to examine posture in conjunction with radiographs to find subluxations. The term 'orthogonal' (which is a geometry term meaning 'having right angles') as applied by the different systems to the upper cervical spine, is special to those techniques, essentially denoting the 'normal' position of vertebrae. Blair used the term 'derinothermographic', undefined in their writings and not comprehensible by context: 'The presence of cervical nerve inter ference is established by observation of both persistent differential paraspinal derinothermographic pattern...' [103] The language of Chiropractic BioPhysics is so special that it protects its name and other terms such as PostureRay [123] with the® registered trademark symbol. Finally, several upper cervical techniques have radiographic views such as the 'nasium', 'base-posterior', and 'vertex', which are used for finding subluxations, and are not found in mainstream radiographic positioning texts.

Combinations of words in unique syntax are also part of the special language used by religions as well as these chiropractic techniques. The words 'holy' and 'see' are commonly understood separately, but when joined and capitalised, Holy See means the ecclesiastical jurisdiction of the Catholic Church in Rome. Nirvana is a word purloined into common English usage, but with the specific meaning of withdrawal from the cycle of rebirth to a Buddhist. In the world of radiographic detection of chiropractic subluxations, some genuinely unique usage of language was developed. Ronald Aragona introduced difficult to decipher definitions of his methods in Applied Spinal Biomechanical Engineering. For example, 'bilateral symmetrical function is secondary to static non-dynamic gravitational dependent equilibrium' [83]. Gonstead developed a complex system for describing subluxations on radiographs [124]. Kale also made statements thick with jargon: 'If the apparent listing does not clear the scan, then the listing will be re-evaluated and changed until the end result is a clear pattern on the scan' [125]. Special language was seen to help define each system, differentiating it from similar systems, and in the case of the techniques that use radiography for subluxation detection, this language may have given patients and practitioners a feeling of being involved in a special group with superior health knowledge to mainstream medical and chiropractic practitioners. See Appendix 5 for additional special language in the technique systems.

Historical links

These findings indicate that a system of belief has operated, and is still present in parts of the chiropractic profession. This belief system demonstrated qualities in common with religion rather than science and a reliance on clinical evidence. This is not to say that these techniques viewed themselves as religions, or that religion was a consciously embedded component during their creation. In fact, quite the opposite was frequently claimed; these techniques often stated that they were scientific [57,83,113,126-129]. Science, though, as has been noted, had a unique definition within some circles of chiropractic [130]. If technique systems displayed characteristics of religion rather than science in their stated application of radiography, an important question is raised. Why would this be so? In addition to the justifications for radiography discussed in the Background section above, there seemed to be a historical connection to early chiropractic justification for radiography. That is, the rationale for the use of the x-ray as given by BJ Palmer seems to have been adopted by technique systems subsequently developed throughout the 20th and into the 21st centuries. Evidence for those historical links will now be elucidated.

First, consideration should be given to the trial of Shegataro Morikubo and how it shaped chiropractic. In 1907, Morikubo was arrested for practicing medicine without a licence. Attorney Tom Morris successfully defended him. Morris invoked the concept that chiropractic was 'separate and distinct' from medicine and osteopathy by reason of chiropractic's unique philosophy, science and art [131]. For the most part, he used evidence of the workings of the profession from Solon Langworthy. Langworthy had been trying to advance the cause of modern science in the profession and was strongly opposed by both BJ and DD Palmer [131]. In Morikubo's defence, Morris referred to Langworthy's assertion that the brain was a source of 'unseen power' in the body, transmitting this power through the nerves to the organs, which could be blocked by out-of-place vertebrae [131]. For an unknown reason, Morris did not call Langworthy as a witness. However, BJ Palmer testified, and supported this refinement of the idea of chiropractic then and in many subsequent trials [131]. It is from this experience that Palmer adopted Langworthy's definition of 'subluxation', the concept of the brain supplying life force through the nerves, which he then fervently promoted [131,132]. So although the emphasis on, and singular importance of, the chiropractic subluxation to general health did not originate with BJ Palmer, Palmer's preeminent influence on the profession until at least 1925 was undeniable [131,133]. Palmer was the major source of the dissemination of these concepts, which he saw the opportunity to reinforce with the advent of diagnostic x-ray technology.

Perhaps additional insight was given by Wilson in his book *Spinatology* (1955), [134] in which he indicated the fear of insignificance as well as the desire to be thought to be working for good:

> Why discuss the question of an inborn intelligence? First, if there were no inborn intelligence, Chiropractic would not make sense. Secondly, and of no little importance, it gives us a feeling of working with a higher power, in which we are helping to make more complete its expression in the human body. Such an idea certainly adds to the dignity of our work and causes us to feel more important. Then we can recognize more fully the real value of our work for suffering humanity [134].

The second argument seems to be simply a longing for belief in the unseen, and the circularity of the first argument is obvious: inborn intelligence (Innate) must exist, otherwise chiropractic cannot exist; therefore Innate must exist because chiropractic exists.

Cyrus Lerner was an attorney commissioned to examine the chiropractic profession with a view to improving its image in the mid-20th century [135]. He produced a report realistically portraying what he found, and the report was buried [136]. In it he noted that chiropractic offered 'highly questionable evidence' regarding 'nerve impulses' and that 'Nearly all the writings examined on the "Story of Chiropractic" gave the feeling of one wandering through a fog' [135]. Perhaps it is not surprising that, building on this foundation, some descendant practitioners demonstrated similar thinking. The public documents examined for this paper indicated that observations and modifications of methods were limited to improving the description or quantification of subluxation radiographically. There was no evidence found of exploration as to how misaligned vertebrae actually caused ill health. As Keating [2] noted, 'BJ's "science" was constrained to support the "truths" of chiropractic that he was promoting' [2].

In discussing cults within chiropractic, CO Watkins, himself a chiropractor, noted:

> Each has accepted a particular system with the same finality that one accepts his religion, and assumes that its methods represent the alpha and omega of chiropractic knowledge. They make no attempt to review other

knowledge, to test their own methods for specific end results, or to compare their methods with others. They develop a faith in their methods which precludes any attempt to examine others; the same attitude of faith removes any necessity in their opinion of critically examining their own methods. Their approach to the patient is that of the cultist. They seek through philosophy and logic to instill in the public their own faith in their methods, at the same time tyring to discredit all other methods of healing the patient may have confidence in [137].

To call these techniques cults may be hyperbolic. But Watkins' observations seem to have a certain merit, at least as represented by systems the examined for this paper.

Two of the characteristics of religion discussed here, claims of supremacy to other techniques and the sacred stories of testimonials could be viewed simply as efforts to obtain business advantage. It is certainly possible that some of the techniques use them in that way. However, the overall context of the writings of these systems conveys a different message. It may be legitimate to view them as religious, or at least bearing a great resemblance to religion. The mysteries of the universe have led people to invent ideas to explain them when they could not yet discover the real explanations. So, too, the mysteries of the human body's structure, function and dysfunction have led people to invent explanations for the as yet inexplicable processes of disease and health. A religion-like thread is visible, woven into the contemplation of such matters, from the earliest days of healthcare development in the United States. Gaucher-Peslherbe noted that in 'the rationalisations that the [theories of healthcare] were based on were often no more than articles of faith which it was heresy to renounce' [40]. Gaucher-Peslherbe quoted Bernard, who also saw evidence of the quasi-religious in non-mainstream health practitioners, as well as a vulnerability in the public at large: 'Believing only in himself and rejecting all authority the empiric can boast of anything he likes, and claim that he can cure all ills. He will always find enough people who believe him to encourage him in his quackery, for men are so made that they have a need to be deceived; the miraculous is preferred to the real, and people would rather believe in inspired than acquired knowledge' [40]. Certainly the path to that belief is streamlined with the modern 'miracles' of technology, like the x-ray to show the subluxation as the cause of disease. Perhaps the subluxation is imaginary, perhaps not, but that makes the radiograph no less powerful a talisman.

Wright [117] noted that it is one thing to create a plausible universe, but quite another to believe it. 'That is the difference between art and religion' [117]. There was no evidence of art, or hucksterism, found. All the advocates of the various techniques seemed sincere in their belief of the usefulness of the radiograph in demonstrating a tiny, but life-endangering misalignment of bones. The friction arises in that health care systems should not be based in belief, but in evidence. They should not be dogmatic, but adaptable to new information. They should not be self-centred, but patient-centred. As Phillips and Mootz noted: 'A complete reliance on a holistic universal intelligence entails dogma and is not acceptable in current chiropractic philosophy or practice' [36].

Fuller [138] observed that a sense of wonder was a principal source of belief in the existence of an unseen order of life [138]. Certainly a personal 'miracle', in this case a cure by unconventional methods, after a period of strife and disillusionment with conventional methods, would engender a sense of wonder. Then the unseen order of life is revealed by the chiropractor providing the treatment, and the patient becomes a believer. Once belief is entrenched, it is exceedingly difficult to change, even when the believer confronted with incontrovertible evidence [139]. So these practitioners' explorations within their beliefs, without questioning the core principles of them seems explicable. But is it acceptable within the profession? Can these methods thrive in a world moving towards evidence-based healthcare?

The idea of healthcare ritual as being similar to religious ritual is not restricted to chiropractic. Welch [140] noted that due to their unique powers to see into human beings, to understand how we functioned and what had gone awry, 'before the priest and physician, we stand individually transparent' [140]. The healing powers of pre-medical practitioners have been partially attributed to ritual and the placebo effect that it brings [140]. A full discussion of this subject is beyond the scope of this paper, but from the evidence gathered herein, it does seem plausible that the ritual of radiography may have played some role in creating the successes claimed by the practitioners.

It may be argued that medical artefacts, such as the white coat, the stethoscope, and the scalpel might also be construed as sacred, that the trappings of any profession create an atmosphere conducive to indoctrination. The difference is that medical writings do not refer to vital energy, or a single cause of disease, or dis-ease. They do not advertise that once magnetic resonance imaging reveals a tumour, subsequently removed by the surgeon, the flow of life force will be restored and other, unrelated ailments may then be healed. The intent of the chiropractor, who uses his or her superior knowledge and the reputation of a learned profession to persuade, cajole, or frighten lay people into belief in a particular system is the differentiating factor. The overall impression from studying the chiropractic systems in this paper was that the intent of the documents was to win new converts by indoctrination. It did not give the impression of educating the public to choose a healthier lifestyle by fully informing themselves of physiological and pathological processes as best understood by science. The tone seemed to be one of conspiracy. The implication was that the practitioner knew a secret to health that was somehow beyond the grasp of mainstream medicine, or perhaps suppressed by it. The idea of limiting healthcare to a single cause, to be fully understood only by one man, the originator of a technique system, transformed into saviour because of his understanding, was a theme that emerged from the characteristics of each system. This environment, with all the characteristics taken together, their denotations and connotations, is what evoked the idea of religion rather than science.

Religion seems to limit the possibilities of the way the world works. By accepting one religion and its views on the machinations of the universe, one must necessarily discount other views, limiting perspective to a certain framework. Life becomes easier. It is satisfying to be part of a community and to be told that the complex, confusing world is actually simple and explicable. This is one of the psychological benefits of religion [141,142]. The chiropractic systems that use radiography for subluxation detection limit the possibilities of the way health and disease work. The claims of supremacy that each technique espouses would seem to indicate that the practitioners thereof derive satisfaction from their understanding of health. However, they limit the potential benefits that could be achieved for their patients if less partisan, more objective research was employed to discover the mechanism of action of chiropractic methods.

Limitations of the study

It is possible that some techniques were inadvertently excluded if they no longer exist, had very small numbers of practitioners, and/or no internet presence. This paper only sampled the publicly available writings from techniques' official websites, papers, and textbooks; nuances and variations would likely be revealed by interviews with the spokespeople for the techniques, for those techniques that are not defunct. Also, because websites are sometimes created or edited by external individuals or companies conversant with information technology but not necessarily the subjects of the sites they design, they may not always accurately reflect information presented to them for publication. Differences would also likely have been found if individual practitioners were interviewed on how they practically applied the techniques in their own practices, rather than just how the techniques officially advocated use of their systems.

Summary

The founders and early pioneers of chiropractic did not benefit from the current understanding of science and research and therefore substituted deductive and inductive reasoning to arrive at conclusions about health and disease in the human body. Some of this thinking and rationalisation demonstrably followed a religion-like pattern, including BJ Palmer's use of radiography. Access to scientific methods and research education became much advanced and more accessible during the past few decades. However, the publicly available documents of technique systems that used radiography for chiropractic subluxation detection employed a historically derived paradigm for radiography that displayed characteristics in common with religion.

Appendix 1: evidence of supernatural concepts in the technique systems

Advanced orthogonal

Vitalism and supernatural calling: 'By God's design, the balanced function of the brain and nervous system is essential to the integrity of health. Our focus is on identifying and correcting the structural causes of this dysfunction, to restore and maintain the health and well-being of all those whom we serve. Too many people are suffering from conditions that are impeding their ability to live fruitful and productive lives. We want to let these people know that there is hope for answers, and opportunities for healing. Finally, we recognize that the human body is fearfully and wonderfully made, and our desire is to honor the Creator of this dynamic body through our approach to health care' [72].

Applied spinal biomechanical engineering

Vitalism: 'A chiropractic doctor detects and corrects these spinal misalignments (vertebral subluxation causing nerve interference), restoring normal nerve impulses to the body allowing the body's own innate healing capabilities to function optimally' [67].

Applied upper cervical biomechanics

AUCB only obliquely references vitalism with phrases like 'neural reintegration' and they are couched in science-like terminology. However, the original chiropractic premise is implied by statements like the following: 'The foundation of the chiropractic profession stands upon the premise that health and disease are nervous system dependent,' 'How can I transcend the practice of pain management to the practice of true health care? We all have been told that chiropractic can effect [sic] the body as a whole, but where is this practice? These are the questions our association is striving to provide objective answers to', and 'If you are ready for a practice that delivers consistent broad-scope health care, then welcome to the IUCCA [International Upper Cervical Chiropractic Association]' [143].

Atlas orthogonality

Vitalism: 'When the atlas bone is properly aligned, that is in the orthogonal—or neutral—position, the rest of the spinal vertebra [sic] come into better alignment allowing the body to heal itself' [144].

Blair

Vitalism: 'The nervous system controls and regulates all parts and functions in the body. When there is nerve interference (subluxation) your body loses the ability to properly self regulate and heal itself. The result can be pain and illness. Blair upper cervical care is often the key to people regaining and maintaining good health' [69].

Supernatural calling: 'There is a verse in the Bible-Chapter 9, Verse 6 in II Corinthians... by changing a few words, we can make this revealing verse read - "He which soweth competence and precision will reap outstanding results, and he which soweth carelessness and inaccuracy will reap guilt and mediocre results"' [112].

Chiropractic BioPhysics

Chiropractic BioPhysics (CBP) makes no explicit references to religion or vitalism however, however their stated goal is to 'correct human spines and alleviate human suffering' [70]. CBP also aligns itself with the International Chiropractic Association (ICA) and World Chiropractic Alliance (WCA) [145].

Cowin upper cervical orthogonal

Vitalism: 'Our procedures are based on the traditional chiropractic concept of vertebral subluxation' [68].

Duff

Vitalism: 'The goal of a Chiropractor is to correct the "Vertebral Subluxations" (misaligned vertebra the cause a disturbance to the nervous system and other systems) for the purpose of restoring the proper communication of nerve energy over nerve pathways that exit the spine' [121]. 'Most of this problem (Subluxation) [sic] exists at the base of the skull or known as the upper cervical region of the spine. It is at this level of the spine that can produce many health problems and is where I often first focus my attention, even if there are lower spine problems, This is because of the likely hood [sic] of Upper Cervical [sic] involvement. It's importance cannot be overlooked both in terms of preve*ntion* [sic] of sickness or disease or correction of dysfunction of the body and its return to optimal health' [121]. Duff's logo is a chiropractic angel, which is common throughout the profession, but with the addition of radiating lines that make it look particularly heavenly [77].

Gonstead

Vitalism: '...compressed nerves often become inflamed and impede the proper transmission of impulses to the section of the body controlled by these nerves. A seemingly endless list of ailments and pain may be brought about by these subluxations' [120]. 'It is the goal of your Gonstead doctor to restore and maintain optimal health by locating and correcting any interference to the nervous system caused by vertebral subluxation' [146]. The picture on the official website shows Gonstead showing him with hands clasped, wearing a white shirt with high, priestly collar, staring beatifically into the distance, a halo emanating from his upper body [75].

Supernatural calling: 'Our Mission is to perpetuate the teachings of Dr. Clarence S. Gonstead, fund chiropractic research, and encourage cooperation and camaraderie amongst all who practice the Gonstead technique' [73]. 'To spread the word about the Gonstead technique, we need to be in the public eye. You can help' [147]. Gonstead chose for his clinic the town of Mount Horeb, [75] named after the Biblical site of Moses' receipt of the Ten Commandments.

Grostic

Vitalism: 'When the vertebrae become misaligned (subluxated) a decrease of innate vital energy between the brain and the body occurs causing malfunction and disease. Chiropractors release the innate power of the body within by detecting and correcting spinal subluxations' [148]. '...misaligned vertebra(e) impinge the flow of innate intelligence and cause illness, or what BJ Palmer later referred to as dis-ease [66]. 'Orthogonally-based upper cervical care is not a treatment for conditions or diseases, however, this subluxation-centered care has been shown to have an associative effect on various conditions' [149]. Christian religion was also directly injected into Grostic seminars, as each day began with a prayer [66].

Kale

Vitalism: 'When one or both of the top two bones (Atlas and Axis) misalign, creating pressure on the "Brain Stem" and causes an interference of nerve flow to all parts of the body. This is what causes the body organs and tissues to malfunction, thus causing disease' [127]. 'The "Specific Chiropractor" ("Brain Stem Specialist") is trained to locate and remove this subluxation (misalignment) and restore the vertebrae to its normal position. The mental impulse, life force, Innate Intelligence, can flow in its full capacity from the "Brain Stem" to its diseased tissue or organ; healing or repair takes place in a natural way and pain and the ravenges [sic] of disease disappear' [97]. 'Mild to moderate [spinal] malfunction results in sickness and disease, while extreme malfunction results in DEATH!!' [emphasis original] [97].

Supernatural calling: 'The Kale Foreign Messenger has been in over 9 countries doing missionary work' [74].

Knee chest upper cervical specific

Vitalism: '**Upper Cervical Specific Chiropractic Care** focuses on removing nerve irritation to restore communication between the brain and the body. Restoring function at the level of the brainstem and upper cervical spine (the control center of the body) is essential so that the body may heal itself and have optimal vitality. With the nervous system functioning at 100% the body has the potential to heal itself from even the most complex of ailments' [127]. 'a significant academic influence running through every KCUCS module. KCUCS finds a good balance between "bringing the Spiz" of Upper Cervical Chiropractic while also bringing the science' [150]. Spiz or spizzerinctum was BJ Palmer's word meaning enthusiasm for chiropractic.

Logan basic

Vitalism: displacement of the sacrum is the root cause of disease. Claims of cures of various organic conditions such as asthma and appendicitis, with pre- and post-treatment full-spine radiographs provided as evidence showing distorted and corrected vertebral and pelvic alignments [151].

Mears

Vitalism: 'The Mears Technique is a specific upper cervical system of X-ray analysis and adjustment that carries on where the H.I.O. concept ends' [152].

National upper cervical chiropractic association

Vitalism: 'The postural rebalancing created by the upper cervical adjustment allows for the body to have less gravitational stress and therefore the person can direct that now unused energy to self-healing, maintenance and thinking' [153].

Orthospinology

Since Orthospinology is essentially inseparable from Grostic; the same vitalistic concepts apply [66].

Supernatural calling: 'I encourage each of you to thank God... for the job that you have... Correcting an atlas misalignment and restoring your patient's body balance, integrity, and health...' [86].

Palmer upper cervical specific (Hole-in-One)

Vitalism: 'That the *sunnum bonum* of all life and death, health or disease issues pivoted around a study of the correct or incorrect position of vertebrae' [39].

Pettibon

Vitalism: 'The purpose of the chiropractic adjustment is to work "with" the innate intelligence of the body to produce a predictable response. Our specific adjusting forces are designed to cause innate to react positively with its environment. An adjustment must be a positive, constructive force that causes the body to predictably react to its environment, correcting the spine so the nerves can function normally resulting in health to be expressed optimally' [101].

Pierce results

Vitalism: 'By correcting subluxations more effectively, Dr. Pierce began to see many things heal faster, even spines that never changed on x-ray were now exhibiting complete corrections in minutes! (Thanks to Innate!)' [154].

Spinal orthopaedic neurological advancement and research

Vitalism: 'God built within us the ability to heal ourselves. If the communication between the brain and body becomes disrupted, this ability degrades. The atlas is the top bone in the neck. It houses and protects the brainstem and upper spinal cord, which is the communication center between the brain and body. When the atlas misaligns, it irritates the delicate nerve tissue' [155]. 'The procedure cures nothing, but it allows the body to cure itself. It restores body balance and proper nerve flow so that organs, limbs, and tissues can resume normal functioning. This is why we see so many different conditions with no apparent relationship responding to the SONAR procedure' [156]. '... [The] result of a misaligned atlas is the restriction or distortion of critical messages at the brainstem and upper-spinal cord, disrupting the brain's communication. Every cell, organ, or tissue that is not receiving adequate nerve energy and communication from the brain will suffer and degenerate' [155].

Supernatural calling: 'Through the grace of God, Dr. Elliott has developed the SONAR instrument' [71].

Spinal stressology

Vitalism: 'When you put subluxations in terms of a disorganized system and the treatment of subluxations as you are trying to release that pattern of disorganization and bring it back into a reorganized format, where it can recover and create its own homeostasis...' [128]. 'Is it possible to read a persons personality or emotional history by an analysis of their spinal alignment and posture? Although from a superficial standpoint it may seem obvious that a depressed person would carry himself differently than a happy one, we have found that a radiographic spine/posture analysis can reveal stresses that correlate to emotional trauma, deep-seated personality characteristics, inherited trauma and relationship issues' [157].

Sutter

Vitalism and supernatural calling: 'That there is a Creative Intelligence in back of all laws and life on earth, call It God, Universal Intelligence or what you will. That we are instruments placed upon this earth for self-development and service... That health is natural and disease is unnatural. That disease is caused by an interference with the Creative Intelligence that wills normality within the body. That such interference is caused by obstruction of nerve impulse flow from the brain to the body due to a subluxated spinal vertebra. That this Chiropractic principle is the greatest boon to suffering humanity and supplies a need for which there is no substitute' [129].

Zimmerman

Vitalilsm: 'All it takes to restore the flow of energy to the sick body is ONE accurate adjustment.' [emphasis original] [56].

Appendix 2: evidence of claims of supremacy to other methods

Advanced orthogonal

- '...the most accurate assessment of spinal misalignment' [158].
- 'Today, Advanced Orthogonal chiropractic stands alone as the most evolved offspring of the upper cervical procedures' [159].
- 'Upper cervical doctors utilizing the Advanced Orthogonal have acquired that additional education' [160].
- 'With the increased accuracy of Orthogonal chiropractic, Advanced Orthogonal doctors have higher expectations for correcting patient subluxations' [160].
- 'Digital x-ray analysis to measure misalignments to the 1/100th of a degree' [81].

Applied spinal biomechanical engineering (ASBE)

- '...doctors discover how little they knew before they started learning these methods and procedures. With this scientific work incorporated in their clinical setting, a new enthusiasm manifests. Practitioners are no longer bored with methods and procedures. They are continuously learning and providing a better service to humanity' [83].
- '...a dependable and proven effective procedure in improving patient's posture that can be added to your current adjusting protocol' [83].
- ASBE provides '...a remarkable advantage over other methods and procedures...' [83]. They claim to base their methods on '...12 volumes of A.S.B.E. research discoveries' [83]. These works seem to be self-published [67].

Applied upper cervical biomechanics (AUCB)

- 'Our association's research into this critical area of the spine has founded a highly effective form of health care that is unique from any other in the world' [161].
- Radiographic landmarks form the foundations of entire systems of analysis; hence their reliability is paramount to the accuracy of the evaluation [162].
- '...AUCB uses a complex and unique form of upper cervical radiographic analysis' [84].
- 'Adjustments based on this system of analysis have consistently produced full body neurophysiologic benefits on patients, which has been objectively substantiated by both high-resolution camera and paraspinal infrared imaging' [84].
- '...15 years of unprecedented research...' [84].

Atlas orthogonality

- 'Improving the health and extending the lives of people around the world' [163].
- It also claims to provide certainty of diagnosis and treatment for the practitioner, 'There is no guess work [sic] in this program' [144].
- '...the most precise atlas correction...' [144].

Blair

- 'This "blue print" of your neck [created from the x-rays] allows the Blair chiropractor to deliver the adjustment that is exactly what your body needs' [69].
- Patients 'enjoy better health, less pain, less illness and greater quality of life' [69].
- '...[it's] possible for a chiropractor to achieve excellent if not outstanding results. This chiropractor will eventually find that he will be able to make the spinographs and give the adjustment with confidence and ease' [112].

Chiropractic BioPhysics (CBP)

- 'Chiropractic BioPhysics®, or CBP®, is, in short, a higher level of chiropractic. It is a more knowledgeable, comprehensive, systematic, scientific approach to chiropractic, that provides predictable results for patients and will contribute to building a more stable and successful chiropractic practice' [126].
- This technique's literature also appeals to the readers' rational inclinations, 'CBP® is the most published named chiropractic Technique [sic] within the Index Medicus in the history of Chiropractic. CBP® has more published papers in peer-reviewed indexed journals than all other techniques' [164].
- Photo of a man tearing open his shirt to reveal a cape and the logo of a business-enhancement company underneath, associated with CBP [165,166].
- CBP® is '...the best technique in chiropractic' [167].

Cowin upper cervical orthogonal

- 'Our methods were observed by Wollongong University mathematicians Aldis and Hill and written up in the Journal and Proceedings of the Royal Society of NSW in 1979' [68].

- Measurements 'as small as 0.75 degrees (or, translated into linear measurements, each as small as 28 thousandths of an inch or 0.7 mm)' [82].

Duff

- 'Dr. Duff's speciality is in aligning the upper top two vertebrae Atlas Axis, C1 and C2 [sic] by using specific X-Ray views ...' [77].
- '...tailor-made, specific adjustment...' [77].

Gonstead

- '...why don't all chiropractors use this technique? Because the analysis takes more time and mastering the art of delivering a specific adjustment takes a LOT of practice and dedication' [emphasis original] [57].
- '...one of the most advanced and scientific methods [of correcting] spinal misalignments, joint dysfunctions and subluxation complexes' [57].
- 'The Gonstead Chiropractor goes beyond what many chiropractors consider a spinal assessment by conducting a thorough analysis of your spine using five criteria to detect the presence of the vertebral subluxation complex' [57].
- 'The focus of the Gonstead adjustment is to be as specific, precise and accurate as possible, addressing only the problem areas (areas of subluxation).' [146]
- 'There is a worldwide referral network of qualified Gonstead chiropractors using the same methods of analysis, the same specific adjusting procedures, and who share the same goal... to correct the subluxations in your spine for the purpose of creating a healthier you!' [168].

Grostic

- '[Grostic is a] method for analyzing and correcting the occipito-atlanto-axial subluxation complex. It is actually a series of steps in the total care of the patient and is therefore a chiropractic procedure and not simply a spinal adjusting technique' [149].
- 'The analysis of your x-ray views will reveal the exact degree of misalignment or imbalance. The mathematical measurements taken from your x-ray films give the doctor the correct formula to realign your spine' [149].

Kale

- The motto of the affiliated TIC (as in ChiropracTIC, from BJ Palmer) Institute is 'Principled, Dedicated, Pure' [169].
- 'Dr. Kale was the world's leading authority on "Upper Cervical Specific" Chiropractic Knee-Chest Technique' [74].
- 'DO I NEED THIS PROCEDURE? Unlike knowing when you are hungry, or when you have to go to the bathroom you DON'T know if you are in SUBLUXATION. A Specific Chiropractor can tell you if and when you need this procedure, using specialized scientific scanning equipment' [emphasis original] [127].
- 'DOES THIS REALLY WORK? YES!!! For 100 years people with all kinds of sickness and diseases have been getting well from this procedure. YES!!! There is research to back up this procedure. YES!!! There are plenty of satisfied patients, over 40 million.' [emphasis original] [127].
- 'This new relationship brings the legacy of Dr. Michael Kale through his son, Dr. B.J. Kale to The Specific Chiropractic Center. Dr. Michael Kale was responsible for the perpetuation of the Knee Chest Upper Cervical Specific work during a vital time in the history of Upper Cervical Specific Chiropractic. Dr. Michael Kale was the only Associate of Dr. Lyle Sherman, who was the Assistant Director of the BJ Palmer Research Center, prior to launching his career as a noted healer and disciplined teacher. His legacy extends throughout the world, having trained almost every noted authority in the Knee Chest Upper Cervical Specific world and having provided care to citizens of numerous countries around the world.
  Today, the tradition of the Kale name is carried forth by his son, Dr. B.J. Kale, who continues to teach around the world and uphold the values instilled in him by his father through The Kale Chiropractic Research Clinic, The Kale Foundation and the Kale teachings at the TIC Institute, an in depth training program for Doctors and Students who desire to learn the methods of his father, and the principled deliverance of the Knee Chest work through the BJ Palmer Research years of 1935-1951 under the direction of Dr. Sherman and Dr. B.J. Palmer. The Kale Chiropractic Research Clinic and Kale Foundation will continue to provide care to the people around the globe' [170].

Knee-chest upper cervical specific

- 6 week 'X-ray Bootcamp' [171].
- 'The misaligned segments are identified through the use of Digital Laser-aligned Radiography. Because the misalignment is very slight (measured in millimeters) it is very important that precise x-ray equipment is used' [127].

Logan basic

- '...the secret of health and longevity has been solved... in Logan Basic Technique more than by all other asserted advances in healing methods since the beginning of time...' [85].

Mears

- '...more reliable points of reference to determine cervical distortion more accurately. This in turn led to the need to modify the adjusting procedure used in the H.I.O. technique' [152].

National upper cervical chiropractic association (NUCCA)

- 'NUCCA has provided the chiropractic profession with more biomechanical data than any other chiropractic entity concerning the atlas subluxation, its effects on the spinal column and human body, how to restore its misalignments to the vertical axis, and has shown acceptable and measurable proof of the benefits of the chiropractic adjustment on the human body' [102].
- 'Defining the basic "problem" in chiropractic has been in dispute since the beginning of the profession. Measuring a "bone out of place" has eluded the vast majority in Chiropractic. While the rest of the profession has essentially walked away from this difficult concept, upper cervical chiropractic has been quietly and accurately measuring and correcting upper cervical misalignments (subluxations) for more than sixty years' [172].
- 'NUCCA's forte, even among the other upper cervical specific groups, has been to deal directly with postural imbalance. Indications when to and when not to intervene are dependent upon postural measurements. The direction of vectored mani pulation, the how to intervene, is dependant [sic] on X-ray analysis and an understanding of biomechanics and patient abnormalities' [122].
- 'NUCCA practitioners in general appear to have a more rigorous system with more pervasive and refined posture measurements, more meticulous X-ray procedures, and consistently better corrections as evidenced by its certification process and standards' [122].
- 'Gregory was able to independently develop or improve upon both the accuracy and precision of all levels of analysis of the "Grostic" system by 1) development of a double-pivot-point system in X-ray analysis (1962)... 5) design of better film analytical instruments... 7) design and development of the Anatometer which reduces the need for X-rays (1978), 8) classification of C-1 subluxations into basic types(1980)...' [122].

Orthospinology

- '...one of the greatest health care procedures in the world' [173].
- '...has helped millions of people overcome countless health problems' [173].
- '...greatest health care procedure in the world' [86].
- '...revolutionary advances by Dr. John F. Grostic to upper cervical chiropractic care in detecting, quan tifying, and correcting the upper cervical sublu xation complex. All of these events have led to what is known as orthospinology and orthogonally based upper cervical care' [66].

Palmer upper cervical specific (HIO, toggle recoil)

- BJ Palmer spent much of his time in self-promotion; examples are replete throughout his writings and speeches [2].

Pettibon

- 'In 1988, Dr. Pettibon was honored for his work as the recipient of the Daniel David Chiropractic Scientific Award' [113].
- 'We have an unwavering passion to help you become the best practitioner that you can be. Our goal is to enable you and your staff to reach new levels of success in delivering patient care while simultaneously maximizing the efficiency and profitability of your clinic' [113].
- 'Dozens of doctors, on the verge of leaving the profession, have reclaimed their calling because of the understanding and protocols which is now known as The Pettibon System' [113].
- 'Most Doctors of Chiropractic laugh at the idea of "hit and hope" or "pop and pray" chiropractic procedures. Unfortunately in the "dark hours" of being alone, they wonder if what they are doing really works. They desire technical certainty. This is what Pettibon Spinal Biomechanics explains' [101].
- 'Conventional chiropractic x-ray procedures don't consider spinal soft tissue injuries. The Pettibon System's x-ray procedures do' [100].
- 'The Pettibon Procedures are an advanced, scientific approach to Chiropractic...' [101].

Pierce results

- 'not a chiropractic technique like any others, but a systematic approach to correcting subluxations using the most advanced tools for spinal analysis and adjusting [154].
- 'consistent and predictable results' [154].

- 'By correcting subluxations more effectively... even spines that never changed on x-ray were now exhibiting complete corrections in minutes!' [154].
- 'We don't simply claim to provide the best chiropractic has to offer... we can back it up!' [154].

Spinal orthopedic neurological advancement and research (SONAR)

- '...far superior to other upper cervical techniques' [71].
- '...[regain] health and wholeness without polluting your body with drugs and chemicals...' [156].
- '...we have patients who come in from around the country to receive upper cervical chiropractic care' [174].

Spinal stressology

- 'I'm kind of a revolutionary scientist...' [128].
- '...when you are introducing something new (Thomas Kuhn has a book on it, called The Structure of Scientific Revolutions) there is always incredible resistance because you can't take the current concepts and explain the revolutionary concepts. You have to go with the revolutionary concepts and you almost have to unlearn so many things that you have learned to understand the new concept' [128].
- '...we have documented more chiropractic cases than any before' [128].
- 'I've been doing this for 25 years' [128].
- 'Dr. Stephen Ward, an experienced Long Beach chiropractor, has a unique approach to pain mana gement and treatment. He pioneered the use of the wall adjustment technique to provide more effec tive, longer-lasting adjustments' [175].
- The official website provides a link to a video of an animated male figure in red and blue tights called ChiroMan doing a dance and some muscle stretches to heavy metal music [176].

Sutter

- 'Specific Atlas Correction deals with the specific location and correction of the cause of such interference within the nervous mechanism. It represents the latest development of scientific exactitude in the location and correction of the cause of disease within the body' [129].
- 'The exact variation of the atlas subluxation in relation to its surrounding structures peculiar to the individual case must be accurately determined. This can only be done through a specialized X-ray technique and analysis' [177].

Zimmerman

- 'Due to the precision of the x-rays and other methods, '[the chiropractor] is trained to place the tip of the machine so accurately as to do that which has never been done before' [56].
- '...opens up a field for practice with absolutely no competition' [56].

Appendix 3: evidence for the rules and rituals

The examples cited below are specifications or additions to the findings that all the technique systems had the rule that chiropractic subluxations were visible on radiographs, and all included the ritual of taking the radiographs as well as analysing them for subluxations.

Advanced orthogonal

- '...consistent clinical procedure for accurate evaluation and reduction of the atlas subluxation complex' [159].
- 'This assessment can only be obtained by looking at very precise x-rays from all 3 dimensions. The views are left (sagittal or side), center (nasium or front) and right taken from above (vertex)' [160].

Applied spinal biomechanical engineering

- 'ASBE utilizes very low radiation dosage static and dynamic spinal radiographs to help with objective pre-treatment and post-treatment diagnostic rational [sic] for the reduction of vertebral subluxations...' [83 p. 2]. 'ASBE starts the analysis with the static weight bearing x-ray views. Then adds intersegmental bilateral lateral flexion biomechanical analysis' [83 p. 2].

Applied upper-cervical biomechanics

- Radiographs must be obtained using the same views for every patient and that they are analysed the same way every time [178].

Atlas orthogonality

- 'The first step of the diagnosis is to determine the degree in which the atlas is misaligned. Very precise x-rays are taken which show the doctor exactly how the atlas is displaced. The x-rays taken are invaluable in making the most precise atlas correction which is as unique to the patient as their own fingerprint' [144].
- 'One of the most important post adjustment steps are post x-rays, which are taken immediately after the initial treatments... These three dimensional x-rays are taken and analyzed to verify that the best

possible correction was rendered. The doctor may then show the patient the comparison between before and after x-rays. Post x-rays are an illustration of the exact change that has taken place because of the atlas orthogonal correction' [144].

Blair

- 'Precise x-rays are taken to custom tailor the neck adjustment to your individual spinal anatomy and condition' [69].
- These x-rays are 'the hallmark of the Blair Upper Cervical Technique' [179].

Chiropractic BioPhysics

- Radiographs are obtained for every patient and analysed in the same way every time, obtaining post-treatment radiographs to verify changes but, uniquely to CBP, comparisons are made to 'ideal' posture calculated with a geometrical formula [180].
- 'CBP® protocols require that the doctor must measure the displacements on spinal radiographs (segmental Subluxation). Both lateral-side view and anterior to posterior (AP) or frontal view CBP® x-ray line drawing procedures [are necessary] ...' [114]. and '...CBP® utilizes standardized x-ray positioning procedures...' [114].
- Ease in applying the rules is available to the computer-savvy with CBPs proprietary x-ray line-drawing software, called PostureRay: 'Sick and Tired [sic] of marking [subluxations on] your x-rays by hand? Most clinicians are! PostureCo offers the latest and most accurate technology for clinical x-ray digitization' [123]. 'PostureRay was released in January 1, 2007. Since this program is already in high demand, you may wish to secure your copy by emailing [address] or calling [phone number]. Only 30 installations per month will be supported so that we can provide the first rate personalized technical support in this first release. Reserve your copy today' [123].

Cowin upper cervical orthogonal

- 'We take X-rays in three planes to see how far the spinal bones have moved from their normal positions. Because the cumulative effects of several upper-neck misalignments, each perhaps as small as 0.75 degrees (or, translated into linear measurements, each as small as 28 thousandths of an inch or 0.7 mm)' [82].
- 'The wire artefacts we place on the skin show up on the X-rays to tell us how far the spinal bones are from the ear and other 'outside' structures, allowing us to map both the locations of the spinal bones and the line of access for the spinal adjustments' [82].
- 'We fuss about positioning patients for X-ray, and about ensuring they keep their eyes closed, because we want the films to show posture the patient has unconsciously adopted to compensate for the spinal malfunction' [82].
- 'Before a patient receives a first adjustment (treatment), we spend an hour or more analysing the X-rays' [82].
- 'The analysis is completed when the chiropractor has decided which of about 36 adjustment categories is most strongly indicated by the initial set of films' [82].
- 'After the first "trial-adjustment", we take two new X-rays and compare them with two of the three initial X-rays to find out what changes in vertebral position may have been achieved by this adjustment attempt. Getting the best adjustment, may require several 'trial-adjustments' over a number of visits' [82].
- 'The other comparison X-ray in the series (sagittal plane natural lateral) is taken about 18 months later in the hope of finding evidence of improved posture. The chiropractors interpret this kind of improvement as resulting from the patient's new self-help activities over this time' [82].

Duff method of analysis

- Upper cervical x-rays are taken on patients [77].

Gonstead

- '...full-spine radiographs are taken in the standing, weight-bearing position to fully substantiate the examination findings' [57].
- 'This is helpful in evaluating posture, joint and disc integrity, vertebral misalignments and ruling out any pathologies...' [57].

Grostic

- 'The procedure employs a method of X-ray analysis that quantifies the lateral and rotational misalignments between atlas and axis as well as atlas and occiput. The analytical procedure examines the spatial orientation of the atlas, the geometry of the articulating surfaces, and the misalignment configuration to arrive at an effective correction vector. In addition to the X-ray analysis, the system contains steps for ensuring the precision of the X-ray analysis, adjusting procedures, and post-adjustment re-evaluation procedures' [149].

- 'The x-ray analysis is the real core of the procedure and is the one area that has remained constant over the last 30 years' [149].
- Seven of twenty-one chapters of the official textbook for this technique pertain to x-ray [66]
- 'Post X-ray assessment was recommended to ascertain that at least 50% correction was achieved after the initial adjustment. Post X-ray assessment is also important to determine if an errant adjustment occurs; and provides information for the doctor to make the appropriate correction(s) for future adjustments' [149].
- Grostic encouraged the chiropractors attending his seminars to arrive early, be radiographed, adjusted personally by him, then re-radiographed, so they could see the change themselves [66] p.24.
- Kale
- 'Three x-ray views are required to determine the subluxation of the Atlas (top cervical vertebra); they are AP open mouth, lateral (through C1), and base posterior' [125].

Knee chest upper cervical specific (KCUCS)

- '6 week intensive course designed to develop you into an expert in Upper Cervical X-ray analysis' [181].
- 'Curvilinear Misalignment of C1 in Subluxation. The foundational basis of this concept is rooted in the work of William Blair, D.C., originator of the Blair technique' [182].

Logan basic

- Full spine radiography is required [183].
- Ten patterns of 'distortion' or what they considered abnormal spinal curvatures, which they marked on the radiographs [49] p.176.

Mears

- 'a new method of X-ray analysis ... which established more reliable points of reference to determine cervical distortion more accurately. This in turn led to the need to modify the adjusting procedure used in the H.I.O. technique. The new X-ray analysis indicated that segment rotation was a major factor in cervical distortion and it became apparent that a method of adjustment had to be devised which would correct rotational as well as lateral displacement. What developed was a new method of adjustment which with the X-ray analysis became the basis for the Mears Technique' [152].

National upper cervical chiropractic association (NUCCA)

- 'Our profession offers a plethora of organizations to belong to and have membership in. Each has their own agenda and to the extent that agenda resonates with how you practice and what you believe in, is the extent that you would support them. No organization will be perfectly aligned with what you know to be true, but our group represents the doctor who makes NUCCA protocol the mainstay of his/her practice. Just think if you suddenly lost your ability to take post x-rays? There is movement to enforce this change. One of the strongest voices and your most consistent ally to not let this happen is the NUCCA organization. We are aware and watching these developments and the UCRF [Upper Cervical Research Foundation] has tooled its focus to publish research to support the need for post x-rays' [184].
- 'Research shows that problems in the cervical spine can cause progressively degenerative structural, neu rological, physiological and pathological symptoms. Yet, when a small but measurable spinal misalignment known as the Atlas Subluxation Complex (ASC) is detected and corrected, a return toward good health and normal activity can be realized' [76].
- 'We are biomechanically based and depend on objective measurements utilizing pre-adjustment and post-adjustment X-rays along with an instrument called the Anatometer for the measurement of body posture and skeletal distortion. It is our long-term clinical experience that postural distortions compromise the functioning of the nervous system and eventually the overall physiology of the human body' [172].
- The Atlas Subluxation Complex and Atlas Subluxation Complex Syndrome are '...progressive and degenerative, are a detriment to human health and well being and pose a burden on our society and the health care providers treating the various symptoms and conditions associated with them' [172].

Orthospinology

- Uses Grostic x-ray analysis [185] including post x-rays [149].
- Outcome measures are radiographic and postural analysis [186].

Palmer upper cervical specific/HIO

- Radiographs are necessary to demonstrate subluxation [1].

- Post-treatment radiographs show correction [43].

Pettibon

- 'The Pettibon Rehabilitation System starts with an x-ray examination. Seven views of the spine are routinely taken, more if necessary' [100].
- 'Pettibon x-ray analysis may involve over 41 lines and 23 angles to specifically locate the displaced vertebra' [101] p.7.
- 'The initial set of examination x-rays are compared to x-rays taken during treatment to assess progress and ultimately to prove the treatment's success. Whether the x-rays are for diagnosis, testing, assessing progress, post-treatment evaluation and/or proof, patients are seated and the x-rays are always taken, marked, and measured the same way, every time' [100].
- 'The initial, interim and post x-rays are specifically analyzed and measured...' [101] p.33.
- 'Prospective patients aren't automatically accepted for care. Doctors need to determine "if" and "how" prospective patients will respond to care. And this requires testing. In one test, prospective patients will wear Pettibon System Weights and have their lateral cervical spine re-x-rayed. Other tests evaluate whether prospective patients' postural muscles are strong enough for the corrective procedures. Typically, as high as 40% lack the strength and endurance they need. So they will be required to go through a rehabilitation program to strengthen their postural muscles before going on to spinal correction' [100].
- 'At the end of acute care, patients are re-x-rayed. The x-rays helps the doctor assess patients' progress and qualification for the next phase of care. Re-x-raying serves another purpose. If patients have been in an accident, it's only after their muscles are no longer in spasm, guarding the spine, that the exact damage can be seen' [187].
- 'Chiropractors claim to "adjust" or "manipulate" the spine. If this is true, the results or changes should be visible on x-rays taken after the adjustment or manipulation. The Pettibon Procedures are one of the few techniques in Chiropractic that cause measurable changes...' [101] p.7.

Pierce results

- Pierce was confounded by inconsistent results and so developed a model of a 'normal spine' and 'true subluxation' and so developed a more rigid system to produce consistent results [188].

Spinal orthopaedic neurological advancement and research (SONAR)

- 'SONAR was developed by Thomas Elliott, Jr., D.C. who was a NUCCA practitioner. SONAR employs procedures for taking and analyzing x-rays' [66].
- '...linear and torque forces in the exact angle and amplitude as determined by x-ray analysis' [152].

Spinal stressology

- 'Standing and seated front-view and side-view full spine x-rays are recommended in severe pain patterns, work related injuries, automobile accidents and degenerative disease conditions. A system analysis consists of standing and seated front-view and side-view full spine x-rays. We can scientifically measure abnormal stress, and predict what specific damage it will cause if not corrected' [189].
- 'First of all, we sit down and tell them what we need to find on x-rays. If we find there is a difference between standing and sitting patterns, and there is a prognosis, then we will accept them. We also say if the spine is degenerative in both standing and sitting positions, that we cannot accept them, or the prognosis is, in fact, poor. Some of our kids, you know, are totally confined to a wheelchair, and it is very difficult to get standing x-rays on them' [128].
- 'A mental-emotional profile is an evaluation based on standing and seated, front and side view, full spine X-rays' [157].
- 'Each [radiographic] measurement allows us to help people understand which emotions are theirs and which emotions are inherited from a previous generation' [157].
- 'People ask if we have to take full spinal X-rays on every patient to gain awareness of their underlying mental-emotional stress issues? The answer is that pain in the body and short leg deficiency will reveal specific information about what specific stressors are taking place within a person's life' [157].
- 'We are saying that we make no cures and can give no guarantees...' [128].
- '...on every patient we record 40 different measurements of critical landmarks of the spine and their variations as to the systemic normals. So each measurement is classified as to whether it is a breakdown component or whether it is in defense. Then the computer makes its analysis and each measurement is then classified as to whether it is mild, moderate, severe, degenerative acute, degenerative severe, or degenerative out of control. We look at this as a way of measuring subluxations on a systemic basis' [128].

- 'We have to evaluate what we've done in order to substantiate what we are doing, and the chiropractic profession doesn't believe in re-evaluation and they haven't put together a subluxation system that would warrant post x-ray analysis. I think this is too bad and is really a short vision type thing' [128].

Sutter specific atlas correction

- Radiographic interpretation is a combination of standard HIO and elements that Sutter invented himself [177].

Zimmerman

- 'Two views taken down through the hole-in-the-head [sic] plus a side view and a front to back view constitute an X-Ray [sic] set. Analysis of these X-Rays provides the information needed to make the proper adjustment' [190].

Appendix 4: sacred stories

Advanced orthogonal

Case reports, patient testimonials, practitioner testimonials, and unsupported extrapolations from basic anatomy: '...in simple terms the human skeleton is "top down design" not "bottom/feet up". This means your posture is driven by the position of your head in space' [160]. Another type of story is related in the concept of 'holding a correction' as determined by radiographic analysis [159].

Applied spinal biomechanical engineering

Practitioner testimonials and patient testimonials, [191] and vague definitions for the practice methods with difficult to decipher language: 'ASBE identifies and reduces spinal distortion through the rehabilitation of normal muscle tissue, restores the normal physiologic dynamics of the spine, and treats within the natural parameters of the individual patient (bilateral symmetrical function is secondary to static non-dynamic gravitational dependent equilibrium)' [83] p. 2. 'Most patients are amazed once they see their X-rays up close' [192].

Applied upper-cervical biomechanics

Essays about the existence of subluxation and its 'correction' proven by the use of thermal (infrared) imaging, as well as case studies that focus on claimed benefits to patients with multiple organic syndromes like cortical blindness, epilepsy, autism, asthma, etc. [193].

Atlas orthogonality

Patient [105] and practitioner testimonials [194]. One case series is cited as well as several case reports. Unsupported extrapolations from basic anatomy with oversimplified analogies are also used: 'The nervous system can be likened to a major super highway. Without problems and all vehicles going the speed limit, travel is smooth and without accident. However, if there is a car crash, traffic slows down and even stops. The highway does not function as it was intended' [144]. 'This one bone can effect [sic] the alignment of the entire spine. The spine is like a chain—when the first link is twisted and turned, each link down to the last turns—thereby disrupting the rest of the chain. Consider the atlas the first and therefore the most important link in that chain' [144].

Blair

[Chiropractic] helped Blair's chronic bronchial asthma so much that he decided to become a chiropractor [66] p.30.

Extrapolations from basic science: 'All nerve messages between the brain and body must pass through the upper cervical area' [69]. Appeal to authority epistemology: 'Dr. Palmer conducted studies in Germany on cadavers and found that the brain stem or medulla, extended into the neural canal down to the level of the lamina of the second cervical vertebrae, at which point it becomes the spinal cord extending downward. The brain stem has been referred to as "Houston Control". It is the area where nerve cell centers are located that control many of the major functions of the body...' [98]. 'If for example the atlas is impinged against the part of the cord that sends messages to the left hand, that individual may experience a numbness, burning or tingling sensation in that hand' [98]. Note: These symptoms are lower motor neuron signs and would be present if a peripheral nerve was impinged, not if the spinal cord or medulla oblongata were. 'If the nerve tracts at the brain stem level go to the heart are being impinged that individual may experience high blood pressure, palpitations or an irregular heartbeat' [98]. 'Any part of the body can be effected [sic] when there is pressure on the brain stem or spinal cord because almost all of the nerves have to pass through this area before reaching the part of the body they innervate'. 'WHEN [sic] we turn the fan off it does not stop immediately because the momentum must ease down and stop. When we turn the fan on it does not reach its maximum r.p.m.'s [sic] immediately because it must pick up or gain momentum. I, [sic] think you appreciate our idea of momentum, and resistance. In applying this to your body, recognize that your body is living under a condition of momentum. Every impression you receive is more or less resisted by the tissue cell. Let's consider a physical force such as a fall. The invasion of force to the body caused by the fall overcomes the resistance of the body internally. These momenta coming together causes a clash of forces. If the invasive force is greater than the internal resistive force, the shock waves or forces cause the vertebral subluxation. Now that the vertebral subluxation has been produced an alteration or interference of life energy (nerve impulses) causes a dis-eased condition to develop in one tissue cell, two cells, then 200, 2,000 and then 2 million. Proportionately, the longer the subluxation exists, the greater becomes the momentum of speed of diseases. The longer it runs, the longer you go down hill, the greater becomes it's [sic] speed and the greater becomes the momentum of disease' [111]. 'A subluxation may be present for months or years before producing any outward signs such as pain or symptoms, causing the body to break down to a state of diseases' [98]. 'The purpose of the Blair Chiropractic technique is not to diagnose or treat diseases or conditions, but to analyze and correct vertebral subluxations in an accurate, precise and specific manner to allow the body's intelligence, (see chiropractic philosophy) to mend, repair and maintain health from within' [98].

Chiropractic BioPhysics

In addition to case reports, CBP utilised case anecdotes: '...studies have shown that many CBP patients have also seen a dramatic improvement of other health issues, including ADD/ADHD, Asthma, Blood Pressure, Chest Pain, Chronic Fatigue, Constipation, Fibromyalgia, Headaches, Hypertension, etc.' [167].

Distorted evidence: 'In CBP® Technique, the use of initial and follow-up spinal x-rays or radiographs is deemed necessary; however, some in chiropractic have condemned the use of follow-radiographs to collect alignment data. Importantly, there is data [sic] to show that the use of medical/chiropractic x-rays constitutes a very minor health risk and in fact has been shown to be of benefit (decreased sickness and cancer mortality rates) in some studies' [114].

Oversimplified analogies: 'In reality, the only way to see what an individual patient's spine alignment looks likes, is to obtain spinal imaging such as Radiography or X-ray. No-one would not [sic] take their car to the mechanic and say: Something's wrong with my engine but don't look under the hood – Would you? Then why would anyone want a Chiropractor to adjust-treat their spine [sic] without having an x-ray to see what the person's spine looked like? Would You?' [114].

Cowin upper cervical orthogonal

Case anecdotes [195] and a single case report [196]. 'A surprising number of stubborn health problems have been helped by chiropractic care over the past 106 years. Current conjectures for the successes reported in the past century include the following component ideas. Most persistent health problems have more than one cause' [68]. 'A frequent contributing cause is somatic disturbance, such as loading distortion on the supporting structures, causing the highly movable spinal bones to lose their proper alignment' [68]. 'The somatic disturbance most frequently assessed and treated by chiropractors, called a subluxation, is a persistent and/or recurring, small alteration in alignment, movement integrity and/or physiological function in one or more spinal motion segments' [68].

Duff method of analysis

Patient testimonials [106] and a mission statement which reads: 'Health and Happiness are Synonymous' [121].

Gonstead

Clarence Gonstead entered the profession on the belief of his own personal rheumatoid arthritis cure at the hands of a chiropractor. The other story about Gonstead personally was that he was somehow superhuman, with claims that while in practice he adjusted 250 patients every day in the 1940s, and even more in subsequent decades, increasing his office hours and often finishing the last patient at 2:30 am [75].

Practitioner testimonials [197] and case reports [198]. Case reports were solicited on the website: 'We are looking for both cases which you successfully helped and those you didn't and might have even referred out [sic]. We are also looking for cases that you might consider ordinary or routine, as these are rarely presented, but we often see patients with these presentations. This is the minimum that we would like if you want to submit a case study for the newsletter and web site. We have removed some parts that are required for peer-reviewed journals and have emphasized some to provide a Gonstead perspective. If you absolutely cannot write, send us whatever you have, and we will work with it' [147].

Oversimplified analogies: 'The Gonstead Concept of chiropractic begins with a basic biomechanical principle of physics. Every engineer, architect, builder and carpenter knows the importance of a proper foundation in constructing a building, for this insures durability and long life. Any slight change or shift in the foundation can cause a great amount of deviation in the top part of the structure and, perhaps, ultimately, its collapse. When the pelvic girdle or any of the vertebrae (bones making up the spinal column) become tilted or rotated out of their proper position, dramatic changes may occur in the body' [120].

Assertion of superiority over upper cervical systems: 'If just the top misaligned vertebra was adjusted, in cases where additional vertebrae are misaligned, only limited relief could result. This would not be getting to the source of the trouble. For complete and lasting results, all of the misaligned vertebrae must be identified and then a program can be initiated to restore them to their normal position' [120].

Grostic

Sacred stories included the above-mentioned tales of Grostic's health and restoration, his superhuman practice schedule, case reports, case anecdotes, and theories on the mechanism of vital energy flow and health [66]. Several paragraphs of the official textbook were a treatment of the concept of spinal irritation; they quoted texts from the 19th century and their discussions of how bones may impinge the flow of nervous energy, leading to derangement of the functions of organs [66] p.2. This information is presented as relevant and is reprinted without questions or clarification.

'The evidence that 'specific' upper cervical chiropractic is effective in promoting wellness is compelling and widespread. You need only look for it' [149].

'...the peer-reviewed literature... shows a documented correlation between orthogonally-based care (Grostic/Orthospinology, NUCCA and Atlas Orthogonality) and the improvement of various patient complaints' [149]. There followed a list of 22 papers claiming resolution of cases of various conditions, including seizure disorders, Tourette's syndrome, and congenital brain malformations, one of which appeared in a peer-reviewed journal that is included in PubMed [149]. The anecdotes continued with broad claims: 'Athletes and people looking to achieve peak potential performance also seek Chiropractic care to have the best possible brain body connection so their reaction time and endurance is at it's best. Many pregnant mothers have experienced the benefits of shorter births, easier labor, and pain free pregnancies while under Chiropractic care' [199]. The stories also included extrapolation of anatomical findings. 'minute amounts of atlas [upper cervical vertebra] laterality or rotation were important from a neurological standpoint...' [66] p.19. 'The two most plausible hypotheses have to do with spinal cord tension and mechanoreceptive dysafferentation' [149].

Kale

'By eliminating nerve interference, Specific Chiropractic, ("Brain Stem Specialist") can correct numerous health problems and help prevent many conditions from developing. This enables the body to maintain its natural, inborn resistance to illness and disease. For you to have a longer, healthier and happier life, it is imperative that you be aware of the fact Subluxation of the top two vertebrae is a serious condition and can easily develop conditions affecting every part of the body. It has been estimated that as much as 90% of the world's population suffers from this type of Subluxation in varying degrees interfering with the normal function of the body, and therefore, interfering with and preventing health. Don't wait for health threatening, or even life threatening conditions to develop. Have a "Brain Stem Specialist" evaluation today' [200].

'The spinal column is intended to protect the delicate Brain Stem [sic] and the nerves leading from it. When it becomes subluxated, the column does not protect. Instead, the misaligned spinal bones of C1 and C2 impinge the Brain Stem. This causes interference with normal nerve function to all parts of the body. When there is interference in normal nerve function, there will be health problems, sickness and disease' [200].

'For you to have a longer, healthier and happier life, it is imperative that you be aware of the fact Subluxation of the top two vertebrae is a serious condition and can easily develop conditions affecting every part of the body. It has been estimated that as much as 90% of the world's population suffers from this type of Subluxation in varying degrees interfering with the normal function of the body, and therefore, interfering with and preventing health. Don't wait for health threatening, or even life threatening conditions to develop. Have a Specific Upper Cervical Chiropractic evaluation today' [201].

'Subluxation of the top two vertebrae, C1 and C2, Atlas-Axis, close down the opening of the neural canal in this area and result in pressure upon the "Brain Stem", thus causing impingement of spinal nerve tracts. This can result in malfunction in all parts of the human body with resulting pathological changes. Mild to moderate malfunction results in sickness and disease, while extreme malfunction results in DEATH!!' [97]. [emphasis original]

'The patients... had positive results and some had complete recovery from such problems as Parkinson's Disease, AIDS, Paralysis, Sight and Hearing disorders [74].

Knee chest upper cervical specific (KCUCS)

'Upper Cervical Care is not new to healthcare; it was first introduced back in the early 1920's. Dr. BJ Palmer began his endeavor back in 1910 when x-ray was introduced and visualization of the spine was made possible. In 1935 the Research Clinic was opened and began seeing patients. From 1935–1942 5,000 cases were seen and of those, 3,856 made a full recovery, 1,013 cases reported improvement, only 49 or 0.9% reported no improvement, with 82 or 1.6% unreported. 97.3% were recovered or improved. Then in 1942 – 1954 they began to only except cases that had no prior success with medicine or otherwise. 139,096 cases were seen, 63.8% (88,743) made a full recovery, 29.4% (40,894) improved, and 6.7% (9,319) no change'. There were also four case reports supporting the KCUCS system, one of which was published in a peer-reviewed journal that is included in PubMed [202] as well as case anecdotes [171].

Logan basic

'We can prove conclusively that the sacrum and coccyx are the primary portion of the primary curvature of the spinal column-"as the sacrum goes so goes the spine"-

and that it is absolutely necessary to restore the sacrum to normal position and relationship with articulating bones to effectively reduce curvatures, subluxations, and disease' [151].

National upper cervical chiropractic association (NUCCA)

Case anecdotes [203,184] and extrapolations from basic anatomical observation [122] were both present.

'It is the experience of upper cervical chiropractors (2-3% of all chiropractors) in general and NUCCA practitioners in particular that there is no anatomical region of the human body that is so commonly a first cause of postural problems as the upper cervical spine. Specifically this first cause is itself often the effect of injury from trauma, surgery, applied mechanical forces, or even age itself. This site of injury can be at any location; either above, at, or below C-1. The C-1 joint, composed of C0-C1-C2, is the focus of upper cervical work. It is well known that at no other location in the spine are the joint mechanoreceptors as dense, motion so allowed, and structures below and probably above so dependent' [122]. 'The design and development of the Anatometer by Dr. Gregory and Peter Benesh, an instrument which measures bodily distortions before and after the C-1 adjustment, providing proof of the effects of a C-1 subluxation' [102].

The Mission Statement includes: 'Maximizing the human health potential associated with the reduction of the Atlas Subluxation Complex (ASC)' and 'Maintaining an effective, passionate, responsible organization contributing to the standards of the measurable, objective and reproducible reduction of the Atlas Subluxation Complex' [204].

'The Atlas Subluxation Complex includes the measurable misalignment of the head, atlas and cervical spine, the contracted spinal musculature, postural distortion and short leg phenomena. The Atlas Subluxation Complex Syndrome includes the ASC and its effects on the central and peripheral nervous system and the relationship to the symptoms and conditions directly related and those associated with this progressive degenerative condition' [76]. Misalignments of less than a degree can cause systemic disorders: '...there is only a very small range of neurological alignments possible...' for example, the atlas must be laterally displaced '...less than 0.75 degrees...' [205,122]. '...UCRF (Upper Cervical Research Foundation) research provides the validation to understand the wide variety of negative effects that a misaligned upper cervical spine has on human well-being, and provides answers on how to best correct the misaligned spine, to determine the practice limits of the upper cervical specialist, to determine the extent that a misaligned upper cervical spine affects the entire human organism, and to establish the necessity for insurance coverage and other support by involved agencies' [206].

Orthospinology

Patient testimonials [207]. 'Spinal misalignments cause abnormal input to the nervous system. This phenomenon is referred to as the Vertebral Subluxation Complex' [186]. 'Abnormal input to the nervous system creates Body Imbalance, resulting in postural distortions that manifest as head, neck and back pain, numbness, tingling, and pain radiating into the arms and legs, and compromised general health'. 'Chiropractic is the science of detecting and correcting spinal misalignments that cause irregular input to the nervous system, restoring balance to the body and its systems. Normal health is the natural result' [186]. 'Because the upper cervical spine connects to the brainstem, a misalignment there may also disrupt brain to body communication leading to symptoms such as headaches and migraines, sinus problems, vertigo and blackouts, seizures, TMJ and facial pain as well as fatigue, immune compromise and general health deterioration. Even before symptoms manifest, this misalignment called the Vertebral Subluxation Complex, may be limiting your bodies' ability to function at the highest level creating an internal environment conducive to the development of disease' [186].

Oversimplified analogies: 'The nervous system works like a telephone network carrying messages between the brain and the body. When the nervous system is working correctly, the body has the proper information to heal itself and maintain balance of all your systems. Static on the telephone line interferes with the messages being sent. If the nervous system has "static" (irregular input), the messages between the brain and the body will be interrupted. A misalignment of the vertebra of the spine may cause distortion, and body imbalance results. When a Vertebral Misalignment causes the nervous system to initiate imbalances of the body systems, it is known as a Vertebral Subluxation Complex, or in simpler terms: loss of body balance. Upper Cervical doctors are trained to determine exactly how the upper cervical spine has misaligned in your neck and the set-up and exact angle necessary to correct it. Once the Vertebral Subluxation Complex is corrected and the "static" removed, the body can return to a state of balance' [186]. A video is provided on the official website, apparently showing an unconscious patient with a known seizure disorder revived by application of this technique [173].

Palmer upper cervical specific/HIO

The writings of BJ Palmer are replete with case anecdotes, [43] as is commonly known.

Pettibon

Case anecdotes [208] as well as patient and practitioner testimonials [107]. 'Our purpose: To energize lives through spine & posture rehabilitation' [209]. Pettibon and Vern Pierce '...discovered how chiropractic students—about 100 from Palmer and Life—who entered college with x-rays showing normal or near normal lordotic cervical curves, on comparison x-rays taken at the end of their schooling, had abnormal military or kyphotic necks, and most had spinal pathology' [113]. Sharon Freese-Pettibon '...did what Dr. Pettibon prescribed and two weeks later was eating solid food for the first time in three months, her bleeding ulcer was starting to heal and she was beginning to feel better.' After a surfing accident, 'In three visits the paralysis was totally gone and she was able to return to Hawaii with her health intact' [113].

Extrapolation from basic science: 'Gravity is an absolute environment to which the upright spine and posture of humans must develop and relate. Since gravity is an absolute, there has to be an absolute optimal position for the upright spine and posture. The skull is a vertebra. It's the only vertebra that knows its neurologically optimal position and has the ability to establish and maintain that posture. The global spine's position relative to gravity is more important than its units or its segments. A less than optimum lateral and A-P spine and posture compromises spinal function' [210].

Distorted evidence: 'Debunking the Myth About X-Rays with Facts: The accepted cumulative dose of ionizing radiation during pregnancy is 5 rads The most sensitive time during pregnancy is between 10 and 17 weeks. Two routine chest x-rays = .00007 rad. Radiation to the fetus shouldn't exceed 10,000 millirads. Annual environmental radiation is 300 millirads/year which equals 12 chest x-rays. The Pettibon X-ray Series (7 views) = 20 millirads. To exceed 10,000 millirads would take 3,124 x-rays' [100]. No references were cited for this information.

Pierce results

'... high quality chiropractic care can not only save the lives of your patients, but your practice as well as our profession!' [188]. 6 case anecdotes, including '100 percent recovery!!!' from headaches, low back pain, heart palpitations, migraines, and degenerative disc disease ('Osteophytic bridge being RESORBED!!!' 'Notice IVD regeneration') [211].

Spinal orthopaedic neurological advancement and research (SONAR)

'Not having your atlas corrected to restore body balance is like continuing to drive a car that is out of alignment. Over time, everything is going to break down. You can keep replacing the tires, but unless you have the car aligned, you'll just be wasting your money. Similarly you can keep taking medication, but if your atlas is out of its proper position, causing the problem, you're not going to get well until you get your atlas corrected' [155]. '...if the atlas has moved out of position even a fraction of a degree very serious things can result' [212]. 'The power that made the body heals the body, it happens no other way' [213].

Spinal stressology

Patient testimonials [214] and case anecdotes [214]. Muscular dystrophy '...is a psychosomatically-induced disorder...We find that usually it is referenced to inherited abortion, inherited abandonment, and inherited adoption processes where something of this nature has occurred in parents, grandparents, or even great grandparents, and the hostility of that is passed on, and we believe that muscular dystrophy becomes a psychosomatically-induced illness wherein the child unconsciously develops a covert disease process that will lead to his death' [128].

'I just lost a son-in-law, 35 years old, whose x-rays showed, back in 1986, that he inherited death wishes... I should not say the x-rays showed; the personality analysis of the psychological coefficients from the x-ray findings would tend to indicate that he had multiple death wishes' [128].

'Well, it's kind of interesting that in the article on "SIDS Death", they found that the average atlas angle was at 30 degrees. Now, when we find 30 standing and 29 sitting, the 29 indicates an intent to commit suicide and the 30 indicates that the person tried to commit suicide, so we feels that even in SIDS death that there is a fetal suicide' [128].

'Comparative radiographs are justified and mandatory for monitoring patient progress and for evaluating treatment effectiveness. -From the comparative x-rays an updated diagnosis and prognosis is ascertained. Documentation establishes objectivity' [215]. 'When you see an X-ray of the entire spine, you start to understand the why' [215]. 'Dr. Ward has found that disease, both physical and mental, shows up in a specific spinal curvature pattern' [176]. 'Maybe we shouldn't be surprised to discover that your spine reflects your personality, or that today's stress was passed down from a previous generation' [216]. 'Each measurement allows us to help people understand which emotions are theirs and which emotions are inherited from a previous generation' [216]. 'When a person is driven in their behavior, the spine always goes forward to normal. The neck goes forward, the mid-back curve goes forward, the lumbar curve reverses. People who are most driven are forward in both the standing and sitting position. A forward spinal curve relates to the driven mother, grandmother and or great grandmother. When the spine begins to go forward, the person will begin to feel exhausted. The more the spine deviates forward the more immune compromised the person will be' [216].

Sutter specific atlas correction

Rejection of scientific enquiry: 'Any attempt to explain how these elements have come to be arranged into this complex, self-regulating "machine", how these elements have come to feel, think, and live as one unified whole, upon a purely material basis, is doomed to failure in advance' [129].

'You will note that our examination is largely confined to the spinal column, and particularly to the topmost part of the spinal column immediately below the head. This is because our research work has proved that practically all of the disturbances of nerve structures which interfere with control of normal body function take place in the region of the first spinal bone or vertebra called the atlas. Our object in making this examination is not to diagnose disease as does the physician, but to gain information regarding the cause of the interference that is preventing Innate Intelligence from curing. When this cause is corrected Innate Intelligence immediately starts the curing process. The disease may be in the stomach, the liver, the heart, the intestines, or any other part of the body, but wherever it is Innate Intelligence knows, and is the only one who knows, exactly what to do about it. The best doctor in existence is the Intelligence that God left in charge of our bodies...' [129].

'The effects of such nerve interference may not show up for some period of time. It is much easier and better to correct the cause of such interferences as they occur and thus prevent the development of some condition than to correct a condition once well established. Should anything unusual in the way of a fall or sudden strain or jar to the head or neck occur, it would be advisable to have the atlas checked as soon as possible. Once a month would be a good average interval for checking the condition of the atlas vertebra under usual circumstances. Develop the once a month check-up habit. It is inexpensive health insurance' [129]. 'Only when symptoms disappear, following the correction of the cause of the condition within the body, as a result of regeneration by the Innate Intelligence within the body has anything really worth while and of lasting benefit been accomplished [129].

Zimmerman

Patient and practitioner testimonials [190]. 'A chiropractor who is skilled in the art of adjusting by machine can free the spinal cord from pressure and get the patient well' [56]. 'The basic natural premise behind the idea is the fact that life depends on a connection from the brain to the body through the central nervous system. This connection is in the form of nerve fibres leading down the spinal cord from the brain to all parts of the body. These fibres (there are about 10 billion of them) are like wires in a telephone cable. They are subject to pressure at the base of the skull when the atlas or axis vertebra is out of its normal alignment' [56]. 'When pressure is removed from the spinal cord, the effect is the same as turning on the electric power to a light bulb. Without the electricity the lamp does not produce any light. When the patient's body is deprived of energy by a nerve pressure, anything can go wrong and death may occur. All it takes to restore the flow of energy to the sick body is ONE accurate adjustment' [56]. 'Trauma is the origin of most subluxations, even back to "birth trauma" including forceps delivery' [56].

Appendix 5: special language

Advanced orthogonal

With this technique, special language includes the term 'orthogonal' meaning 'in normal position'. The standard definition of orthogonal is 'at right angles'. In addition, the x-ray views, 'nasium' and 'vertex' are not standard views taught to or utilised by medical radiographers and so the names can be considered special language. The term 'three dimensional x-rays' is also specially defined here, meaning x-rays taken from three different angles, not the creation of a 3-D image as the term is understood for advanced imaging or modern movies and television.

Applied upper-cervical biomechanics

The non-standard radiographic views of nasium and 'base posterior' [162] as well as 'arthrokinematic radiographic analysis,' and 'neurophysiological imaging' [143].

Atlas orthogonality

'Orthogonal' as used by the technique, as was seen with Advanced Orthogonal technique (above). The term 'three dimensional x-rays' was also the same as that used by Advanced Orthogonal and has the same meaning, that is, x-rays taken from three different angles, not the creation of a 3-D image.

Blair

The names of some of the radiographic views, 'Blair Oblique Protractoviews', 'base-posterior' and the terms for some of the equipment for radiographic imaging and analysis: 'D-arm protractor' and 'Blair Protracto clamp', used in radiography. Another term, undefined, was used in this way: 'The presence of cervical nerve interference is established by observation of both persistent differential paraspinal derinothermographic pattern and functional leg length deficiency' [103]. Although 'derinothermographic' may or may not have been directly related to radiography, it is included here because of its stated close relation to x-ray analysis of the subluxation.

Chiropractic BioPhysics

'PostureRay' software for x-ray subluxation analysis as well as the name of the technique and its acronym, and the names for non-mainstream radiographic views like 'nasium'. The special language of this technique claimed propriety for its name and devices, like PostureRay, which were rarely found without the® registration symbol.

Cowin upper cervical orthogonal
Non-standard x-ray view names (e.g. nasium, vertex, etc.) [82].

Gonstead
Highly detailed vocabulary of subluxation 'listings' [124] or descriptions of perceived spinal misalignments, and was bolstered recently to help bring all practitioners of the system into line. 'The GCSS Gonstead Technique Terminology Project began in response to a highly inaccurate 2002 article on the Gonstead System...' [217].

The terms 'split' or 'gradient' screens: 'In the past, and not uncommonly today, x-ray screens of different sensitivity speeds were used to compensate for the different body densities' [124].

Grostic
The non-standard x-ray view names (e.g. nasium, vertex, etc.), 'cephalocentroscope'.

Kale
The non-standard x-ray view names (e.g. nasium, vertex, etc.).

Knee chest upper cervical specific (KCUCS)
Similar to that used by Blair, as well as 'Spiz'.

Logan basic
X-ray marking system [218].

National upper cervical chiropractic association (NUCCA)
The non-standard x-ray view names (e.g. nasium, vertex, etc.), and 'anatometer' [219].

Orthospinology
The non-standard x-ray view names (e.g. nasium, vertex, etc.), [185] and spiz or spizzerinctum [220].

Pettibon
Non-standard x-ray view names (e.g. base-posterior), and postural change descriptors (e.g. cervical dorsal angle, upper angle, lower angle, etc.) [221].

Pierce results
Subluxation. Atlas 'out of compensation' [211]. 'Spinal visualizer' believed to mean cineradiography [211]. 'Master Level' certification, [222] not through a university.

Sutter specific atlas correction
None found other than 'subluxation' and 'nerve interference' [129].

Zimmerman
None found other than 'subluxation' [56].

Additional files

Additional file 1: List of named techniques that used plain radiography for subluxation detection.

Additional file 2: Summary of religious characteristics in each technique.

Competing interests
The author declares that he has no competing interests.

Acknowledgements
Many thanks to Michael Sturma, PhD and Barclay Bakkum, DC, PhD for manuscript review, and to Bart Green, DC, MSEd, Lawrence Siordia, MD, DC as well as a source that wishes to remain anonymous, for assistance with research.

References
1. Palmer BJ: **Introduction of Spinography: Its Origin, Purpose, Field of Labor and why.** In *Chiropractic Spinography.* 2nd edition. Edited by Thompson EA, Davenport IA. USA: Palmer School of Chiropractic; 1919.
2. Keating JC Jr: *B.J. Of Davenport : The Early Years of Chiropractic.* Davenport, Iowa: Association for the History of Chiropractic; 1997.
3. Ammendolia C, Bombardier C, Hogg-Johnson S, Glazier R: **Views on radiography use for patients with acute low back pain among chiropractors in an Ontario community.** *J Manipulative Physiol Therapeut* 2004, **25**(8):511–520.
4. Scheurmier N, Breen AC: **A pilot study of the purchase of manipulation services for acute low back pain in the United Kingdom.** *J Manipulative Physiol Therapeut* 1998, **21**(1):14–18.
5. Ernst E: **Chiropractors' use of x-rays.** *Br J Radiol* 1998, **71**:249–251.
6. Williams CM, Maher CG, Hancock MJ, McAuley JH, McLachlan AJ, Britt H, Fahridin S, Harrison C, Latimer J: **Low back pain and best practice care: a survey of general practice physicians.** *Arch Intern Med* 2010, **170**(3):271–277.
7. Chou R, Fu R, Carrino JA, Deyo RA: **Imaging strategies for low-back pain: systematic review and meta-analysis.** *Lancet* 2009, **373**(9662):463–472.
8. Isaacs DM, Marinac J, Sun C: **Radiograph use in low back pain: a United States emergency department database analysis.** *J Emerg Med* 2004, **26**(1):37–45.
9. Carey TS, Garrett J: **Patterns of ordering diagnostic tests for patients with acute Low back pain.** *Ann Intern Med* 1996, **125**(10):807–814.
10. Committee to Assess Health Risks from Exposure to Low Levels of Ionizing Radiation: *Health Risks from Exposure to Low Levels of Ionizing Radiation: BEIR VII Phase 2.* Washington, DC: The National Academies Press; 2006.
11. Berrington de Gonzalez A, Darby S: **Risk of cancer from diagnostic X-rays: estimates for the UK and 14 other countries.** *Lancet* 2004, **363**(9406):345–351.
12. Mendelson RM, Murray CPJ: **Towards the appropriate use of diagnostic imaging.** *Med J Aust* 2007, **187**(1):5–6.
13. Sherman R: **Chiropractic x-ray rationale.** *J Can Chiropr Assoc* 1986, **30**(1):33–35.
14. Bussières AE, Peterson C, Taylor JAM: **Diagnostic imaging practice guidelines for musculoskeletal complaints in adults—an evidence-based approach: introduction.** *J Manip Physiol Ther* 2007, **30**(9):617–683.
15. Dixon P: **Chiropractors' use of x-rays.** *Br J Radiol* 1998, **71**:897–900.
16. Ammendolia C, Taylor JAM, Pennick V, Côté P, Hogg-Johnson S, Bombardier C: **Adherence to radiography guidelines for Low back pain: a survey of chiropractic schools worldwide.** *J Manip Physiol Ther* 2008, **31**(6):412–418.
17. Humphreys BK, Peterson CK, Muehlemann D, Haueter P: **Are Swiss chiropractors different than other chiropractors? Results of the job analysis survey 2009.** *J Manip Physiol Ther* 2010, **33**(7):519–535.
18. Haas M, Taylor JAM, Gillette RG: **The routine use of radiographic spinal displacement analysis: a dissent.** *J Manip Physiol Ther* 1999, **22**(4):254–259.

19. Kouri BEP, Parsons RG, Alpert HR: **Physician self-referral for diagnostic imaging: review of the empiric literature.** *Am J Roentgenol* 2002, **179**:843–850.
20. Bronfort G, Haas M, Evans R, Leininger B, Triano J: **Effectiveness of manual therapies: the UK evidence report.** *Chiropr Osteopat* 2010, **18**:3.
21. Clar C, Tsertsvadze A, Court R, Hundt G, Clarke A, Sutcliffe P: **Clinical effectiveness of manual therapy for the management of musculoskeletal and non-musculoskeletal conditions: systematic review and update of UK evidence report.** *Chiropr & Manual Ther* 2014, **22**(1):12.
22. **American chiropractic board of radiology: home page.** [http://www.acbr.org] Accessed August 13, 2014.
23. Poehner WG: **Chiropractic roentgenology.** *The Chiropractic Journal* 1939, **8**(1):14. 48.
24. Bussières AE, Taylor JAM, Peterson C: **Diagnostic imaging practice guidelines for musculoskeletal complaints in adults - an evidence-based approach: part 1: lower extremity disorders.** *J Manipulative Physiol Therapeut* 2007, **30**(9):684–717.
25. Bussières AE, Peterson C, Taylor JAM: **Diagnostic imaging guideline for musculoskeletal complaints in adults—an evidence-based approach—part 2: upper extremity disorders.** *J Manip Physiol Ther* 2008, **31**(1):2–32.
26. Bussières AE, Taylor JAM, Peterson C: **Diagnostic imaging practice guidelines for musculoskeletal complaints in adults—an evidence-based approach—part 3: spinal disorders.** *J Manip Physiol Ther* 2008, **31**(1):33–88.
27. Harrison D, Kent C, Betz J, Harrison D, Oakley P: **Practicing Chiropractors' Committee on Radiology Protocols.** Elko, NV, USA: PCCRP; 2006.
28. Harrison DD, Siskin LA: **Best Practices and Practice Guidelines.** Arlington, VA, USA: International Chiropractors Association; 2008.
29. Keating JC: **Beyond the theosophy of chiropractic.** *J Manip Physiol Ther* 1989, **12**(2):147–150.
30. Cherkin DC, Mootz RD: **A new AHCPR report: "Chiropractic in the United States: training, practice, and research".** *J Am Chiropract Assoc* 1998, **35**(7):16–16.
31. Mirtz T: **Universal intelligence: a theological entity in conflict with Lutheran theology.** *J Chiropr Humanit* 2000, **9**:55–71.
32. Mirtz TA: **The question of theology for chiropractic: a theological study of Chiropractic's prime tenets.** *J Chiropr Humanit* 2001, **10**:48–82.
33. Keating J, Charlton K, Grod J, Perle S, Sikorski D, Winterstein J: **Subluxation: dogma or science?** *Chiropr & Osteopat* 2005, **13**:17.
34. Keating J, Mootz R: **The influence of political medicine on chiropractic dogma: implications for scientific development.** *J Manip Physiol Ther* 1989, **12**:393–398.
35. Phillips RB: **The battle for innate: a perspective on fundamentalism in chiropractic.** *J Chiropr Humanit* **11**:2–10.
36. Phillips RB, Mootz RD: **Contemporary Chiropractic Philosophy.** In *Principles and Practice of Chiropractic.* Edited by Haldeman S. Norwalk, CT, USA: Appleton and Lange; 1992.
37. Brown CG: **Chiropractic and Christianity: the power of pain to adjust cultural alignments.** *Church Hist* 2010, **79**(1):144–181.
38. Moore JS: *Chiropractic in America: the history of a medical alternative.* Baltimore: Johns Hopkins University Press; 1993.
39. Thompson EA: *Chiropractic Spinography.* 2nd edition. Iowa, USA: Davenport; 1919.
40. Gaucher-Peslherbe P-L, Lawrence DJ: *Chiropractic: early concepts in their historical setting.* Lombard, IL: National College of Chiropractic; 1993.
41. Keating JC Jr: **Several pathways in the evolution of chiropractic manipulation.** *J Manip Physiol Ther* 2003, **26**(5):300–321.
42. Quigley WH: **Bartlett Joshua Palmer: toward an understanding of the man, 1881–1961.** *Chiropract Hist* 1995, **15**(2):30–35.
43. Palmer BJ: *The Subluxation Specific –The Adjustment Specific,* Volume XVIII. Palmer School of Chiropractic: Davenport, IA, USA; 1934.
44. Palmer BJ: *Answers,* Volume XXVIII. Davenport, IA, USA: Chiropractic Fountain Head; 1952.
45. Palmer BJ: *Chiropractic Clinical Controlled Research,* Volume XXV. Davenport, IA, USA: Chiropractic Fountain Head; 1951.
46. Palmer BJ: *The Science of Chiropractic,* Volume II. 3rd edition. Davenport, IA, USA: Palmer School of Chiropractic; 1920.
47. Dye AA: *The evolution of chiropractic: its discovery and development.* 1st edition. Philadelphia, PA, USA: A Aug Dye, DC; 1939.
48. Wardwell WI: *Chiropractic: History and Evolution of a new Profession.* St. Louis: Mosby-Year Book; 1992.
49. Cooperstein R, Gleberzon BJ: *Technique Systems in Chiropractic.* 1st edition. Edinburgh: Churchill Livingstone; 2004.
50. Palmer DD: *The Chiropractor.* Los Angeles: Beacon Light Publishing Co.; 1914.
51. Palmer D: *The Chiropractor's adjuster: text-book of the Science, Art and philosophy of chiropractic for students and practitioners.* Portland, OR, USA: Portland Printing HousePortland, OR, USA; 1910.
52. Palmer DD: **Chiropractic as Religion.** Edited by Johnson PW. 1911:1. http://www.chiro.org/Plus/History/Persons/PalmerDD/PalmerDD's_Religion-of-Chiro.pdf.
53. Gibbons RW: **Chiropractic's Abraham Flexner: the lonely journey of John J Nugent, 1935–1963.** *Chiropract Hist* 1985, **5**(1):45–51.
54. Stephenson RW: *Chiropractic Textbook,* Volume 14. 4th edition. Davenport, IA, USA: Palmer School of Chiropractic; 1927.
55. Johnson CB, McKell IJ, Thompson EA: **Locating the cause of disease by x-ray.** Ogden, Utah: The Ogden Standard; 1917:9.
56. Zimmerman AD: **An Adjusting Machine to Correct Subluxation.** In *Digest of Chiropractic Economics,* Volume 5. Ponte Vedra Beach, FL, USA: Chiropractic Economics; 1963:14.
57. Gonstead Clnical Studies Society: **What makes us so special?** [http://www.gonstead.com/index.php?content_type=general_content&content=10] Accessed April 05, 2013.
58. Owens EF Jr: **Line drawing analyses of static cervical X ray used in chiropractic.** *J Manipulative Physiol Ther* 1992, **15**(7):442–449.
59. Alston W: *The Encyclopedia of Philosophy,* Volume 7. New York: Macmillian; 1967.
60. Smart N: *The Religious Experience of Mankind,* Volume 3. New York: Scribner; 1984.
61. Durkheim E: *The Elementary Forms of the Religious Life.* New York: The Free Press; 1995.
62. Yandell KE: *Philosophy of Religion: A Contemporary Introduction.* London: Routledge; 1999.
63. Geertz C: **Religion as a Cultural System.** In *The Interpretation of Cultures: Selected Essays.* Edited by Geertz C. Waukegan, IL, USA: Fontana Press; 1993.
64. Peterson M, Hasker W, Reichenback B, Basinger D: *Reason and Religious Belief: An Introduction to the Philosophy of Religion.* Oxford: Oxford University Press; 1991.
65. Albanese CL: *Nature Religion in America: From the Algonkian Indians to the New Age.* Chicago, USA: University of Chicago Press; 1990.
66. Eriksen K, Rochester R: *Orthospinology Procedures: An Evidence-Based Approach to Spinal Care, Based on the John F Grostic Model and Procedure.* 1st edition. Philadelphia, PA, USA: Lippincott Williams & Wilkins; 2007.
67. **ChiroMatrix - discover wellness: Borges chiropractic - research supports chiropractic.** [http://borgeschiro.com/research-supports-chiropractic.html] Accessed April 07, 2013.
68. **UpCSpine: Upper Cervical Orthogonal - Cowin.** [http://www.upcspine.com/tech1.htm] Accessed May 10, 2013.
69. Blair Chiropractic Society: **Blair Chiropractic Society (home page).** [http://www.blairchiropractic.com] Accessed April 12, 2013.
70. **Chiropractic BioPhysics: Origins of CBP®.** [http://www.idealspine.com/origins-of-cbp/] Accessed April 14, 2013.
71. **Elliott SONAR Chiropractic: Elliott SONAR Chiropractic Doctors.** [http://www.sonarchiropractic.com/sonarchiropracticdocs.htm] Accessed May 07, 2013.
72. **Advanced Orthogonal: mission statement.** [http://www.advancedorthogonal.com/mission-statement/] Accessed April 05, 2013.
73. **Gonstead clinical studies society: what is the gonstead clinical studies society.** [http://gonstead.com/what-is-the-gonstead-clinical-studies-society/] Accessed April 05, 2013.
74. **Kale Chiropractic Center: Dr Kale.** [http://thespecific.com/blog/2011/02/07/kale-chiropractic-research-clinic/] Accessed May 03, 2013.
75. Amman MJ: **Who was Dr. Gonstead? The history of Clarence S. Gonstead, D.C.** [http://gonstead.com/who-was-dr-gonstead/] Accessed January 31, 2013.
76. **Upper Cervical Research Foundation: Home page.** [http://www.ucrf.org] Accessed May 04, 2013.
77. Duff R: **Home page.** [http://www.duffchiropractic.net] Accessed April 21, 2013.
78. Nash J, Keating JC Jr: **Birth of the 'chiropractic angel': a caduceus counterpoint.** *Chiropr Hist* 1993, **13**(2):26–29.
79. Society of Chiropractic Orthospinology: **Orthospinology related videos.** [http://www.orthospinology.org/research/videos] Accessed August 13, 2014.
80. Runzo J: **God, commitment, and other faiths: pluralism vs relativism.** *Faith and Philosophy* 1988, **5**(2):343–364.

81. Advanced Orthogonal: **The advanced orthogonal difference.** [http://www.kcucs.com/category/blog/] Accessed April 07, 2013.
82. Chirocowin.com.au: **PROCEDURES FOLLOWED AT THIS CLINIC: X-rays & type of chiropractic adjustment.** [http://www.chirocowin.com.au/index.php?p=1_4] Accessed May 10, 2013.
83. **American Academy of Clinical Applied Spinal Biomechanical Engineering: Applied Spinal Biomechanical Engineering.** [http://www.asbechiro.com/index.html] Accessed April 07, 2013.
84. International Upper Cervical Chiropractic Association: **Frequently Asked Questions.** [http://www.pacificchiro.com/iucca/iucca_faq_page.htm] Accessed April 12, 2013.
85. Logan HB: **For History.** *Journal of the International Chiropractic Research Foundation* 1937, **1**(10):6.
86. Humber K: **President's Message.** In *The Atlas - The Society of Chiropractic Orthospinology Upper Cervical News.* Society of Chiropractic Orthospinology; 2009. http://www.orthospinology.org/images/orthospinology/Documents/Newsletter/SOCO_July_Newsletter_2009.pdf. 12 April 2013.
87. Himmelstein JS, Andersson GBJ: **Low-back pain - risk evaluation and preplacement screening.** *Occup Med* 1988, **3**(2):255–269.
88. Rockey PH, Fantel J, Omenn GS: **Discriminatory aspects of pre-employment screening: low back x-ray examinations in the railroad industry.** *Am J Law Med* 1979–1980, **5**(3):197–214.
89. Cox JE: **The utility of screening chest radiographs for flight physicals.** *Mil Med* 2000, **165**(9):667–669.
90. Abbott T, Mackay S: **Is plain radiography alive and kicking.** *Synergy* 2010, (11):26–28.
91. van Tulder M, Becker A, Bekkering T, Breen A, del Real M, Hutchinson A, Koes B, Laerum E, Malmivaara A: **Chapter 3 European guidelines for the management of acute nonspecific low back pain in primary care.** *Eur Spine J* 2006, **15**(2):s169–s191.
92. Simmons ED, Guyer RD, Graham-Smith A, Herzog R: **Radiograph assessment for patients with low back pain.** *Spine J* 2003, **3**(3):3S–5S.
93. Henschke N, Maher C, Refshauge K: **Screening for malignancy in low back pain patients: a systematic review.** *Eur Spine J* 2007, **16**(10):1673–1679.
94. Turner VW: **Symbols in African ritual.** In *Symbolic Anthropology: A Reader in the Study of Symbols and Meanings.* Edited by Dolgin JL, Kemnitzer DS, Schneider DM. New York: Columbia University Press; 1977:183–194.
95. Boyer P, Lienard P: **Why ritualized behavior? Precaution Systems and action parsing in developmental, pathological and cultural rituals.** *Behav Brain Sci* 2006, **29**(06):595–613.
96. OpenStax College: **The Sociological Approach to Religion.** In *Introduction to Sociology.* Houston, TX, USA: Rice University; 2013. OpenStax-CNX.
97. **Kale Chiropractic Center: the brain stem.** [http://thespecific.com/blog/2012/10/24/the-neck-bone-is-connected-to-the...everything/] Accessed May 03, 2013.
98. Blair Chiropractic Society: **About the Blair Chiropractic technique.** [http://www.blairchiropractic.com/blair] Accessed April 12, 2013.
99. Sosis R, Alcorta C: **Signaling, solidarity, and the sacred: the evolution of religious behavior.** *Evol Anthropol* 2003, **12**(6):264–274.
100. **The Pettibon System: treatment.** [http://pettibonsystem.com/treatment] Accessed May 06, 2013.
101. Woggon D: *The Science of Pettibon Spinal Biomechanics Systems Adjusting 2001.* St Cloud, MN, USA: Dennis Woggon; 2000.
102. National Upper Cervical Chiropractic Association: **About historical highlights.** [http://www.nucca.org/historical_highlights.php] Accessed May 03, 2013.
103. **Blair Chiropractic Society: X-rays Explained.** [http://www.blairchiropractic.com/the-blair-technique] Accessed April 12, 2013.
104. Snodgrass K: *Stories with Intent: A Comprehensive Guid to the Parables of Jesus.* Grand Rapids, MI, USA: Wm. B. Eerdmans Publishing Co.; 2008.
105. Roy W Sweat Foundation: **Testimonials.** [http://www.atlasorthogonality.com/PatientSite/testimonials.html] Accessed April 12, 2013.
106. Duff R: **Testimonials.** [http://www.duffchiropractic.net/Testimonials.html] Accessed April 21, 2013.
107. The Pettibon System: **Testimonials.** [http://pettibonsystem.com/testimonials] Accessed May 06, 2013.
108. **Advanced Orthogonal: testimonials.** [http://www.advancedorthogonal.com/testimonials/] Accessed August 11, 2014.
109. Greenhalgh T: **How to read a paper. Getting your bearings (deciding what the paper is about).** *BMJ* 1997, **315**(7102):243–246.
110. Petrisor BA, Bhandari M: **The heirarchy of evidence: levels and grades of recommendation.** *Indian J Orthop* 2007, **41**(1):11–15.
111. Blair Chiropractic Society: **Educating the public about Blair Upper Cervical Care.** [http://web.archive.org/web/20130809041628/http://blairchiropractic.com/educating_the_public.htm] Accessed April 12, 2013.
112. Blair Chiropractic Society: **About Dr Blair.** [http://www.blairchiropractic.com/drblair] Accessed April 12, 2013.
113. **The Pettibon System: our history.** [http://pettibonsystem.com/our-history] Accessed May 06, 2013.
114. **Chiropractic BioPhysics: What is CBP®.** [http://www.idealspine.com/what-is-cbp/] Accessed April 14, 2013.
115. Committee to Assess Health Risks from Exposure to Low Levels of Ionizing Radiation: **Health risks from exposure to low levels of ionizing radiation: BEIR VII Phase 2.** In *Biological Effects of Ionizing Radiation.* Edited by Academies NRCotN. Washington, DC: National Academies Press; 2014.
116. National Research Council: **Health Risks from Exposure to Low Levels of Ionizing Radiation.** Washington, DC: National Academies of Science; 2006.
117. Wright L: *Going Clear: Scientology, Hollywood and the Prison of Belief.* 1st edition. New York: Alfred A Knopf; 2013.
118. Fuller RC: *Alternative Medicine and American Religious Life.* New York: Oxford Press; 1989.
119. **Dictionary.com: Subluxation.** [http://dictionary.reference.com/browse/subluxation] Accessed July 02, 2014.
120. **Gonstead Clnical Studies Society: basic principles.** [http://gonstead.com/gonstead-system/basic-principles/] Accessed April 05, 2013.
121. Duff R: **About us.** [http://www.duffchiropractic.net/About-Us.html] Accessed April 21, 2013.
122. Palmer J, Creswell K: **A Brief History of the Modus Operandi of Measuring and Correcting The Atlas Subluxation Complex Syndrome and The Role of Posture in The National Upper Cervical Chiropractic Association (NUCCA) Standard of Care.** unknown.
123. **Chiropractic BioPhysics: PostureRay.** [http://postureanalysis.com] Accessed April 20, 2013.
124. **Gonstead Clinical Studies Society: X-Ray & Listing System Terms.** [http://gonstead.com/gonstead-terminology-project/x-ray-listing-system-terms/] Accessed April 05, 2013.
125. **UpCSpine: Kale Upper Cervical.** [http://www.upcspine.com/tech6.htm] Accessed May 03, 2013.
126. **Chiropractic BioPhysics: CBP seminars.** [http://chiropractic-biophysics.myshopify.com] Accessed April 19, 2013.
127. **TheSpecific: what is specific chiropractic?** [http://thespecific.com/blog/what-is-specific-chiropractic/] Accessed July 11, 2014.
128. Dynamic Chiropractic Editorial Staff: **Lowell Ward, DC, Stressology Pioneer.** In *Dynamic Chiropractic,* Volume 11. onlineth edition. Santa Ana, CA, USA: MPA Media; 1993.
129. Sutter M: **The Master Key to Health: Specific Atlas Correction.** Huntington Park, CA, USA: Max Sutter; 1941.
130. Martin SC: **"The Only Truly Scientific Method of Healing". Chiropractic and American Science, 1895–1990.** *Isis* 1994, **88**:207–227.
131. Rehm WS: **Legally defensible: chiropractic in the courtroom and after, 1907.** *Chiropract Hist* 1986, **6**(1):51–55.
132. Keating JC Jr: **Tom Morris, Defender of Chiropractic, Part I.** In *Dynamic Chiropractic,* Volume 17. 1999. Internet.
133. Keating JC Jr: **Tom Morris, Defender of Chiropractic, Part II.** In *Dynamic Chiropractic,* Volume 18. 1999. Internet.
134. Wilson GA: *Spinatology: The dynamics of the cause and correction of subluxations.* Salt Lake City, UT, USA: The Standard Research Laboratories; 1955.
135. Lerner C: **The Lerner Report: A history of the early years of chiropractic.** Portland, OR, USA: Foundation for Health Research, Inc.; circa; 1952.
136. Keating JC Jr: **A brief history of historical scholarship in chiropractic.** *J Can Chiropr Assoc* 2001, **45**(2):113–136.
137. Watkins CO: **The Basic Principles of Chiropractic Government.** Sunnyvale, CA, USA: 1944.
138. Fuller RC: *Wonder: from emotion to spirituality.* Chapel Hill: University of North Carolina Press; 2006.
139. Nyhan B, Reifler J: **When Corrections Fail: the persistence of political misperceptions.** *Polit Behav* 2010, **32**(2):303–330.
140. Welch JS: **Ritual in western medicine and its role in placebo healing.** *J Relig Health* 2003, **42**(1):21–33.
141. Pollner M: **Divine relations, social relations, and well-being.** *J Health Soc Behav* 1989, **30**(1):92–104.

142. Ellison CG, Gay DA, Glass TA: **Does religious commitment contribute to individual life satisfaction?** *Social Forces* 1989, **68**(1):100.
143. **International Upper Cervical Chiropractic Association: Applied Upper Cervical Biomechanics Post-Graduate Education Program.** [http://www.pacificchiro.com/iucca/aucb_program_page.htm] Accessed April 12, 2013.
144. Roy W Sweat Foundation: **About Atlas Orthogonal.** [http://www.atlasorthogonality.com/PatientSite/aboutAO.html] Accessed April 12, 2013.
145. **Chiropractic BioPhysics: About the Founder.** [http://www.idealspine.com/about-the-founder/] Accessed April 14, 2013.
146. Gonstead Clnical Studies Society: **The Gonstead Adjustment.** [http://gonstead.com/gonstead-system/the-gonstead-adjustment/] Accessed April 05, 2013.
147. Gonstead Clinical Studies Society: **Writing case reports for GCSS.** [http://gonstead.com/writing-case-reports-for-gcss/] Accessed April 05, 2013.
148. Grostic RJ: **Welcome to your health potential.** [http://www.grosticchiro.com/5825.html] Accessed April 25, 2013.
149. Eriksen K: **Orthospinology upper cervical.** [http://www.upcspine.com/tech5.htm] Accessed April 25, 2013.
150. KCUCS: **About KCUCS.** [http://www.kcucs.com/about-kcucs/] Accessed May 03, 2013.
151. Logan HB: *Textbook of Logan Basic Methods.* St Louis, MO, USA: Logan College of Chiropractic; 1950.
152. Sherman College of Chiropractic: **Seventh Annual Subluxation Conference.** [http://www.chiro.org/LINKS/FULL/subcon7.html] Accessed May 07, 2014.
153. National Upper Cervical Chiropractic Association: **Patients Frequently Asked Questions.** [http://www.nucca.org/faq.php] Accessed May 03, 2013.
154. Galgano J, Jaszewski E: **About pierce results.** [pierceresults.com] Accessed July 10, 2014.
155. Elliott SONAR Chiropractic: **Healing Through SONAR.** [http://www.sonarchiropractic.com/sonarchiropractic/healing-through-sonar.htm] Accessed May 07, 2013.
156. Elliott SONAR Chiropractic: **How SONAR Works.** [http://www.sonarchiropractic.com/sonarchiropracticdocs.htm] Accessed May 07, 2013.
157. Ward S: **Mental emotional profiles.** [http://chiroman.com/services/mental-emotional-profiles/] Accessed May 16, 2013.
158. Advanced Orthogonal: **Advanced Orthogonal Chiropractic.** [http://www.advancedorthogonal.com] Accessed April 05, 2013.
159. Advanced Orthogonal: **History of Advanced Orthogonal.** [http://www.advancedorthogonal.com/history-of-advanced-orthogonal/] Accessed April 05, 2013.
160. Buchanan G: **Advanced Orthogonal - Dr Stanley Pierce Sr and Jr.** [http://www.upcspine.com/tech7.htm] Accessed April 05, 2013.
161. International Upper Cervical Chiropractic Association: **Home page.** [http://www.pacificchiro.com/iucca/iucca_home_page.htm] Accessed April 12, 2013.
162. International Upper Cervical Chiropractic Association: **Research page.** [http://www.pacificchiro.com/iucca/iucca_research_page.htm] Accessed April 12, 2013.
163. Roy W Sweat Foundation: **About Us.** [http://www.atlasorthogonality.com/PatientSite/AboutUs.html] Accessed April 12, 2013.
164. Chiropractic BioPhysics: **CBP® Research.** [http://www.idealspine.com/cbp-research/] Accessed April 14, 2013.
165. Chiropractic BioPhysics: **Blog.** [http://www.idealspine.com/news/] Accessed April 14, 2013.
166. MyChiroPractice: **Home page.** [http://mychiropractice.com] Accessed 12/08/2014.
167. Chiropractic BioPhysics: **FAQ.** [http://www.idealspine.com/faq/] Accessed April 14, 2013.
168. Gonstead Clinical Studies Society: **Donate now to the Gonstead Research Fund.** [http://gonstead.com/donate/] Accessed April 05, 2013.
169. (Kale) UCC: **Home page of the TIC Institute.** [http://www.youtube.com/watch?v=GfSb89nx2cc; http://www.youtube.com/watch?v=B4qBkkwdT1g] Accessed May 03, 2013.
170. Kale B: **Upper Cervical Coaching FAQ.** [http://kaleblog.typepad.com/the_tic/2011/02/] Accessed May 03, 2013.
171. Kessinger R: **Dr Robert Kessinger (KCUCS).** [http://www.youtube.com/KCUCS7] Accessed May 03, 2013.
172. UCRF: **Current research/funding.** [http://www.ucrf.org/projects-funding] Accessed May 04, 2013.
173. Society of Chiropractic Orthospinology: **Home page.** [http://www.orthospinology.org] Accessed May 05, 2013.
174. Elliott SONAR Chiropractic: **Welcome to Elliott SONAR Chiropractic.** [http://www.sonarchiropractic.com/index.htm] Accessed May 07, 2013.
175. Ward Chiropractic: **Reviews.** [http://wardchiropractic.localchiropracticreviews.com] Accessed May 16, 2013.
176. Ward Chiropractic: **Home page.** [http://www.chiroman.com] Accessed May 16, 2013.
177. Sutter M: **Sutter specific atlas correction.** [http://www.upcspine.com/tech17.htm] Accessed July 14, 2014.
178. International Upper Cervical Chiropractic Association: **IUCCA clinical equipment.** [http://www.pacificchiro.com/iucca/iucca_clinical_equipment.htm] Accessed April 12, 2013.
179. Blair Chiropractic Society: **The patient experience.** [http://www.blairchiropractic.com/The-Patient-Experience] Accessed July 14, 2013.
180. Chiropractic BioPhysics: **How to use x-ray templates.** [http://www.idealspine.com/how-to-use-x-ray-templates/] Accessed April 14, 2013.
181. (Kale) UCC: **Training.** [http://kneechesttechnique.com/kneechest_training.html] Accessed May 03, 2013.
182. KCUCS: **What makes KCUCS unique.** [http://www.kcucs.com/about-kcucs/what-makes-kcucs-unique/] Accessed May 03, 2013.
183. Young KJ: **WARREN L. SAUSSER, D.C.: INFLUENCE UNRECOGNIZED.** *Chiropr Hist* 1997, **17**(1):75–83.
184. Yardley LG: **President's Letter.** In *NUCCA News. Winter edn.* Minneapolis, MN, USA: NUCCA; 2013.
185. Society of Chiropractic Orthospinology: **Chiropractic Orthospinology Basic I Class.** [http://www.orthospinology.org/seminars/seminar-descriptions/basic-1-outline] Accessed May 05, 2013.
186. Society of Chiropractic Orthospinology: **About Orthospinology.** [http://www.orthospinology.org/patients/what-is-orthospinology] Accessed May 05, 2013.
187. **The Pettibon System: three distinct phases of care.** [http://pettibonsystem.com/three-distinct-phases-care] Accessed May 06, 2013.
188. **Pierce results seminars: about pierce results.** [http://pierceresults.com/index.html] Accessed March 12, 2013.
189. **Ward Chiropractic: About.** [http://www.chiroman.com/about/] Accessed May 16, 2013.
190. Canepa L: **Just Think It! Dr Zimmerman's Specific Adjusting Machine (SAM).** [http://www.just-think-it.com/sam.htm] Accessed May 11, 2013.
191. **ChiroMatrix - Discover Wellness: Borges Chiropractic - Testimonials/Our Patients Speak.** [http://borgeschiro.com/testimonials.html] Accessed April 07, 2013.
192. **ChiroMatrix - Discover Wellness: Borges Chiropractic - Your First Visit.** [http://borgeschiro.com/your-first-visit-to-the-chiropractor.html] Accessed April 07, 2013.
193. International Upper Cervical Chiropractic Association: **Publications.** [http://www.pacificchiro.com/iucca/iucca_publications_page.htm] Accessed April 12, 2013.
194. Roy W Sweat Foundation: **Physician testimonials.** [http://www.atlasorthogonality.com/PatientSite/PhysTestis.html] Accessed April 12, 2013.
195. Chirocowin.com.au: **Clippings.** [http://www.chirocowin.com.au/index.php?p=1_12] Accessed May 10, 2013.
196. Chirocowin.com.au: **Case reports.** [http://www.chirocowin.com.au/index.php?p=1_5] Accessed May 10, 2013.
197. Gonstead Clinical Studies Society: **Testimonials.** [http://gonstead.com/genint/testimonials/] Accessed April 05, 2013.
198. Gonstead Clinical Studies Society: **Field of dreams research fund.** [http://gonstead.com/field-of-dreams-research-fund/] Accessed April 05, 2013.
199. Grostic RJ: **What is chiropractic?** [http://www.grosticchiro.com/7901.html] Accessed April 25, 2013.
200. Kale Chiropractic Center: **The Science behind the Kale Chiropractic Method.** [http://web.archive.org/web/20130517073447/http://kale.com/kaleweb/chiropractic/science.htm] Accessed May 03, 2013.
201. Kale Chiropractic Center: **The Kale Method.** [http://web.archive.org/web/20130924141937/http://kale.com/kaleweb/chiropractic/index.htm] Accessed May 03, 2013.
202. KCUCS: **Research.** [http://www.kcucs.com/research/] Accessed May 03, 2013.
203. National Upper Cervical Chiropractic Association: **Media/News Media Clips and Videos.** [http://www.nucca.org/clips.php] Accessed May 03, 2013.
204. National Upper Cervical Chiropractic Association: **About mission statement.** [http://www.nucca.org/mission.php] Accessed May 03, 2013.
205. UCRF: **News room.** [http://www.ucrf.org/newsroom] Accessed May 04, 2013.

206. UCRF: **FAQS.** [http://www.ucrf.org/faq] Accessed May 04, 2013.
207. Society of Chiropractic Orthospinology: **Testimonials.** [http://www.orthospinology.org/testimonials] Accessed August 13, 2014.
208. **The Pettibon System: Research/Articles.** [http://pettibonsystem.com/institute/research-articles] Accessed May 06, 2013.
209. **The Pettibon System: our mission.** [http://pettibonsystem.com/our-mission] Accessed May 06, 2013.
210. **The Pettibon System: how the pettibon system works.** [http://pettibonsystem.com/about/how-pettibon-works] Accessed May 06, 2013.
211. **Pierce results seminars: case studies.** [http://pierceresults.com/casestudies.html] Accessed March 12, 2013.
212. **Elliott SONAR Chiropractic: the upper cervical procedure.** [http://www.sonarchiropractic.com/sonarchiropractic/healing-through-sonar.htm] Accessed May 07, 2013.
213. **Elliott SONAR Chiropractic: Facebook post 08 April 2013.** [https://www.facebook.com/pages/Elliott-SONAR-Chiropractic/183925001636186] Accessed May 07, 2013.
214. **Ward Chiropractic: video library.** [http://chiroman.com/video-library/] Accessed May 16, 2013.
215. **Ward Chiropractic: X-rays.** [http://chiroman.com/services/x-rays/] Accessed May 16, 2013.
216. **Ward Chiropractic: mind body connection.** [http://chiroman.com/category/mind-body-connection/] Accessed May 16, 2013.
217. Gonstead Clinical Studies Society: **Gonstead terminology project.** [http://gonstead.com/gonstead-terminology-project/] Accessed April 05, 2013.
218. Hutti LJ, Unger-Boyd M: **Structural x-ray marking systems.** In *Textbook of Logan Basic Methods.* 4th edition. Edited by Hutti LJ. Chesterfield, MO, USA: LBM, Inc; 2006:119–126.
219. National Upper Cervical Chiropractic Association: **NUCCA standards of care and practice guidelines.** Edited by NUCCA. Minneapolis, MN, USA: NUCCA; 1992.
220. Society of Chiropractic Orthospinology: **The Atlas - The Society of Chiropractic Orthospinology Upper Cervical News.** Edited by Society of Chiropractic Orthospinology. Society of Chiropractic Orthospinology; 2009. http://www.orthospinology.org/images/orthospinology/Documents/Newsletter/SOCO_July_Newsletter_2009.pdf.
221. **The Pettibon System: X-ray procedures.** [http://pettibonsystem.com/course/x-ray-procedures] Accessed May 06, 2013.
222. **Pierce results seminars: contact us.** [http://pierceresults.com/contactus.html] Accessed March 12, 2013.

Inter-rater agreement, sensitivity, and specificity of the prone hip extension test and active straight leg raise test

Paul A Bruno[1*], David P Millar[2] and Dale A Goertzen[2]

Abstract

Background: Two clinical tests used to assess for neuromuscular control deficits in low back pain (LBP) patients are the prone hip extension (PHE) test and active straight leg raise (ASLR) test. For these tests, it has been suggested examiners classify patients as "positive" or "negative" based on the presence or absence (respectively) of specific "abnormal" lumbopelvic motion patterns. The inter-rater agreement of such a classification scheme has been reported for the PHE test, but not for the ASLR test. In addition, the sensitivity and specificity of such classification schemes have not been reported for either test. The primary objectives of the current study were to investigate: 1) the inter-rater agreement of the examiner-reported classification schemes for these two tests, and 2) the sensitivity and specificity of the classification schemes.

Methods: Thirty participants with LBP and 40 asymptomatic controls took part in this cross-sectional observational study. Participants performed 3–4 repetitions of each test whilst two examiners classified them as "positive" or "negative" based on the presence or absence (respectively) of specific "abnormal" lumbopelvic motion patterns. The inter-rater agreement (Kappa statistic), sensitivity (LBP patients), and specificity (controls) were calculated for each test.

Results: Both tests demonstrated substantial inter-rater agreement (PHE test: Kappa = 0.76, 95% CI = 0.57-0.95, $p < 0.001$; ASLR test: Kappa = 0.76, 95% CI = 0.57-0.96, $p < 0.001$). For the PHE test, the sensitivity was 0.18-0.27 and the specificity was 0.63-0.78; the odds ratio (OR) of "positive" classifications in the LBP group was 1.25 (95% CI = 0.58-2.72; Examiner 1) and 1.27 (95% CI = 0.52-3.12; Examiner 2). For the ASLR test, the sensitivity was 0.20-0.25 and the specificity was 0.84-0.86; the OR of "positive" classifications in the LBP group was 1.72 (95% CI = 0.75-3.95; Examiner 1) and 1.57 (95% CI = 0.64-3.85; Examiner 2).

Conclusion: Classification schemes for the PHE test and ASLR test based on the presence or absence of specific "abnormal" lumbopelvic motion patterns demonstrated substantial inter-rater agreement. However, additional investigation is required to further comment on the clinical usefulness of the motion patterns demonstrated by LBP patients during these tests as a diagnostic tool or treatment outcome.

Keywords: Reproducibility of results, Sensitivity and specificity, Low back pain, Rehabilitation

Background

It is well-established that the coordination of muscle activity around the lumbopelvic region is vital to the generation of mechanical spinal stability [1,2]. Models illustrating mechanisms by which altered motor control strategies in this region serve as a potential cause and/or effect of LBP have been described by Panjabi [3,4] and others [5-7]. Dysfunctional neuromuscular control strategies (e.g. muscle activation levels, coordination of muscle contractions) could therefore result in "clinical instability", which has been defined as the loss of the ability of the spine to maintain its pattern of displacement under physiologic loads resulting in no initial or additional neurological deficit, no major deformity, and no incapacitating pain [4]. People with low back pain (LBP) have been shown to demonstrate a variety of neuromuscular control alterations compared to asymptomatic individuals [8-15]. The neuromuscular control strategies used during specific

* Correspondence: paul.bruno@uregina.ca
[1]Faculty of Kinesiology and Health Studies, University of Regina, 3737 Wascana Parkway, Regina, Saskatchewan S4S 0A2, Canada
Full list of author information is available at the end of the article

postures or tasks can be objectively quantified and used to provide estimates of spinal stability [1,16]. However, these methods involve the use of advanced technology and mathematical modeling that make them of limited use in a routine clinical setting. It would therefore be valuable to develop practical clinical tests that demonstrate sufficient reliability and validity in assessing the neuromuscular control strategies of LBP patients to help facilitate treatment targeted at correcting specific neuromuscular control deficits. Two tests that have been suggested as having potential in this regard are the prone hip extension (PHE) test [17] and active straight leg raise (ASLR) test [18,19].

The PHE test was originally developed as a means of evaluating for a specific neuromuscular control deficit in the lumbopelvic region. During the test, the patient lays prone and alternately lifts each leg off the table to a height of ~20 cm whilst an examiner observes and/or palpates the gluteus maximus (GM), hamstring (HAM), and erector spinae (ES) muscles to determine their relative order of activation [20-22]. Since these original descriptions, however, many studies have demonstrated that there is not a consistent order of activation in LBP patients or asymptomatic individuals [8,23-28]. Although there is a general consensus that the GM becomes active after the HAM and ES during the test [8,23-28], there is some evidence that the onset of the GM is significantly delayed in LBP patients [8] and asymptomatic individuals who demonstrate certain lumbar spine motion patterns [24]. However, the clinical importance of these findings has not been established since the impact of a delayed onset of the GM during the PHE test on the mechanical stability of the lumbopelvic region has not been reported.

An alternative use for the PHE test has also been proposed [17], namely that clinicians should instead observe for three specific "abnormal" lumbar spine motion patterns during the test: 1) rotation of the lumbar spine such that the spinous processes appear to move toward the side of hip extension, 2) a lateral shift of the lumbar spine toward the side of hip extension, and 3) extension of the lumbar spine. The inter-rater agreement of classifying LBP patients as "positive" or "negative" based on the presence or absence (respectively) of these motion patterns has been shown to be good [17].

The ASLR test was originally described as a clinical tool to evaluate the ability of the sacroiliac joints to effectively transfer loads between the pelvis and legs in females with pregnancy-related pelvic pain [29,30]. More recently, researchers have also commented on this test's potential usefulness in the assessment of the neuromuscular control strategies of the lumbopelvic region in the general LBP population [18,19]. The test is similar to the PHE test, with the patient supine (rather than prone) and asked to alternately lift each leg away from the table to a height of ~20 cm [19,31]. It has been suggested that an inability to maintain a neutral alignment of the pelvis during the test indicates the presence of a neuromuscular control deficit [19,31-33]. However, there are no published studies related to the inter-rater agreement of classifying patients as "positive" or "negative" based on their inability or ability (respectively) to maintain a neutral pelvic alignment during the test.

In addition, the sensitivity and specificity of these examiner-reported classification schemes have not been reported for either test.

Therefore, the primary objectives of the current study were to investigate: 1) the inter-rater agreement of the examiner-reported classification schemes for these two tests, and 2) the sensitivity and specificity of the classification schemes.

Methods

Study design and reporting

The design and reporting for the current study conform with the Guidelines for Reporting Reliability and Agreement Studies (GRRAS) [34].

Participants

A convenience sample of 30 participants with LBP and 40 asymptomatic controls were recruited to take part in this cross-sectional observational study. The demographic information for the LBP group and control group is presented in Table 1. LBP participants were recruited from local medical, chiropractic, physiotherapy, and massage therapy clinics. Control participants were recruited from the students, faculty, and staff of

Table 1 Demographic information for the low back pain (LBP) group and control group

		LBP group	Control group
Gender (#)	*Males*	10	20
	Females	20	20
Age (years)	*Mean (SD)*	27.7 (5.9)	27.7 (6.1)
Height (cm)	*Mean (SD)*	171.1 (9.8)	173.3 (10.3)
Weight (kg)	*Mean (SD)*	71.0 (16.4)	71.2 (17.7)
LBP duration (months)	*Mean (SD)*	21.2 (35.1)	-
	Median (range)	6.0 (1–168)	-
NPRS (0–10)	*Mean (SD)*	5.0 (1.5)	-
	Median (range)	5.0 (2–7)	-
ODI (0–100)	*Mean (SD)*	16.7 (8.5)	-
	Median (range)	14.0 (6-36)	-

Abbreviations: NPRS Numerical Pain Rating Scale, *ODI* Oswestry Disability Index.
In addition to the mean and SD, the median and range are also reported for demographic data that did not demonstrate a normal distribution (LBP duration, NPRS, ODI).
No statistically significant ($p < 0.05$) between-group differences were noted for gender, age, height, or weight.

the University of Regina. All participants were naïve to the purpose of the study and provided written informed consent. The study was approved by the University of Regina Research Ethics Board.

A priori exclusion criteria for *all* participants included: adults under 20 years of age or over 40 years of age; history of hip joint injury or trauma, lumbar spine surgery, spinal arthritic disorders, central nervous system disorders, or neuromuscular disorders; unable to perform painless active hip ranges of motion; true leg length inequality > 1 cm; and currently pregnant or recently postpartum (<1 year) females. Additional exclusion criteria for the *LBP group* included: history of significant trauma or unexplained weight loss; LBP not confined to an area between the lower ribs and gluteal folds with or without referral into the lower limbs above the knees; presence of radicular signs (e.g. myotomal motor weakness, deep tendon reflex differences) or nerve root tension tests (e.g. straight leg raise test) in the lower limb; current episode of LBP was not present for at least one month and on most days over the previous month; and average LBP over the previous week < 2/10 on a Numerical Pain Rating Scale (NPRS) [35]. An additional criterion for the *control group* was a history of any spinal or lower limb injury that prevented the performance of normal activities for at least one day in the previous three months.

Examiners

Two of the investigators (DM, DG), both of whom are licensed chiropractors with over 30 years of clinical experience, examined and provided classifications (see Procedure section) for all participants. In order to minimize the bias in the classifications provided during the data collection sessions, the examiners were blinded to the group status (i.e. LBP, control) of each participant. They were also not permitted to confer with each other during the testing procedures and recorded their classifications on separate pieces of paper.

Prior to the initiation of data collection, the examiners underwent a joint training phase. At the first meeting, a consensus was achieved between the two examiners regarding the specific procedure and criteria to be used for each test (see Procedure section paragraphs 4 and 5). Following this, three sessions were conducted during which undergraduate student and faculty volunteers performed the tests whilst the examiners discussed their findings and clarified any discrepancies in classifications. Adequate training has been shown to be more important than the examiners' collective experience with a testing procedure for observation-based clinical tests [36].

Procedures

All data collection sessions took place in the same room in the Faculty of Kinesiology and Health Studies' Neuromechanical Research Centre at the University of Regina. Upon presentation, participants were provided with a study information sheet and asked to complete an intake form and informed consent form. The intake form was used to collect demographic data and confirm their eligibility for the study. The LBP participants were also asked to complete a NPRS [35] related to their average pain over the last week and an Oswestry Disability Index [37,38].

Participants were required to wear a pair of shorts and lay on a treatment bench. Using a standardized protocol and participant positioning, one of the investigators (PB) instructed the participants on the performance of the two testing procedures. For the PHE test, the participants lay prone and were instructed to alternately lift each leg to a height of ~20 cm and return it to the bench after a 1–2 second hold in the elevated position (Figure 1) [17]. For the ASLR test, the participants lay supine and were instructed to alternately lift each leg to a height of ~20 cm and return it to the bench after a 1–2 second hold in the elevated position (Figure 2) [19,31]. Once the participants were sufficiently familiar with each test, they were allowed to rest for ~ 1 minute before the examiners entered the room.

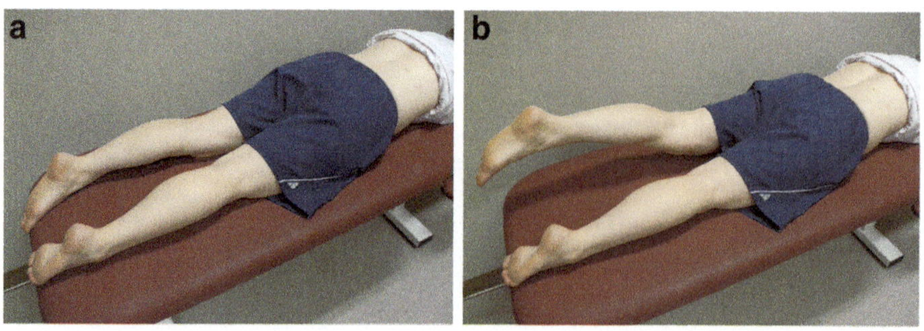

Figure 1 The start (a) and end (b) positions for the prone hip extension (PHE) test. The participant is prone with both legs in contact with the bench in the start position **(a)**. The participant's left leg has been raised off the bench in the end position **(b)**.

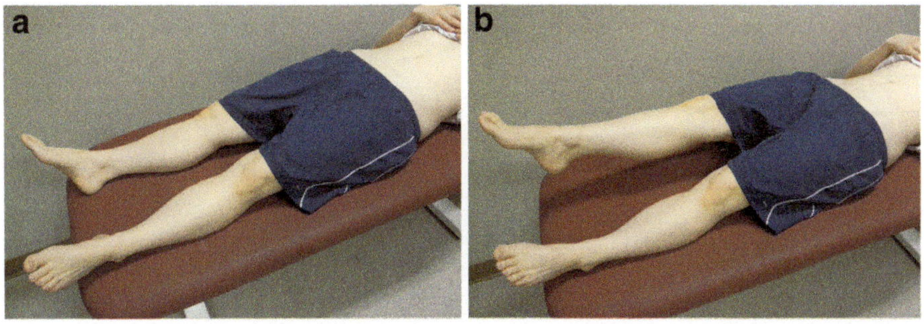

Figure 2 The start (a) and end (b) positions for the active straight leg raise (ASLR) test. The participant is supine with both legs in contact with the bench in the start position **(a)**. The participant's right leg has been raised off the bench in the end position **(b)**.

The participants then performed 3–5 repetitions of each test (performance of the test on both the left and right sides constituted one repetition) whilst the examiners simultaneously observed the performances. The order of test (PHE/ASLR) and leg lifted first (left/right) were randomized to control for order effects and possible fatigue over time. Between each test, the examiners were asked to leave the room and the participants were allowed to rest for ~1 minute.

For the PHE test, the examiners classified each participant as "positive" if one of the following motion patterns was observed during the test: 1) rotation of the lumbar spine such that the spinous processes appear to move toward the side of hip extension, 2) a lateral shift of the lumbar spine toward the side of hip extension, 3) extension of the lumbar spine, or 4) the pelvic girdle raises on the side of hip extension [17]. If none of these motion patterns was observed, the participant was classified as "negative". The examiners recorded a classification for the participant's left leg and a classification for the right leg.

For the ASLR test, the examiners classified each participant as "positive" if the pelvic girdle failed to maintain neutral alignment during the test [31-33]. If the pelvic girdle maintained a neutral alignment, the participant was classified as "negative". The examiners recorded a classification for the participant's left leg and a classification for the right leg.

Statistical analyses

For both tests, 2×2 contingency tables were constructed with the classifications provided by Examiner 1 forming the columns and those provided by Examiner 2 forming the rows. The inter-rater agreement for each test was calculated using the kappa statistic and prevalence-adjusted bias-adjusted kappa (PABAK) statistic [39].

For each examiner's classifications, the sensitivity for both tests was calculated as the "true positive" rate in the LBP group (TP/TP + FN) [40]. The specificity was calculated as the "true negative" rate in the control group (TN/TN + FP) [40]. In addition, the odds ratio (OR) of a "positive" classification (outcome) in the LBP group (exposure) was calculated for both tests.

All statistical analyses were performed using PASW Statistics 18.0 (SPSS Inc, Chicago, IL, USA) and GraphPad InStat 3.10 (GraphPad Software Inc, San Diego, CA, USA) software.

Results

Examiner classifications – LBP group

For the PHE test, Examiner 1 classified 16/60 legs (26.7%) as "positive", and Examiner 2 classified 11/60 legs (18.3%) as "positive" (Table 2). For the ASLR test, Examiner 1 classified 15/60 legs (25.0%) as "positive", and Examiner 2 classified 12/60 legs (20.0%) as "positive" (Table 3).

Examiner classifications – control group

For the PHE test, Examiner 1 classified 18/80 legs (22.5%) as "positive", and Examiner 2 classified 12/80 legs (15.0%) as "positive" (Table 4). For the ASLR test, Examiner 1 classified 13/80 legs (16.3%) as "positive", and Examiner 2 classified 11/80 (13.8%) legs as "positive" (Table 5).

Inter-rater agreement (LBP group)

For each test, there was 91.7% overall agreement between the examiners for the classification of legs as "positive" or "negative" (Table 6). Both tests demonstrated substantial inter-rater agreement (Kappa = 0.61-0.80), with lower

Table 2 Examiner-reported classifications for the prone hip extension (PHE) test for the low back pain (LBP) group

		Examiner 1		
		Positive	Negative	
Examiner 2	Positive	11	0	*11*
	Negative	5	44	*49*
		16	*44*	

Table 3 Examiner-reported classifications for the active straight leg raise (ASLR) test for the low back pain (LBP) group

		Examiner 1		
		Positive	Negative	
Examiner 2	Positive	11	1	*12*
	Negative	4	44	*48*
		15	*45*	

limits (95% CI) that extend into the range of what is considered moderate agreement (Kappa = 0.41-0.60) [41].

Sensitivity, specificity, and frequency of "positive" classifications

Both tests demonstrated relatively poor sensitivity and relatively high specificity (Table 7). The frequency of "positive" classifications was not significantly greater in the LBP group compared to the control group for either test (Table 7).

Discussion

The results of the current study suggest that the classification schemes proposed for the PHE test [17] and ASLR test [31-33] demonstrate substantial inter-rater agreement [41], with calculated Kappa values of 0.76 for each test (Table 6). These findings generally agree with those reported by Murphy and colleagues for the PHE test [17]. In the current study, the prevalence of the "positive" test findings for both tests need to be considered when interpreting these values since the kappa statistic is influenced by the relative proportion of "positive" and "negative" test findings [39]. This effect is quantified as a "prevalence index", which is calculated as the absolute value of the difference between the number of "positive" and "negative" test findings as a proportion of the total number of paired ratings. A very high or very low number of "positive" test findings will result in a "high" prevalence index, which will cause the resulting kappa statistic to be reduced (an effect that is greater for larger kappa values) [39]. The kappa statistic can be adjusted in cases of a high prevalence index by calculating the PABAK statistic [39]. In the current study, the calculated prevalence index for both tests was moderate due to the relatively low number of "positive" test findings in the LBP group. The calculated PABAK statistic values were marginally higher, and moved the reliability of both tests into the "almost perfect" range (Table 6) [41].

Table 4 Examiner-reported classifications for the prone hip extension (PHE) test for the control group

		Examiner 1		
		Positive	Negative	
Examiner 2	Positive	11	1	*12*
	Negative	7	61	*68*
		18	*62*	

Table 5 Examiner-reported classifications for the active straight leg raise (ASLR) test for the control group

		Examiner 1		
		Positive	Negative	
Examiner 2	Positive	10	1	*11*
	Negative	3	66	*69*
		13	*67*	

The frequency of "positive" test findings was not significantly greater in the LBP group compared to the control group for either test (Table 7). However, there was a non-significant trend for the LBP participants to test "positive" more frequently than the control participants, particularly for the ASLR test. However, it should also be highlighted that the 95% CIs of the calculated ORs were relatively large. The specificity of both tests was relatively high, whilst the accompanying sensitivity values were relatively poor (Table 7). These results suggest that there was a relatively low "false positive" rate in the control group and a relatively high "false negative" rate in the LBP group. The low sensitivity values would seem to question whether observing for the "abnormal" motion patterns used in the current study are an effective tool in assessing the neuromuscular control strategies of the lumbopelvic region in LBP patients. However, the sensitivity values may also reflect the non-specific nature of the diagnostic criteria used for our LBP group. Beyond establishing exclusion criteria to rule out a sinister cause of a participant's LBP (e.g. tumour, infection) and potential neurological involvement, we did not attempt to localize the source of the participants' symptoms. Murphy and colleagues [42] have suggested that these two tests may be useful in distinguishing patients with LBP originating in the lumbar spine (PHE test) and the sacroiliac joints (ASLR test). In their study, the participants were divided into sub-groups who met

Table 6 Inter-rater agreement of the prone hip extension (PHE) test and active straight leg raise (ASLR) test for the low back pain (LBP) group

	PHE test	ASLR test
Overall agreement (%)	**91.7%**	**91.7%**
Kappa statistic	**0.76**	**0.76**
95% CI	*0.57-0.95*	*0.57-0.96*
p value	*p < 0.001*	*p < 0.001*
PABAK statistic	**0.83**	**0.83**
Prevalence index	0.55	0.55
Bias index	0.08	0.05

Abbreviation: PABAK Prevalence-Adjusted Bias-Adjusted Kappa.

Table 7 Sensitivity, specificity, and the odds ratio (OR) of "positive" classifications in the low back pain (LBP) group for the prone hip extension (PHE) test and active straight leg raise (ASLR) test

	PHE test		ASLR test	
	Examiner 1	*Examiner 2*	*Examiner 1*	*Examiner 2*
Sensitivity	**0.27**	**0.18**	**0.25**	**0.20**
95% CI	*0.16-0.40*	*0.10-0.30*	*0.15-0.38*	*0.11-0.32*
Specificity	**0.78**	**0.85**	**0.84**	**0.86**
95% CI	*0.67-0.86*	*0.75-0.92*	*0.74-0.91*	*0.77-0.93*
OR	**1.25**	**1.27**	**1.72**	**1.57**
95% CI	*0.58-2.72*	*0.52-3.12*	*0.75-3.95*	*0.64-3.85*

specific criteria to establish the origin of their pain as being either in the lumbar spine or sacroiliac joints. The results indicated that the proportion of "positive" PHE test findings was higher in patients deemed to have pain originating in the lumbar spine, while the proportion of "positive" ASLR test findings was higher in patients deemed to have pain originating in the sacroiliac joints.

It is also possible that the criteria used in the current study to indicate a "positive" test were too general. There may be a sub-group of LBP patients who possess specific neuromuscular control deficits that account for the non-significant increase in "positive" test findings in the current study. The selection of the specific motion patterns used in the current study as being representative of neuromuscular control deficits in the lumbopelvic region during the PHE test [17] and ASLR test [19,31-33] have been based on the clinical observation of LBP patients; however, the clinical importance of an individual's ability or inability to maintain a neutral alignment of the lumbar spine (PHE test) or pelvic girdle (ASLR test) during these tests has not been established. Patients with a clinical diagnosis of sacroiliac joint pain have been shown to demonstrate quantifiable differences in pelvic motion during standing hip flexion compared to asymptomatic individuals [32]. However, it is unknown whether similar (or other) motion pattern differences exist during the ASLR test. In fact, whether LBP patients demonstrate objective quantifiable differences in lumbar spine or pelvic motion during the PHE test or ASLR test has not been reported. Objectively quantifying the lumbopelvic motion patterns used by LBP patients during these tests may elicit specific motion patterns that are better able to distinguish patients with specific neuromuscular control deficits.

The current study has several additional limitations. First, our sample size was relatively small and confined to one geographical location (Regina, Saskatchewan, Canada). In addition, all of our participants were relatively young adults (20–40 years), and our LBP group did not include individuals with co-morbidities (e.g. LBP with radicular involvement, osteoarthritis, diabetes, heart disease). The generalizability of our results to other populations is therefore questionable. Second, neither of our examiners routinely used the PHE test or ASLR test in clinical practice prior to their involvement in the current study. Although it has been reported that adequate training appears to be more important than the examiners' collective experience with a testing procedure for observation-based clinical tests [36], these findings only relate to a test involving the knee. Therefore, the examiners' relative lack of experience with the two tests prior to undergoing the training sessions for the current study may have had an effect on our results. Third, we used a dichotomous scale ("positive" and "negative") to classify the PHE test and ASLR test findings. The examiners in the current study commented that it may have been preferable to use a graded scale (e.g. 3-point scale, 5-point scale) to rate the participants' performance during the tests. The potential value of such non-dichotomous scales has not been investigated for these tests. Fourth, since the examiners performed the two tests in relatively quick succession on each participant, recollection bias may have potentially influenced the results. Analysis of the raw data demonstrated that: 1) when the first test was classified as "positive", the second test was also classified as "positive" 54% of the time (Examiner 1) and 56% of the time (Examiner 2), and 2) when the second test was classified as "positive", the first test had also been classified as "positive" 44% of the time (Examiner 1) and 45% of the time (Examiner 2). Therefore, the influence of recollection bias on the examiners' classifications for the second test would appear to have been minimal. Finally, the clinical significance of motion pattern alterations during the PHE test and ASLR test has not been fully established. It has been suggested that neuromuscular control deficits present during these tests may have functional implications for the stability of the lumbopelvic region during static postures and dynamic activities [20-22,29,30]. However, since there are no published studies that have assessed the association between the neuromuscular control strategies used during these tests and activities such as gait, the functional implications of neuromuscular control deficits during the tests are currently unknown [15,43].

Conclusions

Specific classification schemes for the PHE test and ASLR test based on the presence or absence of certain "abnormal" lumbopelvic motion patterns demonstrate substantial inter-rater agreement. Although the specificity of these schemes also appears to be relatively high, their sensitivity was found to be relatively poor. This may be a reflection of the non-specific nature of the diagnostic criteria used in the current study and/or the presence of a certain sub-group of LBP patients who possess specific neuromuscular control deficits that are detectable using these tests. Additional investigation is required to further comment on the potential clinical usefulness of the motion patterns demonstrated by LBP patients during these tests as either a diagnostic tool or treatment outcome.

Abbreviations

ASLR: Active straight leg raise; FN: False negative; FP: False positive; LBP: Low back pain; NPRS: Numerical pain rating scale; OR: Odds ratio; ODI: Oswestry disability index; PABAK: Prevalence-adjusted bias-adjusted kappa; PHE: Prone hip extension; TN: True negative; TP: True positive.

Competing interests

The authors declare they have no competing interests.

Authors' contributions

PB conceived and designed the study, and drafted the manuscript. All authors were involved in collecting and analyzing the data, as well as reading and approving the final manuscript.

Acknowledgments

Funding for the study was supported through the University of Regina Social Sciences and Humanities Research Council General Research Grant/ President's Fund. The authors wish to acknowledge Christine Meckamalil for her assistance in data collection, as well as the chiropractors, massage therapists, and physiotherapists who assisted in recruiting participants for our LBP group.

Author details

[1]Faculty of Kinesiology and Health Studies, University of Regina, 3737 Wascana Parkway, Regina, Saskatchewan S4S 0A2, Canada. [2]Private Practice, Regina, Saskatchewan, Canada.

References

1. Cholewicki J, McGill SM: **Mechanical stability of the in vivo lumbar spine: implications for injury and chronic low back pain.** *Clin Biomech* 1996, **11**:1–15.
2. McGill SM, Grenier S, Kavcic N, Cholewicki J: **Coordination of muscle activity to assure stability of the lumbar spine.** *J Electromyogr Kinesiol* 2003, **13**:353–359.
3. Panjabi MM: **The stabilizing system of the spine. Part I. Function, dysfunction, adaptation, and enhancement.** *J Spinal Disord* 1992, **5**:383–389.
4. Panjabi MM: **The stabilizing system of the spine. Part II. Neutral zone and instability hypothesis.** *J Spinal Disord* 1992, **5**:390–396.
5. Barr KP, Griggs M, Cadby T: **Lumbar stabilization: core concepts and current literature. Part 1.** *Am J Phys Med Rehabil* 2005, **84**:473–480.
6. Barr KP, Griggs M, Cadby T: **Lumbar stabilization: a review of core concepts and current literature. Part 2.** *Am J Phys Med Rehabil* 2007, **86**:72–80.
7. Hodges PW: **Pain and motor control: from the laboratory to rehabilitation.** *J Electromyogr Kinesiol* 2011, **21**:220–228.
8. Bruno P, Bagust J: **An investigation into motor pattern differences used during prone hip extension between subjects with and without low back pain.** *Clin Chiropr* 2007, **10**:68–80.
9. Hodges PW, Richardson CA: **Inefficient muscular stabilization of the lumbar spine associated with low back pain. A motor control evaluation of transversus abdominis.** *Spine* 1996, **21**:2640–2650.
10. Hodges PW, Richardson CA: **Delayed postural contraction of transversus abdominis in low back pain associated with movement of the lower limb.** *J Spinal Disord* 1998, **11**:46–56.
11. Hungerford B, Gilleard W, Hodges P: **Evidence of altered lumbopelvic muscle recruitment in the presence of sacroiliac joint pain.** *Spine* 2003, **28**:1593–1600.
12. Leinonen V, Kankaanpaa M, Airaksinen O, Hanninen O: **Back and hip extensor activities during trunk flexion/extension: effects of low back pain and rehabilitation.** *Arch Phys Med Rehabil* 2000, **81**:32–37.
13. Newcomer KL, Jacobson TD, Gabriel DA, Larson DR, Brey RH, An KN: **Muscle activation patterns in subjects with and without low back pain.** *Arch Phys Med Rehabil* 2002, **83**:816–821.
14. Scholtes SA, Gombatto SP, Van Dillen LR: **Differences in lumbopelvic motion between people with and people without low back pain during two lower limb movement tests.** *Clin Biomech* 2009, **24**:7–12.
15. Vogt L, Pfeifer K, Banzer W: **Neuromuscular control of walking with chronic low-back pain.** *Man Ther* 2003, **8**:21–28.
16. Howarth SJ, Allison AE, Grenier SG, Cholewicki J, McGill SM: **On the implications of interpreting the stability index: a spine example.** *J Biomech* 2004, **37**:1147–1154.
17. Murphy DR, Byfield D, McCarthy P, Humphreys K, Gregory AA, Rochon R: **Interexaminer reliability of the hip extension test for suspected impaired motor control of the lumbar spine.** *J Manipulative Physiol Ther* 2006, **29**:374–377.
18. Liebenson C, Karpowicz AM, Brown SH, Howarth SJ, McGill SM: **The active straight leg raise test and lumbar spine stability.** *PM R* 2010, **1**:530–535.
19. Roussel NA, Nijs J, Truijen S, Smeuninx L, Stassijns G: **Low back pain: clinimetric properties of the Trendelenburg test, active straight leg raise test, and breathing pattern during active straight leg raising.** *J Manipulative Physiol Ther* 2007, **30**:270–278.
20. Chaitow L, DeLany JW: *Clinical Application of Neuromuscular Techniques. Volume 2. The Lower Body*, Volume 2. Edinburgh: Churchill Livingstone; 2002.
21. Janda V: **Evaluation of muscular imbalance.** In *Rehabilitation of the Spine: A Practitioner's Manual.* Edited by Liebenson C. Baltimore: Lippincott Williams & Wilkins; 1996:97–112.
22. Jull GA, Janda V: **Muscles and motor control in low back pain: assessment and management.** In *Physical Therapy of the Low Back.* Edited by Twomey LT, Taylor JR. New York: Churchill Livingstone; 1987:253–278.
23. Bruno P, Bagust J: **An investigation into the within-subject and between-subject consistency of motor patterns used during prone hip extension in subjects without low back pain.** *Clin Chiropr* 2006, **9**:11–20.
24. Bruno P, Bagust J, Cook J, Osborne N: **An investigation into the activation patterns of back and hip muscles during prone hip extension in non-low back pain subjects: Normal vs. abnormal lumbar spine motion patterns.** *Clin Chiropr* 2008, **11**:4–14.
25. Guimaraes CQ, Sakamoto ACL, Laurentino GEC, Teixeira-Salmela LF: **Electromyographic activity during active prone hip extension did not discriminate individuals with and without low back pain.** *Rev Bras Fisioter* 2010, **14**:351–357.
26. Lehman GJ, Lennon D, Tresidder B, Rayfield B, Poschar M: **Muscle recruitment patterns during the prone leg extension.** *BMC Musculoskelet Disord* 2004, **5**:3.
27. Sakamoto AC, Teixeira-Salmela LF, de Paula-Goulart FR, de Morais Faria CD, Guimaraes CQ: **Muscular activation patterns during active prone hip extension exercises.** *J Electromyogr Kinesiol* 2009, **19**:105–112.
28. Vogt L, Banzer W: **Dynamic testing of the motor stereotype in prone hip extension from neutral position.** *Clin Biomech* 1997, **12**:122–127.
29. Mens JM, Vleeming A, Snijders CJ, Stam HJ, Ginai AZ: **The active straight leg raising test and mobility of the pelvic joints.** *Eur Spine J* 1999, **8**:468–473.
30. Snijders CJ, Vleeming A, Stoeckart R: **Transfer of lumbosacral load to iliac bones and legs.1. Biomechanics of self-bracing of the sacroiliac joints and its significance for treatment and exercise.** *Clin Biomech* 1993, **8**:285–294.
31. Mens JM, Vleeming A, Snijders CJ, Koes BW, Stam HJ: **Reliability and validity of the active straight leg raise test in posterior pelvic pain since pregnancy.** *Spine* 2001, **26**:1167–1171.
32. Hungerford B, Gilleard W, Lee D: **Altered patterns of pelvic bone motion determined in subjects with posterior pelvic pain using skin markers.** *Clin Biomech* 2004, **19**:456–464.
33. Rabin A, Shashua A, Pizem K, Dar G: **The interrater reliability of physical examination tests that may predict the outcome or suggest the need for lumbar stabilization exercises.** *J Orthop Sports Phys Ther* 2013, **43**:83–90.
34. Kottner J, Audige L, Brorson S, Donner A, Gajewski BJ, Hrobjartsson A, Roberts C, Shoukri M, Streiner DL: **Guidelines for reporting reliability and agreement studies (GRRAS) were proposed.** *J Clin Epidemiol* 2011, **64**:96–106.
35. Childs JD, Piva SR, Fritz JM: **Responsiveness of the numeric pain rating scale in patients with low back pain.** *Spine* 2005, **30**:1331–1334.
36. Ageberg E, Bennell KL, Hunt MA, Simic M, Roos EM, Creaby MW: **Validity and inter-rater reliability of medio-lateral knee motion observed during a single-limb mini squat.** *BMC Musculoskelet Disord* 2010, **11**:265.

37. Davidson M, Keating JL: **A comparison of five low back disability questionnaires: reliability and responsiveness.** *Phys Ther* 2002, **82**:8–24.
38. Fairbank JC, Pynsent PB: **The oswestry disability index.** *Spine* 2000, **25**:2940–2952.
39. Sim J, Wright CC: **The kappa statistic in reliability studies: use, interpretation, and sample size requirements.** *Phys Ther* 2005, **85**:257–268.
40. Davidson M: **The interpretation of diagnostic test: a primer for physiotherapists.** *Aust J Physiother* 2002, **48**:227–232.
41. Landis JR, Koch GG: **The measurement of observer agreement for categorical data.** *Biometrics* 1977, **33**:159–174.
42. Murphy DR, Hurwitz EL, Hart B: **Comparison of findings of active straight leg raise test in patients with lumbar versus sacroiliac pain [abstract].** *J Chriopr Educ* 2012, **26**:100.
43. Lewis CL, Sahrmann SA: **Muscle activation and movement patterns during prone hip extension exercise in women.** *J Athl Train* 2009, **44**:238–248.

Reliability of ultrasound measurement of automatic activity of the abdominal muscle in participants with and without chronic low back pain

Amir Massoud Arab[1*], Omid Rasouli[2], Mohsen Amiri[1] and Nahid Tahan[3]

Abstract

Background: Ultrasound (US) imaging has been considered as a non-invasive technique to measure thickness and estimate relative abdominal muscle activity. Although some studies have assessed the reliability of US imaging, no study has assessed the reliability of US measurement of automatic activity of abdominal muscles in positions with different levels of stability in participants with chronic low back pain (cLBP). The purpose of this study was to investigate within-day and between-days reliability of US thickness measurements of automatic activity of the abdominal muscles in asymptomatic participants and within-day reliability in those with cLBP.

Methods: A total of 20 participants (10 with cLBP, 10 healthy) participated in the study. The reliability of US thickness measurements at supine lying and sitting positions (sitting on a chair, sitting on a gym ball with both feet on the ground or lifting one foot off the floor) were assessed. We evaluated within-day reliability in all participants and between-days reliability in asymptomatic participants.

Results: We found high ICC scores (0.85-0.95) and also small SEM and MDC scores in both groups. The reliability of the measurements was comparable between participants with and without LBP in each position but the SEMs and MDCs was slightly higher in patient group compared with healthy group. It indicates high intra-tester reliability for the US measurement of the thickness of abdominal muscles in all positions.

Conclusion: US imaging can be used as a reliable method for assessment of automatic activity of abdominal muscles in positions with low levels of stability in participants with and without LBP.

Keywords: Ultrasound, Reliability, Abdominal muscles, Low back pain

Background

Low back pain (LBP) is one of the most common musculoskeletal complaints in today's societies, affecting up to 70-80% of the population, at least one episode during their lifetime [1]. There is a considerable evidence indicating that dysfunction of abdominal muscles is a key impairment in patients with chronic LBP (cLBP) [2-4], which might affect spinal stability [5].

The abdominal musculature are divided into the anterolateral abdominal wall, consisting of the transversus abdominis (TrA), internal oblique (IO) and external oblique (EO); and the anterior wall, including the rectus abdominis (RA) muscle and associated fascia. The TrA muscle and posterior part of IO muscle are the part of a deep muscle cylinder that play a major role in spinal stability during functional activities [6]. The RA and EO are considered as part of a global muscle system that control spinal orientation, balance the external loads applied to the trunk and transfer load from the thorax to the pelvis [7]. Automatic activation of the abdominal muscles has been considered as a protective mechanism for lumbar spine [8]. Different patterns of abdominal muscle activation have been reported in patients with LBP compared to healthy individuals [9-11]. Ferreira et al. [9] found changes in automatic control of TrA during isometric low load tasks with the limbs suspended in people with LBP. Rasouli et al. [11] showed although the thickness change in TrA and IO increased as the stability of the position

* Correspondence: arabloo_masoud@hotmail.com
[1]Department of Physical Therapy, University of Social Welfare and Rehabilitation Sciences, Evin, Koodakyar Ave, Zip Code: 1985713831 Tehran, Iran
Full list of author information is available at the end of the article

decreased in individuals with and without LBP, the amount of thickness changes were less in participants with LBP.

Assessment and measurement of the activity pattern of abdominal muscles can provide better understanding of pain behavior in patients with cLBP in the clinical environment.

A variety of measurement tools have been used by physical therapists to assess abdominal muscle activity in individuals with or without LBP. Real-time ultrasound (US) imaging has been recently used as a safe, cost-effective and feasible method to evaluate muscle structure, function and activity [12-14]. It allows real time and direct visualization and evaluation of the abdominal muscles while they contract. Changes in the thickness of abdominal muscles is measured and considered as indicator of voluntary or automatic activity of the abdominal muscles during US imaging [9,12,15]. Validity studies found good to high correlation between the muscle thickness measured by US and EMG activity in low force contractions [13,16] or those obtained using magnetic resonance imaging (MRI) [17]. McMeeken et al. [13] found good to high correlation between the needle EMG recordings of the TrA and US changes in thickness of the muscle at all activity level. Hodges et al. [16] compared the thickness changes in the abdominal muscles in real time US and EMG activity. They found that change in thickness and EMG activity of the TrA and IO muscles were linearly correlated at low contraction levels. Accordingly, using US imaging has been considered as a non-invasive technique to measure the thickness and estimate relative abdominal muscles activity.

Reliability is a psychometric property reflecting the degree to which repeated measurements provide similar results and reduction in measurement errors. Demonstrating acceptable reliability is essential for any kind of measurement and for making valid decisions. Considering lower stability, gym ball is frequently recommended in clinical practice to facilitate abdominal muscles activity. Change in the abdominal muscle thickness during sitting on a gym ball has been previously considered as automatic activity of the abdominal muscles to provide more stability [11,18]. Previous studies have investigated the reliability of US imaging in healthy individuals and patients with LBP [9,18-24] but they have mostly assessed the reliability of the antero-lateral abdominal wall muscles thickness, at rest and during voluntary abdominal muscle contraction such as abdominal hollowing manoeuvre [21,23,25-27]. The studies reported good to excellent reliability for single measures of thickness and poor to good reliability for thickness change measurements (reflecting the muscle activity). However, only a few studies evaluated the reliability of US measurements of automatic activation of abdominal muscles [9,12]. Review of the literature showed that there is no research conducted to determine the reliability of US measurement of automatic activity of abdominal muscles in sitting positions with different levels of stability. Considering the fact that gym ball is not a stable condition and during sitting on gym ball the participant's position is instantaneously changing compared with sitting on a stable level such as a chair, abdominal muscles thickness may change in different moments and recording the US thickness measurement may be criticized.

Therefore, the purpose of this study was to evaluate within-day and between-days reliability in obtaining US thickness measurements of all abdominal muscles at supine lying and during different sitting positions (sitting on a chair, sitting on a gym ball with both feet on the ground or lifting one foot off the floor) in participants with and without cLBP.

Methods

Subjects

A total of 20 male volunteers (10 with chronic LBP, 10 without LBP) participated in the study. The population in this study was a sample of convenience made up of participants who were between the ages of 20 and 40 years. Patients were included if they had a history of LBP for more than six weeks before the study or had recurrent LBP and had experienced at least three episodes of LBP, each lasting more than one week, during the year before the study [28]. Asymptomatic participants were evaluated and found to have no complaint of any pain or dysfunction in their low back, pelvis, thoracic and lower extremities. Participants were excluded if they had a history of neuromuscular, musculoskeletal and cardiopulmonary diseases. The study conformed to the Declaration of Helsinki and was approved by the Human Ethics Committee at the University of Social Welfare and Rehabilitation Sciences, Tehran, Iran. All participants signed a consent form before participation in the study.

Ultrasound measurement of the abdominal muscle thickness

A diagnostic US imaging unit set in B-mode (Ultrasonix-ES500, Canada) with a linear array transducer (7.5 MHz) was used to measure the abdominal muscles thickness in four different positions: 1) supine lying, 2) relaxed sitting comfortably on a chair 43 cm high supported against a back rest, with arms folded; hands gently resting on the opposite shoulders and the feet together on the floor, 3) sitting comfortably with a straight back on a 65 cm in diameter, gym ball with arms folded and resting on the opposite shoulders and both feet on the floor and 4) sitting on a gym ball lifting the left foot off the floor by approximately 10 cm [11,18]. Each position was held enough for the examiner to freeze a clear image of the muscle thickness at the end of expiration, usually no more than 2 minutes.

For antero-lateral abdominal wall muscles (TrA, IO, EO), the US transducer was transversely located across the right side of the abdominal wall over the anterior axillary line, midway between the 12th rib and the iliac crest, to obtain a clear image of the deep abdominal layers [13,22]. For anterior abdominal wall muscle (RA), the transducer was placed 2–3 cm above the umbilicus, 2–3 cm from the midline [22,29].

The image was frozen at the end of expiration and a vertical straight line through the center of the US image was used to ensure standardized placement of the measurement line. The cursor points carefully measured the muscle thickness between the inside edge of fascial bands in millimeter (mm). The US transducer was not displaced during the testing procedure.

Procedures

Within-day intra-tester reliability of the US thickness measurements of the abdominal muscles was assessed in all participants (with and without cLBP) while between-day reliability was investigated in asymptomatic participants. To establish within-day reliability, at first the examiner performed measurements in all tested positions in participants and then after 60 minutes repeated the measurements in a blinded fashion and in a random order with the same procedure. The participants testing positions and the order of measurements were randomly selected to reduce the memory effect. For between-days reliability, the US measurements in all positions were repeated after one week in asymptomatic participants (N = 10). All testing procedure was performed in the biomechanics laboratory of the Department of Physical Therapy in the University of Social Welfare and Rehabilitation Sciences, Tehran, Iran.

Data analysis

Kolmogrov-Smirnov test was utilized to assess the normality of distribution for US measurement of muscle thickness at different testing positions. Normal distribution was observed for variables.

Two measurement sessions were implemented in one day for within-day reliability in all participants. Third session of measurement was done one week later in asymptomatic participants for between-days reliability assessment. The intra-class correlation coefficient (ICC) has become the preferred index for test-retest reliability as it reflects both correlation and agreement [30]. The ICC, two way mixed effect model, was used to assess intra-tester reliability of the measurements. We calculated the ICC (3,1) as described by Shrout and Fleiss [31] because only one judge evaluated the same population.

Relative reliability values such as ICC are not sufficient to interpret in the context of an individual score. Therefore, we calculated standard error of measurement (SEM) and minimal detectable change (MDC) to make a judgment about the degree that measurements vary for an individual. The SEM is useful in reliability studies to determine the range of scores that would be expected from one assessment session to the next. The SEM was calculated using the formula: [$SEM = SD \sqrt{1-r}$] where SD is the standard deviation calculated from the measurements and r is the reliability coefficient for that measurement, in this case, the calculated ICC (3,1) value and, then, the coefficient of variation was calculated (CV in %: SEM/mean value for the given parameter × 100) [21].

Power analysis was used to determine the sample size for test. Type I error (α) was set at 0.05 and power of the test was 0.80. Considering this, it seems that calculated sample size in this study was appropriate to test the hypothesis and the results derived from the study are meaningful.

Results

The demographic data for both LBP and healthy control groups are summarized in Table 1.

Table 2 shows the US measurements of the absolute abdominal muscle thicknesses (Mean ± SD) in mm in two groups for different assessments during different testing positions. The smallest absolute abdominal thicknesses were related to supine lying position and the highest values belonged to position 4 when participant sat on the gym ball and lifted his left foot off the floor in both healthy and cLBP groups. The absolute thickness of TrA ranged from 3.5 ± 0.5 mm to 6.6 ± 0.8 during four positions in healthy group and from 3.5 ± 0.8 to 4.9 ± 1 mm in LBP group. The absolute thicknesses of IO,EO and RA ranged from 9.2 ± 1.4 to 12.8 ± 2.1; 5.8 ± 1.1 to 7.5 ± 0.9 and 12.9 ± 2 to 16.9 ± 2.2 mm during mentioned positions in healthy participants respectively, and from 8.3 ± 1.1 to 10.5 ± 2.5; 5.8 ± 1.1 to 7.9 ± 2.6 and 14 ± 3.7 to 17.5 ± 5.4 mm respectively in patients with LBP (Table 2).

Table 3 presents the ICC (3,1), SEM, CV (SEM as % mean) and MDC values for within-day and between-days reliability of US thickness measurements of abdominal muscles were taken during different testing

Table 1 Demographic data of the participants in each group (Mean ± SD)

Variables	Without LBP (n = 10)	With LBP (n = 10)
Age (years)	25 ± 3	26 ± 3
Weight (kg)	75 ± 7	76 ± 8
Height (m)	1.75 ± 0.06	1.75 ± 0.06
BMI (kg/m^2)	24.3 ± 0.9	24.6 ± 0.7

SD Standard deviation, *LBP* Low back pain, *BMI* Body mass index.

Table 2 The (Mean ± SD) scores for the ultrasound thickness measurements (in mm) of the abdominal muscles during different testing positions in both groups

Position	Muscle	Without LBP			With LBP	
		First assessment	Second assessment	Third assessment	First assessment	Second assessment
P 1	TrA	3.6 ± 0.6	3.5 ± 0.5	3.8 ± 0.6	3.5 ± 0.8	3.7 ± 1.0
	IO	9.2 ± 1.4	9.3 ± 1.3	9.2 ± 1.5	8.4 ± 1.5	8.3 ± 1.1
	EO	5.8 ± 1.1	5.9 ± 1.2	5.9 ± 1.0	5.8 ± 1.1	6.1 ± 1.4
	RA	12.9 ± 2.0	13.0 ± 2.3	13.1 ± 2.1	14.0 ± 3.7	14.2 ± 4.3
P 2	TrA	4.0 ± 0.7	3.9 ± 0.8	3.9 ± 0.9	3.6 ± 0.8	3.6 ± 0.8
	IO	9.4 ± 1.5	9.4 ± 1.3	9.5 ± 1.8	8.1 ± 1.2	8.3 ± 1.3
	EO	6.2 ± 1.2	6.0 ± 1.1	5.9 ± 1.2	6.4 ± 2.0	6.7 ± 2.0
	RA	13.1 ± 2.0	13.2 ± 2.1	13.4 ± 2.0	15.8 ± 5.2	15.3 ± 4.8
P 3	TrA	4.4 ± 0.7	4.5 ± 0.6	4.4 ± 0.5	3.8 ± 0.9	4.0 ± 0.7
	IO	10.0 ± 1.6	10.0 ± 1.7	10.3 ± 1.6	8.8 ± 2.2	9.1 ± 2.3
	EO	6.2 ± 1.1	6.54 ± 1.3	6.3 ± 1.1	6.6 ± 2.2	6.9 ± 2.6
	RA	13.9 ± 2.1	14.1 ± 2.4	14.2 ± 2.1	16.2 ± 5.4	16.4 ± 6.0
P 4	TrA	6.6 ± 0.8	6.3 ± 0.6	6.5 ± 0.8	4.9 ± 1.0	4.1 ± 1.0
	IO	12.8 ± 2.1	12.8 ± 2.1	12.6 ± 2.0	10.5 ± 2.5	10.5 ± 2.3
	EO	7.5 ± 0.9	7.4 ± 1.2	7.4 ± 1.0	7.9 ± 2.6	7.9 ± 2.2
	RA	16.5 ± 2.5	16.8 ± 2.8	16.9 ± 2.2	17.2 ± 4.8	17.5 ± 5.4

SD Standard deviation, *LBP* Low back pain, *TrA* Transversus abdominis, *IO* Internal oblique, *EO* External oblique, *RA* Rectus abdominis, *P 1* Supine lying, *P 2* Sitting on chair with both feet on the ground, *P 3* Sitting on gym ball with both feet on the ground, *P 4* Sitting on gym ball lifting the left foot off the floor.

positions in each group. Depending on the muscle (TrA, IO, EO and RA) and participant's position (supine lying or various sitting positions), reliability of thickness measurements ranged from 0.88 to 0.95 for within-day comparisons and from 0.85 to 0.94 for between-days comparisons in healthy group and from 0.89 to 0.94 for within-day comparisons in LBP group which indicated high intra-tester reliability for the US measurement of thickness of abdominal muscles in all positions (Table 3).

Generally we had higher SEM in position 4 than position 1 in both groups and SEMs of patient group (0.25 to 1.27 mm) were rather higher than corresponding SEMs of control group (0.19 to 0.71 mm), and, when expressed as a percentage (CV) of the corresponding mean thicknesses ranged from 1.6 to 9.7% (in healthy participants) and 1.7 to 17.3% (in LBP patients) (Table 3).

Likewise SEM trends in two groups, MDCs were higher in position 4 than supine lying in both groups and MDCs of patient group ranged from 0.69 to 3.50 mm and were slightly higher than corresponding MDCs of control group (0.52 to 1.96 mm) (Table 3).

Discussion

Physical therapists have recently utilized US imaging to evaluate muscle function, structure and activity and change in the thickness of abdominal muscles is measured and considered as indicator of voluntary or automatic activity of the abdominal muscles in this method [12,14,15]. However, like any other measurements demonstrating adequate reliability is a prerequisite for using US measurement as a valid measure of abdominal muscles activity to make decision especially in clinical setting. According to Domholdt [32], the reliability is not a fixed property but it depends on the studied population and testing positions.

To our knowledge, this is the first study to collectively evaluated within-day and between-days reliability of US measurement of automatic activity of abdominal muscles in sitting positions with different stability levels in healthy participants and within-day reliability in patients with cLBP.

The results of this study suggest that there is not only high reliability of muscle thickness in asymptomatic participants but also in patients with cLBP and the results also are consistent with the available literature on the topic, finding high ICC scores and also very small SEM and MDC scores [21,23].

In the patient group, the ICCs were almost the same as the control group during each testing position and it is important for using US to evaluate abdominal muscle activity in patients with LBP in the clinical setting. The ICCs of thickness measurements ranged from 0.85 to 0.95 for within-day and between-days comparisons depending on the muscle and participant's position which indicated high intra-tester reliability for the US

Table 3 ICC, SEM and MDC, CV values for within-day and between-days reliability of the ultrasound measurements at different testing positions

Position	Muscle	Without LBP								With LBP			
		Within-day (Between-trial)				Between-days				Within-day (Between-trial)			
		ICC	SEM	MDC	CV%	ICC	SEM	MDC	CV%	ICC	SEM	MDC	CV%
P 1	TrA	0.92	0.19	0.52	5.4	0.90	0.21	0.58	5.8	0.91	0.25	0.69	6.9
	IO	0.92	0.20	0.55	2.1	0.92	0.20	0.55	2.1	0.92	0.26	0.71	3
	EO	0.90	0.23	0.63	3.9	0.88	0.26	0.71	4.5	0.89	0.34	0.93	5.7
	RA	0.88	0.28	0.77	2.1	0.85	0.31	0.85	2.4	0.93	0.25	0.69	1.7
P 2	TrA	0.95	0.30	0.82	7.6	0.92	0.38	1.05	9.7	0.94	0.37	1.02	10.2
	IO	0.93	0.40	1.10	4.5	0.93	0.40	1.10	4.2	0.93	0.39	1.07	4.8
	EO	0.94	0.38	1.05	6.1	0.91	0.47	1.29	9	0.94	0.53	1.46	8.1
	RA	0.93	0.52	1.43	3.9	0.93	0.52	1.43	3.9	0.94	0.56	1.54	3.6
P 3	TrA	0.90	0.34	0.93	7.7	0.86	0.40	1.10	9	0.90	0.39	1.07	10
	IO	0.92	0.31	0.85	3.1	0.90	0.34	0.93	3.4	0.93	0.49	1.35	5.3
	EO	0.92	0.29	0.80	4.6	0.89	0.33	0.91	5.3	0.92	0.56	1.54	8.3
	RA	0.93	0.22	0.60	1.6	0.87	0.31	0.85	2.2	0.93	0.65	1.79	4
P 4	TrA	0.94	0.40	1.10	6.3	0.89	0.54	1.49	8.3	0.93	0.78	2.15	17.3
	IO	0.94	0.41	1.13	3.2	0.94	0.41	1.13	3.2	0.92	1.27	3.50	12
	EO	0.92	0.52	1.43	7	0.93	0.48	1.32	6.4	0.92	1.23	3.39	15
	RA	0.94	0.55	1.51	3.3	0.90	0.71	1.96	4.3	0.94	0.93	2.57	5.3

SD Standard deviation, *ICC* Intra-class correlation coefficient, *SEM* Standard error of measurement, *MDC* Minimal detectable change, *CV* Coefficient of variation, *LBP* Low back pain, *TrA* Transversus abdominis, *IO* Internal oblique, *EO* External oblique, *RA* Rectus abdominis, *P 1* Supine lying, *P 2* Sitting on chair with both feet on the ground, *P 3* Sitting on gym ball with both feet on the ground, *P 4* Sitting on gym ball lifting the left foot off the floor. All SEM and MDC values are in millimeter.

measurement of abdominal muscle thickness in all positions. Norasteh et al. [22] reported good reliability (ICC: 0.81- 0.97) of abdominal muscles (TrA, IO, EO, RA) assessment by US imaging in asymptomatic participants and patients with acute LBP. In another study, Costa et al. [12] reported high reliability (ICC: 0.75- 0.94) for absolute thickness and moderate reliability (ICC: 0.26-0.72) for thickness changes in US measurements of automatic activity of TrA, IO and EO muscles in patients with cLBP. However, in this study we assessed the reliability of absolute muscles thickness measurements and thickness changes were not analyzed.

In practical terms, the SEM shows more useful information than the ICC [33] and the CV is very good to compare the relative measurement error of variables with differing absolute values or measurement units. In the current study, the SEMs in position 4 were higher than position 1 in both groups and the SEMs of patient group (0.25- 1.27 mm) were rather higher than corresponding SEMs of control group (0.19- 0.71 mm), and, the CVs of the corresponding mean thicknesses ranged from 1.6 to 9.7% (healthy participants) and from 1.7 to 17.3% (cLBP patients). The SEMs were consistent with prior error measurements from other accepted techniques like Teyhen et al. [23] found the SEM of 0.13 to 0.31 mm for the TrA muscle. The CV in this study was similar to the results of previous studies which reported 11–14% for the reliability of TrA thickness and whole abdominal mass thickness [21,23]. All the SEMs and the corresponding CVs were low, so make them promising measures for further studies.

The MDC is especially useful for interpreting the relevance of any changes recorded after an intervention [34]. The MDCs of abdominal muscles were higher in position 4 than supine lying in both groups, the same as SEM values and MDCs of patient group ranged from 0.7 to 3.5 mm and were slightly higher than corresponding MDCs of 0.5 to 1.9 mm in control group. Critchley et al. [35] reported MDC of 0.6 (TrA) and 1.2 (OI) mm in supine position, and Bunce et al. [36] found values ranging from 0.9 to 1.8 mm for TA only in supine, sitting and standing. The differences between our results with previous studies are related to the positions and level of contractions for example if we just exclude the values of position 4, we have a range of 0.5 to 1.8 mm. which are similar to those recorded at rest and hence appear to be acceptable from the perspective of human performance measurements [37].

Reliability can be influenced by several factors such as the participants, examiner and clinical or experimental setting. In addition, there are some sources of error which might affect procedure of US measurement including accuracy of marking the fascial bands, position of patient/transducer and detection of landmarks [12].

The high reliability of our US measurements may be due to the fact that the clear image was frozen on the screen and the muscle thickness between the fascial bands was measured carefully by cursor points. Furthermore, the US transducer was not displaced during the testing procedure as much as possible and the positions were the same for every participant.

This study was not investigated the issue of validity for US imaging. Considering the results of this study and validity studies [16,17], US imaging can be used to assess and compare the automatic activity of the abdominal muscles in positions with different stability level between participants with and without cLBP.

Conclusion

In agreement with previous studies, the results of this study demonstrate high within-day and between-days reliability for US thickness measurements of the abdominal muscles at supine lying and sitting position with different levels of stability in healthy participants and high within-day reliability in patients with cLBP.

These results indicate that real-time US imaging can be reliably used to evaluate and compare the automatic activity of the abdominal muscles between participants with and without cLBP. This might also help to determine the efficacy of prescribed treatments for cLBP patients.

Limitation

This study assessed the reliability of US thickness measurements of the abdominal muscles in men. The results might not be extrapolated to the women. More studies are needed to collectively perform this study in men and women. The other point was that the study was only limited to a younger age group.

Another area of concern is that the between-day reliability was assessed in the asymptomatic participants. For between-days reliability, the US measurements were repeated after one week. It was possible that the pain intensity changed after one week in LBP patients. Change in pain intensity could affect the trunk stabilizer muscles such as abdominal muscles. Since the change in pain could not be completely controlled after one week, we assessed between-day reliability in asymptomatic participants with no LBP. This issue can be considered as a limitation in this study.

It is suggested to assess the within-day and between-day reliability for automatic activation of the abdominal muscles during different tasks in the patients with cLBP.

Clinical implication

US imaging can be used as a reliable method to evaluate and compare the automatic activity of abdominal muscles in different positions with different levels of stability in participants with and without cLBP and this might help to determine the efficacy of prescribed treatments for cLBP patients.

Ethical approval

This research was reviewed and was approved by the Human Subject Committee at University of Social Welfare and Rehabilitation Sciences.

Competing interests

AMA contributed to conception, design, analysis, interpretation of data and drafting the manuscript. OR carried out the data collection and drafting the manuscript. MA participated in design and interpretation of data. NT participated in data collection and helped to draft the manuscript. All authors read and approved the final manuscript.

Authors' contributions

The authors declare that they have no competing interests.

Author details

[1]Department of Physical Therapy, University of Social Welfare and Rehabilitation Sciences, Evin, Koodakyar Ave, Zip Code: 1985713831 Tehran, Iran. [2]Department of Physical Therapy, Faculty of Health Education and Social Work, Sør-Trøndelag University College (HiST), Trondheim, Norway. [3]Department of Physical Therapy, Shahid Beheshti University of Medical Sciences, Tehran, Iran.

References

1. Ehrlich GE: **Low back pain.** *Bull World Health Organ* 2003, **81**:671–672.
2. Hodges PW, Richardson CA: **Inefficient muscular stabilization of the lumbar spine associated with low back pain. A motor control evaluation of transverses abdominis.** *Spine* 1996, **21**:2640–2650.
3. Hodges PW, Richardson CA: **Delayed postural contraction of transverses abdominis associated with movement of lower limb in people with low back pain.** *J Spinal Disord* 1998, **11**:46–56.
4. Jull GA, Richardson CA: **Motor control problems in patients with spinal pain: a new direction for therapeutic exercises.** *J Manipulative Physiol Ther* 2000, **23**:115–117.
5. Cholewicki J, McGill SM: **Mechanical stability of the in vivo lumbar spine: implications for injury and chronic low back pain.** *Clin Biomech* 1996, **11**:1–15.
6. Richardson CA, Jull GA, Hodges PW, Hides JA: *Therapeutic exercise for spinal segmental stabilization in low back pain. Scientific basis and clinical approach.* Edinburgh: Churchill Livingstone; 1999:43–70.
7. Bergmark A: **Stability of the lumbar spine: a study in mechanical engineering.** *Acta Orthop Scand Suppl* 1989, **230**:1–54.
8. Hodges PW, Moseley GL: **Pain and motor control of the lumbopelvic region: effect and possible mechanisms.** *J Electromyogr Kinesiol* 2003, **13**:361–370.
9. Ferreira PH, Ferreira ML, Hodges PW: **Changes in recruitment of the abdominal muscles in people with low back pain: Ultrasound measurement of muscle activity.** *Spine* 2004, **29**:2560–2566.
10. Hides J, Wilson S, Stanton W, McMahon S, Keto H, McMahon K, Bryant M, Richardson C: **An MRI investigation into the function of the transversus abdominis muscle during "drawing-in" of the abdominal wall.** *Spine* 2006, **31**:E175–E178.
11. Rasouli O, Arab AM, Amiri M, Jaberzadeh S: **Ultrasound measurement of deep abdominal muscle activity in sitting positions with different stability levels in subjects with and without chronic low back pain.** *Man Ther* 2011, **16**:388–393.

12. Costa LO, Maher CG, Latimer J, Hodges PW, Shirley D: **An investigation of the reproducibility of ultrasound measures of abdominal muscle activation in patients with chronic non-specific low back pain.** *Eur Spine J* 2009, **18:**1059–1065.
13. McMeeken JM, Beith ID, Newham DJ, Milligan P, Critchley DJ: **The relationship between EMG and changes in thickness of transverses abdominis.** *Clin Biomech* 2004, **19:**337–342.
14. Teyhen DS, Gill NW, Whittaker JL, Henry SM, Hides JA, Hodges P: **Rehabilitative ultrasound imaging of the abdominal muscles.** *J Orthop Sports Phys Ther* 2007, **37:**450–466.
15. Hebert JJ, Koppenhaver SL, Parent EC, Fritz JM: **A systematic review of the reliability of rehabilitative ultrasound imaging for the quantitative assessment of the abdominal and lumbar trunk muscles.** *Spine* 2009, **34:**E848–E856.
16. Hodges PW, Pengel LMH, Herbert RD, Gandevia SC: **Measurement of muscle contraction with ultrasound imaging.** *Muscle and Nerve* 2003, **27:**682–692.
17. Hides JA, Belavý DL, Cassar L, Williams M, Wilson SJ, Richardson CA: **Altered response of the anterolateral abdominal muscles to simulated weight-bearing in subjects with low back pain.** *Eur Spine J* 2009, **18:**410–418.
18. Ainscough-potts AM, Morrissey MC, Critchley D: **The response of the transverse abdiominis and internal oblique muscle to different postures.** *Man Ther* 2006, **11:**54–60.
19. Beazell JR, Grindstaff TL, Magrum EM, Cullaty M, Hart JM, Shen FH: **Comparison of clinical test and real time ultrasound evaluation of muscle contraction in normals and patients with low back pain.** *J Man Manip Ther* 2006, **14:**168–169.
20. Koppenhaver SL, Hebert JJ, Fritz JM, Parent EC, Teyhen DS, Magel JS: **Reliability of rehabilitative ultrasound imaging of the transversus abdominis and lumbar multifidus muscles.** *Arch Phys Med Rehabil* 2009, **90:**87–94.
21. Mannion AF, Pulkovski N, Gubler D, Gorelick M, O'Riordan D, Loupas T, Schenk P, Gerber H, Sprott H: **Muscle thickness changes during abdominal hollowing: an assessment of between day measurement error in controls and patients with chronic low back pain.** *Eur Spine J* 2008, **17:**494–501.
22. Norasteh A, Ebrahimi E, Salavati M, Rafiei J, Abbasnejad E: **Reliability of B-mode ultrasonography for abdominal muscles in asymptomatic and patients with acute low back pain.** *J Bodyw Mov Ther* 2007, **11:**17–20.
23. Teyhen DS, Miltenberger CE, Deiters HM, Del Toro YM, Pulliam JN, Childs JD, Boyles RE, Flynn TW: **The use of ultrasound imaging of the abdominal drawing-in maneuver in subjects with low back pain.** *J Orthop Sports Phys Ther* 2005, **35:**346–355.
24. Costa LO, Maher CG, Latimer J, Smeets RJ: **Reproducibility of rehabilitative ultrasound imaging for the measurement of abdominal muscle activity: a systematic review.** *Phys Ther* 2009, **89**(8):756–769.
25. Pulkovski N, Mannion AF, Caporaso F, Toma V, Gubler D, Helbling D, Sprott H: **Ultrasound assessment of transversus abdominis muscle contraction ratio during abdominal hollowing: a useful tool to distinguish between patients with chronic low back pain and healthy controls? Eur Spine J.** *Suppl* 2012, **6:**S750–S759.
26. Teyhen DS, Childs JD, Stokes MJ, Wright AC, Dugan JL, George SZ: **Abdominal and lumbar multifidus muscle size and symmetry at rest and during contracted States. Normative reference ranges.** *J Ultrasound Med* 2012, **31**(7)1099–1110.
27. Teyhen DS, Rieger JL, Westrick RB, Miller AC, Molloy JM, Childs JD: **Changes in deep abdominal muscle thickness during common trunk-strengthening exercises using ultrasound imaging.** *J Orthop Sports Phys Ther* 2008, **38:**596–605.
28. Nourbakhsh MR, Arab AM: **Relationship between mechanical factors and incidence of low back pain.** *J Orthop Sports Phys Ther* 2002, **32:**447–460.
29. Misuri G, Colagrande S, Gorini M, Iandelli I, Mancini M, Duranti R, Scano G: **In vivo ultrasound assessment of respiratory function of abdominal muscles in normal subjects.** *Eur Respir J* 1997, **10:**2861–2867.
30. Portney LG, Watkins MP: *Reliability of measurements*, Foundations of clinical research: applications to practice. 3rd edition. New Jersey: Pearson Education Inc; 2009.
31. Shrout PE, Fleiss JL: **Intraclass correlation: use in assessing rater reliability.** *Psychol Bull* 1979, **86:**420–428.
32. Domholdt E: *Rehabilitation research: principles and applications.* 3rd edition. Philadelphia: Elsevier Saunders; 2005.
33. Rankin G, Stokes M: **Reliability of assessment tools in rehabilitation: an illustration of appropriate statistical analyses.** *Clin Rehabil* 1998, **12:**187–199.
34. Beaton DE: **Understanding the relevance of measured change through studies of responsiveness.** *Spine* 2000, **25:**3192–3199.
35. Critchley DJ, Coutts FJ: **Abdominal muscle function in chronic low back pain patients.** *Physiotherapy* 2002, **88:**322–332.
36. Bunce SM, Moore AP, Hough AD: **M-mode ultrasound: a reliable measure of transversus abdominis thickness?** *Clin Biomech (Bristol, Avon)* 2002, **17:**315–317.
37. Stokes M: **Reliability and repeatability of methods for measuring muscle in physiotherapy.** *Physiother Theory Pract* 1985, **1:**71–76.

24

Effect of osteopathic manipulative treatment on gastrointestinal function and length of stay of preterm infants: an exploratory study

Gianfranco Pizzolorusso[1*], Patrizia Turi[1], Gina Barlafante[2], Francesco Cerritelli[1], Cinzia Renzetti[2], Vincenzo Cozzolino[2], Marianna D'Orazio[2], Paola Fusilli[3], Fabrizio Carinci[1] and Carmine D'Incecco[3]

Abstract

Background: Organizational improvement of neonatal intensive care units requires strict monitoring of preterm infants, including routine assessment of physiological functions of the gastrointestinal system and optimized procedures for the definition of appropriate discharge timing.

Methods: We conducted a prospective study on the effect of osteopathic manipulative treatment in a cohort of N = 350 consecutive premature infants admitted to a neonatal intensive care unit without any major complication between 2005 and 2008. In addition to ordinary care, N = 162 subjects received osteopathic treatment. Endpoints of the study were differences between study and control groups in terms of excessive length of stay and gastrointestinal symptoms, defined as the upper quartiles in the distribution of the overall population. Statistical analysis was based on crude and adjusted odds ratios from multivariate logistic regression.

Results: Baseline characteristics were evenly distributed across treated/control groups, except for the rate of infants unable to be oral fed at admission, significantly higher among those undergoing osteopathic care (p = .03). Osteopathic treatment was significantly associated with a reduced risk of an average daily occurrence of gut symptoms per subject above .44 (OR = 0.45; 0.26-0.74). Gestational age lower or equal to 32 weeks, birth weight lower or equal to 1700 grams and no milk consumption at admission were associated with higher rates of length of stay in the unit of at least 28 days, while osteopathic treatment significantly reduced such risk (OR = 0.22;0.09-0.51).

Conclusions: In a population of premature infants, osteopathic manipulative treatment showed to reduce a high occurrence of gastrointestinal symptoms and an excessive length of stay in the NICU. Randomized control studies are needed to generalize these results to a broad population of high risk newborns.

Background

Significant improvements in neonatal technology utilized in neonatal intensive care units (NICUs) over the last 2 decades, along with evidence-based care guidelines, have significantly improved hospitalization and survival for both low birth weight (LBW) infants and the residual preterm population, albeit at a high cost. A major proportion of pediatric hospital stays in the United States is attributable to neonatal conditions that rank among the most expensive items in the list of services provided for children [1]. The average cost per infant is highest for preterm newborns with gestational age (GA) between 24-31 weeks, and next highest for those between 32-36 weeks, as opposed to the general population [2]. Costs per surviving infant generally decrease with increasing GA. In the United States, preterm/LBW infants account for half the hospitalization costs of all newborns and one quarter of overall pediatric costs [3].

Length of stay (LOS) in NICUs is strongly associated with GA and birth weight [4]. Infants delivered at the earliest GA have the longest hospital stays, partly because of the higher incidence of medical complications in very low birth weight (VLBW) infants.

* Correspondence: gianfranco.pizzolorusso@gmail.com
[1]EBOM - European Institute for Evidence Based Osteopathic Medicine, viale Unità d'Italia 1, 66100 Chieti, Italy
Full list of author information is available at the end of the article

However, compared to term infants, premature infants are unique in their need to attain not only medical stability but also physiologic maturity, including adequate temperature control, cessation of apnea and bradycardia, and adequate feeding behavior, before they are safely discharged to home [5,6].

Patterns of hospitalization of preterm infants are also associated with the presence of clinical symptoms of abnormal gastrointestinal function. In particular, vomit and regurgitation were found to be associated with increased esophageal acid occurrence among NICU patients [7], as well as gastric residuals (GR) [8], which can be linked to feeding behaviors and definitely improved by targeted feeding strategies.

In VLBW infants, feeding tolerance algorithms are based on pre-prandial GR volume measurement. High pre-prandial volumes of GR are regarded as significant markers of feeding intolerance [9]. Previous studies in NICUs show that neonates under stress have a higher incidence of stress-induced gastric mucosal damage [10,11]. Functional constipation and hard stools are common conditions in both term and preterm infants, usually leading to changes in feeding formulas [12] and use of enemas in specific settings [13].

Non invasive treatments to improve feeding tolerance and to reduce clinical complications of premature infants may represent a convenient option in the absence of standard procedures for specific subgroups of patients.

The present report describes the activity of a research team investigating the effects of Osteopathic Manipulative Treatment (OMT) in preterm infants, including monitoring of physiological functions of the gastrointestinal system and LOS.

Methods

Objective and endpoints of the study

To evaluate the efficacy of OMT on premature infants during hospitalization. Endpoints of the study were differences between study and control groups in terms of changes in gastrointestinal function and LOS.

Primary endpoints were measured over the entire period of NICU hospitalization as follows:

I. High frequency of gut symptoms, defined as the upper quartile of the average number of episodes of vomit, regurgitation, GR and enema per measurement visit per subject.

II. Excess duration of LOS, defined as the upper quartile of LOS in NICU per subject.

Study Design and Population

The study was based on a non randomized, longitudinal observational design investigating outcomes in a cohort of newborns admitted to the NICU of the main public hospital in Pescara, Abruzzo, Italy.

Eligible subjects included all infants consecutively admitted between January 2005 to June 2008 (N = 663). A total of N = 359 passed the following exclusion criteria: GA less than 29 weeks, or greater than 37 weeks; osteopathic treatment performed more than 14 days after birth; newborn transferred to/from other hospital/unit; newborn from an HIV seropositive and/or drug addicted mother; newborn with any of the following clinical conditions: genetic disorders, congenital abnormalities, cardiovascular abnormalities, neurological disorders; proven or suspected necrotizing enterocolitis with or without gastrointestinal perforation; proven or suspected abdominal obstruction; pre- and/or post- surgery patients; pneumoperitoneum and/or atelectasis. Among the 304 subjects excluded, 232 infants had a GA below 29 or above 37, while 78 subjects presented with severe clinical conditions.

After enrollment, 4 additional infants were dropped because of an unrecorded birth weight, and 5 infants (2 from the study group; 3 from the control group) because of complications arising during hospitalization.

The final total number of infants analyzed in this study was 350.

A total of 188 preterm infants were non-randomly assigned to routine neonatal care; while 162 subjects received routine care plus OMT. All patients from both groups were transferred from the delivery and/or operating room to the NICU immediately after birth.

No prior manipulation provided by any physical and/or massage therapist was performed on any infant.

Data collection

Data collection was performed by undergraduate osteopaths from the Accademia Italiana Osteopatia Tradizionale (AIOT). Measurements were recorded twice a week (Tuesdays and Fridays) based upon NICU's clinical charts completed by nursing staff who provided care on the same day.

Additional infant information was included: date of birth, admission/discharge from NICU, GA at birth (based on best obstetrical estimate), birth weight at admission and discharge, formula and/or breast milk intake volume. Gastrointestinal function was measured as regurgitation (defined as the passage of refluxed gastric contents into the oral pharynx), or vomiting (defined as the expulsion of the refluxed gastric contents from the mouth, i.e. feeding tolerance), or GR finding (milky, bilious and bloody; measured only on infants with oro/naso-gastric tube, recorded as present/not present), frequency of stooling and enema administration per patient care encounter. A neurological/developmental evaluation at entry/discharge was not available for this study as it does not constitute part of routine assessment in the NICU.

Data were directly entered on an Excel spreadsheet

Osteopathic Manipulative Treatment

Osteopathic treatment was administered to the intervention group on Tuesdays and Fridays. Subjects in the study arm received osteopathic care within 14 days after birth, regardless of the application of any other procedure (i.e. mechanical ventilation, blood transfusion or phototherapy).

OMT was performed by a group of osteopaths certified by the Registro degli Osteopati d'Italia with at least five years of clinical experience.

Treatment duration ranged between 20-30 minutes. The infant's entire body was evaluated and manipulative procedures were provided as indicated by the osteopathic palpatory structural examination results. Osteopaths performing OMT were trained to use only indirect and fluidic techniques which included: indirect myofascial, sutural spread, balanced membranous tension and balanced ligamentous tension (according to teachings of William Garner Sutherland, DO, and others [14]).

Clinical procedures and discharge strategy

Feeding regimen, feeding strategies and enema administration were based on the application of standard international guidelines to both study arms [13,15]. As distinct from UK/US hospitals, enema prescription used by the study NICU included five percent glucose glycerin enemas (10:1 mixture, 5 mL/kg), administered twice a day, until infants spontaneously expel at least 1 stool per day.

Physiological conditions required for discharge included: maintenance of body heat at room temperature, coordinated sucking, swallowing, and breathing while feeding; sustained pattern of weight gain; and stability of cardiorespiratory function (no episodes of apnea/bradycardia for 2-5 days, free of supplemental oxygen support) [6].

Statistical analysis

Main results are expressed in terms of odds ratios between each level of a potential risk factor and a set reference category (R.C.), with primary endpoints classified as binary outcomes (low/high).

Potential confounders included the following characteristics (categories): gender, GA (≤ 32; > 32- ≤ 35; > 35 weeks), birth weight (≤ 1700; > 1700- ≤ 2200; > 2200 grams), oral feeding at admission (No/Yes).

Univariate statistical tests included formal tests of the differences between study and control groups using chi-square for categorical variables and unpaired t-tests for continuous measurements.

Multivariate logistic regression was used to estimate the independent effect of OMT on primary outcomes, simultaneously adjusting for all potential confounders. Statistical significance was based on a probability level (α) equal to 0.05. Results were expressed in terms of point estimates (odds ratios: OR) and 95% confidence intervals (C.I.). All analyses were performed using the statistical programming language R [16].

Results

Univariate statistical analyses are shown in Table 1. No significant imbalances were found among treated and control groups in terms of main characteristics measured at admission, except for milk at admission (p = 0.03), showing a higher percentage of infants unable to be oral fed at entry into this study among those treated with OMT.

Upper quartiles led to the definition of the following thresholds for the outcomes of interest:

1) average daily occurrence of gut symptoms per subject above .44;

2) LOS of at least 28 days.

Results for gastrointestinal function are shown in Table 2. None of the risk factors considered as potential correlates were found to be associated with an high rate of gut symptoms, except for OMT (OR = 0.45;0.27-0.74). Multivariate logistic regression confirmed OMT to be independently associated with a 55% reduction of gastrointestinal symptoms (Adjusted OR = 0.45;0.26-0.74).

Results for LOS are reported in Table 3. Univariate odds ratios showed the following categories to be associated with increased rates of LOS equal or above 28

Table 1 General characteristics of the study population

	Study Group	Control Group	p value
N	162 (46.3)	188 (53.7)	
Gender			
Females	81 (50.0)	89 (47.3)	
Males	81 (50.0)	99 (52.7)	0.70
Gestational Age			
≤ 32	39 (24.1)	43 (22.9)	
> 32, ≤ 35	69 (42.6)	72 (38.3)	
> 35	54 (33.3)	73 (38.8)	0.56
Weight (grams)			
At Birth			
≤ 1700	27 (16.7)	36 (19.2)	
> 1700, ≤ 2200	62 (38.3)	63 (33.5)	
> 2200	73 (45.0)	89 (47.3)	0.62
At Admission*	2148 (486.7)	2212 (562.3)	0.25
Oral feeding at admission			
No	129 (79.6)	129 (68.6)	
Yes	33 (20.4)	59 (31.4)	0.03

Numbers in Table are N (%), p values from Chi Square test

* = mean, (standard deviation); p value from t test

Table 2 Results for Average Daily Gut Symptoms: Crude and Adjusted Odds Ratios from Multivariate Logistic Regression

	Average Daily Gut Symptoms*		Univariate O.R.		Adjusted O.R	
	≤ 0.44	> 0.44	O.R. (95%CI)	$p > \lvert\chi^2$	O.R. (95%CI)	$p > \lvert\chi^2$
N	262 (74.9)	88 (25.1)				
Gender						
Females [R.C]	129 (75.9)	41 (24.1)	1	-	1	-
Males	133 (73.9)	47 (26.1)	1.11 (0.68-1.80)	0.759	1.08 (0.65-1.79)	0.777
Gestational Age						
≤ 32	57 (69.5)	25 (30.5)	1.20 (0.65-2.21)	0.670	1.02 (0.43-2.40)	0.965
> 32, ≤ 35	112 (79.4)	29 (20.6)	0.71 (0.40-1.25)	0.293	0.72 (0.39-1.32)	0.292
> 35 [R.C]	93 (73.2)	34 (26.8)	1	-	1	-
Birth Weight (grams)						
≤ 1700	39 (67.2)	19 (32.8)	1.54 (0.80-2.96)	0.265	1.39 (0.55-3.46)	0.481
> 1700, ≤ 2200	100 (76.9)	30 (23.1)	0.95 (0.55-1.63)	0.952	1.03 (0.55-1.93)	0.927
> 2200 [R.C]	123 (75.9)	39 (24.1)	1	-	1	-
Oral feeding at admission						
No	192 (74.4)	66 (25.6)	1.09 (0.63-1.90)	0.860	1.18 (0.67-2.13)	0.583
Yes [R.C]	70 (76.1)	22 (23.9)	1	-	1	-
OMT						
No [R.C]	128 (68.1)	60 (31.9)	1	-	1	-
Yes	134 (82.7)	28 (17.3)	0.45 (0.27-0.74)	0.002	0.45 (0.26-0.74)	0.002

R.C. = Reference Category

* No. of episodes of Vomit, Regurgitation, Gastric residual and Enema

days: GA ≤ 32 weeks (OR = 38.10;16.40-88.20; R.C.:GA > 35 weeks), birth weight ≤ 1700 gm vs > 2200 gm (OR = 120.60;42.70-340.60) and birth weight > 1700 gm, ≤ 2200 gm (OR = 5.80;2.40-13.80; R.C.: birth weight > 2200 gm), oral feeding at admission (OR = 2.85;1.44-5.66) and OMT (OR = 0.51;0.30-0.85). Multivariate logistic regression showed similar patterns, confirming an independent effect of OMT, simultaneously adjusted

Table 3 Results for Length of Stay (LOS): Crude Odds Ratios (p value from Cochran Mantel Haenszel Chi Square Test of Zero Correlation) and Adjusted Odds Ratios from Multivariate Logistic Regression (p value from partial test on regression coefficient)

	LOS (days)		Univariate O.R.		Adjusted O.R.	
	< 28	≥ 28	O.R. (95%CI)	$p > \lvert\chi^2$	O.R. (95%CI)	$p > \lvert\chi^2$
N	267 (76.3)	83 (23.7)				
Gender						
Females [R.C]	128 (75.3)	42 (24.7)	1	-	1	-
Males	139 (77.2)	41 (22.8)	0.90 (0.55-1.47)	0.765	1.40 (0.63-3.10)	0.412
Gestational Age						
≤ 32	21 (25.6)	61 (74.4)	38.10 (16.40-88.20)	< 0.001	10.90 (3.53-33.72)	< 0.001
> 32, ≤ 35	128 (90.8)	13 (9.2)	1.33 (0.55-3.22)	0.680	0.76 (0.27-2.15)	0.609
> 35 [R.C]	118 (92.9)	9 (7.1)	1	-		
Birth Weight (grams)						
≤ 1700	9 (15.5)	49 (84.5)	120.60 (42.70-340.60)	< 0.001	43.23 (11.63-160.66)	< 0.001
> 1700, ≤ 2200	103 (79.2)	27 (20.8)	5.80 (2.40-13.80)	< 0.001	3.01 (1.05-8.68)	0.041
> 2200 [R.C]	155 (95.7)	7 (4.3)	1	-	1	-
Oral feeding at admission						
No	186 (72.1)	72 (27.9)	2.85 (1.44-5.66)	0.003	3.11 (1.05-9.25)	0.041
Yes [R.C]	81 (88.0)	11 (12.0)	1	-	1	-
OMT						
No [R.C]	133 (70.7)	55 (29.3)	1	-	1	-
Yes	134 (82.7)	28 (17.3)	0.51 (0.30-0.85)	0.012	0.22 (0.09-0.51)	< 0.001

R.C. = Reference Category

for all factors, corresponding to more than a 75% reduction in excessive LOS (Adjusted OR = 0.22;0.09-0.51)

Discussion

The main objective of this exploratory study was to investigate the effects of OMT in a population of premature infants in terms of gastrointestinal functions and LOS.

The medical literature lacks information of any potential benefits of complementary treatments in this area. To the best of the authors' knowledge, OMT in premature newborns has never been documented by pediatric specialty journals. Studies carried out in pediatric patients suggested positive effects of OMT in very young children [17-19]. In the broader field of manual therapy, specialists of massage therapy and kinesthetic stimulation showed positive results in premature infants [20]. However, such findings were inconsistent and obtained with heterogeneous methods, showing only minimal differences in terms of clinical significance [20,21].

The present study suggests that OMT may reduce the occurrence of frequent symptoms of abnormal gastrointestinal functionality.

Precise mechanisms for such positive effects generated by OMT are difficult to specify, but several hypotheses can be offered on the basis of neurological, tissue and neuroendocrine factors.

In terms of neurology, there is evidence of an association between autonomic nervous system function and OMT, showing a significant direct relation between myofascial release technique and modifications in the autonomic nervous system activity [22].

Regarding the interaction between OMT and tissue modification, in-vitro models highlight a possible decrease in the production of inflammatory factors [23].

A possible role of neuroendocrine factors can be hypothesized as indicated by the evidence of the effect of OMT on pain biomarker modification in patients affected by low back pain [24].

This study also shows that a significantly higher rate of premature infants receiving osteopathic care can be discharged before 28 days regardless of gender, GA, birth weight and oral feeding at admission.

Such a result may have important implications for the optimization of health care in premature infants. Focusing on the percentage of patients discharged before a given threshold, rather than looking at the average reduction in LOS, may be very relevant for health optimization and cost control. Reducing the rate of long stays would reduce the number of patients in the NICU, allowing for more cribs to become simultaneously available for those infants who require specialized care.

From an epidemiological point of view, the potential benefit may also spread beyond discharge, considering that hospitalization can influence nutrition [25] and morbidity of gastrointestinal infections [26].

An understanding of the differential advantage of OMT on specific subgroups, in particular within specified classes of GA, will require ad hoc studies with an adequate sample size. In the present study, it was not possible to perform subgroups analyses on subjects with very low GA, due to the very limited number of patients available for enrollment.

Finally, some intrinsic limitations of the present study need to be outlined.

This report is based on measurements implemented at the local NICU at the start of the study. Additional relevant confounding variables such as maternal/delivery factors (including breast feeding), respiratory support, method of feeding and gastric emptying time could not be included in this study.

Treatment allocation was neither randomized nor structured, as it was based on matters of convenience within the constraints of the proposed two days per week of osteopathic care. Furthermore, due to the current logistics and procedures it was not possible to "blind" nurses and neonatologists to treatment regimen.

This study, which was conducted in only one NICU, cannot capture the intrinsic variability of organizational strategies across multiple clinical centers managing the complexities of the overall population of newborn infants.

From a methodological point of view, sample size was not based on formal power estimation, treatment was not allocated using a random procedure, and the population of preterm infants may not be representative of the entire population of cases.

The above limitations affect our ability to check for bias and duly rely on the precision of our estimates. In other terms, both the size of the effect of OMT (point estimate) and its level of uncertainty (95% confidence interval) are more likely to be inconsistent with further results obtainable under more general conditions.

To evaluate the efficacy of OMT more studies are required using formal experimental methods, such as randomized and placebo controlled clinical trials. The best endpoint of a well designed three armed study would be the difference between the sham and the actual treatment. However, to make it possible, osteopaths should collaborate with NICU managers to revise the application of operational procedures, so that OMT can be smoothly applied on large populations, across multiple clinical sites.

Despite the above limitations, and given the current lack of information on the possible effects of OMT in preterm infants, the finding of this report sets an interesting ground for new developments. Among these, the standard measurement of all relevant parameters represents an essential aspect that deserves attention for future investigations. Key characteristics and outcomes that can be easily monitored on a daily basis by clinicians, nurses and even parents of preterm infants have been identified. Their adoption for the construction of electronic data base registers can offer a sustainable means to improve both analysis and management of NICU activity, allowing to carry out more detailed exploratory studies while providing a basis for ongoing trials.

Conclusion

The study suggests that osteopathic treatment may reduce a high occurrence of gastrointestinal symptoms and the rates of long-term stays.

Randomized control studies are needed to confirm these results and to generalize them to a broader population of high risk newborns.

Abbreviations

NICU: neonatal intensive care unit; VLBW: very low birth weight; LBW: low birth weigh; GA: gestational age; LOS: length of stay; GER: gastroesophageal reflux; GR: gastric residual; OMT: osteopathic manipulative treatment; OR: odd ratio.

Author details

[1]EBOM - European Institute for Evidence Based Osteopathic Medicine, viale Unità d'Italia 1, 66100 Chieti, Italy. [2]AIOT - Accademia Italiana Osteopatia Tradizionale, via Prati 29, 65124 Pescara, Italy. [3]Unità di Terapia Intensiva Neonatale - Ospedale Civile Spirito Santo, Via Renato Paolini 45, 65124 Pescara, Italy.

Authors' contributions

GB and CD conceived the idea of the study. GP, GB, VC, CR and FCE participated in the design of the study and its coordination. GP, PT, MD, FCE and PF coordinated and performed the data collection. GP and FCA drafted the manuscript. FCA performed the statistical analysis. All authors read and approved the final manuscript.

Competing interests

The authors declare that they have no competing interests.

References

1. Owens PL, Thompson J, Elixhauser A, Ryan K: **Care of Children and Adolescents in U.S. Hospitals.**Edited by: Rockville, MD. Agency for Healthcare Research and Quality; 2003:, Report HCUP Fact Book No. 4; AHRQ Publication 04-0004.
2. Clements KM, Barfield WD, Ayadi MF, Wilber N: **Preterm birth-associated cost of early intervention services: an analysis by gestational age.** *Pediatrics* 2007, **119(4)**:e866-74, Epub 2007 Mar 5.
3. Russell RB, Green NS, Steiner CA, Meikle S, Howse JL, Poschman K, Dias T, Potetz L, Davidoff MJ, Damus K, Petrini JR: **Cost of hospitalization for preterm and low birth weight infants in the United States.** *Pediatrics* 2007, **120(1)**:e1-9.
4. Bakewell-Sachs S, Medoff-Cooper B, Escobar GJ, Silber JH, Lorch SA: **Infant functional status: the timing of physiologic maturation of premature infants.** *Pediatrics* 2009, **123(5)**:e878-86.
5. Eichenwald EC, Blackwell M, Lloyd JS, Tran T, Wilker RE, Richardson DK: **Inter-neonatal intensive care unit variation in discharge timing: influence of apnea and feeding management.** *Pediatrics* 2001, **108(4)**:928-33.
6. American Academy of Pediatrics: **Hospital discharge of the high-risk neonate–proposed guidelines.** *Pediatrics* 1998, **102**:411-7.
7. Mezzacappa MA, Rosa AC: **Clinical predictors of abnormal esophageal pH monitoring in preterm infants.** *Arq Gastroenterol* 2008, **45(3)**:234-8.
8. Mihatsch WA, von Schoenaich P, Fahnenstich H, Dehne N, Ebbecke H, Plath C, von Stockhausen HB, Muche R, Franz A, Pohlandt F: **The significance of gastric residuals in the early enteral feeding advancement of extremely low birth weight infants.** *Pediatrics* 2002, **109(3)**:457-9.
9. Bertino E, Giuliani F, Prandi G, Coscia A, Martano C, Fabris C: **Necrotizing enterocolitis: risk factor analysis and role of gastric residuals in very low birth weight infants.** *J Pediatr Gastroenterol Nutr* 2009, **48(4)**:437-42.
10. Mäki M, Ruuska T, Kuusela AL, Karikoski-Leo R, Ikonen RS: **High prevalence of asymptomatic esophageal and gastric lesions in preterm infants in intensive care.** *Crit Care Med* 1993, **21(12)**:1863-7.
11. Kuusela AL, Mäki M, Ruuska T, Laippala P: **Stress-induced gastric findings in critically ill newborn infants: frequency and risk factors.** *Intensive Care Med* 2000, **26(10)**:1501-6.
12. Duman N, Utkutan S, Ozkan H, Ozdoğan S: **Are the stool characteristics of preterm infants affected by infant formulas?** *Turk J Pediatr* 2000, **42(2)**:138-44.
13. Mihatsch WA, Franz AR, Högel J, Pohlandt F: **Hydrolyzed protein accelerates feeding advancement in very low birth weight infants.** *Pediatrics* 2002, **110(6)**:1199-203.
14. Magoun HI: **Osteopathy in the Cranial Field.**Edited by: Kirksville, Mo. Journal Printing Co; , 3 1976.
15. Nutrition Toolkit: 2008 [http://www.cpqcc.org/documents/341/download], Accessed June 24th 2010.
16. The R Development Core Team, R: **A Language and Environment for Statistical Computing.** [http://cran.r-project.org/doc/manuals/refman.pdf], Accessed June 24th 2010.
17. Hayden C, Mullinger B: **A preliminary assessment of the impact of cranial osteopathy for the relief of infantile colic.** *Complement Ther Clin Pract* 2006, **12(2)**:83-90.
18. Vandenplas Y, Denayer E, Vandenbossche T, Vermet L, Hauser B, Deschepper J, Engelen A: **Osteopathy may decrease obstructive apnea in infants: a pilot study.** *Osteopath Med Prim Care* 2008, **19(2)**:8.
19. Philippi H, Faldum A, Schleupen A, Pabst B, Jung T, Bergmann H, Bieber I, Kaemmerer C, Dijs P, Reitter B: **Infantile postural asymmetry and osteopathic treatment: a randomized therapeutic trial.** *Dev Med Child Neurol* 2006, **48(1)**:5-9.
20. Massaro AN, Hammad TA, Jazzo B, Aly H: **Massage with kinesthetic stimulation improves weight gain in preterm infants.** *J Perinatol* 2009, **29(5)**:352-7.
21. Vickers A, Ohlsson A, Lacy JB, Horsley A: **Massage for promoting growth and development of preterm and/or low birth-weight infants.** *Cochrane Database Syst Rev* 2004, **2**: CD000390, Review.
22. Henley CE, Ivins D, Mills M, Wen FK, Benjamin BA: **Osteopathic manipulative treatment and its relationship to autonomic nervous system activity as demonstrated by heart rate variability: a repeated measures study.** *Osteopath Med Prim Care* 2008, **5(2)**:7.
23. Meltzer KR, Standley PR: **Modeled repetitive motion strain and indirect osteopathic manipulative techniques in regulation of human fibroblast proliferation and interleukin secretion.** *J Am Osteopath Assoc* 2007, **107(12)**:527-36.
24. Degenhardt BF, Darmani NA, Johnson JC, Towns LC, Rhodes DC, Trinh C, McClanahan B, DiMarzo V: **Role of osteopathic manipulative treatment in altering pain biomarkers: a pilot study.** *J Am Osteopath Assoc* 2007, **107(9)**:387-400.
25. Kirchner L, Jeitler V, Waldhör T, Pollak A, Wald M: **Long hospitalization is the most important risk factor for early weaning from breast milk in premature babies.** *Acta Paediatr* 2009, **98**:981-984.
26. Kramer MS, Kakuma R: **Optimal duration of exclusive breastfeeding.** *Cochrane Database Syst Rev* 2002, , **1**: CD003517.

Clinical decision rules, spinal pain classification and prediction of treatment outcome: A discussion of recent reports in the rehabilitation literature

Jeffrey J Hebert[1*] and Julie M Fritz[2]

Abstract

Clinical decision rules are an increasingly common presence in the biomedical literature and represent one strategy of enhancing clinical-decision making with the goal of improving the efficiency and effectiveness of healthcare delivery. In the context of rehabilitation research, clinical decision rules have been predominantly aimed at classifying patients by predicting their treatment response to specific therapies. Traditionally, recommendations for developing clinical decision rules propose a multistep process (derivation, validation, impact analysis) using defined methodology. Research efforts aimed at developing a "diagnosis-based clinical decision rule" have departed from this convention. Recent publications in this line of research have used the modified terminology "diagnosis-based clinical decision guide." Modifications to terminology and methodology surrounding clinical decision rules can make it more difficult for clinicians to recognize the level of evidence associated with a decision rule and understand how this evidence should be implemented to inform patient care. We provide a brief overview of clinical decision rule development in the context of the rehabilitation literature and two specific papers recently published in Chiropractic and Manual Therapies.

Keywords: Diagnosis, Clinical prediction rule, Clinical decision making, Low back pain, Neck pain, Back pain

Healthcare has undergone an important paradigm shift toward evidence based practice; an approach thought to enhance clinical decision making by integrating the best available evidence with clinical expertise and the preferences of patients.[1] Ultimately, the goal of evidence based practice is to improve healthcare delivery. However, the translation of scientific evidence into practice has proven a challenging endeavour.

Clinical decision rules (CDRs), also known as clinical prediction rules, are an increasingly common presence in the rehabilitation literature. These are tools designed to inform clinical decision-making by identifying potential predictors of diagnostic test outcome, prognosis or therapeutic response.[2,3] In the rehabilitation literature, CDRs are most commonly used to predict a patient's response to treatment and have been proposed as a means of identifying clinically relevant subgroups of patients presenting with otherwise heterogeneous disorders such as non-specific neck[4] or low back pain[5,6] and this is the perspective on which we intend to focus.

The ability to classify or subgroup patients with heterogeneous disorders such as spinal pain has been highlighted as a research priority[7,8] and consequently, the focus of much research effort. The appeal of such classification approaches is their potential for improved treatment efficiency and effectiveness by matching patients with optimal therapies. In the past, patient classification has relied on implicit approaches founded in tradition or unsystematic observations. The use of CDRs to inform classification is one attempt at a more evidence driven approach, less dependent on unfounded theory.

CDRs are developed in a multistep process involving studies of derivation, validation and analysis of impact with each having a defined purpose and methodological criteria. [2,9] As with all forms of evidence used to make decisions

* Correspondence: J.Hebert@Murdoch.edu.au
[1]Faculty of Health Sciences, Murdoch University, Murdoch, WA, Australia
Full list of author information is available at the end of the article

about patients, attention to appropriate study methodology is critical to assessing the potential benefits of implementation. While a comprehensive discussion of CDR methodology is beyond the scope of this commentary, we seek to present a brief overview of CDR development in the context of the rehabilitation literature and two specific papers recently published in Chiropractic and Manual Therapies.

CDR derivation

The purpose of CDR derivation studies is to identify potentially important predictors of response to therapy and combine important predictors into a preliminary decision rule. Commonly, variables to be considered at this step are included from the history, physical examination and other forms of testing. Multivariate statistical analyses (*e.g.*, logistic regression) are then used to identify relationships between different clusters of variables and the outcome of interest (*e.g.*, decreased pain, increased function).

There has been much discussion and debate regarding the optimal research design of derivation studies.[10-13] Many derivation studies have been single-arm studies, meaning all patients receive the same therapy within the study. A single-arm study design for deriving a CDR has several advantages, foremost among these is that this design requires fewer resources and can generally be completed more rapidly than a two-arm study design such as a randomized trial. The shortcoming of a single-arm design, however, is the inability to distinguish true predictor variables (*i.e.*, effect modifiers) from those generally associated with a favourable prognosis unrelated to the treatment received.

For example, Flynn and colleagues[6] used a single arm design to identify those demographic, historical or physical examination factors associated with a favourable clinical outcome among patients with low back pain undergoing treatment consisting of spinal manipulative therapy and range of motion exercises. The study results identified five variables associated with a favourable treatment response:

1) Pain duration of less than 16 days
2) Fear avoidance beliefs work subscale score less than 19
3) At least one hip with greater than 35° internal rotation range of motion
4) Hypomobility of the lumbar spine
5) No symptoms distal to the knee

When at least 4 of these factors were present (*i.e.*, positive status on the rule), the reported positive likelihood ratio was approximately 24, meaning that individuals with low back pain meeting this criteria had a 95% likelihood of achieving clinical success with spinal manipulative therapy.

However, since an experimental study design was not used to validate these relationships, it was not possible from this derivation study to determine if these variables were predictors of treatment response specific to spinal manipulation (*i.e.*, treatment effect modifiers) or more generally indicative of a patient with a favourable prognosis regardless of management. Therefore, while in some cases it may be appropriate for clinicians to use data from derivation studies to inform clinical decision-making, CDRs must undergo the rigors of full validation (*e.g.*, testing in a randomized clinical trial) prior to widespread implementation.[2]

CDR validation

The validation of a potential CDR is a critical step in its development and is requisite to broad implementation. There are several reasons for this. First, the associations between predictor variables and the outcome of interest identified at the derivation stage could have resulted from chance or may simply represent the identification of positive prognostic factors. Second, the predictor variables may be unique to the participants, clinicians or context of the derivation study and these relationships would therefore not be present in other circumstances. Third, the implementation of the CDR may fail due to problems related to the feasibility of its application.

The appropriate approach for examining the validity of a CDR employs an experimental study design to examine for statistical interaction (*i.e.*, treatment effect modification) between the potential predictor variables and the treatment received. To validate a CDR for predicting treatment response, cohorts of patients who do and do not meet the CDR criteria would be randomly assigned to receive the treatment specific to the CDR or an alternative approach, which could be no treatment. This design permits an assessment of whether the CDR identifies a group of patients who respond to a specific intervention, but not to an alternative treatment.

Returning to our example of the CDR for spinal manipulative therapy, Childs *et al.*[14] examined the validity of the rule using a two-arm randomized trial. The authors investigated the treatment outcomes experienced by patients with low back pain, classified based upon their status on the CDR who were randomly assigned to receive spinal manipulation plus exercise or exercise alone.[14] The results indicated that CDR positive patients experienced a better outcome with spinal manipulation and exercise (*i.e.*, when CDR status was matched to therapy) as compared to those receiving exercise only. Furthermore, the matched patients had better clinical outcomes than CDR negative patients undergoing an exercise program with or without spinal manipulation. These results provided evidence supporting the validity of the CDR criteria. However, as the sample population was similar to that examined in the derivation study, this result was considered evidence of narrow validation. Additional knowledge regarding the validity of this CDR would be gained through a more comprehensive investigation of its validity.

CDR analysis of impact

Ultimately, the usefulness of a CDR lies not with its accuracy but with its ability to improve clinical outcomes and enhance the efficiency of care.[15] Even when a CDR demonstrates evidence of broad validation, this does not ensure that it will change clinical decision making, or that the changes it produces will result in better care. McGinn *et al.*[2] identified three explanations for the failure of a CDR at this stage. First, if clinician judgement is as accurate as a CDR informed decision, there is no benefit to its use. Second, the application of a CDR may involve cumbersome calculations or procedures which discourage clinicians from utilizing the CDR. Third, using the CDR may not be feasible in all environments or circumstances. In addition, we would include the reality that experimental studies may involve patients that are not entirely representative of those seen in routine care and that this may limit the actual value of a CDR. Therefore, to fully understand the utility of a CDR and its ability to improve healthcare delivery, it is necessary to undertake a pragmatic examination of its feasibility and impact when applied in an environment reflecting real world practice. This can be undertaken with different study designs such as randomized trials, cluster randomized trials, or other approaches such as examining the impact of a CDR before and after its implementation.

There has not been an impact analysis of the spinal manipulation CDR. Fritz and colleagues[16] did examine the impact of treatment based on the manipulation CDR by comparing the clinical outcomes (pain and disability) and healthcare utilization (number of treatment sessions, length of stay and healthcare costs) of CDR positive patients undergoing thrust manipulation, nonthrust manipulation or no manipulation. Patients receiving thrust or nonthrust manipulation experienced better clinical outcomes when compared to those receiving no manipulation. While the clinical outcomes did not differ between manipulation groups, patients receiving thrust manipulation utilized less healthcare resources than those receiving nonthrust manipulation. However, the study used a weaker, retrospective, case–control design. Additional impact studies using stronger research designs are needed.

Appropriate interpretation of the diagnosis-based clinical decision rules

Two recent papers published in Chiropractic & Manual Therapies by Murphy and Hurwitz[17,18] highlight the sometimes confusing intersection between decision rules, patient classification and prediction of treatment outcome. The authors have previously published their work describing "diagnosis-based clinical decision rules" for patients with spinal pain.[19,20] As mentioned, the classification of patients with spinal pain is an important and potentially promising area of research activity and this diagnosis-based strategy is a welcome addition to other classification approaches.[21-25]

However, the author's use of the phrase "diagnosis-based clinical decision rule" is noteworthy as it represents a departure from convention. A review of the development of the "diagnosis-based clinical decision rule" reveals no formal derivation, validation or analysis of impact. Instead, the criteria for this rule were derived from non-systematic literature reviews.[19,20] Therefore, the use of the phrase "diagnosis-based clinical decision rule" may be the cause of confusion as it implies the formal derivation and validation of a rule. Consequently, there is concern over the potential for a mistaken belief that the diagnosis-based decision rule represents a high level of evidence, while in its current form, it is an evidence-informed hypothesis. Therefore, it is not appropriate to refer to the criteria defining the diagnosis based classification approach as a clinical decision rule until the appropriately designed studies are undertaken.

In their recent publications, the authors have changed the terminology used to describe the diagnosis-based classification approach from "clinical decision rule" to "clinical decision guide."[17,18] While the former implies a strict methodology of derivation, validation, and impact analysis, the later is an informal term perhaps more appropriate for the current state of the diagnosis-based classification approach and yet it is possible that the significance of this terminology change may be missed by the casual observer.

Moreover, distinctions between "decision rule," "prediction rule," "decision guide," and "prediction guide"[26] can be subtle, and misunderstandings have potential to adversely impact clinical decision making. Although some may find such differences in terminology to be overly pedantic, these issues get to the heart of evidence appraisal and translation of evidence into practice and incorrectly identifying research findings as representing high level evidence (*e.g.*, a fully developed CDR) has potential to mislead clinicians and adversely affect patient care.

This perspective leads to two fundamental questions with respect to the diagnosis based classification approach:

1. What level of evidence does the diagnosis-based approach represent?
2. How should this evidence be used to inform patient care?

In its current state, the diagnosis-based clinical decision guide is a theoretical approach for classifying patients with neck or back pain. The authors have identified the potential classification criteria based upon narrative literature reviews.[19,20] While some of the individual studies identified in these reviews represent a high level of evidence, other studies underpinning the guide represent low level evidence. Furthermore, some aspects of the classification approach are hypothetical. The next logical step in the development of the diagnosis-based classification approach could be to undertake formal CDR derivation studies examining the multivariate relationships between potential predictor variables and treatment outcomes. Subsequently, the potential CDRs should be validated through the rigors of randomized trials. If broad validation of the CDRs were supported by experimental results, analyses of impact could then be undertaken. While it may be appropriate for CDR derivation study results to influence clinical decision making (*e.g.*, when very little evidence is available in a particular area or on a localized level where the impact on patient care can be monitored), widespread implementation of a CDR requires validation. Consequently, given the hypothetical nature of the diagnosis-based clinical decision rule (now termed clinical decision guide), its widespread implementation by clinicians is premature.

Although in its current state the diagnosis-based clinical decision guide represents a preliminary and untested approach, new and innovative developments in neck and back pain classification such as this should be welcomed and their development encouraged. However, it is also important to understand the appropriate context for interpreting this classification approach and recognize its limitations. Despite its potential to inform future efforts of subgrouping patients with neck or back pain who may preferentially respond to one or more forms of therapy, the diagnosis-based classification approach is not ready for clinical implementation. Nevertheless, we are hopeful that future advancements in and additional knowledge of patient classification hold promise for improving the quality of healthcare provided to patients with spinal pain and the diagnosis-based clinical decision approach is no exception.

Competing interests

The authors declare that they have no competing interests.

Author details

[1]Faculty of Health Sciences, Murdoch University, Murdoch, WA, Australia. [2]Department of Physical Therapy, University of Utah and Intermountain Healthcare, Salt Lake City, UT, USA.

Authors' contributions

JH and JF made substantial contributions regarding the conception and drafting of this manuscript. All authors read and approved the final manuscript.

References

1. Sackett DL, Rosenberg WM, Gray JA, Haynes RB, Richardson WS: **Evidence based medicine: what it is and what it isn't.** *BMJ* 1996, **312**(7023):71–72.
2. McGinn TG, Guyatt GH, Wyer PC, Naylor CD, Stiell IG, Richardson WS: **Users' guide to the medical literature XXII: how to use articles about clinical decision rules.** *JAMA* 2000, **284**(1):79–84.
3. Randolph AG, Guyatt GH, Carlet J: **Understanding articles comparing outcomes among intensive care units to rate quality of care.** *Evidence Based Medicine in Critical Care Group. Crit Care Med* 1998, **26**(4):773–781.
4. Cleland JA, Childs JD, Fritz JM, Whitman JM, Eberhart SL: **Development of a clinical prediction rule for guiding treatment of a subgroup of patients with neck pain: use of thoracic spine manipulation, exercise, and patient education.** *Phys Ther* 2007, **87**(1):9–23.
5. Hicks GE, Fritz JM, Delitto A, McGill SM: **Preliminary development of a clinical prediction rule for determining which patients with low back pain will respond to a stabilization exercise program.** *Arch Phys Med Rehabil* 2005, **86**(9):1753–1762.
6. Flynn T, Fritz J, Whitman J, Wainner R, Magel J, Rendeiro D, Butler B, Garber M, Allison S: **A clinical prediction rule for classifying patients with low back pain who demonstrate short term improvement with spinal manipulation.** *Spine* 2002, **27**(24):2835–2843.
7. Borkan JM, Koes B, Reis S, Cherkin DC: **A report from the second international forum for primary care research on low back pain: reexamining priorities.** *Spine* 1998, **23**(18):1992–1996.
8. Henschke N, Maher CG, Refshauge KM, Das A, McAuley JH: **Low back pain research priorities: a survey of primary care practitioners.** *BMC Fam Pract* 2007, **8**:40.
9. Laupacis A, Sekar N, Stiell IG: **Clinical prediction rules: a review and suggested modifications of metodological standards.** *JAMA* 1997, **277**(6):488–494.
10. Hancock M, Herbert RD, Maher CG: **A guide to interpretation of studies investigating subgroups of responders to physical therapy interventions.** *Phys Ther* 2009, **89**(7):698–704.
11. Fritz JM: **Clinical prediction rules in physical therapy: coming of age?** *J Orthop Sports Phys Ther* 2009, **39**(3):159–161.
12. Stanton TR, Hancock MJ, Maher CG, Koes BW: **Critical appraisal of clinical prediction rules that aim to optimize treatment selection for musculoskeletal conditions.** *Phys Ther* 2010, **90**(6):843–854.
13. Fitzgerald GK: **Invited commentary.** *Phys Ther* 2010, **90**(6):855–858. author reply 858.
14. Childs JD, Fritz JM, Flynn TW, Irrgang JJ, Johnson KK, Majkowski GR, Delitto A: **A clinical prediction rule to identify patients with low back pain most likely to benefit from spinal manipulation: a validation study.** *Ann Intern Med* 2004, **141**(12):920–928.
15. Grady D, Berkowitz SA: **Why is a good clinical prediction rule so hard to find?** *Arch Intern Med* 2011, **171**(19):1701–1702.
16. Fritz JM, Brennan GP, Leaman H: **Does the evidence for spinal manipulation translate into better outcomes in routine clinical care for patients with occupational low back pain? A case-control study.** *Spine J* 2006, **6**(3):289–295.
17. Murphy DR, Hurwitz EL: **Application of a diagnosis-based clinical decision guide in patients with low back pain.** *Chiropr Man Therap* 2011, **19**(1):26.
18. Murphy DR, Hurwitz EL: **Application of a diagnosis-based clinical decision guide in patients with neck pain.** *Chiropr Man Therap* 2011, **19**(1):19.
19. Murphy DR, Hurwitz EL, Nelson CF: **A diagnosis-based clinical decision rule for spinal pain part 2: review of the literature.** *Chiropr Osteopat* 2008, **16**:7.
20. Murphy DR, Hurwitz EL: **A theoretical model for the development of a diagnosis-based clinical decision rule for the management of patients with spinal pain.** *BMC Musculoskelet Disord* 2007, **8**:75.
21. Walker BF, Williamson OD: **Mechanical or inflammatory low back pain. What are the potential signs and symptoms?** *Man Ther* 2009, **14**(3):314–320.
22. Delitto A, Erhard RE, Bowling RW: **A treatment-based classification approach to low back syndrome: identifying and staging patients for conservative management.** *Phys Ther* 1995, **75**:470–489.
23. McKenzie R, May S: *The lumbar spine: mechanical diagnosis & therapy.* New Zealand, Limited: Spinal Publications; 2003.
24. Hebert J, Koppenhaver S, Fritz J, Parent E: **Clinical prediction for success of interventions for managing low back pain.** *Clin Sports Med* 2008, **27**(3):463–479. ix-x.
25. Hebert JJ, Koppenhaver SL, Walker BF: **Subgrouping Patients With Low Back Pain: A Treatment-Based Approach to Classification.** *Sports Health: A Multidisciplinary Approach* 2011, **3**(6):534–542.

26. Schneider GM, Jull G, Thomas K, Salo P: **Screening of patients suitable for diagnostic cervical facet joint blocks - A role for physiotherapists.** *Man Ther* 2011, **17**(2):180–183.

Orthosis reduces breast pain and mechanical forces through natural and augmented breast tissue in women lying prone

Karin Ried[1*], Simon Armstrong[1], Avni Sali[1] and Patrick McLaughlin[2]

Abstract

Background: Breast implant displacement or rupture can cause aesthetic problems and serious medical complications. Activities with prone positioning and loading of the anterior chest wall, such as massage, chiropractic or osteopathic therapies may increase the risk of implant failure and can also cause discomfort in women with natural breast tissue. Here we test the effectiveness of a newly developed orthosis on pain, mechanical pressure and displacement of breast tissue in women with cosmetic augmentation, post-mastectomy reconstruction, lactating or natural breast tissue.

Methods: Thirty-two females volunteers, aged 25–56 years with augmented, reconstructed, natural or lactating breast tissue and cup sizes B-F, participated in this open-label clinical trial. We measured pain perception, peak pressure, maximum force, and breast tissue displacement using different sizes of the orthosis compared to no orthosis. Different densities of the orthosis were also tested in a subgroup of women (n = 7). Pain perception was rated using a validated 11-point visual-analogue scale. Peak pressure and maximum force were assessed using a bilateral set of capacitance-pliance® sensor strips whilst participants were load bearing in a prone position, and breast displacement was measured by magnetic-resonance-imaging.

Results: The orthosis significantly reduced pain, breast displacement and mechanical pressures in women with natural and augmented breast tissue in prone position. Greater relief of pain and greater reduction in mechanical forces were found with increased size and density of the orthosis. Use of the orthosis improved overall comfort by 64-100%, lowered peak pressure by up to 85% and maximum force by up to 96%. Medio-lateral displacement of breast tissue was reduced by 16%, resulting in a 51% desirable increase of breast tissue height.

Conclusion: Our study demonstrated that the newly developed orthosis significantly reduced pain, mechanical pressure and breast tissue displacement in women with augmented and natural breast tissue when lying prone. Our findings are of clinical significance, potentially reducing the risk of complication from prone activities in women with breast augmentation or reconstruction, as well as improving comfort whilst undergoing prone procedures.

Trial registration: Australia and New Zealand Clinical Trials Register, ACTRN12613000541707.

Keywords: Breast implant, Breast augmentation, Breast reconstruction, Implant rupture, Lactation, Orthosis, Pain, Mechanical forces, Pressure, Displacement

* Correspondence: karinried@niim.com.au
[1]National Institute of Integrative Medicine, Melbourne VIC 3122, Australia
Full list of author information is available at the end of the article

Background

Clinical and ongoing management following cancer mastectomy and reconstruction, cosmetic augmentation or normal variations in breast tissue structures can present a significant challenge. Some women experience discomfort and potential trauma in clinical settings, when participating in activities that load the anterior chest wall, such as massage, chiropractic or osteopathic therapies. Clinicians need to be aware of altered breast structures and considerations must be given to appropriately manage and accommodate these patients. A new orthosis has been developed to allow women with natural or augmented breast tissue to increase comfort and protection from mechanical forces in the clinical setting or in some recreational activities when lying prone [1].

Breast augmentation has been controversial, especially in light of the French Poly Implant Prothèse (PIP), leading to increased problems and causing anxiety in the perception of this medical field [2,3]. Recent improvements in implant technology and surgical approaches have assisted in improving the outcomes for many individuals. Implants are not for life and will require surgical revision and management [4,5]. Implant rupture rates vary and may be up to 57% at 11 years, with PIP implants rupturing 2–6 times more often than other implants [6]. The biodurability of the implant is of significant concern to patients [7]. In addition, recent court cases on breast implant damage due to manipulation by therapists were decided in favour of the patient [8].

Insertion of a foreign body produces a normal immune response of encapsulation of the object [9]. The body then requires time for the implant to 'settle', which can be an ongoing process when complicated by reconstructive, post mastectomy or radiation treatment [10].

Positioning or undertaking activities where loading through the tissues of the anterior chest wall occurs may alter the state of function of breast tissue and/or implant material. This can be highlighted by imaging techniques. Capsular contracture is the most common complication of breast augmentation and can result in collagen fibres of the implant pocket impacting the breast or implant material, which can lead to hardening and resultant asymmetry [11].

Our study investigated mechanical forces, displacement and subjective pain levels of women with natural and surgically altered breasts in the prone position, with and without an orthosis, of different sizes and densities.

Methods

Study design and participants

Our study comprised of a non-randomised open-label clinical trial of 32 female volunteers, aged 25–56 years, with breast cup sizes ranging from B-F. About two thirds had augmented breast tissues, most for aesthetic purposes (n = 18), and a few had implants after mastectomy (n = 3). About one third of women in the trial had natural breast tissue, with normal (n = 7), lactating (n = 2), after lumpectomy (n = 1), or reconstruction by tram-flap (n = 1). All but one women in the augmented group had bilateral, complete, silicone implants, with no capsular contracture, which were performed by inframammary incision, either with submuscular positioning (n = 13) or subglandular positioning (n = 4). One women in the augmented group had a one-sided reconstruction after mastectomy (n = 1) (Table 1).

All measurements were taken with the participant lying prone for up to 1 hour during a single day of testing. Magnetic Resonance Imaging (MRI) was performed at Medical Imaging Australia (MIA Victoria) in East Melbourne (45 min), and mechanical forces (peak pressure and maximum pressure were tested at the Victoria University biomechanics lab (15 min). Transport was provided between the testing labs. Pain perception, tissue displacement measured by MRI (4 MRIs per participant) and mechanical forces during prone loading through the anterior chest and breast tissue without and with different sizes (sizes 1–3) of the orthosis were assessed in all participants. In addition, mechanical

Table 1 Baseline characteristics, N = 32

Characteristics	Mean	SD	Range
Age (yrs)	36.7	9.7	25-56
Height (cm)	166.7	7.3	150-179
Weight (kg)	64.2	7.1	51-80
BMI (kg/m²)	23.1	2.7	18-31.6
Cup-size	4	1.9	B-F
	N		
B	1		
C; CC	8;5		
D; DD	8;2		
E; EE	4;2		
F	2		
Type			
A) Augmentation[1]:		**Details**	
Primary:	18	For aesthetic purposes (5.2 ± 3.0 yrs)	
Reconstruction:	3	After mastectomy (4.3 ± 1.5 yrs)	
B) Natural:			
Normal	7		
Lactating	2	2-3 months	
Lumptectomy	1	3 months since operation	
Tram flap	1	12 months since operation	

[1]All silicone implants, bilateral, complete, no capsular contracture by inframammary incision, with submuscular positioning (n = 13), subglandular (n = 4), or reconstruction (n = 1).
Abbreviations: mth month, *n* number, *SD* standard deviation, *yrs* year.

forces were tested with different densities (soft, medium, firm) of the orthosis in a subgroup of women.

The study was approved by the Human Research Ethics Committee at the National Institute of Integrative Medicine, Melbourne, Australia.

The orthosis

Made from medical grade thermoplastic elastomer, the orthosis absorbs, deflects and displaces load, protecting the breast structure from trauma and reduces loading of adjacent tissues. The orthosis demonstrates unique elasticity, durability and elastic strain properties, whilst being capable of long term deformation under load. The orthosis is sterilisable in autoclaves and washable with isopropyl, making it suitable for clinical settings and multi-use environments.

The orthosis device loads the sternum, upper and lower rib cage and upper abdomen (Figure 1). Incremental increases in height, depth and width between the sizes of the orthosis provides allowances for different breast sizes and other structural variations and individual preferences. Size-3 of the orthosis is about 60% higher, 9% wider and 6% longer than the smallest size (size-1) (approximate dimensions of size-1 orthosis: W × L × H = 230 × 260 × 35 mm^3).

Pain

Comfort/pain levels were assessed without and with each of 3 sizes of the orthosis. Pain was assessed using a validated 11-point visual-analogue pain rating scale, ranging from 0='no pain' to 10='worst possible pain' [12,13].

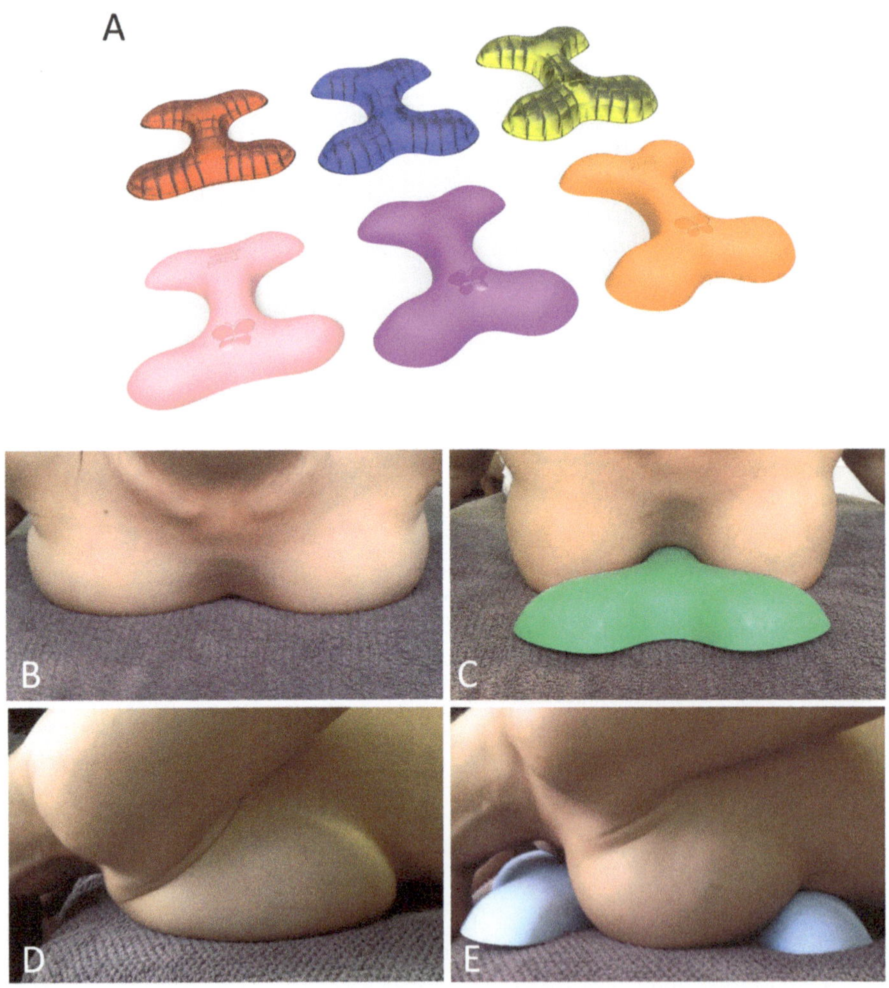

Figure 1 Orthosis in different sizes and densities, the transparent models illustrate the orthosis' ribbing for adjustment of firmness (A); Participant positioning on the orthosis in cephalic view (B), side view (C), lateral view without the orthosis (D) and with the orthosis (E).

Breast displacement and deformation, mechanical force and peak pressure

To measure breast tissue displacement and deformation we used Magnetic Resonance Imaging (MRI) in antero-posterior (AP) and medio-lateral (ML) planes. MRIs were performed to show segmental transverse and para-sagittal mid-breast views, providing linear measurements in millimetres (mm) of breast tissue displacement and compression (Siemens 1.5 T Magnetom Espree) [14].

Following MRI scans, mechanical force assessments were taken with subjects lying prone wearing a 15 kilogram load-vest, simulating therapeutic massage and manipulation loading. Bilateral capacitance pliance® sensor strips were used as a means of measuring force (Newton, N) and pressure (kilo pascal kPa) from the breast tissue. Two 8 × 25 cm sensor strips with sensor resolution of 1 sensor/cm^2 and a total measurement area of 400 cm^2, sensitive to 4 kPa at a sample rate of 50 Hz, were placed onto a standard treatment table under each of the participants' breasts. Sensors were aligned to a standardised scale assuring comparable positioning for all participants.

Sample size and analysis

A sample size of 30 was calculated to detect a difference of 5 ± 2.3 kPa of peak pressure or 25 ± 13 N of maximum force with the orthosis compared to no orthosis with a power of 80% and 95% confidence [1].

Statistical analyses were completed with SPSS Statistics program version 21.0 [15]. Statistical significance was set at $p < 0.05$. All data were analysed descriptively.

Perceived levels of pain using different sizes of the firm density orthosis compared to no orthosis were assessed by ANOVA repeated measures (General Linear Model univariate repeated measures) with Bonferroni adjustment. The ratio between any pain and no pain was tested by chi-square. Analyses were completed for all participants and by subgroups (primary augmentation, reconstruction, natural, lactating).

Maximum force and peak pressure for each breast side were compared between different sizes of the orthosis and no orthosis using the ANOVA Repeated Measures model for all participants and by subgroups. In addition, different densities of the orthosis as well as sizes compared to no orthosis were tested in a subset of patients (total n = 6; augmented n = 5; natural n = 1).

Results

Pain

All women reported a significant reduction of pain with the orthosis compared to no orthosis when lying prone ($p < 0.0001$; Table 2). The larger size orthosis provided generally greater relief than the smaller size, overall reducing pain sensation by 64-100%. In our patient group, the size-3 orthosis provided complete relief and greatest comfort ($p < 0.0001$). Average pain perception with no orthosis was slightly higher in augmented patients compared with natural non-lactating patients. The patient with the tram-flap reconstruction did not have any sensation in the reconstructed breast tissue at all and therefore could not report any pain. Generally, smaller breast cup sizes achieved pain reductions with the smaller devices, compared to the larger breast cup sizes which required the larger devices to achieve adequate pain reduction. Comfort data was not captured with the different densities of the orthosis in the subgroup.

Mechanical forces

Peak pressure, maximum force and displacement of breast tissue were significantly reduced for all patients using the orthosis compared with no orthosis ($p < 0.001$; Table 3A; Figures 2 and 3). The larger size orthosis generally reduced mechanical forces more than the smaller size orthosis (Reduction of forces: Size-3 > Size-2 > Size-1 > no orthosis). The peak pressure reductions observed using the orthosis compared with no orthosis were between 58% and 85% for both breasts for all patients, and maximum force reduction ranged from 73-96%. Breast tissue displacement in the medio-lateral plane was reduced by 14-16%, resulting in a desired increase of 15-51% in the antero-posterior plane.

Table 3B summarises subgroup analysis results on peak pressure, maximum force and displacement by patients with or without implants, and by natural, lactating, primary augmentation or reconstruction. Reductions in peak pressure and maximum forces were similar in women with or without implants using the orthoses, while reduction of displacement was greater in women without implants. The effect of the orthosis on mechanical forces was comparable in all subgroups.

The effect of difference densities of the orthosis on peak pressure was tested in a subgroup of women (n = 7). Mean peak pressure dropped with increasing size and density of the orthosis, with firmer and larger orthosis providing greater decrease in mechanical forces (Figure 4). Almost no peak pressure was observed with the firmer variant of the size-3 orthosis in this group of women.

Table 4 provides a general guide for matching size and density of the orthosis to breast cup-size based on our findings and on clinical practice. Women with A-C cup-size breasts generally require a size-1 orthosis to provide protection. A size-3 orthosis can be used, although there is no functional gain in this group. Women with D-E cup-size require a size-2 orthosis as a minimum, and breast cup-sizes EE and above must only use a size-3 device or larger. Appropriate sizing of the orthosis is crucial as breast tissue and implant material must not load

Table 2 Effect of orthosis on pain scores

All participants (n = 31)[1]	Pain score: Mean (SD)	Pain score: % change vs no orthosis	Orthosis vs no orthosis ANOVA; p-value	Any pain vs no pain Chi-square; p-value
No orthosis	4.8 (1.9)			
Size-1	1.4 (1.0)	−71	<0.0001	0.02
Size-2	0.2 (0.4)	−96	<0.0001	<0.0001
Size-3	0	−100	<0.0001	<0.0001
Primary augmentation (n = 18)				
No orthosis	4.7 (1.8)			
Size-1	1.7 (1.0)	−64	<0.0001	
Size-2	0.2 (0.4)	−96	<0.0001	
Size-3	0	−100	<0.0001	
Reconstruction (n = 3)				
No orthosis	4.3 (0.6)		0.01	
Size-1	1.0 (0)	−77		
Size-1	0.3 (0.6)	−93	0.006	
Size-3	0	−100		
Natural (n = 7)				
No orthosis	4.0 (1.6)			
Size-1	1.3 (1.1)	−68	<0.0001	
Size-2	0.4 (0.5)	−90	<0.0001	
Size-3	0	−100	<0.0001	
Lactating (n = 2)				
No orthosis/Size-1/2/3	8/1.5/0/0	−81,-100		
Lumptectomy (n = 1)	9/0/0/0	−100		
TramFlap (n = 1)[1]	0/0/0/0	no pain sensation		

Participants experienced significantly less pain with the orthosis compared to no orthosis.
[1]The patient with the tram-flap reconstruction did not have any sensation in the breast, therefore did not experience any pain. This patient was excluded from the analysis of all patients.
Ns, not significant; vs, versus.

onto the device but be adjacent to it for correct uses allowing optimal protection (Figure 5).

Discussion

Our study demonstrated that the new orthosis significantly reduced pain, breast displacement and mechanical pressures in women with natural and augmented breast tissue when undergoing activities in prone position. Greatest comfort and complete pain relief was observed with the largest size-3 orthosis in our group of women with B-F cup-sizes. The orthosis allowed peak pressure to be lowered by up to 85%, maximum force by up to 96%, and medio-lateral displacement of breast tissue by up to 16%, which in turn resulted in up to 51% increase of breast tissue in the antero-posterior plane.

Natural breast tissue demonstrated a greater proportional protection from displacement and deformation with the orthosis compared to augmented individuals. This can be attributed to the implant's fixed volume and inability to simulate natural human tissue movement.

The findings of this larger study are in line with our earlier pilot study [1]. Here we provide additional data on bilateral measurements and a variety of densities of the orthosis.

Our findings are clinically important to provide lactating women or women with natural painful breast tissue a safer and more comfortable option when undergoing prone activities, such as massage to relief back pain. Additionally, use of the orthosis in women with augmented breast tissue may reduce the risk of rupture or displacement of implant material during activities involving external pressure and mechanical loading of the breast tissues, often involved in massage, chiropractic, osteopathic, and physical therapy modalities [8].

Stiffness, fluidity, elasticity and density vary between tissue and implant material, causing shear strains parallel to the patient's plane of contact, and when reaching the

Table 3 Effect of orthosis on mechanical forces

Outcome	Participants	Side	No orthosis	Size-1	Size-2	Size-3	Contrast	Change vs no orthosis	ANOVA repeated measures
A)	**All (n = 32)**		**Mean (SD)**	**Mean (SD)**	**Mean (SD)**	**Mean (SD)**		%	**p-value**
Peak pressure (kPa)		left	14.9 (7.4)	6.0 (3.6)	4.5 (3.0)	2.3 (2.1)	S0 vs S1:	−60	<0.001
							S2:	−70	
							S3:	−85	
		right	15.8 (8.4)	6.6 (4.6)	4.8 (3.7)	2.3 (2.1)	S0 vs S1:	−58	<0.001
							S2:	−70	
							S3:	−85	
Max force (N)		left	55.0 (20.4)	14.7 (10.2)	6.9 (5.9)	2.3 (2.6)	S0 vs S1:	−73	<0.001
							S2	−87	
							:S3:	−96	
		right	58.8 (18.7)	15.1 (10.0)	7.3 (6.3)	2.7 (3.0)	S0 vs S1:	−74	<0.001
							S2:	−88	
							S3:	−95	
Displacement (cm)	**All (n = 32)**	ML	14.6 (1.9)	12.5 (1.8)	12.1 (1.7)	12.2 (1.4)	S0 vs S1:	−14	<0.001
		right					S2:	−17	
							S3:	−16	
		AP	4.1 (1.3)	4.7 (1.3)	5.4 (1.1)	6.2 (1.1)	S0 vs S1:	15	<0.001
		right					S2:	32	
							S3:	51	
B)	**Subgroups**								
Peak pressure (kPa)	**Without implant (n = 11)**	left	12.6 (4.6)	4.2 (3.7)	3.2 (3.2)	2.1 (2.5)	S0 vs S1:	−67	0.001
							S2:	−75	
							S3:	−83	
		right	13.2 (4.9)	4.8 (3.9)	3.3 (3.3)	2.0 (2.4)	S0 vs S1:	−64	0.006
							S2:	−75	0.001
							S3:	−85	0.001
	With implant (n = 20-21)[1]	left	16.1 (8.6)	6.6 (2.8)	5.1 (2.7)	2.5 (1.9)	S0 vs S1:	−59	0.002
							S2:	−68	<0.001
							S3:	−84	<0.001
		right	17.1 (9.5)	7.6 (4.8)	5.6 (3.7)	2.5 (2.0)	S0 vs S1:	−56	0.001
							S2:	−67	<0.001
							S3:	−85	<0.001

Table 3 Effect of orthosis on mechanical forces *(Continued)*

Max force (N)	**Without implant (n = 11)**	left	48.8 (14.4)	10.1 (11.9)	4.6 (6.5)	1.9 (3.3)	S0 vs S1:	−79	<0.001
							S2:	−91	
							S3:	−96	
		right	61.4 (20.9)	18.1 (8.2)	8.9 (6.0)	3.0 (2.7)	S0 vs S1:	−71	<0.001
							S2:	−86	
							S3:	−95	
	With implant (n = 20-21)[1]	left	60.4 (20.7)	17.8 (8.0)	8.4 (5.1)	2.7 (2.2)	S0 vs S1:	−71	<0.001
							S2:	−86	
							S3:	−96	
		right	53.6 (12.8)	9.4 (10.6)	4.3 (6.0)	2.0 (3.7)	S0 vs S1:	−82	<0.001
							S2:	−92	
							S3:	−96	
Displacement (cm)	**Without implant (n = 11)**	ML	14.5 (1.8)	12.3 (2.5)	11.4 (2.4)	13.2 (1.6)	S0 vs S1:	−15	0.023
		right					S2:	−21	0.019
							S3:	−9	0.023
		AP	3.1 (1.4)	4.1 (1.6)	5.0 (1.2)	6.4 (1.1)	S0 vs S1:	32	0.023
		right					S2:	61	0.051
							S3:	106	0.002
	With implant (n = 21)	ML	14.6 (1.9)	12.7 (1.0)	12.4 (1.1)	11.9 (1.3)	S0 vs S1:	−13	0.001
		right					S2:	−15	0.002
							S3:	−18	<0.001
		AP	4.6 (0.9)	5.2 (0.9)	5.6 (1.1)	6.1 (1.1)	S0 vs S1:	13	0.002
		right					S2:	22	<0.001
							S3:	33	<0.001
Peak pressure (kPa)	**Natural (n = 7)**	left	13.0 (2.8)	4.3 (4.1)	3.4 (3.4)	2.4 (2.4)	S0 vs S1:	−67	0.014
							S2:	−74	0.006
							S3:	−82	0.002
		right	13.3 (3.6)	5.1 (4.4)	3.4 (3.4)	2.4 (2.4)	S0 vs S1:	−62	0.084
							S2:	−74	0.018
							S3:	−82	0.007
	Lactating (n = 2)	left	15.0 (11.3)	7.0 (0)	5.5 (2.1)	3.0 (4.2)	S0 vs S1:	−53	na
							S2:	−63	
							S3:	−80	

Table 3 Effect of orthosis on mechanical forces *(Continued)*

		right	16.0 (11.3)	7.0 (0)	6.0 (1.4)	2.5 (3.5)	S0 vs S1:	−56	na
							S2:	−63	
							S3:	−84	
	Primary augmentation (n = 18)	left	16.6 (8.9)	6.7 (2.9)	5.1 (2.9)	2.4 (2.0)	S0 vs S1:	−60	0.003
							S2:	−69	0.001
							S3:	−86	<0.001
		right	16.6 (11.3)	7.0 (0)	6.0 (1.4)	2.5 (3.5)	S0 vs S1:	−58	0.003
							S2:	−64	0.001
							S3:	−85	<0.001
	Reconstruction (n = 2-3)[1]	left	11.5 (0.7)	5.5 (0.7)	5.0 (0.7)	3.0 (0)	S0 vs S1:	−52	na
		(n = 2)					S2:	−57	
							S3:	−74	
		right	20.3 (14.4)	12.7 (10.7)	9.0 (7.8)	2.0 (1.7)	S0 vs S1:	−37	na
		(n = 3)					S2:	−56	
							S3:	−90	
	Lumpectomy (n = 1)	left	8	0	0	0	S0 vs all:	−100	na
		right	10	0	0	0	S0 vs all:	−100	
	Tram flap (n = 1)	left	10	2	0	0	S0 vs all:	−80,-100	na
		right	10	3	0	0	S0 vs all:	−70,-100	
Max force (N)	**Natural (n = 7)**	left	52.3 (13.9)	11.6 (13.1)	5.0 (7.0)	2.1 (3.7)	S0 vs S1:	−78	0.005
							S2:	−90	0.001
							S3:	−96	0.001
		right	51.4 (12.0)	10.1 (11.4)	4.0 (5.6)	2.1 (4.1)	S0 vs S1:	−80	0.005
							S2:	−92	0.001
							S3:	−96	<0.001
	Lactating (n = 2)	left	45.5 (17.7)	14.5 (12.0)	8.0 (8.5)	3.0 (4.2)	S0 vs S1:	−68	na
							S2:	−82	
							S3:	−93	
		right	47.0 (15.6)	15.0 (11.3)	9.5 (9.2)	3.5 (4.9)	S0 vs S1:	−68	na
							S2:	−80	
							S3:	−93	

Table 3 Effect of orthosis on mechanical forces *(Continued)*

Primary augmentation (n = 18)	left	59.0 (21.2)	17.5 (8.4)	8.2 (5.2)	2.6 (2.3)	S0 vs S1:	−70	<0.001
						S2:	−86	
						S3:	−96	
	right	60.8 (21.1)	18.1 (8.7)	9.2 (6.4)	2.9 (2.7)	S0 vs S1:	−70	<0.001
						S2:	−85	
						S3:	−95	
Reconstruction (n = 2-3)[1]	left	72.5 (13.4)	20.5 (5.0)	10.5 (5.0)	3.0 (1.4)	S0 vs S1:	−72	na
						S2:	−86	
						S3:	−96	
	right	65.0 (23.6)	18.3 (4.7)	7.3 (2.5)	4.0 (2.6)	S0 vs S1:	−72	na
						S2:	−89	
						S3:	−94	
Lumpecto	left	27	0	0	0	S0 vs all:	−100	na
my (n = 1)	right	70	0	0	0	S0 vs all:	−100	
Tram flap	left	53	1	0	0	S0 vs all:	−98,-100	na
(n = 1)	right	66	2	0	0	S0 vs all:	−97,-100	

A) All participants; B) Subgroups. All orthoses tested were of firm density.[1] One participant had a one sided (right side) implant after mastectomy. Subgroup analysis includes the participant's measures for the right side only.

AP, antero-posterior; kPa, kilopascal; ML, medio-lateral; N, Newton; n, number; na, not applicable; S0, no orthosis; S1, size-1 orthosis; S2, size-2 orthosis; S3, size-3 orthosis; vs, versus

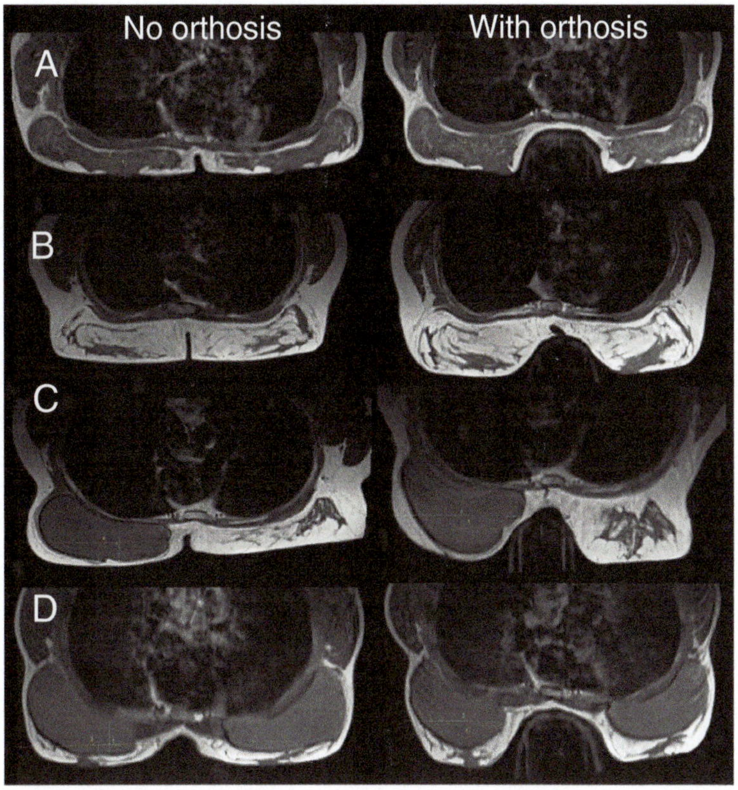

Figure 2 Assessment of breast displacement. MRI transverse view of natural breast C-cup **(A)**; lactating breast EE-cup **(B)**; unilateral reconstruction C-cup **(C)**; primary augmentation DD-cup **(D)**; all without (left panel) and with orthosis (right panel).

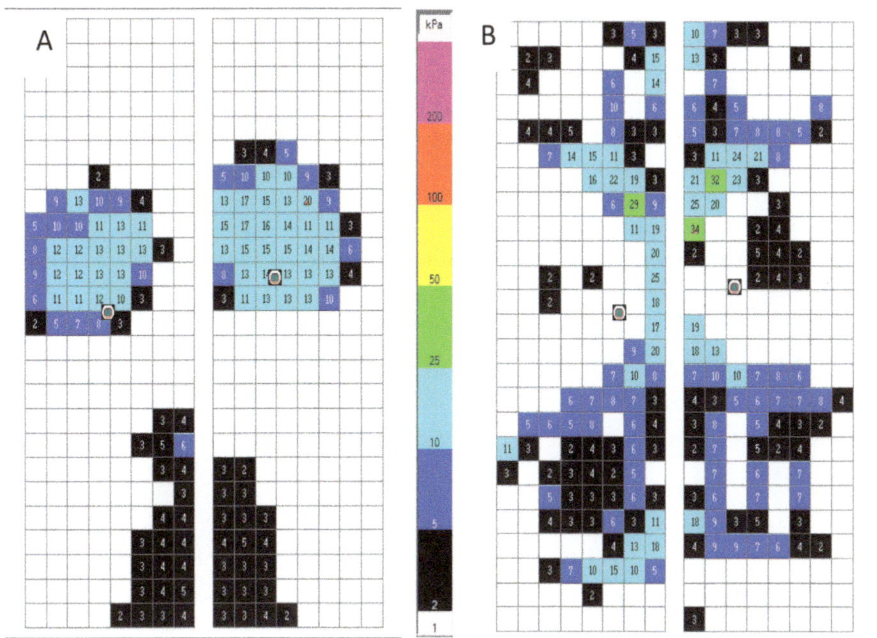

Figure 3 Assessment of mechanical forces. Plane view of loading through breast tissue without **(A)** and with the orthosis **(B)**, where pressure (kPa) is distributed along the orthosis.

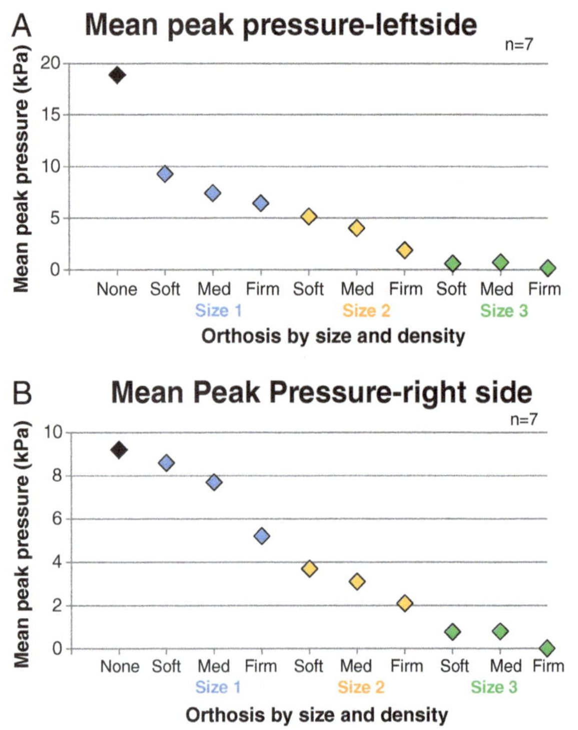

Figure 4 Mean peak pressure by orthosis size (sizes 1–3) and density (soft, medium, firm) on the left (A) or right breast side (B) in a subgroup of participants compared with no orthosis (black diamond).

limits of elasticity the implant material or human tissue may rupture or tear. Patients who have undergone breast reconstruction using implants after breast cancer surgery are likely to have a higher failure rate than primary augmentation patients, as their residual natural tissues are generally more vulnerable [16]. Furthermore, as implant material has no neural innervation the individual may be unaware of the damage, known as silent rupture. Conversely, when human tissue fails and the implant moves, asymmetry such as a symmastia or 'uni-breast' is caused [17].

The newly developed orthosis' structure allows for specificity in load distribution, isolating pressure tolerant areas and relieving sensitive areas (Figure 1a). Further research is needed to capture the breast pain in relation to device density and duration of prone loading. In our study, patients were most comfortable lying prone on the size-3 firm orthosis during the 1 hour testing sessions. Our subgroup study suggests that the softer density device provides less loading protection, but additional studies are needed to ascertain whether softer varieties provide greater rib cage comfort when used for longer periods. In practice lighter subjects generally prefer the softer density device whilst heavier subjects prefer the firmer density device. Comfort and correct fit are key to the orthosis being superior to current methods of using towels, pillows and bolsters. The orthosis is reliable in its capacity, its use is repeatable and results are reproducible, which is important in litigious environments.

Professional fitting by an orthotist or primary healthcare practitioner is recommended to ensure appropriate use and maximum protection (Additional file 1). It is imperative that the altered and 'at risk' breast structures be exposed to minimal loading and therefore must be adjacent to the device. The orthosis should be part of ongoing management when breast tissue has been altered. It is advisable that patient have their own orthosis for use in day to day management.

Future research could test the orthosis in situations other than prone, for example in the upright positioning such as car seat travel to reduce the risk of breast implant rupture by the seat belt during an accident [18]. A light harness or fixation system could hold the orthosis in position against the torso. Further larger long-term

Table 4 Guidelines for size and density choice of orthosis by breast cup-size, as suggested (X), optional (O), and to avoid (white)

	Orthosis size-1				Orthosis size-2				Orthosis size-3			
Breast cup size	SSoft	Soft	Med	Firm	SSoft	Soft	Med	Firm	SSoft	Soft	Med	Firm
A+	X	X	X	X	O	O	O					
B+	X	X	X	X	X	O	O	O				
C+	O	O	X	X	X	X	X	X	O	O		
D+				X	X	X	X	X	X	O	O	O
E+					X	X	X	X	X	X	X	O
F+									X	X	X	X
G+									X	X	X	X
H+										X	X	X

Ssoft, supersoft; Med, medium.
The orthosis of supersoft density was not used in this trial.

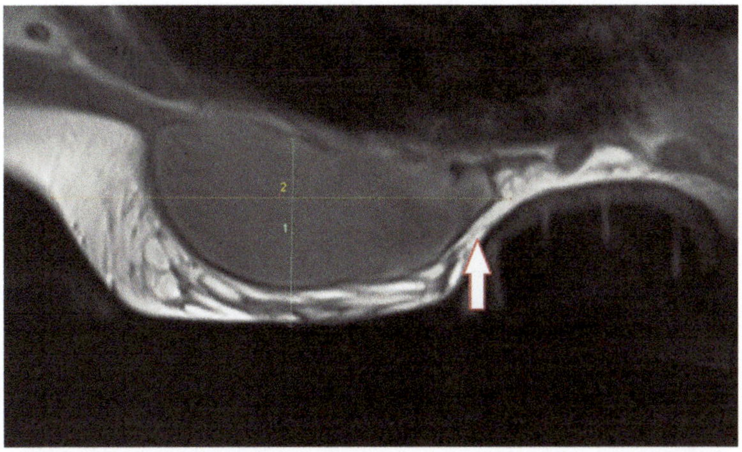

Figure 5 Sagittal MRI view mid-breast of an E-cup primary augmented individual in a size-1 device. The arrow points to the implant loading upon the orthosis, as it is too small. This must be avoided.

studies are needed to determine potential risk reduction in complication rates and breast implant longevity with regular use of the orthosis.

Conclusion

Our research demonstrates the new orthosis to significantly reduce pain, displacement and mechanical pressure in natural and augmented breast tissue in women undertaking prone activities with symmetrical loading across their back. This has significant implications in both clinical settings, and for general activities of the patient in prone position, e.g. massage, orthopaedic treatment. Our study has contributed to developing guidelines for fitting of optimal size and density of the orthosis to reduce loading and increase comfort, also in relation to breast size, and patient weight. In our study, larger and firmer options of the orthosis showed generally greater effectiveness in our group of women with breast cup-sizes B-F. Clinicians placing patients in prone positions are encouraged to use the orthosis. In patients with breast augmentation or reconstruction, to prevent litigation risks, as resultant breast structures are less deformable and may cause greater discomfort in the prone position. Post-operative fitting following breast surgery of any description is advisable to protect the altered tissues and allow for a more safe and comfortable return to activities of daily living.

Consent

Written informed consent was obtained from the participants for the publication of this report and any accompanying images.

Additional file

Additional file 1: Professional fitting guidelines of MammaGard orthosis. Figure S1. The manubrio-sternal joint is lying approximately adjacent to the MammaGard name logo (red circle). The logo is engraved on top of the orthosis (refer to Figure 1A in the main manuscript). **Figure S2.** The xiphoid process is adjacent to the butterfly logo (red circle). The logo is engraved on top of the orthosis (refer to Figure 1A in the main manuscript).

Competing interests
PM is consultant to novel.de, but none of the companies and centres accessed for this study were involved in the study design, data collection, analysis and preparation of the manuscript. No external or industry funding was received. The authors declare no conflict of interest.

Authors' contributions
All authors contributed to the design and planning of the study. SA and PM conceptualised the study, recruited participants, and collected data. KR analysed data and prepared the manuscript for publication with contributions from co-authors. All authors approved the final version.

Acknowledgements
We thank MammaGard Pty Ltd who supplied the orthosis, the Melbourne Specialist Imaging Centre for radiology expertise, College of Health and Biomedicine at Victoria University for biomechanics testing facilities, and the Defence Science and Technology Organisation (Novel.de) for loaning the pliance sensors. We are grateful to all the women who participated in the study.
PM's role in this work was partly supported by the Australian Government funded Collaborative Research Networks Program at Victoria University.

Author details
[1]National Institute of Integrative Medicine, Melbourne VIC 3122, Australia.
[2]College of Health and Biomedicine, Victoria University, Melbourne VIC 3001, Australia.

References

1. Armstrong S, Ried K, Sali A, McLaughlin P: **A new orthosis reduces pain and mechanical forces in prone position in women with augmented or natural breast tissue: a pilot study.** *J Plastic Reconstr Aesthet Surg* 2013, **66:**e179–88.

2. Keogh B: *Poly Implant Prothese (PIP) breast implants: final report of the expert group.* UK: Department of Health, National Health Service (NHS); 2012.
3. Therapeutic Goods Administration: *PIP Breast Implants - TGA Update.* Canberra: Australian Government Department of Health and Ageing; 2012.
4. Therapeutic Goods Administration: *Breast Implant Information Booklet.* 4th edition. Canberra: Australian Government Department of Health and Ageing; 2001.
5. Food and Drug Administration: *FDA update on the safety of silicone gel-filled breast implants.* U.S: Center for Devices and Radiological Health; 2011.
6. Brown SL, Middleton MS, Berg WA, Soo MS, Pennello G: **Prevalence of rupture of silicone gel breast implants revealed on MR imaging in a population of women in Birmingham, Alabama.** *Am J Radiol* 2000, **175:**1057–1064.
7. Daniels A: **Silicone breast implant materials.** *Swiss Med Wkly* 2012, **142:**w13614.
8. Medical Observer: **Judge orders chiro to pay for twisted breast implant.** 2013. http://www.medicalobserver.com.au/news/judge-orders-chiro-to-pay-for-twisted-breast-implant.
9. Granchi D, Cavedagna D, Ciapetti G, Stea S, Schiavon P, Giuliani R, *et al*: **Silicone breast implants: the role of immune system on capsular contracture formation.** *J Biomed Mater Res* 1995, **29:**197–202.
10. Janowsky EC, Kupper LL, Hulka BS: **Meta-analyses of the relation between silicone breast implants and the risk of connective-tissue diseases.** *N Engl J Med* 2000, **342:**781–90.
11. Wong CH, Samuel M, Tan BK, Song C: **Capsular contracture in subglandular breast augmentation with textured versus smooth breast implants: a systematic review.** *Plast Reconstr Surg* 2006, **118:**1224–1236.
12. Farrar JT, Young JP Jr, LaMoreaux L, Werth JL, Poole RM: **Clinical importance of changes in chronic pain intensity measured on an 11-point numerical pain rating scale.** *Pain* 2001, **94:**149–158.
13. Breivik H, Borchgrevink PC, Allen SM, Rosseland LA, Romundstad L, Hals EK, *et al*: **Assessment of pain.** *Br J Anaesth* 2008, **101:**17–24.
14. *Magnetic Resonance Imaging Scanner Siemens 1.5T Magnetom Espree.* USA: Siemens; 2010.
15. IBM Corp: *IBM SPSS Statistics 21.0.* 2012.
16. Handel N, Cordray T, Gutierrez J, Jensen JA: **A long-term study of outcomes, complications, and patient satisfaction with breast implants.** *Plast Reconstr Surg* 2006, **117:**757–767.
17. Spear SL, Bogue DP, Thomassen JM: **Synmastia after breast augmentation.** *Plast Reconstr Surg* 2006, **118:**168S–171S.
18. Nordhoff LS Jr: **Frontal crashes: biomechanics and injuries. Chapter 16 in Motor Vehicle Collision Injuries.** In *Biomechanics Diagnosis and Management.* 2nd edition. MA, USA: Jones and Bartlett Publishers; 2005.

Intra-oral myofascial therapy versus education and self-care in the treatment of chronic, myogenous temporomandibular disorder: a randomised, clinical trial

Allan Kalamir[1*], Petra L Graham[2], Andrew L Vitiello[3], Rodney Bonello[1] and Henry Pollard[4]

Abstract

Background: Myogenous temporomandibular disorders (TMD) are considered to be a common musculoskeletal condition. No studies exist comparing intra-oral myofascial therapies to education, self-care and exercise (ESC) for TMD. This study evaluated short-term differences in pain and mouth opening range between intra-oral myofascial therapy (IMT) and an ESC program.

Methods: Forty-six participants with chronic myogenous TMD (as assessed according to the Research Diagnostic Criteria Axis 1 procedure) were consecutively block randomised into either an IMT group or an ESC group. Each group received two sessions per week (for five weeks) of either IMT or short talks on the anatomy, physiology and biomechanics of the jaw plus instruction and supervision of self-care exercises. The sessions were conducted at the first author's jaw pain and chiropractic clinic in Sydney, Australia. Primary outcome measures included pain at rest, upon opening and clenching, using an eleven point ordinal self reported pain scale. A secondary outcome measure consisted of maximum voluntary opening range in millimetres. Data were analysed using linear models for means and logistic regression for responder analysis.

Results: After adjusting for baseline, the IMT group had significantly lower average pain for all primary outcomes at 6 weeks compared to the ESC group ($p < 0.001$). These differences were not clinically significant but the IMT group had significantly higher odds of a clinically significant change ($p < 0.045$). There was no significant difference in opening range between the IMT and ESC groups. Both groups achieved statistically significant decreases in all three pain measures at six weeks ($p \leq 0.05$), but only the IMT group achieved clinically significant changes of 2 or more points.

Conclusion: This study showed evidence of superiority of IMT compared to ESC over the short-term but not at clinically significant levels. Positive changes over time for both IMT and ESC protocols were noted. A longer term, multi-centre study is warranted.

Trial registration: Australian and New Zealand Clinical Trials Registry ACTRN12610000508077.

Keywords: Myofascial pain syndrome, Trigger points, Craniomandibular disorders, Temporomandibular joint dysfunction syndrome, Musculoskeletal manipulations, Exercise, Education, Self-care, Clinical trial

* Correspondence: thechiro@tpg.com.au
[1]Department of Chiropractic, Faculty of Science, Macquarie University, North Ryde, NSW, Australia
Full list of author information is available at the end of the article

Background

Temporomandibular disorder (TMD) treatment trends in recent decades have leaned toward multi-modal as well as multi-disciplinary management, in line with that of other chronic musculoskeletal conditions [1]. Such strategies often suggest the use of less invasive and reversible interventions, and has been mainly represented by the involvement of psychotherapy (utilising technology such as biofeedback [2], cognitive and behavioural therapies [3,4]); physiotherapy [5-9] (utilising exercises, mobilisation and various electro-medical therapies); and complementary and alternative medicine therapies (chiropractic [10,11], osteopathy [12,13], massage [14-17], relaxation therapy [18], acupuncture [19,20] and others [21-25]). This trend away from more invasive and irreversible treatment is also represented by an increase in the literature pertaining to the use of patient education as well as self-care (relaxation, implementation of cognitive and behavioural therapeutic strategies and exercises) [26].

In the particular case of the various physical therapies, references are broadly made to manual therapy (mobilisation, manipulation, massage) [14,27,28] and also increasingly to self-care activities (less well defined in the literature, but has been reported to include heat packs, self-massage, active range of motion exercise, isometric exercise, and passive self-mobilisation) [29-31]. The more integrated model of treatment in these therapies [6,28] has resulted in a lack of data on the comparative benefits of the various component interventions [29].

The use of intra-oral myofascial therapies (IMT), such as "trigger point releases" has been well entrenched in a wide variety of physical therapy professions, particularly manual medicine, chiropractic, physiotherapy, osteopathy and massage. The authors have previously published the results of a clinical trial comparing IMT to a combined IMT, education and self-care protocol [32,33]. That trial's results suggested that combining education and self-care (ESC) with IMT did not appear to afford any significant superiority in pain outcomes in the short term when compared to IMT alone. The authors therefore decided to directly explore the clinical effectiveness of ESC as a stand-alone therapy as compared to IMT over the short term (6 weeks) utilising similar primary outcome measures of pain at rest, upon opening and clenching (i.e. an 11 point ordinal self reported pain scale). A secondary outcome measure of inter-incisal opening range measured in millimetres was also adopted for the study.

In this paper, we present the results of a short-term randomised clinical trial, conducted within a suburban Sydney chiropractic and TMD clinic, comparing outcomes in pain and opening range in dentist-referred participants suffering from chronic myogenous TMD.

Methods

Design

The study was part of a PhD program undertaken by the first author in the Faculty of Science at Macquarie University, N.S.W., Australia. The design was that of a randomised trial comparing two different conservative care modalities- IMT and ESC. The trial was conducted in accordance with the CONSORT statement, and was registered with the Australian and New Zealand Clinical Trials Registry on the 21st of June 2010, registration number ACTRN12610000508077. The trial was approved by the Macquarie University Human Ethics Committee on the 10th of August 2010, Reference number 5201000771.

Study setting

The trial was conducted at the first author's private TMD and chiropractic clinic in Edensor Park, NSW, Australia. Participants were recruited by referral from several co-operative local dental clinics that already had a well established history of inter-referral and co-management of TMD patients.

Study team

The trial team consisted of a receptionist, an assistant, one practitioner and an assessor. The receptionist answered telephone queries, verbally discussed basic inclusion and exclusion criteria with enquirers, made appointments and prepared files. The assistant was tasked with generating the randomisation schedule using a web-based random number generator and allocate each numbered participant file to one of the two groups until the schedule was exhausted. This schedule was kept off premises by the assistant, who was blinded to the assessments. Group allocation was concealed from all personnel except for the assistant before randomisation. The practitioner role was undertaken by the first author, who performed the interventions. The assessor was previously trained in the administration of the Research Diagnostic Criteria (RDC) for TMD assessment, using video footage as well as practice drills, in order to calibrate for variables such as pressure, location and participant instruction. All baseline and outcome data were collected on-premises by the assessor, who was blinded to the group allocation of participants. The first author was also blinded to the assessment outcomes until the end of the entire data collection.

Subjects

Recruitment occurred between August 2010 and February 2011. Interested parties were invited to phone the clinic for further information and to establish basic inclusion and exclusion criteria. Inclusion criteria consisted of an age restriction between 18 and 50 years old, a daily history of peri-auricular pain (with or without joint sounds) for at least the last three months, and voluntary participation. Participants were not remunerated for their participation. Exclusion criteria screened by the receptionist included the use of dentures; a history of malignancy in the last five years; other physical contra-indications such as active inflammatory arthritides, fractures, dislocations, known instability of the jaw or neck; metabolic , connective tissue, haematologic and rheumatologic diseases.

Enquirers who met these requirements then attended the clinic in person to read and sign their consent forms and to have their baseline assessment. The RDC has been reported to be a valid and reliable bi-axial diagnostic tool for the assessment of myogenous, arthrogenous and mixed trait TMD and is widely used in TMD research [34-39]. The RDC contains both a physical axis of assessment as well as a psychosocial one that was applied to establish specific inclusion criteria which included: a myogenous TMD diagnosis (mixed trait and arthrogenous TMD diagnoses were excluded) and a minimum ordinal pain scale score of 3/10 on each of the three symptom outcome measures included in the study. A further exclusion criterion based on the assessment was a finding of severe depression or somatisation on the psychosocial assessment axis.

Outcome measures

The primary outcome measures used in this trial consisted of the difference between the IMT and ESC groups for each of the three pain measures: jaw pain at rest; jaw pain upon maximal active opening and jaw pain upon clenching. It was hypothesised that these three positional pain measures would give a reasonable interpretation of myofascial pain when the jaw elevator muscles are at a resting physiological tone, undergoing maximal active stretch and maximum isometric contracture. The use of a self reported eleven point numerical rating scale (where zero means "no pain" and 10 represents "pain as bad as could be") provided ease of use for participants, they having familiarised themselves with ordinal pain scales during the administration of the RDC. A difference of 2 or more points between the groups was considered clinically significant, based on previously published studies [32,33].

A secondary outcome measure was that of the difference between groups for maximal voluntary inter-incisal opening range in millimetres, with an increase in opening distance being considered positive. The use of opening range as an outcome measure has been widely reported in the literature, with good support for both its validity and reliability [40] compared to other movements such as lateral deviation, protrusion, retrusion and end-feel stretch pain in these ranges. A 5 mm or more difference between groups was deemed to be clinically significant for measured inter-incisal opening range [41,42].

Interest was also in determining whether each treatment group had declined by a clinically significant about over time for each outcome measure. Reductions in pain of two or more points or increases in opening range of at least 5 mm were deemed clinically significant.

Outcomes were measured during attendance at the clinic at baseline and at six weeks post treatment.

Group allocation

Each consecutively numbered participant file was allocated to a treatment group according to a blocked design randomisation schedule, which was web-generated (www.randomizer.org) and kept off-premises by the assistant.

Interventions

Participants were randomised into one of two treatment groups, IMT or ESC. Each treatment group received two sessions per week for five weeks. The treatments are described as follows:

1. IMT group, whose treatment consisted of several myofascial techniques previously reported in the literature [32,33], and administered by the first author. They were comprised of the following three interventions:

   a) "Intra-oral temporalis release" (Figure 1). This consisted of a gloved index finger intra-oral contact onto the tendonous insertions of the temporalis muscle at the superior aspect of the coronoid process. Light posterior and caudad pressure is applied by the finger within pain tolerance of the patient. Simultaneously, the index and middle fingers of the other hand apply superior pressure longitudinally along the anterior fibres of the temporalis muscle moving gradually anterior to posterior. The patient is asked to

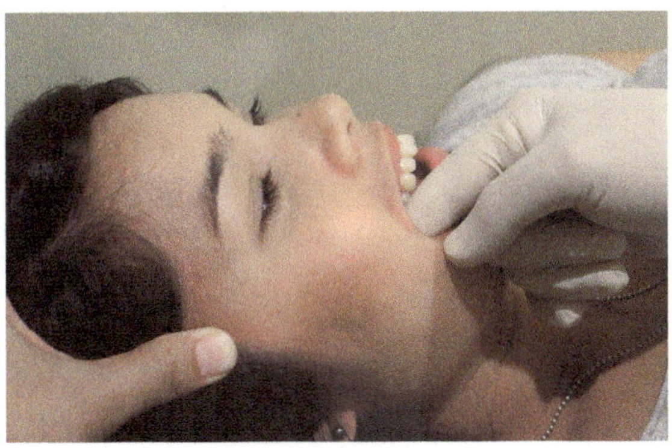

Figure 1 Intra-oral temporalis release.

incrementally open their mouth to its maximum range.

b) "Intra-oral medial and lateral pterygoid (origin) technique" (Figure 2). The practitioner is seated either homolateral or contralateral to the side being treated. A gloved index finger is inserted along the lateral wall of the pharynx, posterior to the last molar. Posterior and cephalad pressure is applied into the pharyngeal mucosal tissues overlying the pterygoid origins arising from the lateral pterygoid plate of the sphenoid. Care is taken to avoid direct contact of the hamulus. The contact is maintained for 5 seconds.
c) "Intra-oral sphenopalatine ganglion technique" (Figure 3). The gloved 5th finger of the caudad hand is slowly inserted along the buccal surface of the lightly occluded teeth. The patient is asked to briefly clench their teeth, and upon relaxing, the practitioner presses their finger deeper posteriorward. This process is repeated until the tip of the finger reaches as close to the anterior aspect of the infratemporal fossa / sphenopalatine fossa as is comfortable to the patient. The patient is then asked to lift their head off the table, pushing into the contact. In this way excessive force by the practitioner is checked by an apprehension response of the patient. After three repetitions, the patient relaxes; resting their head back onto the headrest, and gentle buccal pressure is now applied into medial pterygoid muscle by the practitioner's finger tip before gently being removed from the mouth.

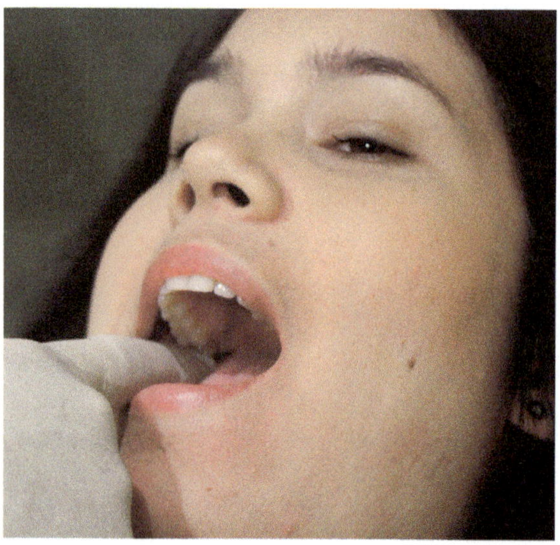

Figure 2 Intra-oral medial and lateral (origin) technique.

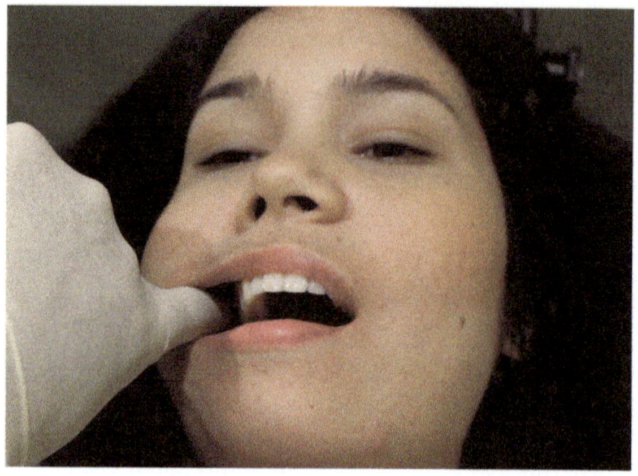

Figure 3 Intra-oral sphenopalatine ganglion technique.

2. ESC group, whose treatment was based on the protocol also previously described by the authors in the literature [32,33], consisted of short scripted lectures on the basic anatomy, biomechanics and pathophysiology of the TMJ, the role of stress; slow, diaphragmatic breathing exercises and general advice on relaxation awareness and avoidance of potentially problematic foods (nuts, chewing gum etc.). This component was partially based on the prior published work by Michelotti et al. [43]; Nicolakis et al. [44] and Dworkin [45]; with further recent work by Jerjes et al. [46]. These ESC sessions also involved the teaching and supervision self-care exercises that were performed both during the session, to ensure proper form, as well as at home by the participant twice a day. The same number of attendances at the clinic and duration of sessions were given to this group. The exercises, which are designed to stimulate and stretch the joint capsule and relax the masticatory muscles are summarised below:

a) Guided and controlled jaw excursions (Figure 4). The patient applies a contact to the TMJ joint of one side with the thenar or pisiform of the ipsilateral hand, while the heel of the other hand is placed on the side of the chin. Both sides exert even pressure upon their contacts, while the patient actively opens and closes their mouth five times. Where tolerable, the patient may increase the pressure exerted by the hand contacts with each successive opening. The contacts are then reversed and repeated on the other side.
b) Post –isometric stretches (lateral deviation and opening, Figures 5 and 6). Placing the heel of one hand on the same side of the chin, the patient exerts and active force of the chin into the hand, which opposes any movement. The contraction is

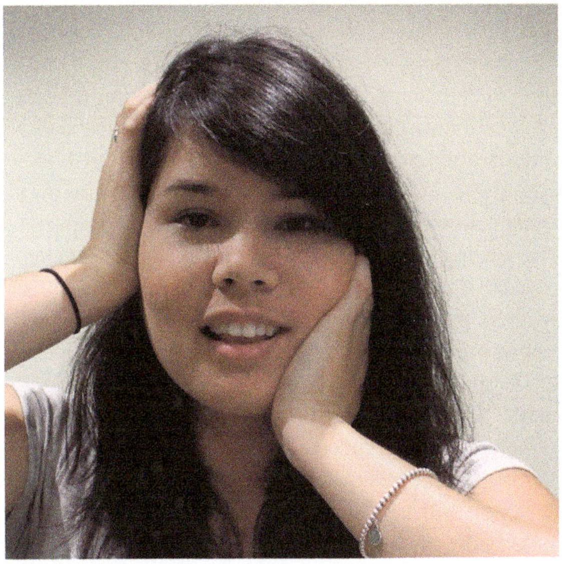

Figure 4 Guided and controlled jaw excursions.

held for up to 10 seconds, depending on the tolerance of the patient. The contraction is then relaxed, while the hand continues to exert some pressure into the chin, deviating it slightly towards the other side. The cycle of isometric contraction is continued at this new point, and repeated in increments until the jaw has deviated to its tolerable limit. The contacts are then reversed and the procedure repeated on the opposite side. A similar process is then applied to incremental opening of the jaw, which is achieved by cupping the chin with both hands and resisting an isometric jaw close contraction, then drawing the jaw into an incrementally greater opening distance.

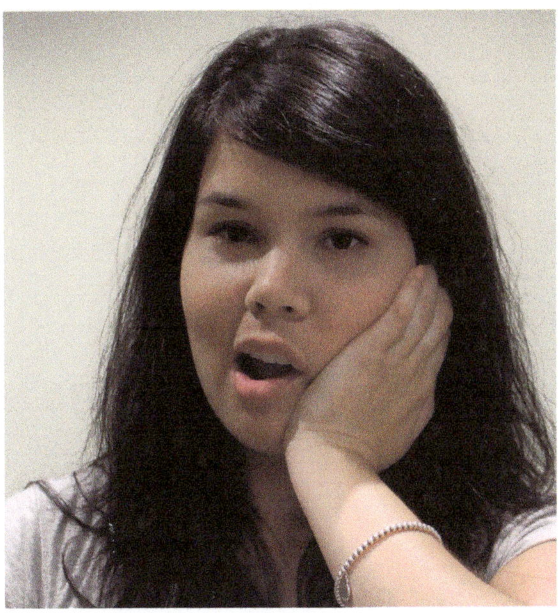

Figure 5 Post-isometric stretches (lateral deviation).

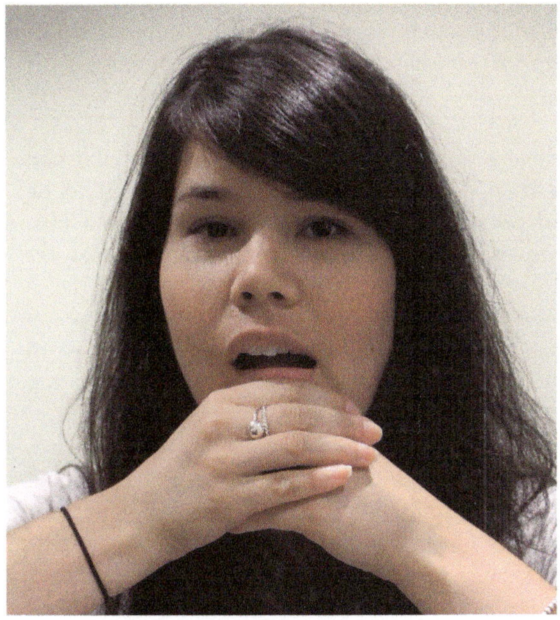

Figure 6 Post-isometric stretches (opening).

Statistical analysis

The data were analysed using linear regression models with pain outcome score at the end of the study as the dependent variable and baseline score as a covariate together with treatment group. For the primary outcomes results are presented as adjusted mean follow-up score with standard deviation and a p-value for the between groups contrast from the associated model. A Bonferroni correction was used whereby a significance level of 0.017 was used to reflect the three comparisons made in the primary outcome (i.e. 0.05 divided by 3).

The secondary outcome measure, opening range in mm, was also analysed using a linear regression model as described above. Results are presented as average adjusted difference in opening range (mm) between groups together with 95% confidence interval (CI).

Remaining within group differences for the pain measures and opening range measurements were presented as the mean change over time with 95% CIs as estimated from a linear model of change over time against treatment group.

Based on the a priori determination of clinical significance, an additional analysis was undertaken whereby for each outcome, change over time was coded as a 1 (success) if it had reached a clinically significant change or better and otherwise it was coded as 0 (failure).

Logistic regression was then used with the new binary variable as the outcome and treatment group and baseline score as covariates. Estimated odds of success for IMT versus ESC are presented for each outcome with 95% CI.

Sample size was estimated according to data published by Dao et al. [47]. Setting the significance level to be 0.05 and the power at 80%, Dao estimated that a 60% difference in pain intensity between groups would require a sample of approximately 42 participants (i.e. a group size of 21 participants per group, depending on the number of groups). The enrolment goal was set to 46 participants, in order to account for a possible ten percent drop-out rate.

For an average two point difference in pain measures (noted earlier as a clinically relevant difference) between the treatment groups using a 0.017% level of significance, power of 80% and estimated standard deviation between groups taken from the main trial [32], only 9 participants would be needed for each group. The larger number initially estimated was retained to increase the power to detect differences between the groups.

The models were fitted using R version 2.15.0. [48].

Results

The study flow chart is presented in Figure 7. Recruitment of participants commenced in August 2010 and concluded in February 2011. There were 71 enquiries, based on local dentist referrals of which 53 met the basic requirements and qualified for an assessment. Of those, 46 met their specific inclusion and exclusion criteria and were consecutively enrolled into the study as participants according to the randomisation schedule, having signed their consent forms. All of the participants accepted their group allocation. Treatments commenced subsequent to baseline assessment and were completed through February 2011. The last of the post-treatment assessments were completed by the end of April 2011. The interventions were successfully administered and the trial concluded without any reports of adverse reactions in any participants. One participant dropped out of the ESC group before the second assessment citing work-related travel prohibiting their continued treatment.

Baseline data, presented in Table 1, showed some differences in baseline scores with the IMT group having higher average pain scores and greater opening range.

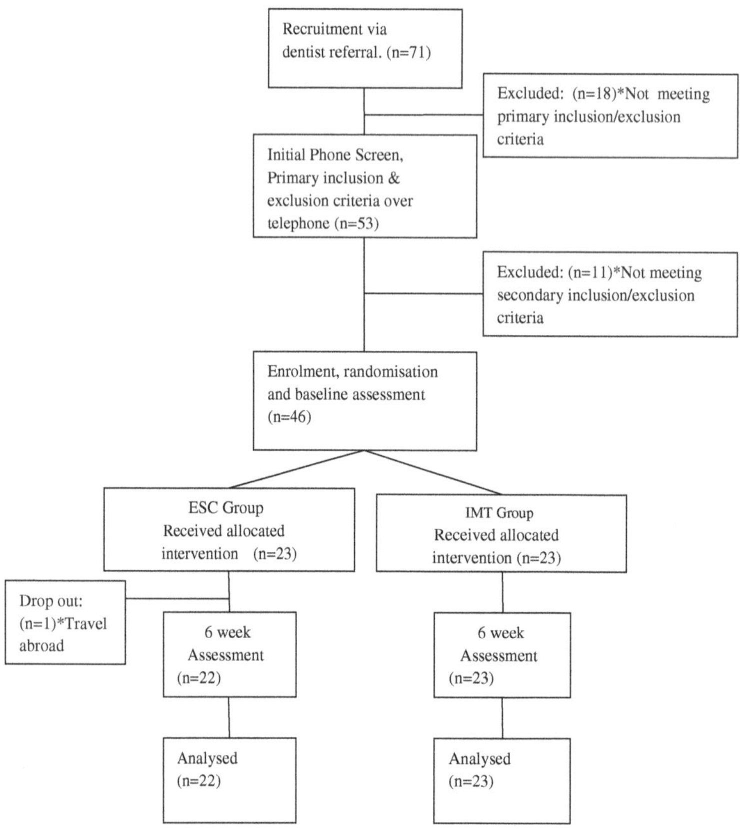

Figure 7 Study flow-chart.

Table 1 Background demographics and baseline characteristics of the participants

Detail	ESC group (n = 23) Mean (SD)	IMT group (n = 23) Mean (SD)
Age in years	26.8 (6.81)	28.2 (9.43)
Gender (m:f)	8:15	9:14
Pain§ at rest	4.09 (0.90)	4.74 (1.36)
Pain§ on opening	4.57 (1.24)	5.17 (1.47)
Pain§ on clenching	5.00 (1.28)	5.87 (1.58)
Opening range mm	37.43 (4.14)	38.83 (4.98)

ESC Education and self-care, *IMT* Intra-oral myofascial therapy, *SD* Standard deviation, § Self reported 11 point ordinal pain scale.

Primary outcomes

Adjusted post treatment results for the pain scores are shown in the final two columns of Table 2. Results indicate strong evidence of a statistically significant difference between groups however this difference was not clinically significant.

Secondary outcome

Results for opening range showed that, at six weeks, the average adjusted difference between groups in opening ranges was not significant (0.66, 95% CI:-0.96, 2.29; p = 0.416). The mean opening range for both the IMT and ESC groups had increased from baseline (p = 0.032 and 0.025, respectively, Table 3). However, from the point of view of clinical significance, neither the between groups nor within groups changes achieved a minimum range change of at least 5 mm post treatment.

For the pain outcomes, Table 3 demonstrates that both groups achieved statistically significant reductions in pain for all three outcome measures at six weeks compared to baseline. The IMT group achieved a clinically significant reduction of at least 2 points for each of the three pain outcomes whereas the ESC group did not.

Table 4 shows that the odds of achieving a two-point decrease was significantly higher for IMT versus ESC for resting pain and similarly for opening pain and clenching pain, respectively although the intervals were very wide.

Table 2 Average adjusted pain scores at 6 weeks and difference between groups

Variable	ESC: Mean (SD)	IMT: Mean (SD)	IMT v ESC (98.3% CI)	P-value
RP	2.87 (0.37)	2.26 (0.55)	−0.88 (−1.44, -0.31)	<0.001
OP	3.22 (0.59)	2.35 (0.70)	−1.16 (−1.80, -0.53)	<0.001
CP	3.39 (0.46)	2.61 (0.57)	−1.10 (−1.81, -0.38)	<0.001

RP Pain at rest, *OP* opening pain, *CP* Clenching pain, *ESC* education and self-care group, *IMT* intra-oral myofascial therapy group, *SD* standard deviation, *P-value* and 98.3% *CI* (confidence interval) is for the between groups difference at six weeks adjusted for baseline score.

Table 3 Average change in pain and opening range over time with 95% confidence interval

Variable	ESC (6 weeks v BL)	IMT (6 weeks v BL)
RP	−1.22 (−1.64, -0.80)	−2.48 (−2.90, -2.06)
OP	−1.35 (−1.81, -0.89)	−2.83 (−3.29, -2.37)
CP	−1.61 (−2.15, -1.06)	−3.26 (−3.81, -2.72)
OR	2.52 (1.37, 3.67)	3.00 (1.85, 4.15)

RP Pain at rest, *OP* opening pain, *CP* Clenching pain, *OR* Opening range (mm), *ESC* education and self-care group, *IMT* intra-oral myofascial therapy group, *BL* baseline.

Odds of a achieving a 5 mm increase in opening range was not significantly different for IMT versus ESC.

Discussion

The results showed that a TMD trial of this nature can be successfully conducted within a private suburban physical therapy clinic, where there is good co-operation with, and referral from local dentists. There was only one drop-out from this short study, which was not typical of other trials that have variably reported rates of up to 30% [43,49]. Studies of drop-out causes have suggested reasons such as environmental obstacles, perceived improvement or dissatisfaction with treatment [43,50] for that figure. The local and de-institutionalised nature of the treatment and assessment facilities and trust in their dentist's referral by patients may account for the good retention rate in this study. In addition, the chronicity; rigorous minimum pain scale and inclusion criteria [51]; benign nature of the interventions, and short duration of the trial may also have contributed.

The main outcome analysis showed that baseline adjusted pain scores were significantly lower for IMT compared to ESC however the difference was not clinically significant over this short term trial. Despite this failure to achieve clinical significance, a secondary responder analysis suggested significantly higher odds of the IMT group achieving a clinically important two-point decrease over the ESC group.

Clinical significance has been described in various ways in the literature. The breadth of change is often

Table 4 Proportion of successes and estimated adjusted odds of success IMT versus ESC

Variable	ESC: Proportion of successes	IMT: Proportion of successes	IMT v ESC OR (95% CI)	P-value
RP	6/23	19/23	27.65 (4.21, 417.52)	<0.001
OP	9/23	19/23	9.90 (1.92, 78.37)	0.012
CP	10/23	19/23	5.20 (1.12, 30.27)	0.045
OR	6/23	5/23	0.84 (0.20, 3.37)	0.805

RP Pain at rest, *OP* opening pain, *CP* Clenching pain, *OR* Opening range, *ESC* education and self-care group, *IMT* intra-oral myofascial therapy group, *SD* standard deviation, *CI* confidence interval.

considered to be an important indicator, with simplified interpretations of self reported 11 point ordinal measures for pain intensity scales suggesting a 2 point shift as being clinically significant [52-54]; and at least a 5 mm shift in opening range scale measures being considered clinically significant [41,42]. A limitation of this study is that it did not employ a comprehensive evaluation of post-treatment disability and patient satisfaction as advocated in TMD guidelines [55].

In light of this, fully evaluating clinical significance means that other factors also need to be taken into account, such as the importance of the change to patients as well as the efficiency of treatment and cost to consumers [56]. A study encompassing broader and more comprehensive outcome measures may be useful and should be conducted over a longer time frame.

The changes observed in pain scores over the course of the trial suggested improvement in pain for both IMT and ESC over the short term though only IMT reached clinically significant improvements. The IMT techniques employed in this study have a long history of being associated to craniomandibular myofascial trigger points-particularly within the chiropractic, osteopathic and physiotherapy / physical medicine professions although the added improvement in this group may be attributable to environmental or other factors not investigated in this study.

Active myofascial trigger points cause clinically perceivable pain complaints, and are tender to palpation. They refer recognizable pain upon contraction, and when compressed, produce referred motor and/or autonomic phenomena. They are also thought to contribute to muscle tension and decreased range of motion [57].

In this study, in spite of the positive trend, there was neither a significant difference between groups nor a clinically significant change in maximum active opening range in either group. It has been suggested that maximal pain free opening range benefits more from a combined treatment approach (such as combining IMT and ESC) than through individual treatment modalities alone [43]. The results of a previous trial by the authors to that effect concur with this idea [32]. However, the modest range of opening findings in this trial may just reflect its short time scale, or just the nature of the participants sampled in this study.

The improvement observed in the ESC group may be explained by several factors. It is thought that the effects of explaining the benign nature of the condition in detail, as well as providing reassurance, are powerful tools for the remission of TMD symptoms [43]. Carefully structured, simple interventions that emphasise self-care are also thought to be of significant benefit to TMD sufferers [58], as are enforcing patient responsibility and simultaneously addressing control factors [59]. Of course, the improvement in this group may also be attributable to factors beyond the ESC therapy that were not considered in this study.

This study was primarily hampered by the limitation that for a chronic condition, it was run over a short time frame (six weeks). It was also run from a single centre, using a single practitioner. This makes generalisation difficult. However, the positive short term results should encourage further, more comprehensive research into patient education and self-care for TMD. They also provide some additional support for the use of IMT protocols already published by the authors.

Conclusion

This study demonstrated significantly lower mean pain scores for IMT versus ESC treatment approaches in myogenous TMD sufferers and significantly higher odds of IMT achieving a two or more point decrease in pain scores over ESC therapy. Both treatments indicated positive effects over time however the short duration of the trial suggests that the results should be interpreted with caution. In light of these findings, we suggest that any further research into myofascial and self-care strategies for TMDs (of any type) use trials of at least one year duration to assess potential benefit.

Competing interests

The authors declare that they have no competing interests.

Authors' contributions

AK being the PhD candidate was involved in the conception, design, ethics and registration, interventions, tabulation, statistical analysis, manuscript write-up. PG was involved in supervising the statistical analysis and manuscript review. AV was involved in the conception and manuscript review. RB was involved in the ethics and manuscript review. HP was involved in the conception of the study and its design. All authors read and approved the final manuscript.

Acknowledgments

The authors would like to thank the anonymous referees whose comments and suggestions greatly improved this paper.

Author details

[1]Department of Chiropractic, Faculty of Science, Macquarie University, North Ryde, NSW, Australia. [2]Department of Statistics, Faculty of Science, Macquarie University, North Ryde, NSW, Australia. [3]Department of Academic Affairs, Anglo-European College of Chiropractic, Bournemouth, Dorset, UK. [4]School of Exercise Science, Faculty of Sports Science, Australian Catholic University, Sydney, NSW, Australia.

References

1. McKinney MW, Londeen TF, Turner SP, Levitt SR: **Chronic TM disorder and non-TM disorder pain: a comparison of behavioral and psychological characteristics.** *Cranio* 1990, **8**(1):40–6.
2. Crider AB, Glaros AG: **A meta-analysis of EMG biofeedback treatment of temporomandibular disorders.** *J Orofac Pain* 1999, **13**(1):29–37.
3. Aggarwal VR, Tickle M, Javidi H, Peters S: **Reviewing the evidence: can cognitive behavioral therapy improve outcomes for patients with chronic orofacial pain?** *J Orofac Pain* 2010, **24**(2):163–71.

4. Orlando B, Manfredini D, Salvetti G, Bosco M: **Evaluation of the effectiveness of biobehavioral therapy in the treatment of temporomandibular disorders: a literature review.** *Behav Med* 2007, **33**(3):101–18.
5. Michelotti A, Parisini F, Farella M, Cimino R, Martina R: **Muscular physiotherapy in patients with temporomandibular disorders. Controlled clinical trial.** *Minerva Stomatol* 2000, **49**(11–12):541–8.
6. Furto ES, Cleland JA, Whitman JM, Olson KA: **Manual physical therapy interventions and exercise for patients with temporomandibular disorders.** *Cranio* 2006, **24**(4):283–91.
7. Sturdivant J, Fricton JR: **Physical therapy for temporomandibular disorders and orofacial pain.** *Curr Op Dent* 1991, **1**(4):485–96.
8. Cetiner S, Kahraman SA, Yucetas S: **Evaluation of low-level laser therapy in the treatment of temporomandibular disorders.** *Photomed Laser Surg* 2006, **24**(5):637–41.
9. Manfredini D, Guarda-Nardini L: **Ultrasonography of the temporomandibular joint: a literature review.** *Int J Oral Maxillofac Surg* 2009, **38**(12):1229–36.
10. De Vocht JW, Long CR, Zeitler DL, Schaeffer W: **Chiropractic treatment of temporomandibular disorders using the activator adjusting instrument: a prospective case series.** *J Manipulative Physiol Ther* 2003, **26**(7):421–5.
11. Gregory TM: **Temporomandibular disorder associated with sacroiliac sprain.** *J Manipulative Physiol Ther* 1993, **16**(4):256–65.
12. Frymann VM: **Cranial osteopathy and its role in disorders of the temporomandibular joint.** *Dent Clin North Am* 1983, **27**(3):595–611.
13. Cuccia AM, Caradonna C, Annunziata V, Caradonna D: **Osteopathic manual therapy versus conventional conservative therapy in the treatment of temporomandibular disorders: a randomized controlled trial.** *J Bodyw Mov Ther* 2010, **14**(2):179–84.
14. Albertin A, Kerppers II, Amorim CF, Costa RV, Ferrari Correa JC, Oliveira CS: **The effect of manual therapy on masseter muscle pain and spasm.** *Electromyogr Clin Neurophysiol* 2010, **50**(2):107–12.
15. Barriere P, Zink S, Riehm S, Kahn JL, Veillon F, Wilk A: **Massage of the lateral pterygoid muscle in acute TMJ dysfunction syndrome.** *Rev Stomatol Chir Maxillofac* 2009, **110**(2):77–80.
16. Capellini VK, de Souza GS, de Faria CR: **Massage therapy in the management of myogenic TMD: a pilot study.** *J Appl Oral Sci* 2006, **14**(1):21–6.
17. Rudrud E, Halaszyn J: **Reduction of bruxism by contingent massage.** *Spec Care Dentist* 1981, **1**(3):122–4.
18. Sherman JJ, Turk DC: **Nonpharmacologic approaches to the management of myofascial temporomandibular disorders.** *Curr Pain Headache Rep* 2001, **5**(5):421–31.
19. Cho SH, Whang WW: **Acupuncture for temporomandibular disorders: a systematic review.** *J Orofac Pain* 2010, **24**(2):152–62.
20. La Touche R, Angulo-Diaz-Parreno S, De-la-Hoz JL, Fernandez-Carnero J, Ge HY, Linares MT, *et al*: **Effectiveness of acupuncture in the treatment of temporomandibular disorders of muscular origin: a systematic review of the last decade.** *J Altern Complement Med* 2010, **16**(1):107–112.
21. Bablis P, Pollard H, Bonello R: **Neuro emotional technique for the treatment of trigger point sensitivity in chronic neck pain sufferers: a controlled clinical trial.** *Chiropr Osteopat* 2008, **16**:4.
22. Vuckovic NH, Gullion CM, Williams LA, Ramirez M, Schneider J: **Feasibility and short-term outcomes of a shamanic treatment for temporomandibular joint disorders.** *Altern Ther Health Med* 2007, **13**(6):18–29.
23. Hakala RV: **Prolotherapy (proliferation therapy) in the treatment of TMD.** *Cranio* 2005, **23**(4):283–8.
24. Ritenbaugh C, Hammerschlag R, Calabrese C, Mist S, Aickin M, Sutherland E, *et al*: **A pilot whole systems clinical trial of traditional chinese medicine and naturopathic medicine for the treatment of temporomandibular disorders.** *J Altern Complement Med* 2008, **14**(5):475–87.
25. Li LC, Wong RW, Rabie AB: **Clinical effect of a topical herbal ointment on pain in temporomandibular disorders: a randomized placebo-controlled trial.** *J Altern Complement Med* 2009, **15**(12):1311–7.
26. List T, Axelsson S: **Management of TMD: evidence from systematic reviews and meta-analyses.** *J Oral Rehabil* 2010, **37**(6):430–51.
27. Bronfort G, Haas M, Evans R, Leininger B, Triano J: **Effectiveness of manual therapies: the UK evidence report.** *Chiropr Osteopat* 2010, **18**:3.
28. Cleland J, Palmer J: **Effectiveness of manual physical therapy, therapeutic exercise, and patient education on bilateral disc displacement without reduction- of the temporomandibular joint: a single-case design.** *J Orthop Sports Phys Ther* 2004, **34**(9):535–48.
29. Kalamir A, Pollard H, Vitiello A, Bonello R: **Manual therapy for temporomandibular disorders: a review of the literature.** *J Bodywork Mov Ther* 2007, **11**(1):84–90.
30. McNeely ML, Armijo Olivo S, Magee DJ: **A systematic review of the effectiveness of physical therapy interventions for temporomandibular disorders.** *Phys Ther* 2006, **86**(5):710–25.
31. Medlicott MS, Harris SR: **A systematic review of the effectiveness of exercise, manual therapy, electrotherapy, relaxation training, and biofeedback in the management of temporomandibular disorder.** *Phys Ther* 2006, **86**(7):955–73.
32. Kalamir A, Bonello R, Graham P, Vitiello AL, Pollard H: **Intra-oral myofascial therapy, education and self care for chronic myogenous temporomandibular disorder: a randomized, controlled trial.** *J Manipulative Physiol Ther* 2012, **35**:26–37.
33. Kalamir A, Pollard H, Vitiello AL, Bonello R: **Intra-oral myofascial therapy for chronic myogenous temporomandibular disorders: a randomized, controlled pilot study.** *J Man Manip Ther* 2010, **18**(3):139–46.
34. Dworkin SF, Huggins KH, Wilson L, Mancl L, Turner J, Massoth D, *et al*: **A randomized clinical trial using research diagnostic criteria for temporomandibular disorders-axis II to target clinic cases for a tailored self-care TMD treatment program.** *J Orofac Pain* 2002, **16**(1):48–63.
35. Dworkin SF, Sherman J, Mancl L, Ohrbach R, LeResche L, Truelove E: **Reliability, validity, and clinical utility of the research diagnostic criteria for temporomandibular disorders axis II scales: depression, non-specific physical symptoms, and graded chronic pain.** *J Orofac Pain* 2002, **16**(3):207–20.
36. Lobbezoo F, van Selms MK, John MT, Huggins K, Ohrbach R, Visscher CM, *et al*: **Use of the research diagnostic criteria for temporomandibular disorders for multinational research: translation efforts and reliability assessments in the netherlands.** *J Orofac Pain* 2005, **19**(4):301–8.
37. Lobbezoo F, Visscher CM, Naeije M: **Some remarks on the RDC/TMD Validation Project: report of an IADR/Toronto-2008 workshop discussion.** *J Oral Rehabil* 2010, **37**(10):779–83.
38. Look JO, John MT, Tai F, Huggins KH, Lenton PA, Truelove EL, *et al*: **The research diagnostic criteria for temporomandibular disorders. II: reliability of Axis I diagnoses and selected clinical measures.** *J Orofac Pain* 2010, **24**(1):25–34.
39. Manfredini D, Chiappe G, Bosco M: **Research diagnostic criteria for temporomandibular disorders (RDC/TMD) axis I diagnoses in an Italian patient population.** *J Oral Rehabil* 2006, **33**(8):551–8.
40. de Wijer A, Lobbezoo-Scholte AM, Steenks MH, Bosman F: **Reliability of clinical findings in temporomandibular disorders.** *J Orofac Pain* 1995, **9**(2):181–91.
41. Kropmans T, Dijkstra P, Stegenga B, Stewart R, de Bont L: **Smallest detectable difference of maximal mouth opening in patients with painfully restricted temporomandibular joint function.** *Eur J Oral Sci* 2000, **108**(1):9–13.
42. Kropmans TJ, Dijkstra PU, van Veen A, Stegenga B, de Bont LG: **The smallest detectable difference of mandibular function impairment in patients with a painfully restricted temporomandibular joint.** *J Dent Res* 1999, **78**(8):1445–9.
43. Michelotti A, Steenks MH, Farella M, Parisini F, Cimino R, Martina R: **The additional value of a home physical therapy regimen versus patient education only for the treatment of myofascial pain of the jaw muscles: short-term results of a randomized clinical trial.** *J Orofac Pain* 2004, **18**(2):114–25.
44. Nicolakis P, Erdogmus B, Kopf A, Djaber-Ansari A, Piehslinger E, Fialka-Moser V: **Exercise therapy for craniomandibular disorders.** *Arch Phys Med Rehabil* 2000, **81**(9):1137–42.
45. Dworkin SF: **Behavioral and educational modalities.** *Oral Surg Oral Med Oral Path Oral Radiol Endod* 1997, **83**(1):128–33.
46. Jerjes W, Madland G, Feinmann C, El Maaytah M, Kumar M, Hopper C, *et al*: **Psycho-education programme for temporomandibular disorders: a pilot study.** *J Negat Results Biomed* 2007, **6**:4.
47. Dao TT, Lavigne GJ, Feine JS, Tanguay R, Lund JP: **Power and sample size calculations for clinical trials of myofascial pain of jaw muscles.** *J Dent Res* 1991, **70**(2):118–22.
48. R_Development_core_team. R: *A language and environment for statistical computing.* Vienna: R Foundation for Statistical Computing; 2012.
49. De Boever JA, Van Wormhoudt K, De Boever EH: **Reasons that patients do not return for appointments in the initial phase of treatment of temporomandibular disorders.** *J Orofac Pain* 1996, **10**(1):66–72.

50. Yatani H, Kaneshima T, Kuboki T, Yoshimoto A, Matsuka Y, Yamashita A: **Long-term follow-up study on drop-out TMD patients with self-administered questionnaires.** *J Orofac Pain* 1997, **11**(3):258–69.
51. Turk DS: **Biospychosocial perspective on chronic pain.** In *Psychological approaches to pain management*. Edited by Gatchel RJ, Turk DS. New York: Guildford Press; 1996:3–32.
52. Hurst H, Bolton J: **Assessing the clinical significance of change scores recorded on subjective outcome measures.** *J Manipulative Physiol Ther* 2004, **27**(1):26–35.
53. Flor H, Fydrich T, Turk DC: **Efficacy of multidisciplinary pain treatment centers: a meta-analytic review.** *Pain* 1992, **49**(2):221–30.
54. Kamper SJ, Maher CG, Mackay G: **Global rating of change scales: a review of strengths and weaknesses and considerations for design.** *J Man Manip Ther* 2009, **17**(3):163–70.
55. Dworkin RH, Turk DC, Farrar JT, Haythornthwaite JA, Jensen MP, Katz NP, *et al:* **Core outcome measures for chronic pain clinical trials: IMMPACT recommendations.** *Pain* 2005, **113**(1–2):9–19 [see comment].
56. Turk DC, Rudy TE, Sorkin BA: **Neglected topics in chronic pain treatment outcome studies: determination of success.** *Pain* 1993, **53**(1):3–16.
57. Simons DG, Travell JG, Simons LS, Cummings BD: *Travell & Simons' Myofascial Pain and Dysfunction: The trigger point manual.* 2nd edition. Baltimore: Lippincott: Williams and Wilkins; 1998:5–44. 103–64.
58. Dworkin SF, Turner JA, Mancl L, Wilson L, Massoth D, Huggins KH, *et al:* **A randomized clinical trial of a tailored comprehensive care treatment program for temporomandibular disorders.** *J Orofac Pain* 2002, **16**(4):259–76.
59. Feine JS, Lund JP: **An assessment of the efficacy of physical therapy and physical modalities for the control of chronic musculoskeletal pain.** *Pain* 1997, **71**(1):5–23.

Management of people with acute low-back pain: a survey of Australian chiropractors

Bruce F Walker[1], Simon D French[2,3*], Matthew J Page[2], Denise A O'Connor[2], Joanne E McKenzie[2], Katherine Beringer[2], Kerry Murphy[2], Jenny L Keating[4], Susan Michie[5], Jill J Francis[6] and Sally E Green[2]

Abstract

Introduction: Chiropractors commonly provide care to people with acute low-back pain (LBP). The aim of this survey was to determine how chiropractors intend to support and manage people with acute LBP and if this management is in accordance with two recommendations from an Australian evidence-based acute LBP guideline. The two recommendations were directed at minimising the use of plain x-ray and encouraging the patient to stay active.

Methods: This is a cross sectional survey of chiropractors in Australia. This paper is part of the ALIGN study in which a targeted implementation strategy was developed to improve the management of acute LBP in a chiropractic setting. This implementation strategy was subsequently tested in a cluster randomised controlled trial. In this survey phase of the ALIGN study we approached a random sample of 880 chiropractors in three States of Australia. The mailed questionnaire consisted of five patient vignettes designed to represent people who would typically present to chiropractors with acute LBP. Four vignettes represented people who, according to the guideline, would not require a plain lumbar x-ray, and one vignette represented a person with a suspected vertebral fracture. Respondents were asked, for each vignette, to indicate which investigation(s) they would order, and which intervention(s) they would recommend or undertake.

Results: Of the 880 chiropractors approached, 137 were deemed ineligible to participate, mostly because they were not currently practising, or mail was returned to sender. We received completed questionnaires from 274 chiropractors (response rate of 37%). Male chiropractors made up 66% of respondents, 75% practised in an urban location and their mean number of years in practice was 15. Across the four vignettes where an x-ray was not indicated 68% (95% Confidence Intervals (CI): 64%, 71%) of chiropractors responded that they would order or take an x-ray. In addition 51% (95%CI: 47%, 56%) indicated they would give advice to stay active when it was indicated. For the vignette where a fracture was suspected, 95% (95% CI: 91%, 97%) of chiropractors would order an x-ray.

Conclusion: The intention of chiropractors surveyed in this study shows low adherence to two recommendations from an evidence-based guideline for acute LBP. Quality of care for these patients could be improved through effective implementation of evidence-based guidelines. Further research to find cost-effective methods to increase implementation is warranted.

Introduction

Low back pain (LBP) is a common and costly problem in high income countries like Australia. At any one time, approximately one in five Australians has LBP, and four out of five Australians will experience it at some time in their lives [1]. The direct and indirect cost of LBP in 2001 was estimated to total AUD$9,175 million [2]. Chiropractors provide a significant proportion of the care for people with LBP in Australia [3].

In 2004, an evidence-based clinical practice guideline for acute LBP [4] was sent to all primary healthcare providers in Australia, including chiropractors. The guideline provided evidence-based recommendations for the diagnosis, prognosis and treatment of acute non-specific LBP in primary care settings. Two relevant key messages were (i) that plain x-rays of the lumbar spine are not routinely recommended for people with acute non-specific LBP as

* Correspondence: s.french@unimelb.edu.au
[2]School of Public Health and Preventive Medicine, Monash University, Level 6, The Alfred Centre, 99 Commercial Road, Melbourne, Victoria 3004, Australia
Full list of author information is available at the end of the article

they are of limited diagnostic value and provide no benefits in pain, function or quality of life, and (ii) advising these patients to stay active produces a beneficial effect on pain, rate of recovery and function [4]. Although the guideline was released in 2004, more recent systematic reviews of randomised trials still support these two recommendations [5,6], and a review of LBP guidelines showed that more recent guidelines made similar recommendations [7].

This paper reports on one phase of the ALIGN study. The ALIGN study explored barriers and enablers to the uptake of the Australian acute LBP guideline in order to develop a targeted implementation strategy for use in a chiropractic setting which was subsequently tested in a cluster randomised controlled trial [8]. Other aspects of the ALIGN study will be reported elsewhere. The aim of this part of the study was to determine the intended practices of chiropractors in the management of acute LBP and whether they are in accordance with two recommendations in the Australian evidence-based acute LBP guideline [4] and more generally how chiropractors intend to support or manage people with acute LBP.

Methods

Design

This study is a cross sectional survey of chiropractors in Australia.

Sample size and participants

The sample size was calculated to address the primary aim of the survey which was to identify factors (e.g. knowledge) that were predictive of intention to perform a particular behaviour, and then to use this information to develop the ALIGN implementation strategy. The sample size was calculated to detect a 0.5 difference in intention to perform a particular behaviour, measured on a 7-point Likert scale, between dichotomised factors (assuming an equal distribution of participants in each dichotomy), with 90% power. To detect this difference, a sample of 440 chiropractors was required, assuming a 5% significance level and standard deviation of 1.6 (estimated from a similar survey our study group had undertaken with general medical practitioners [9]). We allowed for a 50% response rate, and therefore approached 880 chiropractors to participate.

Chiropractors were randomly sampled from three strata, defined by States in Australia, with the same proportion of chiropractors approached in each state. The entire sample frame of 1760 was obtained from the Chiropractic Registration Boards. The numbers approached in Victoria, South Australia, and Western Australia were, respectively, 553, 165, and 162. These States were chosen as other Australian States' Registration Boards would not release contact details of their registrants for research purposes.

Survey instrument

Five patient vignettes (Additional File 1) were adapted from another study in a general medical practice setting [10]. The vignettes were designed to reflect people with acute LBP who would typically present to chiropractors. Elements of each vignette were drawn from the acute LBP guideline, from another study in Victoria that evaluated a media campaign for LBP [11] and from the North-East X-ray Utilisation (NEXUS) study, which evaluated the effectiveness of audit and feedback and educational reminders on United Kingdom general practitioners' ordering of lumbar spine and knee x-rays [12]. The chiropractor's role and patient elements that were included in each vignette were designed to contextualise the vignettes. These elements were chosen because they have been recognised in previous research as potential barriers to practitioners making decisions consistent with guideline recommendations [12].

Four of the five vignettes represented people who would not require a plain lumbar x-ray and would benefit from being advised to stay active as per the recommendations from the Australian guideline [4], and one vignette represented someone with a suspected vertebral fracture who would require a plain x-ray. From a selection of response options respondents were asked to indicate which investigation(s) they would order for the patient described in each vignette, and which intervention(s) they would recommend or undertake (see Additional File 2 for options given). The investigations or treatments offered as options in the responses were developed by two experienced chiropractors who were investigators on the project team. They were chosen by the chiropractic investigators (BW and SF) as those investigations or treatments most likely to be used or recommended by chiropractors. Chiropractor respondents also had three "other" response options and could write free text to describe their intention. The five patient vignettes were pre-tested in a pilot study using six (of eight randomly sampled) Victorian chiropractors. These chiropractors had previously been interviewed about LBP management in a separate phase of the ALIGN study [8]. The pilot results led to minor changes.

Survey administration

The Modified Total Design Method [13] was used for chiropractor recruitment. The sample initially received an invitation letter to participate in the study. This letter was accompanied by a plain language statement, consent form, and reply-paid envelope (for returning an individual's decision to opt-in [or opt-out] by mail). A reminder letter was sent to non-respondents every two weeks for up to a total of eight weeks after the initial letter was sent. Both the fourth and eighth week reminder letters were accompanied by a plain language statement, consent form, survey document and reply-paid envelope.

The Total Design Method usually includes the use of a return mail card to signify that the respondent has opted-in to the study. The return mail card can also be used by individuals to indicate that they do not wish to participate in the study. In this study we replaced the return mail card with an option on the consent form for individuals to indicate they did not wish to participate (i.e. opt-out) in the study (and not be contacted further about this study). It was therefore considered that a return mail card, as per the Total Design Method, was not necessary in this study.

Analysis

Double data entry was performed independently by two researchers (MP and KB) and discrepancies were resolved via discussion with a third researcher.

Descriptive statistics were used to describe demographic details of the chiropractic respondents. The percentage of chiropractic respondents indicating which investigation(s) and which intervention(s) they would undertake for each vignette was calculated. Confidence intervals were calculated adjusting for the stratification variable. Exact binomial confidence intervals were calculated when the normal approximation was not valid [14]. Confidence intervals calculated for the percentage of respondents indicating which investigation(s) and which intervention(s) they would undertake across multiple vignettes (e.g. recommending advice to stay active across vignettes 1 to 4) were adjusted to allow for the correlation of responses within chiropractor. Analyses were undertaken using the svy commands in the statistical package Stata (StataCorp. 2007. Stata Statistical Software: Release 10.1. College Station, TX: StataCorp LP) with Taylor series approximations for the estimation of standard errors.

Human research ethics approval for this study was granted by Monash University (CF07/1060 - 2007000274).

Results

The survey was administered in April 2009. One-hundred and thirty seven (16%) chiropractors approached were deemed ineligible to participate, mostly because they were not currently practising, or mail was returned to sender. We received completed questionnaires from 274 of 743 eligible chiropractors, resulting in a response rate of 37%. Male chiropractors made up 66% of respondents, 75% practised in an urban location and their mean number of years in practice was 15 (Table 1).

Across the four vignettes where an x-ray was not indicated according to the guideline, 68% (95% CI: 64%, 71%) of chiropractors responded that they would order or take an x-ray, and 51% (95% CI: 47%, 56%) indicated they would give advice to stay active. For the vignette where a fracture was suspected, 95% (95% CI: 91%, 97%) of chiropractors would order an x-ray (Table 2). In addition, across all five vignettes, 25% (95% CI: 20%, 29%) of chiropractors would take, or order, a full spine plain x-ray.

Regarding treatment and management options that the chiropractors would employ 76% (95% CI: 72%, 79%) of chiropractors indicated that they would perform spinal manipulation/adjustment for vignettes 1 to 4 (range 63% to 92%), and 51% (95%CI: 47%, 56%) of chiropractors indicated they would give advice to stay active when it was indicated. Other treatments and care that chiropractors indicated they would provide for each vignette are detailed in Table 3. Around one third of chiropractors surveyed (35%; 95% CI: 29%, 40%) indicated that they would perform spinal manipulation of the spine in a patient with a likely fracture for vignette 5.

Discussion

The aim of this survey was to determine if management intended by chiropractors is in accordance with two key recommendations in the Australian evidence-based acute LBP guideline [4] and more generally how chiropractors intend to support or manage people with acute LBP. Ours is the first study undertaken in Australia, that we are aware of, that has investigated these two key recommendations for people with acute LBP in chiropractic practice.

X-ray usage

Where an x-ray was not recommended according to the guideline 68% of chiropractors responded that they would order or take an x-ray, indicating an overall x-ray guideline adherence of 32%. It has been reported previously that chiropractors use plain x-rays at a high frequency for people with acute non-specific LBP, with rates varying from 12% to 63% [15-22]. Our findings are consistent with these studies and suggest that a high proportion of chiropractors who responded to this survey are not complying with the guideline on the use of plain x-ray for acute LBP. Some chiropractors order or take plain x-rays to rule out pathology, screen for contraindications to manipulation, assist in the selection and delivery of treatment, and monitor patient progress [23]. A post-hoc review of the literature found no substantive evidence of harm from chiropractic manipulation because plain x-ray had not been used nor enhanced efficacy.

Across all five vignettes approximately 25% (95% CI: 20%, 29%) of chiropractors would take, or order, a full spine plain x-ray. This was despite the lack of information in the vignettes about any symptoms or examination findings at the other regions of the spine. There is no evidence that full spine x-rays are warranted in these vignettes and this finding is troubling considering the radiation dose that the patient would receive [24,25].

Table 1 Demographic details of chiropractor survey respondents

Variable	Category	Chiropractors (N = 274)
Sex (n, %)	Male	181 (66)
Age (Mean, SD) (Median, IQR)		41 (12) 40 (32, 49)
Practice location (n, %)	Urban	206 (75)
	Rural	64 (23)
	Remote	4 (1)
Practice type (n, %)	Group	173 (63)
	Solo	101 (37)
Years in clinical practice (Mean, SD) (Median, IQR)		15 (11)† 13 (7, 21)
Hours practicing/week (Mean, SD) (Median, IQR)		30 (12) 30 (25, 35)
Total patients/week (Mean, SD) (Median, IQR)		104 (69)‡ 90 (60, 140)
Acute LBP patients/week (Mean, SD) (Median, IQR)		23 (24)* 15 (5, 30)
Involvement in teaching (n, %)	Yes	33 (12.1)
Formal postgraduate training relevant to LBP (n, %)	Yes	96 (35)†
Access to bulk-billing radiology service (n, %)	Yes	245 (89)
Take own x-rays (n, %)	Yes	52 (19)
Gonstead practitioner (n, %)	Yes	31 (11)

SD = standard deviation; IQR = interquartile range; LBP = low back pain; Gonstead practitioner: A type of chiropractor known to use plain x-ray more frequently.
† N = 273; ‡ N = 269; * N = 264

Around one third of chiropractors surveyed (35%; 95% CI: 29%, 40%) would perform spinal manipulation of the spine in a patient with a likely fracture. We did not investigate the reasons for this, however it may be that a) the potential for fracture diagnosis in the vignette was not considered, or b) the chiropractor intended to apply manipulation to regions above or below the fracture site.

The findings above have implications for patients' safety and health resource use. First, a full spine x-ray will expose the patient to needless ionising radiation, and manipulation of a spinal fracture may worsen the fracture with potentially serious consequences. Second, the findings have implications for third party payments for these extensive and expensive diagnostic imaging.

Giving advice to stay active

Over half the chiropractors (51%; 95% CI: 47%, 56%) indicated that in the first four vignettes they would advise the patient to stay active, while 60% (95% CI: 57%, 64%) responded they would give exercises (back specific or general) to people seen who were similar to

Table 2 Percentage (95% confidence interval) of chiropractic respondents ordering, undertaking, or recommending investigations

Investigation	Vignette 1		Vignette 2		Vignette 3		Vignette 4		Vignette 5*	
N = 274										
Lumbosacral plain x-ray	40	(34, 46)	52	(46, 58)	47	(41, 53)	40	(34, 46)	67	(62, 73)
Lumbosacral CT scan	0	(0, 2)†	2	(1, 4) †	18	(13, 22)	10	(7, 14)	4	(2, 7) †
Lumbosacral MRI	1	(0, 3) †	1	(0, 4) †	9	(5, 12)	4	(2, 7) †	2	(1, 5) †
Full spine plain x-ray	24	(19, 29)	32	(27, 38)	14	(10, 18)	25	(20, 30)	28	(23, 33)
None	34	(28, 39)	14	(9, 18)	20	(15, 25)	28	(23, 34)	3	(1, 6) †
Overall x-ray guideline adherence	37	(31, 43)	16	(12, 20)	39	(33, 45)	37	(31, 43)	95	(91, 97) †‡

* The only vignette where guideline recommends plain x-ray and not advice to stay active

Note: For Vignettes 1-4, x-ray guideline adherence is defined as the number of participants not ordering any type of x-ray (e.g., lumbosacral, full spine, AP lateral, pelvic)

Note: For Vignette 5, x-ray guideline adherence is defined as the number of participants ordering some type of x-ray (e.g., lumbosacral, full spine, AP lateral, pelvic)

† Exact binomial confidence calculated [14]

‡ Based on 273 participants.

Table 3 Interventions undertaken or recommended by chiropractic respondents - n (%)

Response options	Vignette 1	Vignette 2	Vignette 3	Vignette 4	Vignette 5
Bed rest*	1 (0)	1 (0)	3 (1)	47 (17)	36 (13)
Bed rest outside guideline recommendations[†]	0 (0)	0 (0)	2 (1)	12 (4)[‡]	NA
Paracetamol	18 (7)	21 (8)	18 (7)	53 (19)	99 (36)
NSAIDs	38 (14)	21 (8)	65 (24)	125 (46)	48 (18)
Back exercises	79 (29)	97 (35)	133 (49)	41 (15)	14 (5)
General exercise	135 (49)	213 (78)	130 (47)	94 (34)	62 (23)
Advice to stay active	143 (52)	183 (67)	134 (49)	101 (37)	68 (25)
Advice regarding alternate ways of moving	184 (67)	168 (61)	141 (51)	169 (62)	131 (48)
Advice to avoid pain provoking movements	196 (72)	181 (66)	134 (49)	191 (70)	155 (57)
Work modification	105 (38)	113 (41)	119 (43)	132 (48)	28 (10)
Spinal manipulation/adjustment	251 (92)	219 (80)	189 (69)	173 (63)	95 (35)
Mobilisation	84 (31)	96 (35)	66 (24)	93 (34)	55 (20)
Massage	155 (57)	162 (59)	120 (44)	131 (48)	106 (39)
Lumbar supports	10 (4)	10 (4)	29 (11)	42 (15)	23 (8)
Spinal traction	6 (2)	5 (2)	21 (8)	23 (8)	4 (1)
Acupuncture	15 (5)	13 (5)	29 (11)	22 (8)	11 (4)
Electrotherapy	22 (8)	20 (7)	24 (9)	31 (11)	25 (9)
Thermal modalities	135 (49)	105 (38)	74 (27)	151 (55)	120 (44)
Printed information	29 (11)	29 (11)	15 (5)	19 (7)	4 (1)
Referral to another health care provider	6 (2)	25 (9)	84 (31)	28 (10)	35 (13)

N = 274 chiropractors unless otherwise specified.

* Advising bed rest (irrespective of the number of days).

† Advising bed rest for more than 2 days.

‡ N = 268

the first four vignettes. In this sample of chiropractors, there appears to be a need to encourage the giving of advice to patients with acute LBP to stay active, regardless of any exercises they would recommend to the patient in order to bring chiropractic management in line with evidence-based practice.

Study limitations

The response rate was low (37%) and therefore the results have an increased potential for selection bias where those who choose to participate differ in important characteristics with those who do not choose to participate [26]. It may be speculated that those who responded were more likely to comply with the guideline, in which case we have calculated underestimates of guideline compliance. If this is the case the problem may be greater than our results demonstrate. It also may be speculated that those who responded were less likely to comply with the guideline, in which case we have calculated overestimates of guideline compliance. Regardless, we can only conclude for the respondents to this survey and are not able to generalise to the broader population of chiropractors in these three States of Australia. No data were available for the broader chiropractic population at the time we undertook this study, so we were unable to compare the characteristics of the respondents to the characteristics of the broader Australian chiropractic population to investigate non-response bias. The response rate is lower than those seen in other surveys of health professionals where a mean of 58% has been reported, however it has also been demonstrated that response rates of health professionals are decreasing over time [26]. Recently published surveys of chiropractors have reported response rates ranging from 38% to 88% [27-31].

Patient vignettes are limited by a lack of detail that may be gleaned during a patient consultation, including visual cues relating to pain during an examination. Further, patient vignettes may not be sensitive enough to pick up the fine nuances of practice that would better guide the practitioner [32]. Therefore, our conclusions are based on a measure of proxy behaviour rather than real behaviour. More research is needed to establish the extent to which proxy measures of behaviour can predict actual behaviour.

Conclusion

The current intention of a significant number of Australian chiropractors who responded to this survey and who manage people with acute LBP is not in accordance with evidence-based recommendations. Quality of care for these patients could potentially be improved through effective implementation of evidence-based guidelines. Further research to find cost-effective methods to increase implementation is warranted.

Additional material

Additional file 1: Patient vignettes. This file contains the five patient vignettes that were used in the survey.

Additional file 2: Investigations and intervention options for the five patient vignettes. This file shows the options available to the survey respondents for investigations and interventions for each of the patient vignettes.

Acknowledgements
This project was funded by an Australian National Health and Medical Research Council (NHMRC) Project Grant (436767). SDF and DOC are supported by NHMRC Fellowships. The NHMRC has had no involvement in the study design, preparation of the manuscript, or the decision to submit the manuscript. We acknowledge the contribution provided by the ALIGN study group, in particular Jeremy Grimshaw and Duncan Mortimer who were Investigators on the project.

Author details
[1]School of Chiropractic and Sports Science, Murdoch University, Murdoch, 6150, Western Australia. [2]School of Public Health and Preventive Medicine, Monash University, Level 6, The Alfred Centre, 99 Commercial Road, Melbourne, Victoria 3004, Australia. [3]Primary Care Research Unit, University of Melbourne, 200 Berkeley St, Carlton, Victoria, 3010, Australia. [4]Department of Physiotherapy, School of Primary Health Care, Faculty of Medicine Nursing and Health Science, Monash University, PO Box 527 Frankston, Victoria, 3199 Australia. [5]Centre for Outcomes Research and Effectiveness, Department of Clinical, Educational and Health Psychology, University College London, WC1E 7HB, London, UK. [6]Health Services Research Unit, Health Sciences Building, University of Aberdeen AB25 2ZD, UK.

Authors' contributions
All authors contributed to the design and conduct of the study. SF wrote the first draft of this manuscript with comments from BW. JM undertook the statistical analysis. BW undertook further revisions of the manuscript with feedback from all authors. All authors agreed to the final manuscript.

Competing interests
Bruce Walker is Editor in Chief and Simon French is an Associate Editor of Chiropractic & Manual Therapies. All decisions on this manuscript were made by another editor. All other authors declare that they have no competing interests.

References

1. Walker BF, Muller R, Grant WD: **Low back pain in Australian adults: prevalence and associated disability.** *J Manipulative Physiol Ther* 2004, **27(4)**:238-244.
2. Walker BF, Muller R, Grant WD: **Low back pain in Australian adults: the economic burden.** *Asia-Pacific Journal of Public Health* 2003, **15(2)**:79-87.
3. Walker BF, Muller R, Grant WD: **Low back pain in Australian adults. health provider utilization and care seeking.** *J Manipulative Physiol Ther* 2004, **27(5)**:327-335.
4. Australian Acute Musculoskeletal Pain Guidelines Group (AAMPGG): **Evidence-based management of acute musculoskeletal pain.** Brisbane: Australian Academic Press; 2003.
5. Chou R, Fu R, Carrino JA, Deyo RA: **Imaging strategies for low-back pain: systematic review and meta-analysis.** *Lancet* 2009, **373(9662)**:463-472.
6. Liddle S, Gracey J, Baxter G: **Advice for the management of low back pain: A systematic review of randomised controlled trials.** *Manual Therapy* 2007, **12(4)**:310-327.
7. Dagenais S, Tricco AC, Haldeman S: **Synthesis of recommendations for the assessment and management of low back pain from recent clinical practice guidelines.** *Spine J* 2010, **10(6)**:514-529.
8. McKenzie JE, O'Connor DA, Page MJ, Mortimer DS, French SD, Walker BF, Keating JL, Grimshaw JM, Michie S, Francis JJ, *et al*: **Improving the care for people with acute low-back pain by allied health professionals (the ALIGN trial): A cluster randomised trial protocol.** *Implement Sci* 2010, **5**:86.
9. O'Connor D, Green S, French S, King S, Francis J, Grimshaw J, Michie S, McKenzie J, Spike N, Schattner P, *et al*: **Identifying general practitioner beliefs, intentions and behaviour toward uptake of an evidence-based guideline for acute low back pain using the theory of planned behaviour.** *International Forum IX: Primary Care Research on Low Back Pain* Palma de Mallorca, Spain.; 2007.
10. McKenzie JE, French SD, O'Connor DA, Grimshaw JM, Mortimer D, Michie S, Francis J, Spike N, Schattner P, Kent PM, *et al*: **IMPLEmenting a clinical practice guideline for acute low back pain evidence-based manageMENT in general practice (IMPLEMENT): Cluster randomised controlled trial study protocol.** *Implement Sci* 2008, **3**:11.
11. Buchbinder R, Jolley D, Wyatt M: **2001 Volvo Award Winner in Clinical Studies: Effects of a media campaign on back pain beliefs and its potential influence on management of low back pain in general practice.** *Spine* 2001, **26(23)**:2535-2542.
12. Bonetti D, Eccles M, Johnston M, Steen N, Grimshaw J, Baker R, Walker A, Pitts N: **Guiding the design and selection of interventions to influence the implementation of evidence-based practice: an experimental simulation of a complex intervention trial.** *Social Science & Medicine* 2005, **60(9)**:2135-2147.
13. Dillman DA: **Mail and internet surveys: the tailored design method: with new internet, visual, and mixed-mode guide, 2nd ed. 2007 update.** Hoboken, N.J., Chichester: John Wiley & Sons, Inc; 2007.
14. Clopper C, Pearson S: **The use of confidence or fiducial limits illustrated in the case of the binomial.** *Biometrika* 1934, **26**:404-413.
15. Assendelft WJ, Pfeifle CE, Bouter LM: **Chiropractic in The Netherlands: a survey of Dutch chiropractors.** *J Manipulative Physiol Ther* 1995, **18(3)**:129-134.
16. Aroua A, Decka I, Robert J, Vader JP, Valley JF: **Chiropractor's use of radiography in Switzerland.** *J Manipulative Physiol Ther* 2003, **26(1)**:9-16.
17. Ammendolia C, Bombardier C, Hogg-Johnson S, Glazier R: **Views on radiography use for patients with acute low back pain among chiropractors in an Ontario community.** *J Manipulative Physiol Ther* 2002, **25(8)**:511-520.
18. Ammendolia C, Cote P, Hogg-Johnson S, Bombardier C: **Do chiropractors adhere to guidelines for back radiographs? A study of chiropractic teaching clinics in Canada.** *Spine* 2007, **32(22)**:2509-2514.
19. Carey TS, Garrett J: **Patterns of ordering diagnostic tests for patients with acute low back pain. The North Carolina Back Pain Project.** *Ann Intern Med* 1996, **125(10)**:807-814.
20. Cherkin DC, MacCornack FA, Berg AO: **Managing low back pain–a comparison of the beliefs and behaviors of family physicians and chiropractors.** *West J Med* 1988, **149(4)**:475-480.
21. Kent PM, Keating JL, Taylor NF: **Primary care clinicians use variable methods to assess acute nonspecific low back pain and usually focus on impairments.** *Man Ther* 2009, **14(1)**:88-100.
22. Pedersen P, Breen AC: **An overview of European chiropractic practice.** *J Manipulative Physiol Ther* 1994, **17(4)**:228-237.
23. Ammendolia C, Hogg-Johnson S, Pennick V, Glazier R, Bombardier C: **Implementing evidence-based guidelines for radiography in acute low back pain: a pilot study in a chiropractic community.** *J Manipulative Physiol Ther* 2004, **27(3)**:170-179.
24. Berrington de Gonzalez A, Darby S: **Risk of cancer from diagnostic X-rays: estimates for the UK and 14 other countries.** *Lancet* 2004, **363(9406)**:345-351.
25. National Research Council of the National Academies: **Health risks from exposure to low levels of ionizing radiation: BEIR VII Phase 2.** The National Academies Press, Washington, D.C.; 2006, Available: http://www.nap.edu/catalog.php?record_id = 11340.
26. Cook JV, Dickinson HO, Eccles MP: **Response rates in postal surveys of healthcare professionals between 1996 and 2005: an observational study.** *BMC health services research* 2009, **9**:160.
27. Malmqvist S, Leboeuf-Yde C: **Chiropractors in Finland–a demographic survey.** *Chiropractic & osteopathy* 2008, **16**:9.
28. Schwarz I, Hondras MA: **A survey of chiropractors practicing in Germany: practice characteristics, professional reading habits, and attitudes and perceptions toward research.** *Chiropractic & osteopathy* 2007, **15**:6.
29. Stuber KJ, Grod JP, Smith DL, Powers P: **An online survey of chiropractors' opinions of Continuing Education.** *Chiropractic & osteopathy* 2005, **13**:22.

30. Page SA, Grod JP, McMorland DG: **The perspectives and practices of alberta chiropractors regarding the sale of health care products in chiropractic offices.** *J Manipulative Physiol Ther* 2011, **34(7)**:476-482.
31. Russell ML, Verhoef MJ, Injeyan HS, McMorland DG: **Response rates for surveys of chiropractors.** *J Manipulative Physiol Ther* 2004, **27(1)**:43-48.
32. Hrisos S, Eccles MP, Francis JJ, Dickinson HO, Kaner EF, Beyer F, Johnston M: **Are there valid proxy measures of clinical behaviour? A systematic review.** *Implement Sci* 2009, **4**:37.

Co-presentation of unilateral femoral and bilateral sciatic nerve variants in one cadaver: A case report with clinical implications

Patrick J Battaglia[1*], Frank Scali[2] and Dennis E Enix[1]

Abstract

Objective: To present a group of anatomical findings that may have clinical significance.

Design: This study is an anatomical case report of combined lumbo-pelvic peripheral nerve and muscular variants.

Setting: University anatomy laboratory.

Participants: One cadaveric specimen.

Methods: During routine cadaveric dissection for a graduate teaching program, unilateral femoral and bilateral sciatic nerve variants were observed in relation to the iliacus and piriformis muscle, respectively. Further dissection of both the femoral nerve and accessory slip of iliacus muscle was performed to fully expose their anatomy.

Results: Piercing of the femoral nerve by an accessory iliacus muscle combined with wide variations in sciatic nerve and piriformis muscle presentations may have clinical significance.

Conclusions: Combined femoral and sciatic nerve variants should be considered when treatment for a lumbar disc herniation is refractory to care despite positive orthopedic testing.

Keywords: Sciatic nerve, Femoral nerve, Disc, Variant

Background

The recurrence of leg pain from lumbar disc herniations is a common post treatment clinical finding. Certain muscular and peripheral nerve variants may represent an unrecognized etiology in these cases and may affect the outcome of specific treatments. Recognition of these variations in normal anatomy may be useful to the clinician when treating the patient with refractory leg pain. The femoral nerve, derived from the second to fourth lumbar dorsal divisions, is one of the terminal branches of the lumbar plexus [1]. Multiple studies have reported variant slips of the psoas and iliacus muscles which may split the femoral nerve causing a potential risk for nerve entrapment [2-9]. In a large study of 121 cadavers, Vazquez et al. reported variations of iliacus and psoas muscles piercing the femoral nerve, piercing of the femoral nerve by a muscular slip, or a muscular slip/sheet covering the femoral nerve as it lay on the iliacus in 19 specimens (7.9%) [3]. Several entities exist which may cause femoral neuropathy [10], however, owing to the lack of anatomic protection, entrapment of the nerve is most likely to occur immediately distal to the inguinal ligament [10]. No clinical finding is pathognomonic for femoral neuropathy, as similar findings of absent or diminished patellar reflex, quadriceps weakness or wasting, weakness in hip flexion and adduction as well as sensory symptoms such as pain in the iliac fossa, inguinal region, anterior thigh and medial calf may also indicate radiculopathy, plexopathy, or combined lesions of the femoral and obturator nerves [11].

The sciatic nerve, formed from the ventral rami of the fourth lumbar to third sacral spinal nerves, leaves the pelvis passing both anterior and inferior to the piriformis or sometimes through the muscle [1]. A 2010 literature review reported that the prevalence of piriformis and sciatic nerve variants in a large sample size of 6,062 cadaveric specimens was 16.9% [12]. The relationship of the piriformis and sciatic nerve causing piriformis

* Correspondence: patrick.battaglia@logan.edu
[1]Division of Research, Logan College of Chiropractic, 1851 Schoettler Rd, Chesterfield, MO 60317, USA
Full list of author information is available at the end of the article

syndrome remains a controversial condition. Most commonly, sciatic neuropathy is iatrogenic, occurring after total hip arthroplasty [13]. Yuen, commenting on numerous studies, estimated the frequency of sciatica neuropathy after total hip arthoplasty to be between 0.7% and 3.7% [13]. Numerous other etiologies for sciatic neuropathy and sciatica pain exist [13,14]. Clinical exam findings of observed foot drop, and motor, sensory and reflex deficits in the sciatic nerve distribution are non-specific for sciatic neuropathy and mimic lesions to the lumbosacral nerve roots or plexus [13].

Piercing of the femoral nerve by an accessory iliacus muscle in combination with bilateral variations in both sciatic nerve and piriformis muscle anatomy exemplifies the wide variability that exists within the lumbar and lumbosacral plexus. The clinical implications of these combined variants are discussed.

Case presentation

During routine cadaveric dissection, bilateral sciatic and unilateral femoral nerve variants were detected. The course and muscular relationships of both sciatic nerve variants were studied. The femoral nerve variant was further dissected and was examined to determine its nerve root contributions and its branching pattern. Also, the accessory muscular slip of the iliacus muscle that was piercing the femoral nerve was dissected to determine both its origin and insertion points.

On the right side, the sciatic nerve was split into the common fibular and tibial divisions proximal to the piriformis muscle, with the common fibular division passing above and superficial to the piriformis muscle and the tibial division passing inferior and deep to the muscle. On the left side, the sciatic nerve was also divided proximal to the piriformis muscle. However, the piriformis muscle was pierced and subdivided into two discrete bellies by the common fibular division, while the tibial division passed inferior and deep to the most caudal border of the piriformis muscle [Figure 1]. The right piriformis was one discrete muscle. On both sides the remaining course and distribution of the tibial and common fibular nerves was considered normal.

In the left iliac fossa, the femoral nerve emerged both lateral and deep to the psoas major muscle between the psoas major and iliacus muscles covered in iliac fascia. It was then pierced and divided into two separate divisions by an accessory slip of the iliacus muscle. Just proximal to the inguinal ligament, these two separate divisions rejoined and the femoral nerve passed as one under the inguinal ligament and then divided into its usual anterior and posterior branches [Figure 2]. The accessory slip of iliacus muscle was then dissected proximally up to its origin on the inferior aspect of the iliac crest. It was detached from its origin confirming it had no attachment to the iliolumbar ligament. The muscular slip was then followed distally until it blended into other iliacus and psoas major fibers to incorporate into the iliopsoas muscle which inserted on the lesser trochanter of the femur. The psoas minor and major muscles were then reflected to expose the lumbar plexus. The femoral nerve was found to be formed from the posterior division of the L2, L3 and L4 ventral nerve roots and was

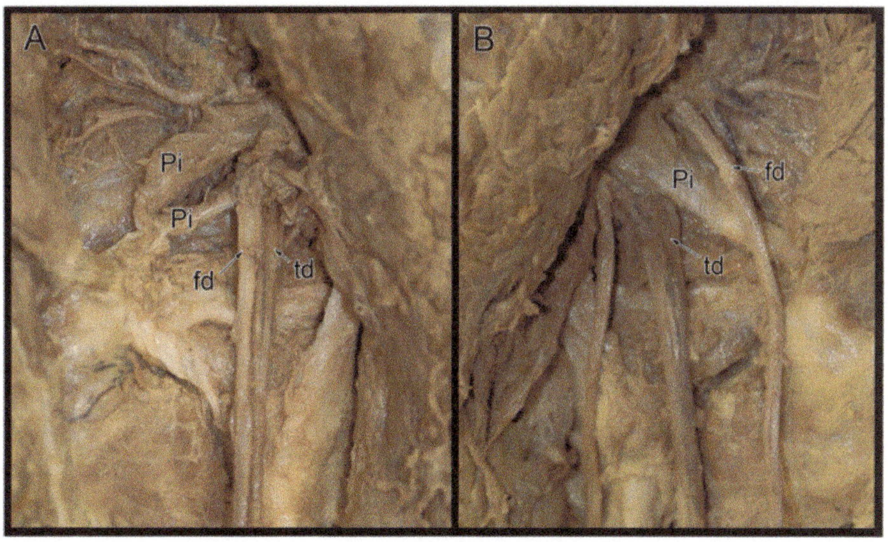

Figure 1 Photograph reveals bilateral sciatic nerve variants on a single cadaveric specimen. The left side (**A**) revealed that sciatic nerve divided proximal to the piriformis muscle. The left common fibular division (fd) divided the piriformis (Pi) into two distinct bellies while the left tibial division (td) passed inferior and deep to the most caudal border of the piriformis muscle. On the right side (**B**), the sciatic nerve was split into the right common fibular (fd) and tibial (td) divisions proximal to the piriformis muscle (Pi). The right common fibular division passed superficial while the tibial division passed deep to the piriformis muscle.

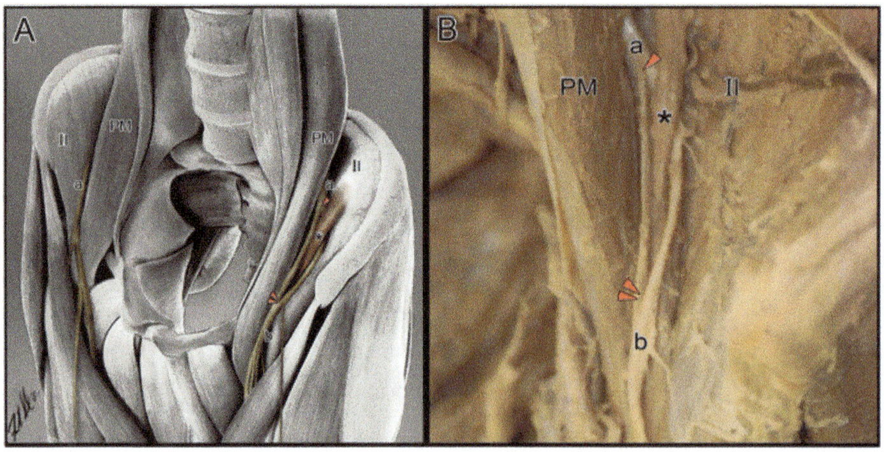

Figure 2 Illustration (A) and photograph (B) reveals unilateral (left side) femoral nerve variant. The femoral nerve (**a**) emerged bilaterally lateral and deep to the psoas major muscle (PM). While the right femoral nerve maintained its usual path, the left femoral nerve was pierced (arrowhead) and divided into two separate divisions by an accessory slip of the iliacus muscle (*). These two separate divisions of the femoral nerve converged (double arrowheads) into a single division (**b**) and divided into its usual branches. Also labeled bilaterally is the iliacus muscle (Il). (Original anatomical illustration by Frank Scali, DC).

fully formed prior to being pierced by the accessory slip of the iliacus muscle. No other lumbar plexus variations were detected. The femoral nerve on the right side of the specimen followed a routine course.

Conclusions

The sciatic and femoral nerves represent the two largest peripheral collections of lumbar and sacral nerve roots [1]. There have been other cadaveric reports of variance in sciatic and femoral nerve as well as piriformis and iliopsoas complex muscle anatomy similar to what is described in this case [2-9,12,15]. However, to the authors' knowledge, these variants have yet to be reported in one single specimen, and thus the potential clinical significance of these sole variants may be enhanced when possessed together.

Straight leg raise and femoral nerve traction tests are commonly performed orthopedic maneuvers done to ascertain the presence of a lumbar disc herniation [16,17]. Femoral nerve traction testing has a reported sensitivity of 50% and specificity of 100% for the diagnosis of midlumbar nerve root impingement, and appears to be insensitive and only 50% specific for lower lumbar nerve root impingement [18]. Straight leg raise testing has sensitivity and specificity characteristics of 16% and 31% respectively for midlumbar nerve root impingement. For the diagnosis of lower lumbar nerve root impingement, straight leg raise testing is 69% sensitive and 84% specific [18]. Reproduction of radicular leg pain in both sciatic and femoral nerve distributions with nerve traction testing is a common sign of lumbar disc herniations [16-18], and variations in both the course of the sciatic and femoral nerves as well as the surrounding musculature may affect the results of these nerve traction tests [2,4]. Recovery from radicular symptoms is often problematic and may be due to diagnostic problems in challenging cases. In a retrospective study conducted by Suri et al. in 2012, 81% of patients who sought conservative care for their leg pain associated with a lumbar disc herniation experienced resolution of symptoms in an average of 6 months. However, within 1 year post resolution, 25% had experienced a recurrence in their leg pain [19]. Patients who are refractory to care may warrant a reexamination, keeping in mind the many variations in anatomy, dermatomal patterns, and false positive/negatives of certain orthopedic tests [18,20-22]. A study of the distribution of dermatomal pain patterns by Murphy et al. showed 64.1% of the 169 lumbar spine pain patients presented with non-dermatomal pain distributions [23]. The sensitivity and specificity of lumbar spine dermatomal pain patterns associated with radiculopathies is too low to be useful in the identification of a specific nerve root level [23]. This is likely due to the communications between posterior collateral sensory ganglia and preganglionic neurons of different nerve root levels, creating variations in cutaneous sensations [22,24]. Several authors have concluded that variant femoral or sciatic nerve anatomy may produce a clinical picture analogous to that of a lumbar or lumbosacral radiculopathy [2,4,5,7,14]. Consideration of these anatomical variants, especially combined femoral and sciatic nerve variants, may prompt earlier or more focused diagnostic tests when a suspected lumbar spine disc herniation is refractory to care. One such test that may prove helpful to clinicians would be needle electromyography, as it can assist in the differentiation of radiculopathy and entrapment neuropathies [11].

Variants in lumbar and lumbosacral plexus anatomy should be considered when a symptomatic lumbar disc herniation is refractory to care. Recognition of these anatomical variants may lead to earlier intervention of physiologic testing, better treatment outcomes and improved patient satisfaction. Future studies examining the prevalence of these combined variants in the general population would be of interest to clinicians.

Consent

Written informed consent was obtained from the deceased prior to the gift of body donation. All handling of anatomical specimens was in accordance with the institutions ethical policy for body donation for anatomical study and scientific purposes. A copy of the written consent is available for review by the Editor-in-Chief of this journal.

Competing interests

The authors declare that they have no competing interests.

Authors' contributions

PB conceived of the case report, assisted in reviewing the literature and drafting the manuscript. FS provided anatomical artwork, assisted in reviewing the literature and drafting the manuscript. DE assisted in reviewing the literature, drafting the manuscript and provided critical review. All authors read and approved the final manuscript.

Acknowledgements

The authors would like to thank Robbyn Keating for her assistance in reviewing the literature.

Author details

[1]Division of Research, Logan College of Chiropractic, 1851 Schoettler Rd, Chesterfield, MO 60317, USA. [2]Independent Researcher, 1272 Dutch Broadway, Valley Stream, NY 11580, USA.

References

1. Standring S: *Gray's Anatomy. The Anatomical Basis of Clinical Practice*. 40th edition. New York: Elsevier Churchill Livingstone; 2008.
2. Spratt JD, Logan BM, Abrahams PH: **Variant Slips of Psoas and Iliacus Muscles, With Splitting of the Femoral Nerve.** *Clin Anat* 1996, **9**:401–404.
3. Vazquez MT, Murillo J, Maranillo E, Parkin IG, Sanudo J: **Femoral Nerve Entrapment: A New Insight.** *Clin Anat* 2007, **20**:175–179.
4. Fabrizio PA: **Anatomic variation of the iliacus and psoas major muscles.** *Int J Anat Var* 2011, **4**:28–30.
5. D'Costa S, Ramanathan LA, Madhyastha A, Nayak SR, Prabhu LV, Rai R, Saralaya W, Prakash: **An accessory iliacus muscle: a case report.** *Rom J Morphol Embryol* 2008, **49**(3):407–409.
6. Anloague PA, Huijbregts P: **Anatomical variation of the lumbar plexus: A descriptive anatomy study with proposed clinical implications.** *J man manip ther* 2009, **17**(4):107–114.
7. Rao TR, Vanishree, Kanyan PS, Rao S: **Bilateral variation of iliacus muscle and splitting of femoral nerve.** *Neuroanatomy* 2008, **7**:72–75.
8. Jelev L, Shivarov V, Surchev L: **Bilateral variations of the psoas major and the iliacus muscles and presence of an undescribed variant muscle – accessory iliopsoas muscle.** *Ann Anat* 2005, **187**:281–286.
9. Astik RB, Dave UH: **Anatomical variations in formation and branching pattern of the femoral nerve in iliac fossa: A study of 64 human lumbar plexuses.** *People's Journal of Scientific Research* 2011, **4**(2):14–19.
10. Chhabra A, Faridian-Aragh N: **High resolution 3-T MR neurography of femoral neuropathy.** *Am J Roentgenol* 2012, **198**:3–10.
11. Busis NA: **Femoral and obturator neuropathies.** *Neurol Clin* 1999, **17**(3):633–653.
12. Smoll NR: **Variations of the piriformis and sciatic nerve with clinical consequence: a review.** *Clin Anat* 2010, **23**(1):8–17.
13. Yuen EC, Yuen TS: **Sciatic neuropathy.** *Neurol Clin* 1999, **17**(3):617–631.
14. Stafford MA, Peng P, Hill DA: **Sciatica: a review of history, epidemiology, pathogensis, and the role of epidural steroid injection in management.** *Br J Anaesth* 2007, **99**:461–73.
15. Khan YS, Khan TK: **A rare case of bilateral high division of sciatic nerve (of different types) with unilateral divided piriformis and unusual high origin of genicular branch of common fibular nerve.** *Int J Anat Var* 2011, **4**:63–66.
16. Cram RH: **Sign of sciatic nerve root pressure.** *J Bone Joint Surg* 1953, **35-B**:192–5.
17. Dyck P: **The femoral nerve traction test with lumbar disc protrusions.** *Surg Neurol* 1976, **3**:163–6.
18. Suri P, Rainville J, Katz JN, Jouve C, Hartigan C, Limke J, Pena E, Li L, Swaim B, Hunter DJ: **The Accuracy of the Physical Examination for the Diagnosis of Midlumbar and Low Lumbar Nerve Root Impingement.** *Spine* 2011, **36**(1):63–73.
19. Suri P, Rainville J, Hunter DJ, Li L, Katz JN: **Recurrence of radicular pain or back pain after nonsurgical treatment of symptomatic lumbar disc herniation.** *Arch Phys Med Rehabil* 2012, **93**:690–5.
20. van der Windt DA, Simons E, Riphagen II, Ammendolia C, Verhagen AP, Laslett M, Devillé W, Deyo RA, Bouter LM, de Vet HC, Aertgeerts B: **Physical examination for lumbar radiculopathy due to disc herniation in patients with low-back pain.** *Cochrane Database Syst Rev* 2010, **17**(2):CD007431.
21. Lee MWL, McPhee RW, Stringer MD: **An Evidence-Based Approach to Human Dermatomes.** *Clin Anat* 2008, **21**:363–373.
22. Greenberg SA: **The history of dermatome mapping.** *Arch Neurol* 2003, **60**:126–131.
23. Murphy DR, Hurwitz EL, Gerrard JK, Clary R: **Pain patterns and descriptions in patients with radicular pain: Does the pain necessarily follow a specific dermatome.** *Chiro & Osteo* 2009, **17**:9.
24. Cramer G, Darby S: *Basic and Clinical Anatomy of the Spine, Spinal Cord, and ANS*. 2nd edition. St. Louis: Elsevier Mosby; 2005.

Permissions

All chapters in this book were first published in CMT, by BioMed Central; hereby published with permission under the Creative Commons Attribution License or equivalent. Every chapter published in this book has been scrutinized by our experts. Their significance has been extensively debated. The topics covered herein carry significant findings which will fuel the growth of the discipline. They may even be implemented as practical applications or may be referred to as a beginning point for another development.

The contributors of this book come from diverse backgrounds, making this book a truly international effort. This book will bring forth new frontiers with its revolutionizing research information and detailed analysis of the nascent developments around the world.

We would like to thank all the contributing authors for lending their expertise to make the book truly unique. They have played a crucial role in the development of this book. Without their invaluable contributions this book wouldn't have been possible. They have made vital efforts to compile up to date information on the varied aspects of this subject to make this book a valuable addition to the collection of many professionals and students.

This book was conceptualized with the vision of imparting up-to-date information and advanced data in this field. To ensure the same, a matchless editorial board was set up. Every individual on the board went through rigorous rounds of assessment to prove their worth. After which they invested a large part of their time researching and compiling the most relevant data for our readers.

The editorial board has been involved in producing this book since its inception. They have spent rigorous hours researching and exploring the diverse topics which have resulted in the successful publishing of this book. They have passed on their knowledge of decades through this book. To expedite this challenging task, the publisher supported the team at every step. A small team of assistant editors was also appointed to further simplify the editing procedure and attain best results for the readers.

Apart from the editorial board, the designing team has also invested a significant amount of their time in understanding the subject and creating the most relevant covers. They scrutinized every image to scout for the most suitable representation of the subject and create an appropriate cover for the book.

The publishing team has been an ardent support to the editorial, designing and production team. Their endless efforts to recruit the best for this project, has resulted in the accomplishment of this book. They are a veteran in the field of academics and their pool of knowledge is as vast as their experience in printing. Their expertise and guidance has proved useful at every step. Their uncompromising quality standards have made this book an exceptional effort. Their encouragement from time to time has been an inspiration for everyone.

The publisher and the editorial board hope that this book will prove to be a valuable piece of knowledge for researchers, students, practitioners and scholars across the globe.

List of Contributors

Michael H Carstensen
Department of Medical Imaging, St Joseph's Hospital London, Ontario, Canada

Mashael Al-Harbi
Department of Medical Imaging, St Joseph's Hospital London, Ontario, Canada

Jean-Luc Urbain
Department of Medical Imaging, St Joseph's Hospital London, Ontario, Canada

Tarik-Zine Belhocine
Department of Medical Imaging, St Joseph's Hospital London, Ontario, Canada

Peter Kent
Research Department, Spine Centre of Southern Denmark, Lillebaelt Hospital, Institute of Regional Health Services Research, University of Southern Denmark, Middelfart, Denmark

Andrew M Briggs
School of Physiotherapy and Curtin Health Innovation Research Institute, Curtin University, Perth, Australia

Hanne B Albert
Research Department, Spine Centre of Southern Denmark, Lillebaelt Hospital, Institute of Regional Health Services Research, University of Southern Denmark, Middelfart, Denmark

Andreas Byrhagen
Odense Physiotherapy Sports and Fitness, Odense, Denmark

Christian Hansen
Quick Care, Odense, Denmark

Karina Kjaergaard
Southwest Jutland Hospital, Esbjerg, Denmark

Tue S Jensen
Research Department, Spine Centre of Southern Denmark, Lillebaelt Hospital, Institute of Regional Health Services Research, University of Southern Denmark, Middelfart, Denmark

Isabelle Pagé
Département des sciences de l'activité physique, Université du Québec à Trois-Rivières, Trois-Rivières, G9A 5H7, Canada

Martin Descarreaux
Département de chiropratique, Université du Québec à Trois-Rivières, Trois-Rivières, G9A 5H7, Canada

Alice Kongsted
Nordic Institute of Chiropractic and Clinical Biomechanics, University of Southern Denmark, Odense. Part of Clinical Locomotion Network, Denmark
Research Department, Spine Centre of Southern Denmark, Hospital Lillebaelt Middelfart, Institute of Regional Health Research, University of Southern Denmark. Part of Clinical Locomotion Network, Denmark

Else Johannesen
Master of Science in Public Health, Institute of Public Health, University of Southern Denmark, Esbjerg, Denmark

Charlotte Leboeuf-Yde
Research Department, Spine Centre of Southern Denmark, Hospital Lillebaelt Middelfart, Institute of Regional Health Research, University of Southern Denmark. Part of Clinical Locomotion Network, Denmark

Cecilie D Testern
Nordic Institute of Chiropractic and Clinical Biomechanics and Institute of Sports Science and Biomechanics, University of Southern Denmark, Odense, Denmark

Lise Hestbæk
Nordic Institute of Chiropractic and Clinical Biomechanics and Institute of Sports Science and Biomechanics, University of Southern Denmark, Odense, Denmark

Simon D French
General Practice and Primary Health Care Academic Centre, University of Melbourne, Melbourne, VIC, Australia
School of Rehabilitation Therapy, Faculty of Health Sciences, Queen's University, Kingston, Ontario,Canada

Cid André Fidelis de Paula Gomes
Postgraduate Program in Biophotonics Applied to Health Sciences, Universidade Nove de Julho (UNINOVE), Av. Dr. Adolfo Pinto,109, Água Branca, 05001-100 São Paulo, SP, Brazil
Department of Physical Therapy, Universidade Nove de Julho (UNINOVE), Av. Dr. Adolfo Pinto,109, Água Branca, 05001-100 São Paulo, SP, Brazil

Yasmin El Hage
Postgraduate Program in Rehabilitation Sciences, Universidade Nove de Julho (UNINOVE), Av. Dr. Adolfo Pinto,109, Água Branca, 05001-100 São Paulo, SP, Brazil
Department of Physical Therapy, Universidade Nove de Julho (UNINOVE), Av. Dr. Adolfo Pinto,109, Água Branca, 05001-100 São Paulo, SP, Brazil

Ana Paula Amaral
Postgraduate Program in Rehabilitation Sciences, Universidade Nove de Julho (UNINOVE), Av. Dr. Adolfo Pinto,109, Água Branca, 05001-100 São Paulo, SP, Brazil

Fabiano Politti
Postgraduate Program in Rehabilitation Sciences, Universidade Nove de Julho (UNINOVE), Av. Dr. Adolfo Pinto,109, Água Branca, 05001-100 São Paulo, SP, Brazil
Department of Physical Therapy, Universidade Nove de Julho (UNINOVE), Av. Dr. Adolfo Pinto,109, Água Branca, 05001-100 São Paulo, SP, Brazil

Daniela Aparecida Biasotto-Gonzalez
Postgraduate Program in Rehabilitation Sciences, Universidade Nove de Julho (UNINOVE), Av. Dr. Adolfo Pinto,109, Água Branca, 05001-100 São Paulo, SP, Brazil
Department of Physical Therapy, Universidade Nove de Julho (UNINOVE), Av. Dr. Adolfo Pinto,109, Água Branca, 05001-100 São Paulo, SP, Brazil

Lisa Zaynab Killinger
Director of Diagnosis and Radiology, Palmer College of Chiropractic, 1000 Brady Street, 52803, Davenport, IA, USA

Jonathan Field
Private practice Back2Health, 2 Charles Street, Petersfield, Hants, UK

Dave Newell
Anglo-European College of Chiropractic, 13-15 Parkwood Rd, Bournemouth, UK

Iris Sun Rudy
Macquarie University, Sydney, Australia

Alexandra Poulos
Macquarie University, Sydney, Australia

Laura Owen
Macquarie University, Sydney, Australia

Ashlee Batters
Macquarie University, Sydney, Australia

Kasia Kieliszek,
Macquarie University, Sydney, Australia

Jessica Willox
Macquarie University, Sydney, Australia

Hazel Jenkins
Macquarie University, Sydney, Australia

Sara Glithro
McTimoney College of Chiropractic, Abingdon, UK

David Newell
Anglo European College of Chiropractic (AECC) and Bournemouth University, Dorset, UK

Lorna Burrows
Salisbury NHS Foundation Trust, Salisbury, UK

Adrian Hunnisett
McTimoney College of Chiropractic, Abingdon, UK

Christina Cunliffe
McTimoney College of Chiropractic, Abingdon, UK

Donald R Murphy
Rhode Island Spine Center, 600 Pawtucket Avenue, Pawtucket, RI 02860 USA
Department of Health Services, Policy and Practice, Alpert Medical School of Brown University, Providence, RI USA
Department of Research, New York Chiropractic College, Seneca Falls, NY USA

Eric L Hurwitz
Department of Public Health Sciences, John A. Burns School of Medicine, University of Hawaii at Mānoa, Hawaii USA

Alice Kongsted
The Nordic Institute of Chiropractic and Clinical Biomechanics, Campusvej 55, 5230 Odense, M, Denmark
Department of Sports Science and Clinical Biomechanics, University of Southern Denmark, Odense, Denmark

Benedicte Aambakk
Department of Sports Science and Clinical Biomechanics, University of Southern Denmark, Odense, Denmark

Sanne Bossen
Department of Sports Science and Clinical Biomechanics, University of Southern Denmark, Odense, Denmark

Lise Hestbaek
The Nordic Institute of Chiropractic and Clinical Biomechanics, Campusvej 55, 5230 Odense, M, Denmark
Department of Sports Science and Clinical Biomechanics, University of Southern Denmark, Odense, Denmark

Rikke K. Jensen
Research Department, Spine Centre of Southern Denmark, Hospital Lillebaelt, Institute of Regional Health Research, University of Southern Denmark, Oestre Hougvej 55, 5500 Middelfart, Denmark

Peter Kent
Research Department, Spine Centre of Southern Denmark, Hospital Lillebaelt, Institute of Regional Health Research, University of Southern Denmark, Oestre Hougvej 55, 5500 Middelfart, Denmark
Department of Sports Science and Clinical Biomechanics, University of Southern Denmark, Campusvej 55, 5230 Odense M, Denmark

Mark Hancock
Faculty of Human Sciences, Macquarie University, Balaclava Rd, North Ryde 2113NSW, Australia

Silvano Ferrari
Master of Manual Therapy and Musculoskeletal Rehabilitation, Department of Molecular Medicine, University of Padova, Padova, Italy

Tiziana Manni
Physical Therapy Private Practice, Treviso, Italy

Francesca Bonetti
Physioup Physical Therapy Private Practice, Rome, Italy

Jorge Hugo Villafañe
IRCCS Don Gnocchi Foundation, Milan, Italy

Carla Vanti
Master of Manual Therapy and Musculoskeletal Rehabilitation, Department of Molecular Medicine, University of Padova, Padova, Italy

Eirik Johan Skeie
MChiro, MSc, Ulriksdal 2, 5009 Bergen, Norway

Jan Arve Borge
DC, MSc, Ulriksdal 2, 5009 Bergen, Norway

Charlotte Leboeuf-Yde
Department Spincenter of Southern Denmark Hospital Lillebælt, Østre Hougvej 55, DK-5500 Middelfart, Denmark

Jenni Bolton
Anglo European College of Chiropractic. Research Department, 13-15 Parkwood Road, Bournemouth BH5 2DF England, UK

Niels Wedderkopp
Orthopaedic Department, Center for Spine Surgery, Hospital of Lillebaelt, Institute of Regional Health Service Research and Center for Research in Childhood Health, University of Southern Denmark, Østre Hougvej 55, DK5500 Middelfart, Denmark

Barbara I Polus
Division of Chiropractic, School of Health Sciences, RMIT University, Plenty Rd Bundoora, Melbourne, Australia

Amanda J Kimpton
Division of Chiropractic, School of Health Sciences, RMIT University, Plenty Rd Bundoora, Melbourne, Australia

Max J Walsh
Division of Chiropractic, School of Health Sciences, RMIT University, Plenty Rd Bundoora, Melbourne, Australia

Michael D Reife
Private Practice, 8 Independence Drive, Marlborough, CT 06447, USA
Basic and Clinical Sciences, University of Bridgeport College of Chiropractic, 75 Linden Ave, Bridgeport, CT 06604, USA

Christopher M Coulis
Department of Veterans Affairs Connecticut Healthcare System, West Haven, CT 06516, USA
Shoreline Spine & Pain Associates, PC, 2415 Boston Post Rd., Guilford, CT 06437, USA
Clinical Sciences, University of Bridgeport College of Chiropractic, 75 Linden Ave., Bridgeport, CT 06604, USA

Charles W Gay
Rehabilitation Science Doctoral Student, University of Florida, Gainesville, Florida, USA

Mark D Bishop
Associate Professor, Department of Physical Therapy, University of Florida, Gainesville, Florida, USA
Center for Pain Research & Behavioral Health, University of Florida, Gainesville, Florida, USA

Michael S Swain
The George Institute for Global Health, Sydney Medical School, University of Sydney, Missenden Rd, PO Box M201, 2050 Sydney, Australia
Department of Chiropractic, Faculty of Science, Macquarie University, 2109 Sydney, Australia

Nicholas Henschke
The George Institute for Global Health, Sydney Medical School, University of Sydney, Missenden Rd, PO Box M201, 2050 Sydney, Australia
Institute of Public Health, University of Heidelberg, 69120 Heidelberg, Germany

Steven J Kamper
The George Institute for Global Health, Sydney Medical School, University of Sydney, Missenden Rd, PO Box M201, 2050 Sydney, Australia
Department of Epidemiology and Biostatistics, EMGO + Institute, VU University Medical Center, 1081BT Amsterdam, Netherlands

Aron S Downie
The George Institute for Global Health, Sydney Medical School, University of Sydney, Missenden Rd, PO Box M201, 2050 Sydney, Australia
Department of Chiropractic, Faculty of Science, Macquarie University, 2109 Sydney, Australia

Bart W Koes
Department of General Practice, Erasmus MC, University Medical Centre, 50 3015 GE Rotterdam, Netherlands

Chris G Maher
The George Institute for Global Health, Sydney Medical School, University of Sydney, Missenden Rd, PO Box M201, 2050 Sydney, Australia

Stacie A Salsbury
Palmer College of Chiropractic, Palmer Center for Chiropractic Research, 741 Brady Street, Davenport, IA 52803, USA

James W DeVocht
Palmer College of Chiropractic, Palmer Center for Chiropractic Research, 741 Brady Street, Davenport, IA 52803, USA

Maria A Hondras
Institute of Sports Science and Clinical Biomechanics, University of Southern Denmark, Odense, Denmark

Michael B Seidman
Palmer College of Chiropractic, Palmer Center for Chiropractic Research, 741 Brady Street, Davenport, IA 52803, USA

Clark M Stanford
The University of Illinois, 801 South Paulina Street, 102c (MC621), Chicago, IL 60612, USA

Christine M Goertz
Palmer College of Chiropractic, Palmer Center for Chiropractic Research, 741 Brady Street, Davenport, IA 52803, USA

Kenneth John Young
School of Arts; Senior Lecturer, School of Health Professions, Murdoch University, South Street, Murdoch 6150, Australia

Paul A Bruno
Faculty of Kinesiology and Health Studies, University of Regina, 3737 Wascana Parkway, Regina, Saskatchewan S4S 0A2, Canada

David P Millar
Private Practice, Regina, Saskatchewan, Canada

Dale A Goertzen
Private Practice, Regina, Saskatchewan, Canada

Amir Massoud Arab
Department of Physical Therapy, University of Social Welfare and Rehabilitation Sciences, Evin, Koodakyar Ave, Zip Code: 1985713831 Tehran, Iran

Omid Rasouli
Department of Physical Therapy, Faculty of Health Education and Social Work, Sør-Trøndelag University College (HiST), Trondheim, Norway

Mohsen Amiri
Department of Physical Therapy, University of Social Welfare and Rehabilitation Sciences, Evin, Koodakyar Ave, Zip Code: 1985713831 Tehran, Iran

Nahid Tahan
Department of Physical Therapy, Shahid Beheshti University of Medical Sciences, Tehran, Iran

Gianfranco Pizzolorusso, Patrizia Turi, Francesco Cerritelli and Fabrizio Carinci
EBOM - European Institute for Evidence Based Osteopathic Medicine, viale Unità d'Italia 1, 66100 Chieti, Italy

Gina Barlafante, Cinzia Renzetti, Vincenzo Cozzolino and Marianna D'Orazio
AIOT - Accademia Italiana Osteopatia Tradizionale, via Prati 29, 65124 Pescara, Italy

Paola Fusilli and Carmine D'Incecco
Unità di Terapia Intensiva Neonatale - Ospedale Civile Spirito Santo, Via Renato Paolini 45, 65124 Pescara, Italy

Jeffrey J Hebert
Faculty of Health Sciences, Murdoch University, Murdoch, WA, Australia

Julie M Fritz
Department of Physical Therapy, University of Utah and Intermountain Healthcare, Salt Lake City, UT, USA

Karin Ried, Simon Armstrong and Avni Sali
National Institute of Integrative Medicine, Melbourne VIC 3122, Australia

Patrick McLaughlin
College of Health and Biomedicine, Victoria University, Melbourne VIC 3001, Australia

Allan Kalamir and Rodney Bonello
Department of Chiropractic, Faculty of Science, Macquarie University, North Ryde, NSW, Australia

Petra L Graham
Department of Statistics, Faculty of Science, Macquarie University, North Ryde, NSW, Australia

Andrew L Vitiello
Department of Academic Affairs, Anglo-European College of Chiropractic, Bournemouth, Dorset, UK

Henry Pollard
School of Exercise Science, Faculty of Sports Science, Australian Catholic University, Sydney, NSW, Australia

Bruce F Walker
School of Chiropractic and Sports Science, Murdoch University, Murdoch, 6150, Western Australia

Simon D French
School of Public Health and Preventive Medicine, Monash University, Level 6, The Alfred Centre, 99 Commercial Road, Melbourne, Victoria 3004, Australia
Primary Care Research Unit, University of Melbourne, 200 Berkeley St, Carlton, Victoria, 3010, Australia

Matthew J Page, Denise A O'Connor, Joanne E McKenzie, Katherine Beringer, Kerry Murphy and Sally E Green
School of Public Health and Preventive Medicine, Monash University, Level 6, The Alfred Centre, 99 Commercial Road, Melbourne, Victoria 3004, Australia

Jenny L Keating
Department of Physiotherapy, School of Primary Health Care, Faculty of Medicine Nursing and Health Science, Monash University, PO Box 527 Frankston, Victoria, 3199 Australia

Susan Michie
Centre for Outcomes Research and Effectiveness, Department of Clinical, Educational and Health Psychology, University College London, WC1E 7HB, London, UK

Jill J Francis
Health Services Research Unit, Health Sciences Building, University of Aberdeen AB25 2ZD, UK

Patrick J Battaglia and Dennis E Enix
Division of Research, Logan College of Chiropractic, 1851 Schoettler Rd, Chesterfield, MO 60317, USA

Frank Scali
Independent Researcher, 1272 Dutch Broadway, Valley Stream, NY 11580, USA